Critical Care

Critical Care

Standards, Audit and Ethics

Edited by

JACK TINKER BSc MB FRCP FRCS DIC

Dean of Postgraduate Medicine, University of London, and previously
Director of the Intensive Therapy Unit,
The Middlesex Hospital,
London, UK

DOREEN RG BROWNE MB BS MSc FRCA

Consultant Anaesthetist and
Director of Intensive Care Therapy,
Royal Free Hospital, London, UK

WILLIAM J SIBBALD MD FRCPC

Coordinator, Critical Care Trauma Unit,
Victoria Hospital, London, Ontario, Canada

A member of the Hodder Headline Group
LONDON • SYDNEY • AUCKLAND
Co-published in the USA by
Oxford University Press, Inc., New York

First published in Great Britain 1996 by
Arnold, a member of the Hodder Headline Group,
338 Euston Road, London NW1 3BH

Co-published in the United States of America by
Oxford University Press, Inc.,
198 Madison Avenue, New York, NY10016
Oxford is a registered trademark of Oxford University Press

Whilst the advice and information in this book is believed to be true and
accurate at the date of going to press, neither the author[s] nor the publisher
can accept any legal responsibility or liability for any errors or omissions
that may be made. In particular (but without limiting the generality of the
preceding disclaimer) every effort has been made to check drug dosages;
however it is still possible that errors have been missed. Furthermore,
dosage schedules are constantly being revised and new side-effects
recognized. For these reasons the reader is strongly urged to consult the
drug companies' printed instructions before administering any of the drugs
recommended in this book.

British Library Cataloguing in Publication Data
A catalogue record for this book is available from the British Library

Library of Congress Cataloging-in-Publication Data
A catalog record for this book is available from the Library of Congress

0 340 55424 X

1 2 3 4 5   96 97 98 99

Typeset in Times and Optima by
Fakenham Photosetting Limited, Fakenham, Norfolk
Printed and bound in Great Britain by
The Bath Press, Bath, Avon

Contents

List of contributors vii
Preface ix

PART I   Critical Care

1. **Critical care today** *Marko Noc, Max Harry Weil* 3
2. **The development, utilization and cost implications of intensive care medicine: strategies for the future** *Teik E Oh* 11

PART II   Resource Standards

(a) Care Provision

3. **Primary and mobile care: land, sea and air** *P Mulrooney* 21
4. **General care units** *Rowland Bennett Hopkinson* 36
5. **Specialist care units** *Malcolm Wright* 56

(b) Technological Provision

6. **Noninvasive monitoring** *ML Price* 70
7. **Invasive hemodynamic monitoring** *Rinaldo Bellomo, Michael R Pinsky* 82
8. **Imaging** *DJ Tawn, SN Jones* 105
9. **Intensive care laboratory** *R Naidoo, DJA Cox* 123
10. **Respiratory support** *William T Peruzzi, Barry A Shapiro* 133
11. **Cardiac support for acute cardiac failure** *Gina Price Lundberg, JE Calvin* 156
12. **Renal support** *Hugh S Cairns, Guy H Neild* 178

(c) Staffing and Training

13. **Medical staffing and training**
    United Kingdom *AR Webb* 193
    Australia *Geofrey J Dobb* 197
    United States of America *David R Gerber, Carolyn E Bekes* 202
    Canada *Brian P Egier, Cindy M Hamielec, John R Hewson* 207
14. **Nursing staffing and training**
    United Kingdom *Mandy Sheppard* 212
    Australia *Michelle Kelly, Frances Monypenny* 217
    Europe *A M Timmermann* 222
15. **Respiratory and physical therapy**
    Physical therapy, USA *Nancy D Ciesla* 226

Respiratory care, USA *Anthony L Bilenki*   231

Canada *Margaret E Fielding, H Ronald Wexler*   234

Education and training of respiratory therapists in Canada *Paul Robinson, H Ronald Wexler*   236

Australia *Jill C Nosworthy, Linda Denehy, Rosemary P Moore*   239

Physiotherapy EC/UK, *Bernadette Henderson, Diana Davis*   244

16. **Education, training and role of the clinical engineer and the clinical scientist in patient care**
Shyam VS Rithalia   255

PART III   Audit

17. **The process of clinical audit: with special reference to critical care** *Robert J Byrick*   265
18. **Quantifying critical illness** *JF Bion*   276
19. **Selection of patients for intensive care** *Alasdair IK Short*   289
20. **Results of critical care and the quality of survival** *Marvin L Birnbaum, Sally Kraft*   297
21. **Evaluating the cost and consequences of critical care: critical appraisal of health technology**
Kevin J Inman, William J Sibbald   315

PART IV   Ethics

22. **Establishing health care priorities** *June Dales*   331
23. **Withholding and withdrawing** *Jean-Louis Vincent*   344
24. **Ethical issues of organ donation** *CJ Hinds, CH Collins*   350
25. **Clinical research in intensive care medicine: ethics in clinical research** *Bara Ricou,
Peter M Suter*   360
26. **Medico-legal aspects of critical care**
United Kingdom *Jenny L Urwin*   367
United States of America *Marshall B Kapp*   382
27. **Moral and religious dilemmas** *K Boyd*   391

Index   400

Contributors

Carolyn E Bekes MD FCCM
Vice President/Medical Affairs, Cooper Hospital/ University Medical Center, One Cooper Plaza, Camden, New Jersey, USA

Rinaldo Bellomo MD
Intensive Care Unit, Austin Hospital, Heidelberg, Victoria, Australia

Anthony L Bilenki RRT
Technical Director, Respiratory Care Services, The Johns Hopkins Hospital, Baltimore, Maryland, USA

Julian F Bion MB BS MRCP FRCA MD
Senior Lecturer in Intensive Care Medicine and Director of Intensive Care, Queen Elizabeth Hospital, Birmingham

Marvin L Birnbaum MD PhD
Director, Emergency Medical Services Program, Editor, Prehospital and Disaster Medicine, Associate Professor of Medicine and Physiology, University of Wisconsin Hospital and Clinics, Madison, Wisconsin, USA

Robert J Byrick MD FRCPC
Professor and Chairman, Department of Anaesthesia, University of Toronto, Toronto, Canada

Hugh S Cairns MD MRCP
Consultant Nephrologist, King's College Hospital, London, UK

JE Calvin MD FRCPC FACC
Associate Professor, Department of Medicine, Section of Cardiology, Rush-Presbyterian-St Luke's Medical Center, Chicago, Illinois, USA

Nancy D Ciesla PT
Clinical Instructor, University of Maryland at Baltimore and Director of Physical Therapy, Maryland Institute for Emergency Services Systems, Baltimore, Maryland, USA

Charles H Collins MB BS FRCA DTMH
Consultant Anaesthetist and Director of Intensive Care, Royal Devon and Exeter Hospitals, Exeter, UK

Dominic JA Cox MSc BSc
Clinical Scientist, Intensive Therapy Unit, The Royal Free Hospital, London, UK

June Dales BA MPhil
Assistant Director (London), Trust Unit, NHS Executive South Thames Regional Office, London, UK

Diana Davis Grad Dip Phys MCSP
Senior Lecturer in Physiotherapy, Division of Physiotherapy, University of Hertfordshire, Hatfield, UK

Linda Denehy B App Sc, Grad Dip Phty
Lecturer, School of Physiotherapy, Faculty of Medicine, Dentistry and Health Sciences, University of Melbourne, Carlton, Victoria, Australia

Geoffrey J Dobb BSc MB BS MRCP FRCA FANZCA FICANZCA
Senior Specialist in Intensive Care and Clinical Senior Lecturer, Department of Medicine, Royal Perth Hospital, Perth, Western Australia

Brian P Egier BSc MD FRCPC
Associate Professor, Department of Anaesthesia, McMaster University, Departments of Critical Care, Anaesthesia, Medicine and Hyperbaric Medicine, Hamilton Civic Hospitals, Hamilton, Ontario, Canada

Margaret E Fielding MCSP MCPA
Manager, Rehabilitation Services, University Hospital, London, Ontario, Canada

David R Gerber DO FCCP
Assistant Professor of Medicine and Anesthesia, University of Medicine and Dentistry of New Jersey, Robert Wood Johnson Medical School, Camden, New Jersey, USA

Cindy M Hamielec MD FRCPC
Chief, Department of Critical Care Medicine, Chedoke-McMaster Hospitals, Hamilton, Ontario, Canada

Bernadette Henderson
Superintendent Physiotherapist, Barnet General Hospital, Barnet, London, UK

John R Hewson MD CM MSc FRCPC
Chairman, Regional Critical Care Program, McMaster University, Chief, Department of Critical Care, Hamilton Civic Hospitals, Hamilton, Ontario, Canada

Charles J Hinds FRCP FRCA
Director of Intensive Care, St Bartholomew's Hospital, London, UK

Rowland B Hopkinson MBBS FRCA
Consultant Anaesthetist and Clinical Director of Intensive Care, Birmingham Heartlands Hospital, Birmingham, UK and Honorary Clinical Lecturer, University of Birmingham

Kevin J Inman MSc
Director, Critical Care Trauma Center, Victoria Hospital, London, Ontario, Canada

Simon N Jones MRCP FRCR
Consultant Radiologist, The Royal Bournemouth Hospital, Bournemouth, UK

Marshall B Kapp JD MPH
Professor of Community Health, Wright State University of Medicine, Dayton, Ohio, USA

Michelle Kelly RN IC Cert, BSc
Nurse Educator, Intensive Therapy Unit, Royal North Shore Hospital, Sydney, Australia

Sally Kraft MD
Department of Pulmonary Critical Care Medicine, Physicians Plus Medical Group, Madison, Wisconsin, USA

Gina Price Lundberg MD
Department of Medicine, Section of Cardiology, Rush-Presbyterian-St Luke's Medical Center, Chicago, Illinois, USA

Frances Monypenny RN CM IC Cert BEd(Nurs)
Nurse Educator, Graduate Diploma in Intensive Care Nursing, Northern Sydney Area Health Service and University of Technology, Sydney, Australia

Rosemary P Moore B App Sc Grad Dip Phty
Senior Clinical Cardiothoracic Physiotherapist, Alfred Hospital, Pahran, Victoria, Australia

P Mulrooney MB ChB FRCA
Walsgrove Hospital NHS Trust, Coventry, UK

Rohini Naidoo MSc BSc
Clinical Scientist, Intensive Therapy Unit, The Royal Free Hospital, London, UK

Guy H Neild MD FRCP
Professor of Nephrology, University College London Medical School, London, UK

Marko Noc MD
Center of Intensive Internal Medicine, University Clinical Center, Ljubljana, Slovenia

Jill C Nosworthy AUA Grad Dip Phty M App Sc
Chief Physiotherapist, St Vincent's Hospital, Melbourne, Australia

Teik E Oh MB BS MD FRCP FRCPE FRACP FRCA FANZCA FFICANZCA FHKAM
Professor and Chairman, Department of Anaesthesia and Intensive Care, The Chinese University of Hong Kong, Hong Kong

William T Peruzzi MD
Associate Professor of Anaesthesia and Chief, Section of Respiratory and Critical Care, Northwestern University Medical School, Chicago, Illinois, USA

Michael R Pinsky CM
Professor of Anesthesiology, Critical Care Medicine and Medicine, University of Pittsburgh, USA

Martin L Price MB BS, BSc FRCA
Department of Anaesthetics, St Mary's Hospital, Praed Street, London, UK

Bara Ricou MD
Surgical Intensive Care Unit, University Hospital of Geneva, Geneva, Switzerland

Shyam VS Rithalia PhD
Scientific Officer, Department of Orthopaedic Mechanics, University of Salford, Salford, UK

Paul Robinson
Department of Anaesthesia, University Hospital, London, Ontario, Canada

Barry A Shapiro MD
Professor and Vice-Chairman, Department of Anaesthesia, Northwestern University Medical School, Chicago, Illinois, USA

Amanda Sheppard
ITU/HDU Manager, Bromley Hospitals NHS Trust, Farnborough Hospital, Orpington, Kent, UK

Alasdair IK Short FRCP FRCP(Ed) FRCPC
Consultant Physician, Intensive Care Unit, Broomfield Hospital, Chelmsford, Essex, UK

William J Sibbald MD FRCPC CHE
Coordinator, Critical Care Trauma Center and Acting Chief, Department of Medicine, Victoria Hospital, London, Ontario, Canada

Peter M Suter MD
Surgical Intensive Care Unit, University Hospital of Geneva, Geneva, Switzerland

Julian Tawn MB CLB FRCR
Consultant Radiologist, The Royal Bournemouth Hospital, Bournemouth, UK

AM Timmermann RN
Chief of Nursing, Intensive Care Units, University Hospital of Liege, Belgium

Jenny L Urwin MA LLM(Cantab)
Lecturer in Law, Faculty of Law, University of Manchester, Manchester, UK

Jean-Louis Vincent MD PhD
Professor, Department of Intensive Care, Erasme University Hospital, Free University of Brussels, Belgium

Andrew R Webb MD MRCP
Consultant Physician and Clinical Director of Intensive Care, University College London Hospitals, Mortimer Street, London, UK

Max Harry Weil MD PhD
Distinguished University Professor and President, Institute of Critical Care Medicine, Palm Springs, California, USA

H Ronald Wexler BA MD FRCPC
Medical Director, Intensive Care Unit and Associate Professor, Department of Anaesthesia, University Hospital, London, Ontario, Canada

Malcolm Wright MB ChB FRCP FRACP FRCA FANZCA
Emeritus Consultant in Intensive Care, Princess Alexandra Hospital, Brisbane, Australia

Preface

Critical Care Standards, Audit and Ethics brings together the important issues of standards of care of the critically ill, the assessment and measurement of quality of that care, the cost effectiveness of care and the legal and ethical issues which are challenging us as we move towards the twenty-first century. The authors have been specially chosen as experts in their field. The editors have been particularly anxious to obtain world wide views and they feel that this book is timely now that technology is no longer the limiting factor in the management of the critically ill patient.

This book is concerned with the adult patient who requires organ support on the *general* intensive care unit. It does not include specialized areas such as coronary care and pediatrics. It is divided into four main sections: an overview of critical care; resource standards; audit; and ethics.

The section on resource standards is subdivided into core provision, technical provision and provision for staffing and training in each of the various disciplines. Core provision has chapters on transport of the critically ill, and the design of general and specialist care units. Technological provision covers monitoring techniques, the intensive care laboratory, and organ support systems. Staffing and training involves the medical, nursing, respiratory, physiotherapy, scientific and technical disciplines which are all involved in intensive care. The chapters within each of these disciplines convey various international approaches to the subject.

This section on resource standards sets the stage for the subsequent two sections devoted to audit and ethics, respectively.

The section on audit looks at the process of clinical audit, quantification of critical illness and the evaluation of costs and benefits. The section on ethics addresses the establishment of health care priorities, withholding and withdrawing life support, organ donation, research and the medico-legal aspects of these issues. Some of the moral and religious dilemmas involved in the care of the critically ill are also discussed, such as, when should hopes of cure with intensive therapy become the acceptance of noninterventional care as the preferable more humane alternative.

It is hoped that at least some aspect of this book will appeal to everyone concerned with the management and care of the critically ill. This includes the members of the multidisciplinary ITU team, students and trainees, carers and the appropriate relatives' support groups, lawyers, theologians and hospital managers.

The editors are particularly grateful to Yvonne Perks for her organizational expertise, patient forbearance and good humor. Without her help and generous spirit this book would never have been compiled.

Jack Tinker
Doreen RG Browne
William J Sibbald

PART I

Critical Care

CHAPTER 1

Critical Care Today

MARKO NOC, MAX HARRY WEIL

Introduction   3
Intensive care unit   3
Leadership   4
Intensive care unit team   4
Medical technology   5
Utilization of critical care services   6
Demography of patient population   6
Dynamic disease patterns   6
Moral, ethical and economic implications   7
Conclusion   8
References   8

Introduction

Critical care is a recently evolved specialty discipline which addresses the life-saving and life-sustaining medical management of patients at risk of imminent death from acute illness or injury. It is a multidisciplinary service specialty, tightly allied with the conventional disciplines of internal medicine, surgery, anesthesiology, and pediatrics, and their respective subspecialties, including pulmonary, renal, cardiovascular, neurological and infectious diseases. The basic science of critical care medicine may be regarded as life-support biology. Its clinical practice encompasses multiple system failures: cardiovascular, respiratory, renal, metabolic, and neurological. It is a relatively new specialty discipline which maintains cognitive and interventional skills for management of life-threatening crises, whether due to illness or traumatic injury.

Critical care medicine evolved in parallel with advances in invasive surgical and medical procedures. The physical development of intensive care units may be traced to the postoperative recovery units, thence to the respiratory care units, subsequently to shock and trauma units, and finally to units that provided comprehensive medical support for medical and surgical patients with immediate life-threatening crises. Today, critical care medicine has gained wide acceptance and even the smallest of full-service hospitals is likely to have specialized facilities for critically ill or injured patients.[1]

Intensive care unit

Critical care is optimally delivered to patients by a team of highly trained personnel who are provided with the physical facilities, equipment, and organizational structure that will enable them to fulfill their life-saving and life-preserving function and to do so effectively and efficiently. The intensive care unit has therefore been looked on as the 'hospital's hospital'.

The organization of intensive care units for a given hospital reflects a skillful blend of general concepts of management of acutely ill or injured patients together with modifications which reflect the needs and restraints related to the demographic uniqueness of the patients and their diseases. The organization further reflects the availability, composition, and priorities of professional staff and unusual demands for care specific settings.

Issues of space and funding are of great import in smaller hospitals, where only one intensive care unit can typically be supported and this usually serves as a multipurpose medical/surgical/coronary care unit. Such multidisciplinary units may provide more optimal utilization of available technology, beds and critical care personnel.[2]

The number and specialization of units typically increases with the overall bed capacity of the hospital.[3] The broad range of specialized units reduces reliance on multidisciplinary units and enhances the operational integrity of specific clinical services (Table 1.1). This may justify the separation of general medical, surgical and cardiac care units. Pediatric and neonatal units, both historically and pragmatically, are separated from adult units. They have special requirements for a unique patient population. As a rule, there is justification for other subspecialty units like cardiothoracic, trauma, burns, neurosciences and respiratory care units only when the demands for such specialized care, and specifically the number of patients and the comprehensiveness of service, make this administratively and financially feasible.

Table 1.1 Percentage of hospitals with designated 'special care units'

Hospital bed capacity:	<100	100–300	300–500	>500
Med/Surg/CCU (%)	75.6	53.9	13.1	5.6
Med/Surg (%)	11.5	14.9	17.6	7.8
Medical (%)	2.7	4.9	11.9	17.8
Surgical (%)	–	4.9	17.6	28.4
CCU (%)	2.5	7.8	16.1	11.7
Neurology (%)	–	0.6	2.7	6.0
Pediatric (%)	0.6	5.1	6.9	8.9
Neonatal (%)	0.9	5.6	11.3	11.4
Other (%)	5.7	2.0	2.1	2.0

Med = medical; Surg = surgical; CCU = coronary care unit.
Adapted from ref. 3.

The number of beds for each specialized intensive care unit is contingent on local, regional and national precedents and requirements, together with more unique local considerations including demography of diseases and injuries and therefore number of admissions, length of stay, admission and discharge practices, total hospital bed capacity, and the availability of specialized services such as cardiac catheterization facilities and cardiac surgery teams or burns services. They also reflect the special services and bed capacities of neighboring hospitals. Of greatest current importance in the US setting is cost-effectiveness of special care units.

Multidisciplinary medical, coronary and pediatric units in the USA have an average capacity of 10 beds.

Surgical units average 12 beds. Neonatal units maintain a much larger bed capacity, averaging 21 beds per unit.[3] Because there are major differences among western countries in the number of beds that constitute an intensive care unit, the number of admissions per bed per year, the duration of stay in the unit and the occupancy rate of those beds, the North American experience is not likely to be directly applicable to other countries. The number of beds for each unit averages 19 in Belgium and varies from 10 to 14 in other western European countries and in the USA. Smaller units with an average capacity of only six to eight beds are typically provided in the UK and in Japan.[4–7]

There is also great variability in the proportion of total hospital beds which are committed to critical care. In the USA, approximately 8% of hospital beds are reserved for critical care.[3] In western European countries, the percentage of intensive care beds varies from 4.1 in Denmark to 2.6 in the UK. In New Zealand and Japan, only 2% of hospital beds are so committed and this represents the smallest allocation among industrialized nations.[7,8]

Leadership

The professional direction of the intensive care unit is delegated to a conventional clinical department in the majority of US hospitals. More than one third of intensive care units in the USA are professionally administered by the hospital's Department of Medicine. Twelve per cent are administered by the Department of Pediatrics, and 10% by Department of Surgery. Only 3% of units are currently operated by a named Department of Critical Care Medicine, independently of traditional departments, and only 1% by the Departments of Anesthesiology.[3] The US model, however, differs from that of the European model in which one-half of intensive care units are operated by the Department of Anesthesiology.[6] Remarkably, approximately one-fourth of American intensive care units have no defined departmental affiliation and operate as specialized medical surgical beds with responsibility for care totally assigned to a visiting attending clinician or surgeon.[3]

Intensive care unit team

The team which has responsibility for the care of the critically ill or injured patient includes clinicians, nurses and allied health personnel and especially respiratory therapists, dieticians and clinical pharmacists. Unpredictable changes in the clinical condition of the critically ill or injured patient have increasingly called for the professional attendance of clinicians to maintain both a continuum of critical care services and immediate availability for life-saving or life-sustaining interventions.[9] This perceived need for on-site expert medical care was the impetus, at least in part, for the formal board certification of clinical specialists in the USA.[10] Clinicians, surgeons, anesthesiologists and pediatricians, who are trained and qualified as critical care specialists, are now avidly recruited for such full-time posts in hospital practice.

The first examination and certification in Critical Care Medicine was sponsored in 1986 by the American Board of Anesthesia. Today, there are approximately 6000 certified specialists and more than 150 fully accredited formal American training programs in critical care medicine. In Europe, a somewhat less authoritative recognition process of postgraduate training and certification in critical care medicine has been sponsored by the European Society of Intensive Care Medicine. The Society awards a European Diploma of Critical Care Medicine, based on completion of training as defined by a core curriculum and successful completion of written and oral examinations.

The responsibilities of specialist critical care nurses include direct nursing care in addition to expert clinical observation and patient care. These nurse specialists have responsibility for data gathering of both non invasive and invasive measurement and interpretation of laboratory values. They have an important shared responsibility for immediate assessment and emergency interventions. The American Association of Critical Care Nurses established a certification program for nurse specialists in 1973 based on formal examination. Successful candidates are designated Critical Care Registered Nurses and authorized to identify themselves as 'CCRN'. The patient to nurse ratio is typically 2 : 1 in the USA. In western European countries, it varies from 1.9 : 1 in France and Denmark to 4.2 : 1 in the UK (Table 1.2).[6]

With impressive advances in the techniques for enteral and parenteral nutrition for critically ill or injured patients, dietitians have become an important part of the intensive care unit team. The clinical pharmacist is also an important resource as a team member. This professional is a major resource on indications, selection, modes of administration, compatibility, drug interactions and adverse reactions. Such clinical pharmacists are increasingly present at the bedside. The clinical pharmacist has participated in the full care of the patient with special effectiveness during life-threatening crises including those of cardiac arrest.[11] The role of respiratory therapist has been expanded for they are the primary specialists responsible for the technical component of mechanical ventilation.[12]

In the critical care setting in which both patient

Table 1.2 Number of admissions to each bed each year, duration of stay, per cent occupancy and patient to nurse ratio in western European countries

Country	Admission (bed/year)	ICU stay (days)	Occupancy (%)	Patient:nurse ratio
Sweden	124 ± 54	3.0	99	1.9
Holland	93 ± 40	3.5	78	3.0
Germany	83 ± 38	4.4	95	2.1
Denmark	74 ± 7	2.9	59	1.2
Switzerland	74 ± 21	3.0	60	3.1
Belgium	67 ± 18	4.6	89	2.4
UK	65 ± 47	3.5	68	4.2
France	58 ± 35	5.6	83	1.9
Spain	50 ± 17	5.9	73	2.2
Austria	46 ± 10	5.3	68	2.2

Adapted from ref. 6.

monitoring and life support are dependent on electronic and mechanical devices, the clinical (biomedical) engineers and technologists have an essential function. In larger centers, such engineering talents secure operability of the equipment by in-house experts.[1,13]

Medical technology

Almost all units in the USA provide facilities for continuous electrocardiogram monitoring, pulse oximetry, mechanical ventilation and invasive arterial pressure monitoring.[3] Pulmonary artery catheterization, intra-aortic counterpulsion, bronchoscopy, capnography, hemodialysis and/or hemofiltration, and transvenous cardiac pacing are routinely performed in the majority of medical and surgical intensive care units. The indications for and frequency of use are typically quite different in pediatric and neonatal intensive care units in which the principal focus is on respiratory life support, fluid management and environmental temperature. Monitoring of intracranial pressure has revolutionized neurological intensive care.

To fulfill the need for the rapid availability of laboratory measurements in support of clinical decision-making at the bedside of a critically ill or injured patient, the concept of a dedicated laboratory, situated at or near the site of an intensive care unit, has evolved. The 'stat laboratory' provides for automated blood gas measurements and routine emergency measurements on blood, urine and other body fluids.[14] Remarkable advances have been made also in imaging procedures including ultrasound, radionuclear scanning, computed tomography and magnetic resonance imaging. These procedures are coming closer to the bedside, bringing substantial increases in efficiency. There is also substantial opportunity for automation, including capabilities for computer-assisted decision making and record keeping.[15]

The introduction of sophisticated monitors and invasive measurements and related technologies into intensive care units has been at a relatively high cost, not only monetary, but also the cost of iatrogenic complications. Iatrogenic complications of central venous catheterization exceed 4%.[16,17] This complication rate increases when a catheter is advanced into the pulmonary artery. The incidence of pulmonary embolism is estimated to be 2%[18] and that of right-sided endocarditis on autopsy as high as 7%.[19] Arterial catheterization has a risk of complications exceeding 8%.[20,21] Tracheostomy is followed by major complications in more than 17% of patients, and is the likely cause of death in 2% of these patients.[22] Serious complications are associated with intra-aortic counterpulsation in approximately 16% of patients.[23] We can therefore not escape the reality that the benefits of invasive procedures for critically ill patients are counterbalanced by a substantial risk of iatrogenic complication for such patients.[13,24]

Utilization of critical care services

Few other inpatient units have the large fluctuations in census that are likely to occur in the intensive care units. When maximum capacity is too small, availability of critical care services may be critically constrained. When capacity is unduly large, occupancy may be too small to financially support such units, which have disproportionately high fixed operational costs. Constraints stemming from low usage are not only monetary. They also include suboptimal staff preparedness and lesser professional satisfaction of the nursing and technical staff.

The number of admissions per bed per year, the duration of stay in intensive care unit and the occupancy rate vary considerably (Table 1.2). Annual admission numbers for each bed range from 124 patients in Sweden to 46 patients in Austria. The occupancy rate of intensive care units is almost 100% in Sweden, which contrasts with Denmark where occupancy rate averages only 59%. The duration of patient stay in the intensive care unit is longest in Spain with an average of 5.9 days, and shortest in Denmark with an average of only 2.9 days.[6]

Demography of patient population

The patient population in the intensive care units is typically heterogeneous. The age of patients in medical intensive care units varies from less than 20 years to more than 90 years. The majority range in age between 50 and 80 years. Male patients predominate except for ages more than 80 years (Table 1.3).[25] The ages of

Table 1.3 Admissions to medical intensive care unit during five year period by age and sex of patient

Age (years)	Number of admissions	Male (%)	Female (%)
0–19	52	63.5	36.5
20–29	354	52.8	47.2
30–39	375	69.9	30.1
40–49	687	70.9	29.1
50–59	1298	65.8	34.2
60–69	1705	57.6	42.4
70–79	1443	52.0	48.0
80–89	622	43.2	56.8
90+	104	42.3	57.7

Adapted from ref. 25.

patients admitted to medical and to surgical intensive care units are similar. Medical patients have more generalized, less reversible problems which are more likely to result in the syndrome of multiple organ dysfunction. Surgical patients are provided with more monitoring and therapeutic interventions but, as a rule, these patients have greater likelihood of better outcome.[26]

Dynamic disease patterns

Disease patterns changed strikingly after the late 1950s when intensive care units first emerged. The better understanding of acutely life-threatening diseases and injuries, and more particularly the advances in medical technology, surgery and pharmacology, accounted for more successful management of previously fatal conditions. Increases in survival are unequivocal for neonates, who have survived with significantly lower birthweights. This followed remarkable advances in neonatal and perinatal critical care. More specifically, the survival of premature neonates has been doubled between 1955 and 1975.[27] However, this success has been at the expense of major increases in the duration of hospital stay together with greater risk of late death due to pathophysiological syndromes associated with physical underdevelopment and iatrogenic complications.[28]

For adults, circulatory shock was the greatest threat to immediate survival in the 1930s. An understanding of the role of blood loss and the introduction of blood-banking techniques in the mid 1930s was followed by the saving of many patients after massive blood loss, especially when due to traumatic injury.[29] After the end of World War II, acute renal failure following trauma emerged as a fatal condition, limiting survival of war victims. The introduction of hemodialysis secured survival of such patients.[30] In the 1960s, coronary care units evolved in an attempt to prevent otherwise fatal cardiac arrhythmias. The utilization of electrical defibrillation in such units allowed for the resuscitation of patients who previously had fatal ectopic dysrhythmic events. Insertion of transvenous cardiac pacemakers also precluded a significant number of 'electrical' cardiac deaths due to otherwise fatal cardiac bradyarrhythmias.[31] Also in the 1960s, endotracheal intubation and volume-controlled mechanical ventilation replaced the iron lung that had barricaded the patient who was dependent on a mechanical ventilator.[32] Techniques for parenteral alimentation with the use of central venous catheters were evolved at the same time such that nutrition could be sustained in patients who were deprived of gastrointestinal function.

With the advent of potent antibiotic therapy during that era, which was initially directed against Gram-positive organisms and tuberculosis, Gram-negative sepsis emerged as the major threat to patient survival. This brought focus on septic shock and the hemodynamic manifestations of invasive hematogenous infections.[33,34]

Subsequent advances in hemodynamic monitoring and supportive care allowed some patients to survive the circulatory shock state associated with sepsis, only to succumb to metabolic and immunologic complications and the consequent syndrome of multiple organ dysfunction. Indeed, multiple organ dysfunction is now well recognized as a precursor to death. Adult respiratory distress syndrome, progressive metabolic failure and especially renal and liver failure, were first recognized in the late 1960s, but they now constitute major complications that follow initial resuscitation of the critically ill and injured.[35,36] The major threat to the survival of critically ill patients therefore stemmed not only from the underlying illness and typically from a single organ system, but from a process of progressive physiologic failure of interdependent organ systems. The incidence of multiple organ dysfunction syndrome in intensive care units has continuously increased and may now exceed 50% in some medical intensive care units.[37-39] We view this, in part, as an outgrowth of the substantially more effective life support interventions which prolong but do not necessarily 'cure' the progressive life-threatening process. For practical purposes, it also reflects the application of life-sustaining interventions to an increasingly older and higher-risk patient population.

With the emergence of HIV infections in the 1980s and increasing success with life-prolonging interventions in pneumocystic and mycotic infections, the intensive care unit has had an increasingly important role in the management of these unfortunate and typically younger patients.[40,41] The challenges are profound, not only in terms of medical and nursing care, but also economic and, most of all, ethical.

Moral, ethical and economic implications

Critical care medicine is professionally demanding, technologically sophisticated and utilizes invasive devices and expensive drugs and biologicals. It is therefore an inordinately expensive component of health care delivery, and especially so near the end of life. The expansion of critical care services and the increase in the number of patients who are the beneficiaries of critical care has been far more rapid than the expansion of the health care system as a whole. In the 1960s, only 10% of hospitals with more than 200 beds in the USA had intensive care units, whereas today 99% provide such facilities.[42] The number of intensive care beds in the USA increased from 36 000 to 71 000 between 1974 and 1983. Total expenditures for health care in the USA increased to 12% of the gross national product in 1991. It is estimated that approximately 20% of all hospital costs represent intensive care units costs.[13] Since only a small proportion of the population receive critical care services, the cost per patient is extremely high. Consequently, there is much social pressure on the profession to justify such expenditures. This has intensified the demand for objective proof that critical care services reduce mortality and morbidity and preserve meaningful life for the beneficiaries of such care.[13]

Aged and chronically ill patients are the largest consumers of intensive care.[43,44] Patients aged 70 years or older consume 32% of all services. More than 40% of these patients have substantial limitations in function and therefore in quality of life during the month preceding admission to the intensive care unit. Moreover, patients with disorders that regularly require major interventions for support of respiratory, renal or hepatic function or following cardiac arrest, require the largest expenditure and yet have the highest mortality rates. Although these patients constituted only 4% of patients admitted to the intensive care unit in the year 1980, they incurred 9% of total charges and accounted for 21% of hospital deaths.[43]

These considerations notwithstanding, some patients may be monitored and managed in hospital beds other than intensive care without compromise of outcome. Thibault and coworkers[43] concluded that approximately 80% of the patients admitted to an intensive care unit could be competently monitored with noninvasive methods. Only 10% of these noninvasively monitored patients required major interventions. In another survey, 40% of medical and 30% of surgical intensive care patients never received any active interventions and were admitted only for purposes of monitoring.[26] These data suggest that a step-down unit which provides intermediate care may be an appropriate alternative for a large number of patients in the USA.

The challenge is therefore to identify more precisely the level of intensiveness required for patients in relation to outcome of critical care. Accordingly, we concern ourselves increasingly with outcome measurements and address the human and social implications of what we do.[15] Indeed, there is such a paucity of objective data with which to document the ultimate benefits of diagnostic and therapeutic interventions, especially in adults, that unbridled expansion of critical care services cannot be recommended.[13] To some observers, it represents a costly experiment on an unproven model rather than secure progress.[24, 28]

The Development of APACHE systems,[45, 46] the Therapeutic Intervention Scoring System[47] and the Mortality Prediction Models[48] represent constructive efforts to achieve more objective outcome measurements. These are avidly sought to clarify not only what can and therefore might be done, but what should be done to secure significant benefits and minimize risks of sustaining what is perceived to be meaningful life. Inevitably more objective measurements of benefit will be essential for hospitals which are financially constrained, and especially so if the availability of high-cost critical care services is to be secured.

Conclusion

Critical care medicine is a recently evolved special discipline which addresses the life-saving and life-sustaining medical management of patients at risk of imminent death from acute illness or injury. It is a multidisciplinary service specialty, tightly allied with the conventional disciplines of internal medicine, surgery, anesthesiology, pediatrics and their respective subspecialties.

Critical care services are delivered to patients by a team of highly trained personnel who are provided with physical facilities, sophisticated technology, costly drugs and biologicals, and an organizational structure with leadership that secures immediate preparedness for life-sustaining interventions. The design of intensive care units for a given hospital reflects a skillful blend of general concepts of patient management together with modifications which reflect the needs and restraints related to the demographic uniqueness of patients, their

diseases, the availability, composition and priorities of professional staff, and unusual demands for care in this specific setting. The team which has responsibility for the care of the critically ill or injured patient includes clinicians, nurses and allied health personnel and especially respiratory therapists, dietitians and clinical pharmacists. The critical care team is equipped with highly advanced technology for patient monitoring and therapeutic interventions, but with the restraints stemming from high monetary and human costs. The human cost involves relatively high risks of iatrogenic complications. With increasing effectiveness of life-sustaining interventions, new disease states have emerged. The most prominent of these is the progressive failure of interdependent organ systems now termed the multiple organ dysfunction syndrome. The high cost of critical care for a relatively small proportion of the population has prompted much social pressure on the profession to justify such expenditures. Unfortunately, objective proof of reduced mortality and morbidity with meaningful life salvage for the beneficiaries of such care is as yet scant except for pediatric patients. The challenge is therefore to identify more precisely the appropriate intensiveness of critical care in relation to meaningful outcome.

References

1. Weil MH, von Planta M, Rackow EC. Critical care medicine: introduction and historical perspective. In: Shoemaker WC (ed.) *Textbook of Critical Care Medicine.* Philadelphia: WB Saunders, 1988: 1–5.
2. Cady LD, Whitson CW, Weil MH. Optimizing the use of critical care beds. *Hospitals* 1972; **46**: 58–60.
3. Groeger JS, Strosberg MA, Halpern NA *et al.* Descriptive analysis of critical care units in the United States. *Crit Care Med* 1992; **20**: 846–63.
4. Knaus WA, Wagner DP, Loriat P *et al.* A comparison of intensive care in the USA and France. *Lancet* 1982; **ii**: 642–6.
5. Zimmerman JE, Knaus WA, Judson JA *et al.* Patient selection for intensive care: A comparison of New Zealand and United States hospitals. *Crit Care Med* 1988; **16**: 318–26.
6. Miranda DR, Spangenberg JFA. Aspects of critical care organizations in Europe. In: Hall JB, Schmidt GA, Wood LDH (eds) *Principles of Critical Care.* New York: McGraw-Hill Inc., 1992: 2300–2.
7. Sirio CA, Tajimi K, Tase C *et al.* An initial comparison of intensive care in Japan and the United States. *Crit Care Med* 1992; **20**: 1207–15.
8. Miranda DR, Langrehr D (eds). *The ICU: A Cost-Benefit Analysis. International Congress Series 709.* Amsterdam: Excerpta Medica, 1986.
9. Task Force on Guidelines, Society of Critical Care Medicine. Recommendations for service and personnel

for delivery of care in a critical care setting. *Crit Care Med* 1988; **16**: 809–11.

10. Grenvik A, Leonard JJ, Arens JF, Carey LC, Disney FA. Critical care medicine: certification as a multidisciplinary subspecialty. *Crit Care Med* 1981; **9**: 117–25.

11. Gonzales ER. Providing pharmaceutical care during cardiopulmonary resuscitation. *J Pharm Technol* 1992; **8**: 145.

12. Barach AL, Segal MS. The indiscriminate use of IPPB. *J Am Med Assoc* 1975; **231**: 1141–2.

13. NIH Consensus Development Conference Statement on Critical Care Medicine. In: Parrillo JE, Ayers SM (eds) *Major Issues in Critical Care Medicine*. Baltimore: Williams & Wilkins, 1984: 277–89.

14. Weil MH, Michaels S, Puri VK, Carlson RW. The stat laboratory. Facilitating blood gas and biochemical measurements for the critically ill and injured. *Am J Clin Pathol* 1981; **76**: 34–42.

15. Weil MH, Weil CJ, Rackow EC. Guide to ethical decision-making for the critically ill: the three R's and Q.C. *Crit Care Med* 1988; **16**: 636–41.

16. Bernard RW, Stahl WM. Subclavian vein catheterizations: (1) Noninfectious complications. *Ann Surg* 1971; **173**: 184.

17. Goldfarb G, Lebrec D. Percutaneous cannulation of the internal jugular vein in patients with coagulopathies: an experience based on 1,000 attempts. *Anesthesiology* 1982; **56**: 321–3.

18. Foote GA, Schabel SI, Hodges M. Pulmonary complications on the flow directed balloon-tipped catheter. *New Engl J Med* 1974; **290**: 927–31.

19. Rowley KM, Clubb KS, Smith GJW, Cabin HS. Right sided infective endocarditis is a consequence of flow directed pulmonary artery catheterization. *New Engl J Med* 1984; **311**: 1152–6.

20. Gardner RM, Schwartz R, Wong HC, Burke JP. Percutaneous indwelling radial-artery catheters for monitoring cardiovascular function: prospective study of the risk of thrombosis and infection. *New Engl J Med* 1974; **290**: 1227–31.

21. Puri VK, Carlson RW, Bandler JJ, Weil MH. Complications of vascular catheterization in the critically ill: a prospective study. *Crit Care Med* 1980; **8**: 495–9.

22. Meade JW. Tracheotomy – its complications and their management: a study of 212 cases. *New Engl J Med* 1961; **265**: 519–23.

23. Lefemine AA, Kosowosky B, Madoff I, Black H, Lewis M. Results and complications of intra-aortic balloon pumping in surgical and medical patients. *Am J Cardiol* 1977; **40**: 416–20.

24. Robin E. Critical look at critical care. *Crit Care Med* 1983; **11**: 144–8.

25. Thibault GE. The medical intensive care unit: a five-year perspective. In: Parrillo JE, Ayers SM (eds) *Major Issues in Critical Care Medicine*. Baltimore/London: Williams & Wilkins, 1984: 9–15.

26. Henning RJ, McClish D, Daly B, Nearman H, Franklin C, Jackson D. Clinical characteristics and resource utilization of ICU patients: implications for organization of intensive care. *Crit Care Med* 1987; **15**: 264–9.

27. Teberg AJ, Wu PYK, Hodgman JE *et al*. Infants with birth weight under 1,500 g: physical, neurological, and developmental outcome. *Crit Care Med* 1982; **10**: 10–14.

28. Caroline NL. Quo vadis intensive care: More intensive or more care? *Crit Care Med* 1977; **5**: 256.

29. Fantus B. Therapy of Cook County Hospital; blood preservation. *J Am Med Assoc* 1937; **109**: 128.

30. Kolff WJ. *New Ways of Treating Uremia*. London: Churchill Livingstone, 1947.

31. Day HW. An intensive coronary care area. *Dis Chest* 1963; **44**: 423–6.

32. Lassen HCA. A preliminary report on the 1952 epidemic of poliomyelitis in Copenhagen with special reference to the treatment of acute respiratory insufficiency. *Lancet* 1953; **i**: 37–41.

33. Weil MH, Shubin H, Biddle M. Shock caused by Gram-negative micro-organisms: analysis of 169 cases. *Ann Intern Med* 1964; **60**: 384–400.

34. Altemeier WA, Todd JC, Inge WW. Gram-negative septicemia: a growing threat. *Ann Surg* 1967; **166**: 530–42.

35. Skillman JJ, Bushnell LS, Goldman H. Respiratory failure, hypotension, sepsis and jaundice: a clinical syndrome associated with lethal hemorrhage from acute stress ulceration of the stomach. *Am J Surg* 1969; **117**: 523–30.

36. Tilney NL, Batley GL, Morgan AP. Sequential system failure after rupture of abdominal aortic aneurysms. An unsolved problem in postoperative care. *Ann Surg* 1973; **178**: 117–22.

37. Machiedo GW, LoVerme RJ, McGovern PJ, Blackwood JM. Patterns of mortality in a surgical intensive care unit. *Surg Gynecol Obstet* 1981; **152**: 757–9.

38. Wilkinson JD, Pollack MM, Glass NL, Kanter RK, Katz RW, Steinhart CM. Mortality associated with multiple organ system failure and sepsis in pediatric intensive care unit. *J Pediatr* 1987; **111**: 324–8.

39. Darling GE, Duff JH, Mustard RA, Finlay RJ. Multiorgan failure in critically ill patients. *Can J Surg* 1988; **31**: 172–6.

40. Friedman Y, Franklin C, Rackow EC, Weil MH. Improved survival in patients with AIDS, *Pneumocystis carinii* pneumonia, and severe respiratory failure. *Chest* 1989; **96**: 862–6.

41. Rogers PL, Lane HC, Henderson DK, Parrillo J, Masur H. Admission of AIDS patients to a medical intensive care unit: causes and outcome. *Crit Care Med* 1989; **17**: 113–17.

42. Knaus WA, Wagner DP, Draper EA, Lawrence DE, Zimmerman JE. The range of intensive care services today. *J Am Med Assoc* 1981; **246**: 2711–16.

43. Thibault GE, Mulley AG, Barnett GO *et al*. Medical intensive care: indications, interventions, and outcomes. *New Engl J Med* 1980; **302**: 938–42.

44. Tran DD, Groeneveld BJ, van der Meulen J, Nauta JJP, Strack van Schijndel RJM, Thijs LG. Age, chronic disease, sepsis, organ system failure, and mortality in a medical intensive care unit. *Crit Care Med* 1990; **18**: 474–9.

45. Knaus WA, Zimmerman JE, Wagner DP, Draper EA, Lawrence DE. APACHE-acute physiology and chronic health evaluation: a physiologically based classification system. *Crit Care Med* 1980; **9**: 591–7.

46. Knaus WA, Wagner DP, Draper EA *et al*. The APACHE III prognostic system: risk prediction of hospital mortality for critically ill hospitalized adults. *Chest* 1991; **100**: 1619–36.

47. Keene AR, Cullen DJ. Therapeutic intervention scoring system: Update 1983. *Crit Care Med* 1983; **11**: 1–3.

48. Eiseman H, Beart R, Norton L. Multiple organ failure. *Surg Gynecol Obstet* 1977; **144**: 323–6.

CHAPTER 2

The Development, Utilization and Cost Implications of Intensive Care Medicine: Strategies for the Future

TEIK E OH

Development of critical care medicine   11
Organization of ICUs   12
Utilization of ICUs   12
Costs of intensive care   13
Strategies for quality assurance and standardization   14
Summary   17
References   17

Critical care or intensive care medicine is the management and support of patients with established or threatening severe organ dysfunction. These patients in general are the most seriously ill in the hospital and are managed in a specialized ward, the intensive care unit (ICU). Intensive care medicine is now an established and important specialty, ICUs are used heavily but unfortunately they are high consumers of health resources, which are likely to become more scarce in the future. This chapter reviews the development of intensive care medicine and discusses strategies to improve the utilization and quality of service, so as to set the priority of intensive care in the demands for future funding of health care.

Development of critical care medicine

Intensive care medicine started over 40 years ago in Europe and the USA, when ventilatory support was given to polio victims with respiratory failure. Prolonged artificial ventilation of the lungs reduced mortality and complication rates were markedly reduced when such patients were managed together in one ward. This was the start of respiratory care units which became established in many centers in various countries in the late 1950s and 1960s. These respiratory care units gradually evolved into ICUs offering care for a spectrum of problems other than respiratory failure alone.

The development of intensive care was also helped by the advent of postoperative recovery rooms. In the 1940s a few institutions had implemented recovery rooms within the operating theater suite, and the resultant benefits in reducing morbidity and mortality of postoperative patients were reported in 1947.[1] Recovery rooms became universally accepted and then proliferated in the 1960s, when advances in anesthesia and surgery enabled more major surgical procedures to be undertaken. This concept of close monitoring of unstable patients in the recovery room was then extended to the development of further designated areas for care of the critically ill – the ICU.

The 1960s also saw the use of continuous electro-cardiogram (ECG) monitoring for patients with myocardial infarction. This, with the introduction of advances in cardiology such as cardiac pacing and cardioversion, saw the organization of specialized wards for cardiac patients called coronary care units (CCUs),[2] which added impetus to the development of intensive care and other such specialized units.

Organization of ICUs

ICUs evolved one by one, over the last three decades, to support surgical and medical patients with organ failure, and special care techniques also evolved for pediatric (including neonatal) patients. However, the rapid establishment of ICUs and intensive care services worldwide has not followed specific criteria or guidelines on organization. No fundamental differences in monitoring and life support interventions can be made between medical and surgical patients, but the development of multidisciplinary ICUs was resisted by doctors in some countries. Specialists in certain disciplines did not wish to relinquish control of their patients by handing over their management to another team. Consequently, ICUs in North America and parts of Europe developed along specialty lines with separate medical, surgical, cardiothoracic, neurosurgical and burns ICUs. In Australia, New Zealand, the UK and Scandinavia, however, the development of multidisciplinary ICUs became more common.

The control of the ICU varies by unit and institution, and has obviously evolved from territorial battles between specialists, case mix and local resources. Anesthetists have traditionally taken a major role in the development of intensive care because many patients are postoperative with respiratory failure and hemodynamic derangement. Significant contributions have also been made by physicians, surgeons, and pediatricians, especially with the establishment of single discipline ICUs. At present intensive care can be provided by dedicated full-time intensivists headed by the ICU director. Advice from specialists of other disciplines is available by consultation, a model often referred to as the *closed ICU*. An *open ICU* model is one in which patient care is delivered by more than one group of doctors. There is often a team of attending part-time clinicians, usually anesthetists, who co-manage the patients with the referring doctors. Much less common now, fortunately, is intensive care given by the patients' own specialty clinicians without any attending ICU medical staff. With different models of organization and control of ICUs, the case mix and standard of care must inevitably vary. The cost and utilization implica-

tions from a dissimilarity of ICUs must also be significant.

Utilization of ICUs

Consolidation of intensive care in the 1970s and 1980s was accompanied by a growth of ICUs and increased utilization of intensive care services. New hospitals planned for ICUs and old hospitals created ICUs from existing wards. This proliferation of ICUs did not follow any overall national health care planning. Instead, ICUs were usually created according to local perceptions of need, available finances, and interest shown by particular doctors. A number of factors contributed to the expansion of intensive care services. Firstly, overall expenditure in health increased in some developed countries. For example, between 1960 and 1980 the cost of US health care rose from 5.2% to 9.4% of the gross national product (GNP), an increase in cash terms of 11.7% annually.[3] The growth in intensive care was also fed by the belief by both the medical profession and the public[4] that intensive care services are effective and necessary and should not be denied to any patient. New technologies in invasive monitoring and in procedures such as transplantion and cancer surgery demanded care that was more sophisticated than could be given on an average ward. Intensive care no longer remained the sole domain of general hospitals as small hospitals and private hospitals established their own ICUs. New training programs produced intensivists who promoted utilization of intensive care services. ICUs themselves allowed survival of patients who would otherwise have died, and thus propagated the role of intensive care services. Finally, services increased because of incentives in health care systems, such as payment to doctors on a fee for service basis and by more than one paymaster.

Data on intensive care utilization are imprecise but are available for some countries. ICU utilization appears to be the greatest by far in the USA. In 1986, there were 108 ICU patient days per 1000 population.[5] Use of ICUs increased by an average of 8% annually from 1979 to 1982, when the increase levelled off at a rate of under 2% per year. By the 1980s, ICU beds made up 6–15% of total hospital beds and 15–20% of all medical patients received a portion of their hospital care in an ICU.[6] In comparison, ICU utilization in Canada grew by an average 4.8% annually from 1969 to 1986, with an increase in ICU patient days per 1000 population from 17 to 42.[5] ICU beds in Canada take up 4% of hospital beds, and use of intensive care on a population basis is 2.5 times less than the USA.[5] In Europe, utilization of ICUs varies greatly but about 1–4% of hospital beds are ICU beds, which represent 10–15% of total health care costs.[7] Australia and New Zealand have about 1.5% of hospital beds given to ICU beds.[8] In Japan, ICU beds increased from 12 760 in 1984 to 14 789 in 1987, with ICU beds constituting 1.2% of general hospital beds in 1987.[9]

It is obvious that intensive care utilization in terms of provision of beds and use of ICU services increased most markedly in the 1970s. The growth in intensive care utilization slowed down in the 1980s, as the costs of ICU beds were realized. This was probably related in the USA to the introduction of a new prospective payment system (see below).

Costs of intensive care

The growth in intensive care services must inevitably involve consideration of costs. Much has been written on the matter but useful research is relatively sparse because of the difficulties in identifying and comparing true costs. There are *fixed costs* in any ICU which are irrelevant to the workload and the outcome of patients. Salaries make up the bulk of fixed costs (usually at least 60%)[10] and the services of nurses represent the largest resource consumed by an ICU. *Variable costs* depend on the numbers of patients admitted and the extent and variety of services rendered (e.g. investigations, monitoring and procedures). In both fixed and variable costs, there are components which can be related to patient care (*direct costs*) and those which do not, such as 'hotel' or administration expenditures (*indirect costs*). The factors which dictate the costs of providing intensive care services relate to economic considerations of *supply* and *demand*.

SUPPLY

The supply of resources to ICUs through hospital administrators may come from a single source of government funding or from multiple sources, e.g. federal and state grants, private fees and insurance reimbursements. Obviously, resources are limited if the hospital is funded only from government allocations such as those of the UK's National Health Service or Australia's Federal and State governments. The growth in intensive care services suggests that the supply of resources has been responsive to demand. However, rising costs, especially with the recent downturn of many countries' economies, have resulted in restrictions on supply mediated through rationing of fixed hospital budgets ('implicit rationing')[11] and payments for services ('explicit rationing').[11] For example, a prospective payment system for hospital care based on diagnosis-related groups (DRGs) was introduced by the

US government in 1983, and reimbursements for certain patients treated in ICUs can fall short of actual costs.[12,13]

DEMAND

ICUs will always have a 'captive consumer market' of critically ill patients, as there are no alternatives for this care. Nonetheless, the demand for ICU services can be largely doctor generated. Demand is reflected by admissions and services, and with supply, are related to demography, economy and technology. New technological advances nearly always increase health costs, even in times of economic recession. The declining birth rates and increasing elderly population in most developed nations will have implications on intensive care services in the future. Due to the aging of the post World War II 'baby boomers', the proportion of older people will increase. By the next decade, people over 55 years will constitute over one-fourth of the population of many developed countries. Society's productivity and economic growth may stagnate with a shrinking workforce having to support an enlarging group of dependants. A changing case mix, with possibly less trauma admissions but more diseases of the elderly (especially heart disease, cancer, stroke), may increase the average length of stay in ICU, adding to increased ICU costs. Future ICU utilization and costs will also be profoundly increased if the global spread of the acquired immune deficiency syndrome (AIDS) undergoes a rampant upsurge.

How an ICU is organized will also have implications on demand. An *open* ICU with access by multiple doctors is likely to generate more admissions than a *closed* unit with full time intensivists who act as triage 'gatekeepers'. After admission, the clinical services rendered to patients in an ICU will be dependent on the practice patterns of its doctors. There is undoubtedly a great variation in the use of resources by different ICUs, but so far little attention has been paid to the link between ICU utilization and organization.

REPORTED COSTS

How much then does intensive care cost? Most studies published have been from the USA, based on retrospective analyses of data from late 1970s and early 1980s, a period which reflected the fastest growth rate of intensive care. Close scrutiny of the costs of ICU care was necessitated by the introduction of prospective payments based on DRGs. Different methods and estimations were used to deduce costs, and most studies were retrospective. The actual numerical costs would, of course, be higher today if adjustments were made for inflation. Apart from inflation, higher costs of intensive care and health care stemmed from fee incentives, oversupply of specialists with access to high technological services, health administrative costs, and poor coordination of purchasing of services.[14] Costs of intensive care can be considered at a *microeconomic*, hospital level or on a *macroeconomic*, national or population basis.

Microeconomic

The cost of managing an individual patient in an ICU of course varies with the diagnosis, severity of illness, doctors and type of ICU, and individual costs may vary as much as 1000-fold.[15] Nonetheless, average costs per patient can be examined from a pool of consecutive ICU patients. In 1978, 199 critically ill surgical patients averaged US$22 000 per ICU stay.[16] Ventilated patients in an ICU in one US institution in 1976 cost US$16 930 per patient.[17] A daily ICU bed cost almost seven times that of an acute care bed in 1978 has been reported,[18] but a commonly accepted estimated ratio for the daily ICU bed:acute care bed cost is 3 : 1.[5] Later US figures (for 1984/85) reported a mean daily cost of US$100 per therapeutic intervention scoring system (TISS)[19] point, with patients having a daily range of 18.5 to 26.9 points.[20]

Elsewhere, an European study in 1985 found that half the total hospital costs of 238 patients in a surgical ICU were generated during the ICU stage, which accounted for 17.5% of the hospitalization period.[21] An Australian study in 1986[10] on 100 consecutive patients admitted to a teaching hospital ICU, found that the mean *total* admission cost was A$1357 (approximately US$1000) but for over 70% of patients, costs were less than A$1000 each, considerably less than US costs.

Macroeconomic

On a national scale, the cost of ICUs in the USA since the 1970s has been estimated to be 14–20% of global hospital costs.[5, 22, 23] In cash terms, US ICU costs in 1986 totalled US$33.9 billion or 0.8% GNP. Even so, ICU costs in the USA are believed to be underestimated as hospital charges for intensive care services are reported to be less than real incurred costs.[24] Canada, with its single payer system (by the Provinces), had ICU costs at 8% of total hospital costs or 0.2% GNP.[5] In Holland, 10–15% of total health care costs are consumed by intensive care services.[25] Data for other countries are not readily available, but intensive care would also constitute a significant portion of their health costs.

Thus intensive care providers now need to be cost conscious, and to focus on cost-effectiveness and productivity in order to bid competitively for future resources. At the same time, strategies must also be developed to implement quality assurance and standardize health care norms.

Strategies for quality assurance and standardization

Since there is relative paucity of information on the costs, utilization, efficiency and benefits of intensive care, an important strategy is to collect explicit and complete data and conduct research into these areas. Benefits of intensive care can be demonstrated and appropriate levels of funding can also be derived. Each ICU should start to keep data on its utilization, manpower, resources consumed (e.g. investigations, disposable items and drugs), case mix and patient outcome. Other major strategic approaches to achieve adequate funding and cost efficiency include restructuring the organization of ICUs, steps to increase resource supply and rationalize demands on ICU services, as well as ongoing audits of both the cost and quality of intensive care given to patients.

REORGANIZATION OF ICUs

Planning and distribution of adequate resources for intensive care should be made at a national or state level and then at regional levels.[25] An ICU must have its role defined, both with respect to its region, as well as to its hospital. Within the region, its role should be one to serve the region best. It may be a main tertiary referral ICU or a supporting one. It may be a specialized ICU if its hospital is a regional referral centre for a specialized activity such as trauma, neurosurgery, cardiac surgery, obstetrics or pediatrics. In this way, resources are rationalized and expensive duplication is avoided. The community is thus best served. Within the hospital itself, the role and function of the ICU will depend on the hospital structure, staff qualifications and resources. Reorganization should be aimed at rationalizing the levels of intensive care, number of beds and types of ICUs.

Levels of ICUs

Effective regionalization of intensive care services can only be made possible by establishing different standards or levels of ICUs. Different patients require different levels of intensive care; the more critically ill patients require a higher level of ICU with a higher investment of resources. The minimal requirements of a lower level of ICU are the ability to resuscitate patients and to support vital functions for limited periods. Three levels of ICUs have been identified in Australia and New Zealand and in Europe.[26, 27]

- *Level I* ICUs cater for basic monitoring. There are no full-time specialists and no 24-hour on-site doctor.

Essentially, it offers better nursing observations than in the wards, i.e. 'high dependency' care, otherwise called 'intermediate' or 'step-down' units. Typical of these units are those of small hospitals such as the private hospitals.

• *Level II* ICUs offer general intensive care services but not in specialized areas like neurosurgery and renal dialysis. There is usually a full-time specialist director with a doctor on-site after hours. However, after-hours support services may not be complete. These Level II units apply to district hospitals.

• *Level III* ICUs offer full services. A specialist intensivist is always available and there is always a doctor on-site. Radiology and pathology provide 24-hour support. These should be the ICUs of major teaching hospitals.

By defining the levels of ICUs, the most appropriate intensive care services can then be offered to patients, matching organization and resources with particular needs for intensive care. Level I and Level II ICUs should be available at a reasonable time and distance from the population they serve, but Level III ICUs should only be located at tertiary referral centres. Better purchasing of intensive care services is achieved and appropriate expertise better accorded; less proficient doctors and small hospitals are dissuaded from delivering intensive care services beyond their competence or means.

Number of ICU beds

The number of beds dedicated to intensive care should be re-examined at both regional and institutional levels. ICUs in Australia, New Zealand, the UK and other countries have beds numbering 1.5–2.0% of total acute hospital beds, in sharp contrast to the USA with up to 15%. The quality of intensive care and outcome of ICU patients have not been shown to be any different despite a large difference in bed availability between ICUs.[8,28] Thus many patients admitted into US ICUs would not warrant admission into Australasian ICUs. These are mostly postsurgical or less severely ill medical 'high dependency' patients who are admitted for monitoring. There is no evidence to show that these patients have a worse outcome if managed in general wards than if admitted to ICUs. Singer *et al.* reported that when their medical ICU/CCU reduced their beds from 18 to 8 in 1981 because of nurse shortages, the proportion of patients admitted primarily for monitoring decreased.[23] While more patients with myocardial infarction were admitted to non intensive care wards, there was no increase in mortality.[23]

Reducing the number of ICU beds will reduce the cost of intensive care without influencing the availability or quality of care, provided the ICU beds comprise a significant proportion of hospital beds. This is different from reducing admissions to an ICU, which is not likely to reduce costs to any notable extent, as staffing and capital outlays on equipment will remain unchanged. Thus, there is no convincing evidence to support allocating ICU beds for all levels of intensive care at more than, say, 3% of the hospital's total acute beds.

Multidisciplinary ICUs

Many countries such as Australia, New Zealand, the UK, Japan and Scandinavia, have multidisciplinary ICUs in the main, although separate CCUs and neonatal ICUs are also common. Other countries follow the US organization of separate single discipline ICUs, in particular medical (MICU) and surgical ICUs (SICU) which admit patients specific to their specialties and are managed by specialists in that particular field. However, the problems of critically ill patients are not confined solely to their primary disease. For example, MICU patients may develop surgical complications, and conversely, SICU patients will often have concomitant medical problems. With the complexities of multiple organ failure, doctors in specialized ICUs do not have the wide-ranging experience and expertise to deal with problems outside their trained specialty. Critically ill patients with organ failure develop the same pathophysiological processes no matter whether they are classified as medical or surgical patients, and they require the same approaches to support vital organs.

Why, then, do we need multiple, single discipline ICUs in the same hospital? A case can be made for having a separate CCU and neonatal ICU in a hospital, and even for a separate pediatric ICU if children make up a large proportion of admissions. However, there is no good argument against amalgamating all other ICUs in the same institution as a single, multidisciplinary ICU with a reduced number of beds. Some beds from existing single discipline ICUs could be redesignated as Level I intermediate ICUs with less resource requirements. A leaner, more efficient intensive care service would result in cost savings to the hospital.

Dedicated full-time intensivists

Present day training programs in intensive care are able to produce specialist intensivists capable of managing all patients in a closed model multidisciplinary ICU, with support when necessary, through consulting specialists in other departments.[29] If intensive care is now recognized as a separate specialty, it follows that ICUs should be managed by dedicated intensivists rather than by other specialists who devote only a part of their time to the ICU. Also, *closed* ICUs managed by full-time intensivists are likely to be more cost efficient than *open* models with access by different and many more specialists. Indeed, objective evidence on quality of care favoring dedicated doctors in the ICU have been reported.[30, 31]

COST CONTROL STRATEGIES

To control and analyze the cost of ICUs it is important to recognize control at two levels of operation: (i) resource allocation at a national or regional *macro* level; and (ii) at the hospital and department *micro* level. At the *macro* level, any implicit rationing of intensive care resources is imposed by society, and is already present in countries like the UK and Australia, where many tertiary hospitals are already overburdened. Although 'the die is already cast' with implicit rationing, clinicians must define or show limits of rationing beyond which adequate care cannot be given. Also at a national level, cost control measures can be better achieved if there are fewer paymasters for intensive care services and if payments for services can be audited. However, it is hard to see how a prospective payment system, such as by DRGs, can benefit intensive care. Apart from introducing more administrative bureaucracy, it can influence diagnoses and treatment by clinicians.

At the *micro* level, intensivists must strive for enough funds to provide the safest care within the system. Tighter control of resources given to hospitals will not automatically result in lower operating costs. Management initiatives, such as incentives to reward hospitals and ICUs able to show improvements in cost efficiency, also need to be implemented. *Quality assurance* (QA), which measures standards of care by clinical staff, is an essential and integral component of health care, and QA programs will promote quality of care and use of resources. Other strategies in cost control at the *micro* level include establishing an ICU cost management system, increasing supply, and decreasing demand for services. The objective is to rationalize rather than to ration services.

ICU cost management system

A cost management centre for the ICU should be set up in the hospital and lines of financial responsibility clearly defined. Policy decisions must be made by the hospital on the number of ICU beds, case mix, staffing, and overall annual budget, and should be complemented by longer-term 3- to 5-year forecasts. The ICU director is given a greater leadership role and, with his deputies, assumes responsibility and accountability for the total ICU budget. Assistance from finance managers must be readily available. The cost center will track all expenditures incurred in providing intensive care services, such as salaries and the cost of equipment, drugs, disposable items, and pathology and imaging investigations. In this way, the cost of each service becomes

transparent, rather than unknown and out of mind. Staff education programs such as cost awareness programs and protocols in relation to ordering drugs, diagnostic tests and blood can be recommended, but may not achieve a lasting effect.[32]

Increase supply

While the concept of spending extra new resources on intensive care runs contrary to cost containment, additional resources are required with any development requiring the introduction of useful new technologies, and replacement of expensive capital equipment. The annual and future business plans submitted by the ICU director should present data to justify needs and to demonstrate efficient management of resources. For example, an increased workload can be supported by figures showing increased ICU and hospital admissions and increased ICU patient bed-days. Requests for additional resources can be backed up by data showing a case mix of patients with more severe illness and increasing mean APACHE II scores. TISS points and examples of critical incidents can be presented to promote requests for additional nurses and junior doctors. Requests for new drugs and devices need to be backed up by reasonably convincing arguments of better care and earlier patient recovery, with the best form of argument being published clinical trials.

Increase in supply can also be achieved by shifting resources from less cost-efficient areas. There should be incentives, for example, to allow some savings from reducing the number of ICU beds and curtailing less useful investigations to be channelled back to the ICU. An increase in the 'supply of beds' by increasing the availability of ICU services to more patients, can be achieved by early discharge of patients who no longer require, or benefit from, intensive care. This can be effected by clear admission and discharge policies.

Rationalize or decrease demand

Demand can be decreased by formal rationing policies based on:

1. *equality* (every patient is entitled to a fixed equal allotment of intensive care);
2. *equity* (every patient has access to a minimal level of intensive care);
3. *utilitarianism* (social factors govern allocation of services);
4. *distribution according to medical need.*[33]

However, *suitability* for intensive care, which regards both need and eventual outcome, is probably the most appropriate consideration. Also, the first approach to decrease demand is to reduce overuse or inappropriate use of intensive care.

ICUs should not admit patients who are too 'well' or too sick to benefit. A study of 2072 MICU/CCU patients at the Massachusetts General Hospital in 1977–79[34] reported that 77% required only noninvasive monitoring of whom only 10% required major interventions. Between 10 and 50% of patients in a sample of US ICUs never received active intensive care.[35] Only 23% of patients admitted to ICUs in four areas of the USA examined by the General Accounting Office had less than a 10% chance of active treatment.[20] Hence, many patients admitted to ICUs require only monitoring and can be managed in a high dependency unit or in normal wards.

At the other end of the spectrum, a relatively small proportion of ICU patients (around 10%) consume as much resources as the remainder.[20] This high-cost group includes many patients who die. Thus, massive resources can be spent to treat inappropriate patients to save only a few for discharge from hospital. The difficulty lies in identifying high-cost patients who will die. Severity of illness does not necessarily reflect cost. Costs tend to rise with severity and then fall with the upper levels of severity, presumably because of shorter stays in ICU due to early deaths.[20] Unfortunately, prediction of outcome is still imprecise. High cost patients tend to be patients who have outcomes opposite to those predicted by their doctors.[20, 36] Although there appears to be a crude relationship between TISS points and resource consumption,[10, 20] TISS and APACHE II scores cannot guide resource allocation for individual patients.

Intensivists thus have to filter admissions and rank by priorities the requests for admission at times of bed shortage, acting as advocates for both the patient and society. They have to use their trained clinical skills to judge the suitability of patients for admission. The traditional 'first come first served' admission principle must be abandoned. In times of acute bed shortage, selected patients in the unit may need to be discharged earlier in order to admit more appropriate patients, and any elective major surgery which requires ICU post-operative care should be postponed.

It is important that clear guidelines regarding termination of intensive care be developed. This decision concerning brain (stem) dead patients should no longer present ethical or legal problems in developed countries today. Problems have arisen due to the confusion of doctors themselves on the definition of brain death, often calling patients in the vegetative state 'brain dead'. With all other patients, treatment which has been optimally given but without benefit, should be withdrawn when death is inevitable. Under the same circumstances, no treatment should be started if judged to offer no benefit. This approach is already practiced by many ICUs.[28, 37] A recent enquiry into dying in Australia stated that 'the nonapplication of medical treatment, does not in itself constitute the cause of death, where a medical practitioner is acting in good faith'.[38] The term 'passive euthanasia' which has been applied to this situation is misleading and misrepresentative and must be deplored, because euthanasia has no place in the ICU. Similar ICU guidelines should also be developed to handle issues such as 'living wills', 'health proxies', and the rights of minors. Good communication with families is paramount. The intensivist has a responsibility to inform relatives of the clinical situation, treatment given, and judged prognosis.

Summary

Intensive care medicine is now an established branch of medicine. It developed in the 1950s and 1960s, and expanded rapidly in the 1970s and 1980s without proper planning or appropriate appraisal of benefits. Increased utilization, with inflation, new technologies, incentives to overservice, and fragmented payment systems have contributed to high costs. The aging of the population and possible rampant spread of AIDS will add to future costs. Strategies to improve utilization and quality of intensive care service include gathering useful data on use and benefits, reorganization of ICU beds, standards and management, and development of hospital initiatives to monitor costs, increase supply and rationalize demand.

References

1. Ruth HS, Hawgen FP, Grave DD. Anesthesia Study Commission: findings of eleven years' activity. *J Am Med Assoc* 1947; **35**: 881–6.
2. Day HW. An intensive coronary care area. *Dis Chest* 1963; **44**: 423–5.
3. Public Health Service. *Health, United States: 1981.* Hyattsville, MD: DHHS publication no. (PHS)82–1232, 1981.
4. Davis M, Patrick DL, Southerland LI, Green ML. Patients' and families' preferences for medical intensive care. *J Am Med Assoc* 1988; **260**: 797–802.
5. Jacobs P, Noseworthy TW. National estimates of intensive care utilization and costs: Canada and the United States. *Crit Care Med* 1991; **18**: 1282–6.
6. Consensus Conference. Critical Care Medicine. *J Am Med Assoc* 1983; **250**: 798–804.
7. Miranda DR, Langrehr D (eds). *The ICU: A Cost-Benefit Analysis. International Congress Series 709.* Amsterdam: Excerpta Medica, 1986.
8. Zimmerman JE, Knaus WA, Judson JA *et al.* Patient selection for intensive care: a comparison of New Zealand and United States hospitals. *Crit Care Med* 1988; **16**: 318–26.

9. Aikawa N. International perspectives on critical care: Japan. In: Hall JB, Schmidt GA, Wood LDH (eds). *Principles of Critical Care*. New York: McGraw-Hill Inc., 1992: 2285–90.

10. Slatyer MA, James OF, Moore PG, Leeder SR. Costs, severity of illness and outcome in intensive care. *Anaesthesia Intensive Care* 1986; **14**: 381–9.

11. Mechanic D. Rationing of medical care and the preservation of clinical judgement. *J Family Practice* 1980; **11**: 431–3.

12. Bekes C, Fleming S, Scott WE. Reimbursement for intensive care services under diagnosis-related groups. *Crit Care Med* 1988; **16**: 478–81.

13. Ahmad M, Fergus L, Stothard P, Harrington D, Sivak E, Farmer R. Impact of diagnosis-related groups' prospective payment on utilization of medical intensive care. *Chest* 1988; **93**: 176–9.

14. Dixon J. US health care II: the cost problem. *Br Med J* 1992; **305**: 878–80.

15. Bendixen HH. The cost of intensive care. In: Bunker JP, Barnes BA, Mosteller F (eds). *Costs, Risks and Benefits of Surgery*. New York: Oxford University Press, 1984: 372–84.

16. Cullen DJ, Keene R, Waternoux C *et al.* Results, changes, and benefits of intensive care for critically ill patients: update 1983. *Crit Care Med* 1984; **12**: 102–6.

17. Schmidt C, Elliott CG, Carmelli D *et al.* Prolonged mechanical ventilation for respiratory failure: a cost benefit analysis. *Crit Care Med* 1983; **11**: 407–11.

18. Parno JR, Teres D, Lemeshow S, Brown RB. Hospital charges and long-term survival of ICU versus non ICU patients. *Crit Care Med* 1982; **10**: 569–74.

19. Keene AR, Cullen DJ. Therapeutic intervention scoring system: update 1983. *Crit Care Med* 1983; **11**: 1–3.

20. Oye RK, Bellamy PE. Patterns of resource consumption in medical intensive care. *Chest* 1991; **99**: 685–9.

21. Bams JL, Miranda DR. Outcome and costs of intensive care. A follow up study on 238 ICU patients. *Intensive Care Med* 1985; **11**: 234–41.

22. Knaus WA, Thibault GE. Intensive care units today. In: McNeil BJ, Cravalho EG (eds). *Critical Issues in Medical Technology*. Boston: Auburn House Publishing, 1982: 193–215.

23. Singer DE, Carr PL, Mulley AG, Thibault GE. Rationing intensive care – physician responses to a resource shortage. *New Engl J Med* 1983; **309**: 1155–60.

24. Mulley AG. The allocation of resources for medical intensive care. In: *President's Commission for the Study of Ethical Problems in Medicare and Biomedical Research: Securing Access to Health Care*. Washington DC: Government Printing Office, 1983; **3**: 285–311.

25. Miranda DR. Management of resources in intensive care. *Intensive Care Med* 1991; **17**: 127–8.

26. Miranda DR, Williams A, Loirat PH (eds). *Guidelines For Better Resource Use. European Society of Intensive Care Task Force*. Amsterdam: Kluwer Academic Publishers, 1990.

27. Australian and New Zealand College of Anaesthetists. *Standards for Intensive Care Units*. Melbourne: ANZCA document P10, 1985.

28. Oh TE, Hutchinson RC, Short S, Buckley TA, Lin ES, Leung D. Verification and use of the acute physiology and chronic health evaluation scoring system in a Hong Kong intensive care unit. *Crit Care Med* 1993; **21**: 698–705.

29. Byth PL, Harrison GA. A survey of successful FFARACS candidates in Australasia. *Crit Care Med* 1986; **14**: 583–6.

30. Knaus WA, Draper EA, Wagner DP, Zimmerman JE. An evaluation of outcome from intensive care in major medical centers. *Ann Intern Med* 1986; **104**: 410–18.

31. Li TC, Philips MC, Shaw L, Cook EF, Nathanson C, Goldman L. Staffing in a community hospital intensive care. *J Am Med Assoc* 1984; *252*: 2023–7.

32. Soumerai SB, Avorn J. Efficacy and cost-containment in hospital pharmacotherapy: state of the art and future directions. *Milbank Memorial Fund Quart* 1984; **62**: 447–74.

33. Kalb PE, Miller DH. Utilization strategies for intensive care units. *J Am Med Assoc* 1989; **261**: 2389–95.

34. Thibault GE, Mulley AG, Barnett GO *et al.* Medical intensive care: Indications, interventions, and outcomes. *New Engl J Med* 1980; **302**: 938–42

35. Wagner DP, Knaus WA, Draper EA. Identification of low-risk monitor admissions to medical-surgical ICUs. *Chest* 1987; **92**: 423–8.

36. Detsky AS, Stricker SC, Mulley AG, Thibault GE. Prognosis, survival and the expenditure of hospital resources for patients in an intensive care unit. *New Engl J Med* 1981; **305**: 667–72.

37. Smedira NG, Evans BH, Grais LS *et al.* Withholding and withdrawal of life support from the critically ill. *New Engl J Med* 1990; **322**: 309–15.

38. Parliament of Victoria Social Development Committee. *Report upon the Inquiry into Options for Dying with Dignity*. Second and Final Report. Melbourne: Government Printer, 1987.

PART II

Resource Standards

CHAPTER 3

Primary and Mobile Care: Land, Sea and Air

P MULROONEY

Primary care in the field   22
Primary patient transfer   26
Initial treatment at receiving hospital   28
Problems of the transport environment   30
References   32

Medical emergencies in the community requiring intervention by trained personnel with subsequent transfer to a hospital broadly fall into two categories: cardiorespiratory collapse and major trauma. In the UK cardiovascular disease is the main cause of death in the age group 45–54 years (7456 in 1986)[1] and over 500 000 trauma victims are admitted to hospital each year.[2] In principle there is the choice of 'scoop and run' if the specialist treatment center is deemed to be close enough, or alternatively stabilization at the scene of the incident. A number of authors suggest that stabilization at the scene of the incident prior to transport is preferable.[3–5] Furthermore, it has been suggested that the quality of prehospital care is a major factor in the outcome of the seriously injured patient. Two main requirements have been identified for the improvement of management of these patients:

1. improvement in the quality of prehospital care;
2. centralization of hospital services for the injured (trauma centers) with greater medical involvement by medical staff in the training and running of the ambulance service (in line with the French Service d'Aide Médicale Urgente (SAMU) system).[6]

There is agreement amongst a number of experts as to the necessity of providing a pool of medical specialists to provide immediate care to victims, though there is no unanimity as how best to provide this.[7,8] A French retrospective study comparing two series of multiply injured patients before and after the creation of SAMU showed that between 1969 and 1979 survival rate increased from 52 to 81%,[9] although the reasons for this are probably multifactorial. The German experience showed that by 1972 a 20–30% improvement in patient survival was achieved through the institution of prehospital medical care.[10] Further German data between 1972 and 1984 showed a decrease in the number of victims dying in transport.[11] These same data were re-evaluated in 1981 when two groups of patients with similar severity of injury were retrospectively studied. Sixty-three per cent of patients who had received medical attention at the accident site had been transferred from the intensive care unit (ICU) to routine ward care within 3 days of admission compared with 14% of those who had not received medical attention at the accident site.[12] Relating mortality to injury severity score (ISS), it was found that when ISS was greater than 35, those not receiving prehospital physician care had a significantly higher mortality rate.[13]

Reviewing a series of cardiorespiratory emergencies between 1981 and 1988, a French SAMU team attended 628 asthma patients. Fifty per cent of patients were less than 40 years old; 16.3% of these were suffering life-threatening acute asthma and half of these were intubated and ventilated immediately. This was regarded as a potent argument for the early involvement of a doctor in the field.[14] A similar conclusion was drawn in a survey taken between 1985 and 1987 in patients suffering from status asthmaticus.[15]

Primary care in the field

In the field the fundamental approach is no different from that in the hospital environment, namely that of diagnosis and resuscitation. The principal difference lies in the level of equipment and expertise available at the site of the incident.

The ability of a medical team in the field to cope with an emergency is dependent on the drugs and equipment available to them and there should be a system designed to cope with most if not all eventualities. There should be a bag or a box containing drugs and equipment for resuscitation and field anesthesia (Fig. 3.1 and Table

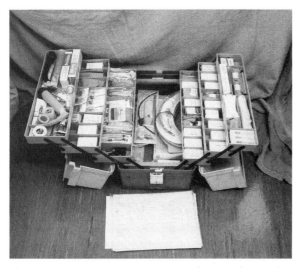

Fig. 3.1 Bag containing emergency drugs and resuscitation equipment with chart showing location of contents. From ref. 95, with permission.

3.1). The template suggested in Table 3.1 is chosen so that there is a permanently available pack with drugs suitable for most situations, as the condition of the patient may bear no relation to that anticipated. The reasons for choosing most of the drugs is self-explanatory, however, explanation of individual drugs may be necessary. These include doxapram, which may be used to stimulate respiration in the event of field anesthesia (in the absence of pathological causes); droperidol, which in low doses can be used as an antiemetic and in higher doses to supplement anesthesia; labetalol in addition to propranolol because of its dual alpha and beta sympathetic blocking action; nalbuphine because it is an opioid which is not a controlled drug and hence can be left in the bag and does not need to be signed out; naloxone because in the event of trauma other personnel may have treated the patient with opiates and the respiratory depressant effects of these may require reversal (especially if intramuscular doses have been given in a shocked patient who is then resuscitated);

Table 3.1 Contents of resuscitation/field anesthesia bag

Drugs
Adrenaline, atropine, calcium gluconate/chloride, chlorpheniramine, dexamethasone, 50% dextrose, digoxin, doxapram, droperidol, etomidate, frusemide, hydrocortisone, isoprenaline, ketamine, labetalol, lignocaine 2%, lignocaine 1 g, metoclopramide, midazolam, nalbuphine, naloxone, neostigmine, propranolol, salbutamol, sodium bicarbonate 8.4%, sodium chloride 0.9%, suxamethonium, vecuronium

Intubating equipment
Laryngoscope (with spare batteries and bulb), endotracheal tubes (sizes 5, 6, 7, 8, 9), airways (sizes 1, 2, 3, 4), introducer, Magill forceps, catheter mount, lubricating jelly, tie, artery forceps, Minitrac™, humidification filter, self-inflating bag and mask

Intravenous equipment
Intravenous cannulae, needles, alcohol swabs, syringes (1, 2, 5, 10 and 20 ml)

Miscellaneous
Chest drains, Heimlich valves, scalpel, adhesive tape, sutures, ECG electrodes

suxamethonium bromide is available as a powder for reconstitution. This bag should be checked daily and drugs and equipment replaced or cleaned as they are used. If specific problems are anticipated, then extra drugs or equipment can be added. In the patient transport, be it helicopter or road ambulance, there should be a ventilator, suction apparatus and appropriate monitoring. The choice of ventilator will depend on power sources available and the amount and source of oxygen available. Most aircraft have either 28 or 110 V DC power supply, though DC/AC converters are available which can provide 240 V AC supply (equivalent to UK domestic supply).[16] British ambulances have 13 V DC supply. It is possible to use a compressor-driven ventilator, but for work in the field a small portable robust gas-driven, fluid-logic ventilator is the ideal. Examples include the VentiPAC (Fig. 3.2) and the Dräger Oxylog. When cylinders are in use it is essential to be aware of the contents of the cylinders and the gas requirements of these ventilators as the oxygen cylinder provides both the driving force and the fresh gas flow. The calculation of gas requirements should assume the worst case scenario i.e. 100% oxygen (Tables 3.2 and 3.3). Within the helicopter or road ambulance the problems of oxygen cylinders may be obviated by the development of liquid oxygen (LOX) systems, e.g. 30 000 liters in a single container developed by Puritan Bennett to drive ventilators, suction apparatus and membrane oxygenators.[16] Suction apparatus can be hand- or foot-driven, electrically driven or gas-driven (Fig. 3.3). The latter are probably the most

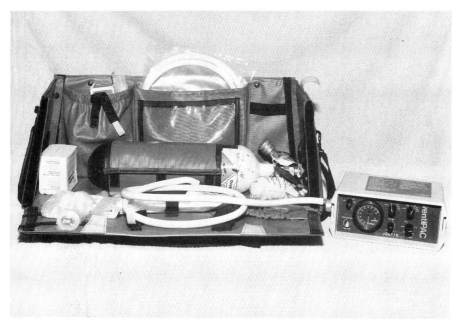

Fig. 3.2 VentiPAC gas-driven fluid-logic ventilator showing humidification filter. From ref. 95, with permission.

Table 3.2 Gas consumption of gas-powered ventilators

Model	Consumption
PneuPAC 2	Maximum of 2 liters in excess of minute volume
TransPAC	No air mix: minute volume + 20 ml/cycle Air mix: 30% minute volume + 20 ml/cycle
VentiPAC	No air mix: minute volume + 20 ml/cycle Air mix: 30% minute volume + 20 ml/cycle
Dräger Oxylog	No air mix: minute volume + 800 ml/min Air mix: 50% minute volume + 800 ml/min

From ref. 95, with permission.

Table 3.3 Gas consumption per minute of gas-powered ventilators for a 70 kg adult receiving 700 ml tidal volume at 10 breaths per minute for both 100% and 45% oxygen

Ventilatory	Consumption (l/min)	Oxygen (%)
PneuPAC 2	9	100
TransPAC	7.2	100
VentiPAC	2.3	45
Dräger Oxylog	7.8	100
	4.3	45

convenient. An electrically powered syringe driver can be invaluable in the transport environment.

Monitoring should be comprehensive as it has been shown that potentially fatal complications have occurred during the transfer of critically ill patients (up to 14% incidence in one series).[17] In the field, however, there are obviously limitations in terms of equipment held and time available for setting up invasive monitoring, therefore, pulse oximetry, noninvasive blood pressure monitoring and electrocardiography should be available. To this should be added temperature measurement, as mortality has been shown to increase in trauma victims when there is a fall in core temperature.[18] Temperature is best measured electrically as it should be noted that mercury-in-glass thermometers are potentially hazardous and are defined as dangerous air cargo. It is possible to monitor all of these with a single unit such as the Propaq[TM] monitor or the Marquette[TM] TRAM monitoring system. In addition to the monitoring, a defibrillator should be carried. End-tidal carbon dioxide monitoring would be ideal in the event of a difficult endotracheal intubation to confirm correct placement of the endotracheal tube. At present, there is a limited capability for portable electronic end-tidal carbon dioxide analysis, although a simple single-use device produced by FENEM Airway Management Systems is available to confirm correct placement of the endotracheal tube.

In addition to the equipment requirements, there is a very real requirement for the attending medical personnel to be appropriately trained and experienced. In the UK the last decade has seen the widespread introduc-

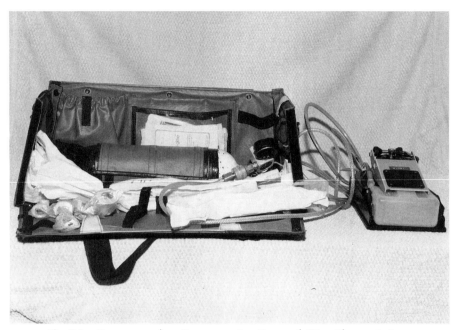

Fig. 3.3   Gas-powered suction apparatus. From ref. 95, with permission.

tion of paramedical training in the various ambulance services. Additionally specific training in trauma management for medical staff has been introduced in the form of the Advanced Trauma Life Support (ATLS) course, although this approach has been criticized as being too didactic.[19] Specialized knowledge in the problems of the different modes of transport is required, for instance how to cope with loading a patient onto a helicopter with the engines running and the rotors turning or how to cooperate with a helicopter winching operation.

In the event of being confronted by an emergency the attending personnel should have a common protocol to follow. One based on the ATLS course would seem logical in as much as it would be likely that personnel from different sources would then have a common 'language'. Such a protocol for initial diagnosis and resuscitation in the field would include a primary survey with assessment and appropriate management of the airway, breathing, circulation, neurological deficit and exposure of any hidden injuries. Following resuscitation a second survey should be completed in order to check the adequacy of resuscitation and whether any injuries have been missed. Further surveys are carried out repeatedly in order to ensure optimum patient management.

AIRWAY MANAGEMENT

There are three peaks in the mortality of trauma victims.[20] The first is immediate due to the nature of the injuries, such as massive penetrating trauma to the brain or heart. The second is at 1–2 hours due to, for example, intra-abdominal, intrathoracic or pelvic bleeding. The third occurs approximately 2 weeks post injury and is due to sepsis, multiple organ failure and irremediable brain damage. A potentially avoidable loss of life immediately after the injury, providing help is at hand, is that due to the loss of airway. Relatively simple maneuvers may be all that are necessary, such as clearing the airway with perhaps the insertion of an oropharyngeal airway, and this is true not just of trauma but also of cardiorespiratory collapse. One study reported that in the event of a cardiac arrest the chances of successful resuscitation were improved if the initial resuscitation by bystanders occurred within 4 minutes and if properly trained personnel restored adequate spontaneous perfusion in 10–15 minutes.[21,22]

Table 3.4   Cylinder duration for gas-powered ventilators for a 70 kg adult receiving 700 ml at 10 breaths per minute

Ventilator		Size E cylinder: 680 liters	Size F cylinder: 1360 liters
PneuPAC 2		75 min	150 min
TransPAC VentiPAC	100% oxygen	94 min	188 min
TransPAC VentiPAC	45% oxygen	295 min	590 min
Dräger Oxylog	100% oxygen	87 min	174 min
	45% oxygen	158 min	316 min

Securing the airway can be relatively straightforward in the field in the majority of cases, despite less than ideal conditions, providing that the person performing this is sufficiently experienced and has the appropriate equipment. The method of choice is orotracheal intubation with a cuffed endotracheal tube (uncuffed, in a child of less than approximately 10–12 years of age). The difficulty arises when orotracheal intubation proves difficult or impossible. In this situation there would be a number of options open to the medical practitioner in the hospital environment, however, in the field lack of equipment, lack of trained assistance and poor environment reduces these options. One option is to perform a cricothyroidotomy with, for example, a Portex Mini-trac™. There is, however, a 31% complication rate reported when this technique is used in the field.[23] This implies that experience of this technique is necessary. Recently the Brain laryngeal mask airway has been reported as having been used in trauma victims where other methods of airway control proved impossible until the patients had been extricated from their vehicles.[24] This technique does not guarantee the airway against aspiration, but it does have a limited ability to protect the airway from blood in the pharynx.[25]

It should not be forgotten that in the trauma victim there is always the possibility of cervical or other vertebral fracture. The majority of injuries occur between C3 and C7.[26] The standard intubating position results in relative stability of the lower cervical spine with relatively horizontal cervical vertebrae and with increasing extension from C1 to C4. This becomes maximal at the atlanto-axial complex. Any trauma victim should be assumed to have a cervical injury, especially in the event that intubation is required. It has been suggested that in the event of the requirement of urgent intubation without definitive diagnosis of cervical damage, that nasal intubation, with the head in a neutral position and without axial traction, should be performed.[27] In the field, however, this would prove impractical. There are also a number of other objections to nasal intubation in trauma victims. Some authors suggest that orotracheal intubation with immobilization or in-line traction resulted in no neurological sequelae.[28–30] The ideal force is not documented but it is likely that an equal amount of force is required to be applied against the force generated by the intubator.[31] Traction should be applied in the axial plane only, however, excessive force may cause significant distraction of a cervical fracture and hence trigger or exacerbate spinal cord injury.[27] This approach has been accepted by the American College of Surgeons as part of the ATLS protocol for emergency intubation.[32] Where possible preoxygenation and cricoid pressure should be applied.[30, 33] In the event of the trauma victim being conscious and requiring intubation, it has been commented that the appropriate use of thiopentone and suxamethonium in rapid sequence induction in spinal

injuries resulted in no serious hemodynamic or neurological sequelae.[34] Suxamethonium suffers from the potential of raising intracranial, intraocular and intragastric pressures along with the possibility of raising serum potassium levels, especially with burns, crush injuries and, at a later stage, with spinal cord injuries. The reason for its use is its rapid onset and short action.

Laryngoscopy during endotracheal tube placement in patients with head injury may cause further damage due to the hypertensive response as the cerebral autoregulatory capacity may be attenuated. This is possibly overemphasized as this autoregulation may remain intact in the first few days post injury.[35, 36]

BREATHING

In the event of a patient requiring ventilation, this may be achieved by a self-inflating bag or preferably by a portable gas-powered fluid-logic ventilator.[37] The patient may need hyperventilation to reduce carbon dioxide tension, thus reducing intracranical pressure. Supplementary oxygen should be supplied as it has been shown that apart from the effects of hypovolemia or any associated injuries, there is an increase in alveolar–arterial oxygen difference in patients during transport.[38]

It is essential to drain a pneumothorax prior to transport, especially if it is under tension, if the medical facility is some distance away or if the patient is to be transferred by air. An underwater seal for the chest drain is unwieldy and a one-way valve such as the Heimlich valve is preferable, although it should be noted that there is the potential for the valve to stick open if draining fluid.

CIRCULATORY MANAGEMENT

Hypotension and poor tissue perfusion may be due to either hypovolemia or pump failure. In the field the medical attendant has limited time and capacity for definitive diagnosis.

In the event of trauma with significant hemorrhage, the patient requires rapid intravascular volume expansion in order to restore tissue perfusion.[39] The longer vital organs remain hypoperfused, the greater the chances of sepsis and multiple organ failure at a later date. There is no good evidence for choosing between crystalloid or colloids provided the volume of the infused fluid is appropriate to its diffusion space.[40–43]

The choice of colloid solution is somewhat more complicated than the choice of crystalloid solution. In the USA modified polygelatins are criticized for having a relatively high incidence of anaphylactoid reactions.[44] The polygelatins have at least three beneficial aspects in that they do not effect cross-matching or hemostasis and they cause an osmotic diuresis.[45] Synthetic starch solutions are available. Hetastarch has an intravascular half-life of approximately 24 hours. This, however, results in a prolonged hemodilution and after large volumes levels of factor VIII can fall by up to 50% (more than can be explained by dilution alone).[46] In addition, larger particles of the hetastarch are taken up by the reticuloendothelial system where they accumulate. The long-term effects of this are unknown.[42] A newer starch solution is pentastarch. This has a plasma volume expansion effect lasting less than 12 hours. A 10% solution produces an initial plasma volume expansion of approximately 1.5 times the administered volume.[47] Pentastarch also has minimal effects on coagulation.[48,49]

It has been observed that ambulance personnel have been unable to infuse sufficient volume through the cannulae available to them to replace losses,[50] stimulating interest in the use of hypertonic saline. Animal studies have shown that in hemorrhagic shock infusion of as little as 10% of the total blood loss with 7.5% saline resulted in marked, though short-lived, improvement in mean arterial blood pressure and cardiac output.[51-53] Addition of a crystalloid markedly increased survival.[54] The addition of 6% dextran 70 results in significantly higher survival rates and improved hemodynamics in comparison to isotonic saline.[55]

Injured hypotensive patients treated in the field with 7.5% saline/dextran 70 (250 ml) prior to Ringer's lactate increased their blood pressure by an average of 49 mm Hg compared to an increase of 19 mm Hg in those receiving Ringer's lactate only.[56] This regime has been used with no reported complications in the prehospital management of patients with hypotension with penetrating injuries.[57] Theoretically the dangers of hypertonic saline solutions include hypernatremia, hyperchloremia, hyperosmolarity, hypokalemia and phlebitis. The small boluses used do not appear to have caused any of these, but care should probably be taken in the elderly.[58] These hypertonic solutions provide transient improvement only and must be followed by volume replacement.

Intraosseous infusions have been shown to be effective in children in whom intravenous access has been difficult.[59-61] An intraosseous infusion device with a self-tapping screw has been designed capable of delivering 200 ml of hypertonic saline/dextran into the sternum of sheep in hypovolemic shock, resulting in a rapid return to normal mean arterial pressure.[62] This device could be of practical value in the field.

The use of Military Anti-Shock Trousers (MAST) in acute hypovolemia is controversial. MAST elevate the systemic blood pressure by autotransfusion and a vasoconstrictor effect to increase afterload and improve organ perfusion. Pelvic and extremity fractures are also stabilized. Possible contraindications to MAST include raised intracranial pressure, thoracic injury and cardiac tamponade.[63] Some question the use of MAST because of potential delay and lack of clinical evidence of efficacy.[64] If MAST is used, adequate intravascular filling is necessary to avoid a precipitate fall in blood pressure on deflation (which should be slow).

In the community, trauma is not the only potential problem. As mentioned in the introduction, cardiovascular disease is a significant cause of mortality in the UK.[1] As increasing numbers of ambulance staff have been trained in the paramedical role in the UK, defibrillation has become available in the community. The task has been made safer with the development of defibrillators with a diagnostic facility. The Resuscitation Council of the United Kingdom has agreed recommendations for the approach to cardiovascular collapse.

Primary patient transfer

The patient may be transferred by a variety of methods. In the UK at present the most common method will be road ambulance. There is increasing use of helicopters in the suburban environment[16] and in the sparsely populated areas such as the highlands and islands of Scotland fixed-wing aircraft may be required. Each method of transport has its problems.

Road ambulances have the advantage of easy loading of the patient. The amount of space inside varies according to the make of vehicle. Some makes are totally inadequate for the job, particularly the converted 'estate' vehicles. Lighting remains a problem and cyanosis is difficult to diagnose clinically,[65] especially in the case where blood loss has been considerable or where the patient is cold (cord injuries, especially cervical fractures, result in a decreased ability to maintain body temperature because of inability to sweat or vasoconstrict, making the body temperature critically dependent on ambient temperature). Pulse oximetry can be extremely helpful in this situation. The smoothness of the ride depends on the road surface and the skill of the driver; spinal injuries require particular care.

For transfer by air the problems will vary according to whether the aircraft is fixed- or rotary-winged, and if fixed-wing, the size and type of aircraft. The transferring team should be familiar with the layout of the aircraft, as carrying the patient onto a small executive aircraft (Fig. 3.4) can be remarkably difficult. The position of the stretcher and whether the patient should be head- or feet-first is the subject of some discussion. In fixed-wing aircraft it has been shown that sagittal sinus pressure in anesthetized animals can increase by up to 30% on maximum power take-offs when positioned head-aft.[66] This may be of importance to head

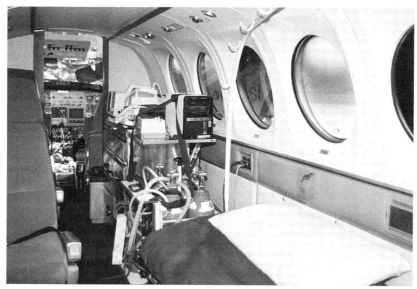

Fig. 3.4 View of the cabin of a Beech King air ambulance.

injuries as a fixed-wing aircraft has limited opportunity to modify take-off power. The dominant attitude of fixed-wing aircraft is nose-up, therefore head-forward position ensures that head-down posture is avoided. An argument against head-forward position is that braking and thrust-reversal would increase intracranial pressure. However, depending on aircraft type and length of runway, braking can be modified. In larger aircraft it has been suggested that cross-plane orientation may be preferable.[66] A further factor to be considered is the restraint of patients in the event of an accident. It is more practical, and indeed kinder, to prevent sudden forward motion by shoulder restraint in the head-forward position than by groin restraint in the head-aft position.

In rotary-wing aircraft it has been argued that positioning the patient head-aft ensures that as the nose tilts forward on acceleration the linear accelerational force is compensated for. Similarly the linear force in deceleration is compensated for by the fact that the aircraft tilts nose-up.[16] In reality this is not so important as the acceleration and deceleration of rotary-wing aircraft can be varied according to the patients' requirements. Often in smaller rotary-wing aircraft the position of the patient is dictated by the size and design of the aircraft rather than by any clinical indication.

Particular problems may be faced in the event of loading the patient onto an aircraft with the engines running. The reasons for having the engines running include the fact that some aircraft require external battery power to start engines and the loading site may not have the appropriate equipment; electrical power for lighting and heating or cooling the aircraft interior may lead to an excessive drain on battery reserves in the absence of external power source, especially if internal power is required to restart the engines. Other problems include rotating propellers and rotors (especially tail rotors); a jet exhaust (hot gases) can lead to direct trauma or may propel foreign bodies into eyes; the airstream from propellers may cause marked cooling when the ambient temperature is low. A number of guidelines will help to minimize these problems:

1. Never approach the aircraft unless instructed by the crew to do so.
2. Always approach in a direction that ensures that the crew can see you.
3. Never approach a helicopter's tail rotor.
4. Do not walk under propellers.
5. Beware of jet exhausts (helicopters are generally powered by jet engines).
6. Do not wear loose head gear.

Patient transfers involving winching operations have their own particular hazards (Fig. 3.5). These transfers will occur usually in situations where restricted access is a problem such as from cliffs or from boats or ships. The first hazard is that since the helicopter contains electrically conducting material and the helicopter moves in a magnetic field (the earth's magnetic field), an electrostatic charge is induced. This charge is sufficient to render an individual unconscious. To obviate this problem the winchman trails a 2 m length of thin wire in order to discharge this before he touches any structure. If the winch is lowered without a winchman, then the winch is lowered onto the ground or dipped into the sea before being available for use. The other hazard is that the winchman on the end of the wire, especially in high winds, becomes a projectile. It is essential, both for this reason and that of the electrostatic charge, that no-one attempts to 'help' the aircrew and winchman. They will be in control and will be making their own adjustments.

Initial treatment at receiving hospital

Once the patient has arrived at the receiving facility the capacity for therapeutic intervention is much greater than in the field. The principles remain the same, i.e. airway, breathing, circulation, deficit, exposure. However, other options become available.

AIRWAY

There is some debate as to the best method of airway control. The ATLS recommendations are as follows:

1. Apneic patient with no X-ray studies – orotracheal intubation. If unable to intubate orally, a surgical airway (tracheostomy or equivalent) should be established.
2. Spontaneous respiration with time for X-ray – if cervical injury excluded, proceed with oral intuba-

tion. If cervical injury confirmed, attempt blind nasal intubation. If unable to intubate nasally, proceed with orotracheal intubation or establish surgical airway.
3. Spontaneous respiration with no time for X-ray – blind nasal intubation. If unable to intubate nasally, proceed with orotracheal intubation or establish surgical airway.

This protocol implies that there are dangers associated with orotracheal intubation in the presence of cervical injury. However, a recent review suggests that the objections to the use of the orotracheal route for intubation in cervical spine injuries remain unproven.[67] Blind nasal intubation itself has significant problems. A comparison of blind nasal versus oral intubation in drug overdose patients showed oral intubation to be superior in terms of success rate (100 versus 65%), time to accomplish (64 versus 276 seconds) and mean number of attempts (1.3 versus 3.7). The blind nasal group had a complication rate of 86% (69% epistaxis, 17% vomiting, 10% aspiration).[68] Attempted nasal intubation may be very difficult in an uncooperative patient. It may result in further damage in cervical injuries because of coughing or retching and vomiting resulting in raised intracranial pressure. Coughing may be controlled by translaryngeal anesthesia, but this may increase the risk

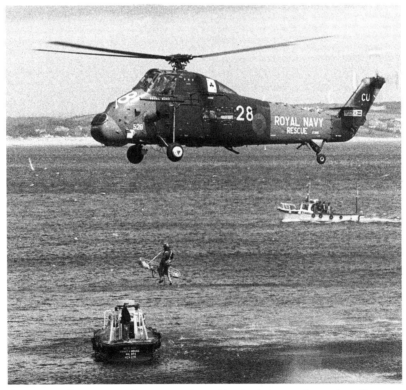

Fig. 3.5 Helicopter winching operation with winchman and stretcher. Courtesy of Barnaby's Picture Library, Barnaby House, 19 Rathbone Street, London W1P 1AF, UK.

of aspiration.[69] Nasotracheal intubation in the presence of a basal skull fracture may result in intracranial insertion[70] and the introduction of bacteria.[71] Apnea increases the difficulties associated with blind nasal intubation although there are devices designed to help in this situation such as the Ballistic Airway Airflow Monitor™.[72] Ultimately the clinician should proceed with the technique with which he/she is practiced.[73].

BREATHING

The problems in the emergency room are potentially the same as in the field, but as with the airway the options are greater. The indications for siting chest drains are the same, however, in the hospital environment there are indications for subsequent thoracotomy. These include bleeding from the chest drain of greater than 300–500 ml/h for 2–3 hours or greater than 200 ml/h for 5 hours, because the likely cause is damage to a systemic artery.[74] Thoracotomy is also indicated if there is an increasing hemothorax on chest X-ray or if there was a large volume of blood on initial insertion of the chest drain.

CIRCULATION

Hypotension in multiple trauma is likely to be secondary to blood loss. However, pump failure should always be considered (tension pneumothorax, cardiac tamponade, myocardial contusion or cardiogenic shock secondary to acute ischemia).

ATLS recommendations are that surgical cutdown should be performed if percutaneous access to forearm or antecubital veins is not possible. In UK hospitals skilled anesthesiologists are available to site central venous lines and a recent study has shown that percutaneous subclavian vein catheterization is faster than surgical cutdown and has a similar complication rate.[75] It can be argued that the internal jugular vein is preferable to the subclavian route as it is less likely to cause a pneumothorax. It is useful additionally to place a large-bore, short-sheath cannula in the femoral vein. This allows greater rates of flow than standard cannulae,[76–79] and ensures that there is access via both vena cavae in case return from one or other is disrupted. Special wide-bore intravenous administration sets are available which, with infusor pumps, allow high rates of administration.[77, 80, 81]

Rapid infusion of intravenous fluid carries the risk of hypothermia which, as commented on previously, carries an increased danger of mortality.[18] As blood temperature decreases, viscosity increases and hence flow decreases. Prewarmed saline added to units of packed red blood cells increases flow.[81] Blood warmers in routine use are unable to warm to more than 35°C at flow rates exceeding 100 ml/min.[82] Specialized blood warmers are available. The Level 1™ will supply blood at over 35°C at flow rates of 500 ml/min[83, 84] and the Rapid Infusion System™ can deliver blood under normothermic conditions at up to 1500 ml/min. To prevent unnecessary addition of resistance to this system the use of standard three-way taps should be avoided and if a pulmonary artery introducer catheter is used, one without a side arm will give higher flow rates.[85]

INVESTIGATIONS AND MONITORING

Whilst the assessment and resuscitation is proceeding comprehensive monitoring should be instituted. Some units may monitor intracranial pressure at this stage.

As lines are inserted blood should be sent for arterial blood gases, cross-matching and other investigations. A full skeletal X-ray survey will be required. Computed tomography (CT) scanning is likely to be required, but only when resuscitation has been completed.

PREPARATION FOR TRANSFER

Deterioration during transfer has been described.[86–88] In one series of 50 patients transferred within a hospital group, seven suffered life-threatening complications during the journey.[17] Of these 50, only 34 were accompanied by an anesthesiologist. It has been shown that hypovolemic dogs tolerate movement poorly.[89] Special care should therefore be used to ensure that optimal fluid loading is maintained in patients being prepared for transport. Manipulation of the cardiovascular system with inotropes and/or antiarrhythmic drugs may be necessary. An increased oxygen concentration should also be supplied to patients in transport and if necessary intermittent positive pressure ventilation with or without positive end expiratory pressure should be instituted.[90] Hand ventilation has been shown to be unsatisfactory even for short journeys and powered ventilators should be used.[35] As mentioned above, full monitoring during the transfer is essential. Recent studies have shown substantial inaccuracies in indirect blood pressure measurement in transit and suggest the use of invasive blood pressure monitoring.[91, 92] One review has shown that in 25% of transfers of critically ill patients from wards, preparation time exceeded 2 hours.[90] The same review showed that for transfers by ambulance the ratio of preparation time to journey time was 2 : 1. The multitudinous problems that may be encountered in the transport of critically ill patients with different pathologies and the potential problems of the different transport environments strongly suggest that experience in the field of 'transport medicine' and intensive care is necessary. It has been stated that the responsibility for transfer of the patient lies with the receiving hospital.[93,94] This is by no means always a practical proposition.

Problems of the transport environment

In addition to the problems already mentioned, there are further problems associated with the different modes of transfer.

LAND

A road ambulance suffers from a number of problems. The electrical power available may be inadequate or incompatible with the equipment. Medical gases, especially oxygen at present carried in cylinders, may take up a considerable amount of room if extra is carried for prolonged journeys. There tends to be no method of carrying extra cylinders safely and they are generally stored beneath the stretchers from where they can roll out, especially when cornering. The environment is obviously mobile and the amount of extraneous motion depends on the road surface, the speed and the skill of the driver. If procedures are necessary the ambulance

may have to stop in order to prevent damage to the patient and/or the medical escort. This amply illustrates the necessity of following the principle that if an intervention, such as endotracheal intubation is considered prior to transfer, then this should be carried out rather than waiting and seeing if it will be required later.[95] The mobility of the environment will result in various forces being applied to equipment attached to the patient, e.g. endotracheal tubes and intravenous giving sets. These should be secured with extra care for transport. Medical equipment if not secured may become projectiles, threatening both patient and staff. Vibration and noise may make diagnosis impossible, again emphasizing the necessity for stabilization prior to transfer with adequate monitoring during the transfer.

SEA

The seaborne environment depends on the size and type of the vessel and the sea conditions. The larger the vessel, the more stable it is likely to be. Electrical power is unlikely to be a problem. The artificial lighting on-board ship leads to similar drawbacks in diagnosis as in the road ambulance. Noise levels tend to be less of a problem. Transferring a patient within the vessel may lead to extra problems if there are no lifts and if there are many water-tight doors (particularly in military vessels). Unless the vessel has full hospital facilities

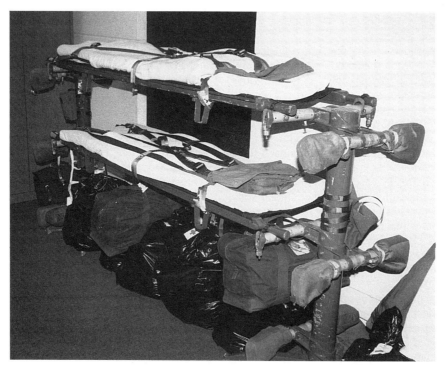

Fig. 3.6   Standard Royal Air Force stretcher harness and stretcher supports which can be fitted in a variety of different aircraft. From ref. 95, with permission.

with appropriate staffing, the requirement will be to transfer the patient to an appropriate facility ashore unless the condition is fairly trivial. The standards of medical care in the adjacent land mass must also be considered. The transfer will be most efficiently effected by helicopter.

AIR

The airborne environment has a number of factors common to land and sea transfer. The limitation of space in smaller aircraft is such that the escort should be familiar with the aircraft. Loading a stretcher onto a small executive aircraft can be remarkably difficult. Equipment should be positioned so that it is readily accessible. The positioning of the patient is a compromise between the space available and maintaining access to the airway and chest. The airborne environment is noisier than either that at sea or on land; this is especially so in helicopters, where normal conversation

and the use of stethoscopes are impossible. Vibration is again a particular problem in helicopter operations. Adult patients have been shown to deteriorate when subjected to vibration below 28 Hz.[96] It has been suggested that resonant frequencies can promote bleeding. However, the importance of this factor is difficult to assess and may be overemphasized. Problems with lighting are similar if not worse than in road ambulances. Restraint of the patient against accelerational and decelerational forces is essential (Fig. 3.6). Additional hazards result from encountering turbulence.

Problems peculiar to the airborne environment are those associated with the effects of altitude. Modern fixed-wing aircraft are pressurized to fly with a cabin altitude of between 5000 and 8000 ft. Helicopters do not tend to be pressurized. The three effects of importance associated with increasing altitude are a decrease in partial pressure of oxygen, a decrease in ambient pressure and a decrease in temperature (Fig. 3.7). In most circumstances the decrease in oxygen availability can be compensated for by increasing the inspired oxygen concentration. The shape of the oxygen dissociation curve is such that the hemoglobin saturation tends to be maintained (Fig. 3.8). Occasionally it will not be possible to maintain oxygenation despite raising the inspired oxygen to 100%. In this situation it would be necessary to request the crew to fly the aircraft at sea level cabin altitude, i.e. to maintain the cabin pressure at 760 mm Hg (1 atmosphere at sea level). The aircraft will therefore need to fly lower in order to maintain the pressure differential between the inside and the outside of the aircraft (Fig. 3.9). This results in increased flying

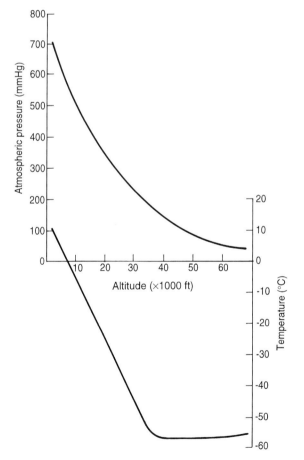

Fig. 3.7 Graph showing the relationship between altitude, atmospheric pressure and temperature. From ref. 95, with permission.

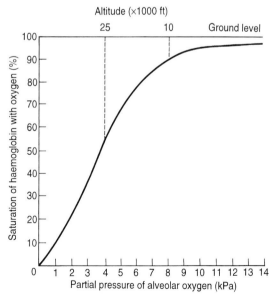

Fig. 3.8 Graph showing the relationship between altitude, partial pressure of alveolar oxygen and percentage saturation of hemoglobin. From ref. 95, with permission.

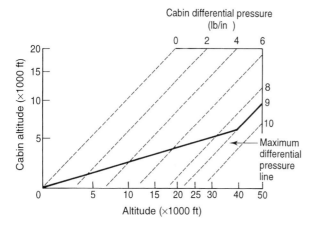

Fig. 3.9 Graph illustrating the ability of an aircraft to maintain pressurization within the cabin. From ref. 95, with permission.

time, fuel consumption and possibly turbulence. On long-distance flights refuelling stops may be necessary.

As ambient pressure decreases any collection of gas will increase and this will be detrimental to the patient in certain conditions. These include gas in the cranium, surgical emphysema of the neck, pneumomediastinum, bowel obstruction (or recent bowel surgery) or pneumothorax. The latter two conditions can be improved prior to transfer. Gas in the abdomen can be diminished by giving the patient 100% oxygen[97] and a pneumothorax can be drained with a one-way valve *in situ* (e.g. Heimlich valve). If the patient has a plaster cast this should be split prior to transfer to allow for expansion. If the collection of gas cannot be drained or sufficiently diminished, sea level cabin altitude may need to be requested. The cuff of an endotracheal tube, if filled with air, will expand on ascent and shrink on descent. This problem can be obviated by filling the cuff with saline or water. Air in a pneumatic splint will expand with increasing altitude and so increase the pressure on the underlying limb. Residual air in a vacuum mattress will also expand, so diminishing its effectiveness. Exposure of a subaqua diver to decreased ambient pressure soon after a dive increases the chances of decompression sickness, therefore, flying less than 24 hours after a dive is inadvisable.[98] The effects of changing ambient pressure when unable to equalize middle ear pressure should be remembered for patient and doctor alike.

The decrease in temperature with altitude is not usually a problem with pressurized aircraft in flight but is a problem more usually associated with helicopters. Another problem associated with pressurized aircraft operations is the fact that the supplied air within the cabin is dry and therefore humidification is required,

especially on longer journeys. A condenser humidifier is ideal for intubated patients.[99]

A potential problem in aircraft operations is interaction between the aircraft's electrical systems and the medical electrical apparatus. With the development of fly-by-wire technology this problem theoretically will become greater. However, on closer inspection this has not proved to be a problem.[100]

References

1. Mortality statistics: death by cause (DH4 No. 4). *Office of Population Census Survey*. London: Her Majesty's Stationery Office, 1987.
2. Working party report. *Management of Patients with Major Injuries*. London: Royal College of Surgeons of England, 1988.
3. Aprahamian C, Thompson BM, Towne JB, Darin JC. The effect of a paramedic system on mortality of major intra-abdominal vascular trauma. *J Trauma* 1983; **23**: 687–90.
4. Cwinn AA, Pons PT, Moore EE, Marx JA, Honigman B, Dinerman N. Prehospital advanced trauma life support for critical blunt trauma victims. *Ann Emergency Med* 1987; **16**: 399–403.
5. Jacobs LM, Sinclair A, Beiser A, D'Agostino RB. Prehospital advances life support: benefits in trauma. *J Trauma* 1984; **24**: 8–13.
6. Royal College of Surgeons. *Royal College of Surgeons of England Report of the Working Party on the Management of Patients with Major Injuries*. London: The Royal College of Surgeons of England, 1988.
7. Buck N, Devlin HB, Lunn JN. *The Report of a Confidential Enquiry into Perioperative Deaths*. London: Nuffield Provincial Hospitals Trusts and King's Fund Publishing Office, 1987.
8. Redmond AD. Reply to disaster management. *Br Med J* 1989; **298**: 962.
9. Huguenard P, Niemeyer E, Hervé C, Métrot J, Desfemmes C, Hrouda P. Justification de l'aide médicale urgente. *Convergences Médicales* 1984; **3**: 113–16.
10. Lent V. Ergebnisse nach erster ärtlicher Hilfe am Unfallort. *Bruns Beitr Klin Chir* 1972; **219**: 757.
11. Tscherne H, Kalbe PM, Wisner DH. Pre-hospital care of the polytrauma patient: the role of the physician. In: Border JR (ed.) *Blunt Multiple Trauma: Comprehensive Pathophysiology and Care*. Boston: Little Brown, 1990: 295–309.
12. Berner W, Brueggermann H, Snakker A. Die Bedeutung des Primaereinsatzes von Rettungshubschraubern für die Prognose Schwerverletzter. In: *Die Luftrettung, ADAC Schriftten Strassenverkehr, Bd 25*. München: ADAC Luftrettung GmbH, 1981.
13. Kalbe P. Probleme der Koordination und Effektiviaet beim Einsatzvon RTH/NAW. In: *Tagungsbericht 8, RTH-Fachtagung*. München: ADAC Luftreittung GmbH, 1983.
14. Mathieu F, Poisot D, Cardinaud JP. Place du SAMU dans le pronostic de l'asthme: experience du SAMU 33

à propos de 628 observations. *La revue des SAMU* 1989; **6**: 257–9.

15. Gaubert Corbery C, Campominosi P. L'asthme aigu grave: expérience pré-hospitalière du SMUR d'Eaubonne. *La revue des SAMU* 1989; **6**: 260–3.

16. Jeffries NJ, Bristow A. Long distance inter-hospital transfers: helicopter transport for IC patients. *Br J Intensive Care* 1991; **5**: 197–204.

17. Bion JF, Wilson IH, Taylor PA. Transporting critically ill patients by ambulance: audit by sickness scoring. *Br Med J* 1988; **296**: 170.

18. Jurkovich GJ, Greiser WB, Luternan A, Curreri PW. Hypothermia in trauma victims: an ominous predictor of survival. *J Trauma* 1987; **27**: 1019–24.

19. McConachie I. American style trauma centres in the UK. *Todays Anesthetist* 1992; **7**: 64–5.

20. Trunkey DD. Trauma. *Scient Am* 1983; **249**: 28–35.

21. Cummins RO, Eisenberg M. Cardiopulmonary resuscitation – American style. *Br Med J* 1985; **291**: 1401–3.

22. Anderson IWR, Black RJ, Ledingham IMcA, Little K, Robertson LE, Urquhart JD. Early emergency care study: the potential and benefits of advanced prehospital care. *Br Med J* 1987; **294**: 228–31.

23. Spaite DW, Joseph M. Prehospital cricothyroidotomy: an investigation of indications, technique, complications and patient outcome. *Ann Emergency Med* 1990; **19**: 279–85.

24. Greene MK, Roden R, Hinchley G. The laryngeal mask airway. Two cases of prehospital trauma care. *Asaesthesia* 1992; **47**: 688–9.

25. John RE, Hill S, Hughes TJ. Airways protection by the laryngeal mask. A barrier to dye placed in the pharynx. *Anaesthesia* 1991; **46**: 366–7.

26. Bohlman HH. Acute fractures and dislocation of the cervical spine. *J Bone Joint Surg* 1979; **61A**: 1119–42.

27. Bivins HG, Ford S, Bezmalinovic Z, Price HM, Williams JL. The effect of axial traction during orotracheal intubation of the trauma victim with an unstable cervical spine. *Ann Emergency Med* 1988; **17**: 25–9.

28. Rhee KJ, Green W, Holcroft JW, Mangili JAA. Oral intubation in the multiply injured patient; the risk of exacerbating spinal cord damage. *Ann Emergency Med* 1990; **19**: 511–14.

29. Stellin GP, Barker S, Murdock M, Waxman K. Oral-tracheal intubation in trauma patients with cervical fractures. *Crit Care Med* 1989; **17**: S37.

30. Grande CM, Barton CR, Stene JK. Appropriate techniques for airway management of emergency patients with suspected spinal cord injury. *Anaesthesia Analgesia* 1988; **67**: 714–15.

31. Grande CM, Barton CR, Stene JK. Emergency airway management in trauma patients with a suspected cervical spine injury: in response. *Anaesthesia Analgesia* 1989; **68**: 416–18.

32. Committee on Trauma. The Advanced Trauma Life Support Program, *Instructors Manual*. Chicago: American College of Surgeons, 1989.

33. Lawes EG, Campbell I, Mercer D. Inflation pressure, gastric insufflation and rapid sequence induction. *Br J Anaesthesia* 1987; **59**: 315–18.

34. Talucci RC, Shaikh KA, Schwab CW. Rapid sequence induction with oral endotracheal intubation in the multiply injured patient. *Am Surgeon* 1988; **54**: 185–7.

35. Eneroldsen EM, Jensen FT. Autoregulation and CO$_2$ responses of cerebral blood flow in patients with acute severe head injury. *J Neurosurg* 1978; **48**: 689–703.

36. Minzelaar JP, Ward JD, Marmaron A, Newlon PG, Wachi A. Cerebral blood flow and metabolism in severely head injured children. Part 2: autoregulation. *J Neurosurg* 1989; **71**: 72–6.

37. Braman SS, Dunn SM, Amico CA, Millman RP. Complications of intrahospital transport in critically ill patients. *Ann Intern Med* 1987; **107**: 469–73.

38. Ridley S, Carter R. The effects of secondary transport on critically ill patients. *Anaesthesia* 1989; **44**: 822–7.

39. Giesecke AH Jr, Grande CM, Whitten CW. Fluid therapy and the resuscitation of traumatic shock. *Crit Care Clinics* 1990; **6**: 61–72.

40. Moss GS, Gould SA. Plasma expanders: an update. *Am J Surg* 1988; **155**: 425–34.

41. Haupt MT. The use of crystalloidal and colloidal solutions for volume replacement in hypovolaemic shock. *Crit Rev Clin Lab Sci* 1989; **27**: 1–26.

42. Davies MJ. Crystalloid or colloid: does it matter? *J Clin Anesthesiol* 1989; **1**: 464–71.

43. Fourth French Consensus Conference on Intensive Care and Emergency Medicine. Selection of a fluid for vascular expansion in the treatment of hypovolaemia in adult patients. *Vox Sanguinis* 1990; **58**: 150–1.

44. Klotz U, Kroemer H. Clinical pharmacokinetic considerations in the use of plasma expanders. *Clin Pharmacokinetics* 1987; **12**: 123–35.

45. Ramsay G. Intravenous volume replacement: indications and choices. *Br Med J* 1988; **296**: 1422–3.

46. Stump DC, Strauss RG, Henriksen RA *et al*. Effects of hydroxyethyl starch on blood coagulation, particularly Factor VIII. *Transfusion* 1985; **25**: 349–54.

47. Köhler H, Zschiedrich G, Clasen R *et al*. Blood volume, colloid osmotic pressure and kidney function after infusion of 10% medium molecular weight hydroxyethyl starch 200/0.5 and 10% dextrab 40 in human volunteers. *Anaesthetist* 1982; **31**: 61–7.

48. Strauss RG, Stansfield C, Henricksen RA, Vilhauer PJ. Pentastarch may cause fewer effects on coagulation than hetastarch. *Transfusion* 1988; **28**: 257–60.

49. Rackow EC, Mecher C, Astiz Me *et al*. Effects of pentastarch and albumin infusion on cardiorespiratory function and coagulation in patients with severe sepsis and systemic hypoperfusion. *Crit Care Med* 1989; **17**: 394–8.

50. Smith JP, Bodai BI, Hill AS, Frey CF. Prehospital stabilization of critically injured patients: a failed concept. *Trauma* 1985; **25**: 65–70.

51. Velasco IT, Pontieri V, Rocha M *et al*. Hyperosmotic NaCl and severe hemorrhagic shock. *Am J Physiol* 1980; **239** (Suppl. 18): H664–73.

52. Nakayama S, Sibley L, Gunther RA *et al*. Small-volume resuscitation with hypertonic saline (2400 mOsm/litre) during hemorrhagic shock. *Circulatory Shock* 1984; **13**: 149–59.

53. Betterman H, Triolo J, Lefer AM. Use of hypertonic saline in the treatment of hemorrhagic shock. *Circulatory Shock* 1987; **21**: 271–83.

54. Stanford GG, Patterson CR, Payne L, Fabian TC. Hypertonic saline resuscitation in a porcine model of severe hemorrhagic shock. *Arch Surg* 1989; **124**: 733–6.

55. Chudnofsky CR, Dronen SC, Syverud SA *et al.* Intravenous fluid therapy in the prehospital management of hemorrhagic shock: improved outcome with hypertonic saline/6% dextran 70 in a swine model. *Am J Emergency Med* 1989; **7**: 357–63.

56. Holcroft JW, Vassar MJ, Turner JE *et al.* 3% NaCl and 7.5% NaCl/Dextran 70 in the resuscitation of severely injured patients. *Ann Surg* 1987; **206**: 279–88.

57. Maningas PA, Mattox KL, Pepe PE *et al.* Hypertonic saline–Dextran solutions for the prehospital management of traumatic hypotension. *Am J Surg* 1989; **157**: 528–34.

58. Matter JA. Hypertonic and hyperoncotic solutions in patients. *Crit Care Med* 1989; **17**: 297–8.

59. Spivey WH. Intraosseous infusions. *J Pediatr* 1987; **111**: 639–43.

60. McNamara RM, Soivey WH, Unger HD, Malone DR. Emergency applications of intraosseous infusion. *J Emergency Med* 1987; **5**: 97–101.

61. Fiser DH. Intraosseous infusion. *New Engl J Med* 1990; **322**: 1579–81.

62. Halvorsen L, Bay BK, Perron PR *et al.* Evaluation of an intraosseous infusion device for the resuscitation of hypovolemic shock. *J Trauma* 1990; **30**: 652–9.

63. Palafox BA, Johnson MN, McEwan K, Gazzaniga AB. Intracranial pressure changes following application of the MAST suit. *J Trauma* 1981; **21(1)**: 55–9.

64. Pepe PE, Bass RR, Mattox KL. Clinical trials of the pneumatic antishock garment in the urban prehospital setting. *Ann Emergency Med* 1986; **15(12)**: 1407–10.

65. Snook R. Medical aspects of ambulance design. *Br Med J* 1972; **iii**: 574–8.

66. McNeil EL. Regulations and operations. In: McNeil EL (ed.) *Airborne Care of the Critically Ill and Injured.* New York: Springer-Verlag Inc., 1983: 66.

67. Wood PR, Lawler PGP. Managing the airway in cervical spine injury. A review of the Advanced Trauma Life Support protocol. *Anaesthesia* 1992; **47**: 792–7.

68. Dronen SC, Merigian KS, Hedges JR, Hoekstra JW, Borron SW. A comparison of blind nasotracheal and succinylcholine-assisted intubation in the poisoned patient. *Ann Emergency Med* 1987; **16**: 650–2.

69. Claeys DW, Lockhart CH, Hinke JE. The effects of translaryngeal block and Innovar on glottic competence. *Anesthesiology* 1973; **38**: 485–6.

70. Bouzarth WF. Intracranial nasogastric tube insertion. *J Trauma* 1978; **18**: 818–19.

71. Dimner M, Tjeuw M, Artusio JF. Bacteremia as a complication of nasotracheal inturbation. *Anesthesiology* 1987; **66**: 460–2.

72. Grande CM. Airway management of the trauma patient in the resuscitation area of a trauma center. *Trauma Quart* 1988; **5**: 30–49.

73. Crosby ET, Lui A. The adult cervical spine: implications for airway management. *Can J Anaesthesia* 1990; **37**: 77–93.

74. Kirsch MM, Sloan H. *Blunt Chest Trauma, General Principles of Management.* Boston: Little Brown, 1977.

75. Arrighi DA, Farnell MB, Mucha P Jr *et al.* Prospective randomized trial of rapid venous access for patients in hypovolemic shock. *Ann Emergency Med* 1989; **18**: 927–30.

76. Hoelzer MF. Recent advances in intravenous therapy. *Emergency Med Clin Am* 1986; **4**: 487–500.

77. Dutky A, Stevens SL, Maull KI. Factors affecting rapid fluid resuscitation with large-bore introducer catheters. *J Trauma* 1989; **29**: 856–60.

78. Haynes BE, Carr FJ, Niemann JT. Catheter introducers for rapid fluid resuscitation. *Ann Emergency Med* 1983; **12**: 606–9.

79. Millikan JS, Cain TL, Hansbrough J. Rapid volume replacement for hypovolaemic shock: a comparison of techniques and equipment. *J Trauma* 1984; **24**: 428–31.

80. Landow L, Shahnarian A. Efficiency of large-bore intravenous fluid administrations sets designed for rapid volume resuscitation. *Crit Care Med* 1990; **18**: 540–3.

81. Zorko MF, Polsky SS. Rapid warming and infusion of packed red blood cells. *Ann Emergency Med* 1986; **15**: 907–10.

82. Russell WJ. A review of blood warmers for massive transfusion. *Anaesthesia Intensive Care* 1974; **2**: 109–30.

83. Flancbaum L, Trooskin SZ, Pedersen H. Evaluation of blood warming devices with the apparent thermal clearance. *Ann Emergency Med* 1989; **18**: 355–9.

84. Kruskall MS, Pacini DG, Malynn ER, Button LN. Evaluation of a blood warmer that utilizes a 40°C heat exchanger. *Transfusion* 1990; **30**: 7–10.

85. Rothen HU, Lauber R, Mosiman M. An evaluation of the Rapid Infusion System. *Anaesthesia* 1992; **47**: 597–600.

86. Gentleman D, Jennett B. Hazards of inter-hospital transfer of comatose head-injured patients. *Lancet* 1981; **ii**: 853–5.

87. Gentleman D, Jennett B. Audit of transfer of unconscious head-injured patients to a neurosurgical unit. *Lancet* 1990; **335**: 330–4.

88. Armitage JM, Pyne A, Williams SJ, Frankel H. Respiratory problems of air travel in patients with spinal cord injuries. *Br Med J* 1990; **300**: 1498–9.

89. Waddell G, Douglas IHS, Ledingham IMcA. Cardiovascular effects of movement in haemorrhagic shock dogs. *Crit Care Med* 1974; **2**: 68–72.

90. Runcie CJ, Reeve WR, Wallace PGM. Preparation of the critically ill for interhospital transfer. *Anaesthesia* 1992; **47**: 327–31.

91. Runcie CJ, Reeve W, Reidy J, Dougall JR. A comparison of measurements of oxygenation, heart-rate and blood pressure during inter-hospital transport of the critically ill. *Intensive Care Med* 1990; **16**: 317–22.

92. Runcie CJ, Reeve W, Reidy J, Dougall JR. Blood pressure measurement during transport – a comparison of direct and oscillometric readings in critically ill patients. *Anaesthesia* 1990; **45**: 659–65.

93. Association of Anaesthetists of Great Britain and Ireland. *Provision of Intensive Care*, 1st edn. London: Association of Anaesthetists, 1988.

94. Joint Commission of Accreditation of Hospitals.

Accreditation Manual for Hospitals 2nd edn. Chicago: Joint Commission for Accreditation of Hospitals, 1986.

95. Mulrooney P. Aeromedical patient transfer. *Br J Hospital Med* 1991; **45**: 209–12.

96. Grabosch A. Ten years experience in helicopter rescue in West Germany. *Proceedings of the First International Assembly on Emergency Medical Services.* US Department of Transportation, 1982: 223–8.

97. Loder RE. Use of hyerbaric oxygen in paralytic ileus. *Br Med J* 1977; **i**: 1448–9.

98. Furry DE, Reave E, Beckman E. Relationships of SCUBA diving to the development of aviation decompression sickness. *Aerospace Med* 1967; **38**: 825–8.

99. Mapleson WW, Morgan SG, Hilliard EK. Assessment of condenser humidifiers with special reference to a multiple gauze model. *Br Med J* 1963; **i**: 300.

100. Mulrooney P. Monitoring during aeromedical transfer. *Anaesthesia* 1990; **45**: 256.

CHAPTER 4

General care units

ROWLAND BENNETT HOPKINSON

Introduction   36
History   36
What is intensive care?   37
Number of beds   38
A survey of intensive care in the United Kingdom   38
Location   39
Accommodation   40
Fire safety   44
Bedside services   44
Cross-infection   44
Equipment   44
Medical records   45
Staffing   45
Unit management   51
Conclusion   53
Appendix. Definition of organ system failures   54
References   54

Introduction

This chapter reviews the management, organization and design of 'general' intensive care units of the type in existence in large District General Hospitals in the UK. The philosophy of intensive care is considered in the context of its history and development in the UK. Reference is made to similar work in the USA.

The factors that have influenced the design of purpose-built intensive care units (ICUs) since the specialty evolved are reviewed with reference to three key documents.[1-3] Deficiencies in the design of such units are identified, as is the impact of these deficiencies on their function. Particular consideration is given to the number of ICU beds required by an acute hospital and to the size of the unit. Comparative data, obtained from a postal survey of ICUs,[4] are presented to assist in the derivation of more general conclusions.

Parallel developments in the USA are considered and illustrated with reference to the Society of Critical Care Medicine's (SCCM) recommendations for critical care unit design.[5]

History

It was in 1967 that the British Medical Association's Working Party on Intensive Care produced its Report on Intensive Care in the United Kingdom.[1] The introduction to the Report commented that 'many hospitals throughout the country are at present considering the setting up of intensive therapy units ...'. The Report maintained that the establishment of an intensive therapy unit within a hospital would not only improve the chances of a patient with a desperate illness, but was also likely to promote an improvement in the general level of medical and nursing care. While few members of the profession or public doubt this assertion, nearly a quarter of a century on, there is little objective evidence to support the claim and the use of such expensive resources for a numerically small group of patients.

In his foreword to the Report the Chairman of the British Medical Association (BMA) Planning Unit, Dr Henry Miller, commented on the age of most British hospitals and that 'the provision of a safe and appropriate environment for intensive therapy will usually mean a new building.' In many hospitals in the UK and Europe this has yet to be realized although colleagues in North America fare better. Adequate staffing (both medical and nursing) for such units is particularly hard to obtain in the UK.

At that time the advantages of establishing ICUs were said to be:

1. The patient can be given nursing and medical attention more closely related to their needs.
2. Nursing staff, space and equipment can be more economically employed.
3. Medical, nursing and ancillary care are not subject to diurnal fluctuations.
4. Continuity of care can be more easily maintained.
5. Equipment is grouped at one site where it can be promptly used by experienced staff.
6. More space can be provided.
7. Training of medical and nursing staff in the care of very sick patients is more efficient.
8. Care is improved by having a common ground for attention by staff of all disciplines.
9. Concentration of experience leads to an increase in the skill and responsibility of the nursing staff.
10. More intensive observation may enable simple measures to be taken in time and thus forestall the need for more complicated measures later.
11. These units save lives.

At the same time a number of disadvantages were recognized:

1. It is unsettling for patients to be moved about and to be cared for by different people.
2. Continuity of medical responsibility is interrupted.
3. Such a unit is disliked by nurses because of the difficulty in arranging the right balance of staff and experience.
4. Technique and equipment, rather than the patient, become the center of attention.
5. The use of nursing staff is extravagant so that care elsewhere suffers; it never saves staff.
6. Overenergetic treatment is encouraged.
7. The unit becomes a substitute for, and inhibits the improvement of, care and facilities in the traditional ward system.

8. Segregation of very sick patients makes it difficult to provide a balanced training for junior medical and nursing staff.
9. Work on such units is an emotional strain on the staff.
10. Such a unit makes unfair claims on the hospital budget.
11. There is a tendency for the unit to develop into an elite organization, separate from the hospital, with unfavorable consequences.
12. The claim that it saves lives, which would not have been saved in a well-organized ward service, rests on anecdotal evidence and is not proven.

In 1988 the Kings Fund convened a multidisciplinary panel to review the benefits, costs and perceived dangers of intensive care.[6] The discussions included consideration of the patients potential loss of dignity, privacy and autonomy. Five questions were posed:

1. Has it been clearly demonstrated that ICUs decrease mortality and morbidity?
2. What admission and discharge criteria are available?
3. What groups of patients will most benefit from intensive care?
4. What extra does this cost?
5. What is the extent of provision needed in the UK and how should it be organized?

Notwithstanding the passage of a quarter of a century, the Kings Fund was addressing again the problems and disputes reflected in the original BMA document and which recur in any debate about the value of intensive care. What is of more concern, is that the panel concluded that the data to answer these questions were not available in the UK: instead a report was produced summarizing the current state of knowledge about the benefits or otherwise of intensive care and proposing a substantial program of research.

What is intensive care?

In its definition of intensive care:

> a service for patients with potentially recoverable diseases who can benefit from more detailed observation and treatment than is generally available in the standard wards and departments

the Kings Fund was making minor changes to that of the BMA Working Party 25 years earlier. They laid emphasis on intensive care being a place, not a form of therapy, and providing special skills and experience for the care of patients suffering one or more organ system failure. The report returns to the unproven assumption that this concentration of special facilities and expertise gives better results and reduces costs. This latter point becomes more contentious as the average age of admissions rises.

Outcomes will reflect many differing aspects of medical practice, not least the skills, knowledge and timing of the admitting practitioners. The case mix of different ICUs makes comparison very difficult and the Kings Fund panel lays emphasis on the heterogeneity of admissions.

In the USA Cullen[7] grouped critical care functions under two categories:

1. monitoring a patient's vital functions and his or her maintenance at levels as close to normal as possible; and
2. provision of definitive therapy to patients with acute but reversible life-threatening dysfunction of vital systems.

The Intensive Care Society (ICS) has published a series of definitions which refine these requirements, relating them to organ system failures.[8]

Intensive Care (or Intensive Therapy)

This is usually reserved for patients with potential or established organ failure. The ICU should offer the facilities for diagnosis, prevention and treatment of multiple organ failure. The most commonly supported organ is the lung but an ICU should offer a wide range of facilities for organ support. This will require a multi-disciplinary team approach and the highest possible standards of nursing and medical care. A nurse/patient ratio of 1:1 should be the minimum and the services of a full-time medical resident are essential.

It is a matter of great concern that many units are unable to meet the staffing requirements detailed above; a survey, undertaken by the Association of Anaesthetists of Great Britain and Ireland in 1988,[9] noted that nearly one-third of units failed to achieve such a nurse to patient ratio.

There is considerable variation in the definition of organ system failure but an example is given in the Appendix. The average sickness level of patients managed in an ICU will reflect the medical practice in the hospital and any other provision for the seriously ill. The Association of Anaesthetists[9] commented that in some intensive care units as many as 50% of admissions were in fact 'high dependency'. Again, the ICS has provided a definition of such high dependency care.

High Dependency Step-Down or Intermediate Care

A High Dependency Unit (HDU) is an area offering a standard of care intermediate between the general ward and full intensive care. The HDU should not manage patients with multi-organ failure but should provide monitoring and support to patients at risk of developing organ system failure. An HDU should be able to undertake short term resuscitative measures and might provide ventilator support for a short time (less than 24 hours) prior to transfer of the patient to an ICU.

The HDU does not need and should not provide a full range of support services. It would normally function with a nurse/patient ratio of 1:2 and does not require the exclusive services of a full-time resident doctor.

Many ICUs in the UK are required to serve both functions because the development of high dependency care is embryonic. The presence of a 24-hour recovery unit may also influence the demands for intensive care.

Number of beds

In 1967 the BMA Working Party estimated that 1% of patients admitted to a district hospital would need intensive care at some time, and that the best size for a unit was 6 to 8 beds. Experience at that time suggested that less than four beds was uneconomic, while more than ten beds was unwieldy. It also concluded that intensive care resources for a number of small hospitals should be concentrated on one site and that a bed occupancy rate of 60% was acceptable in order that beds should be available for emergencies.

By 1974 the Hospital Building Note (HBN) 27 was recommending that 'between one and two per cent of the total acute beds' should be allocated for intensive care, with supplements for large numbers of regional specialties.[2] This number is now thought insufficient,[6] a view supported by experience in North America. The SCCM Guidelines suggest a maximum of 12 beds per module, though six to eight beds[5] is preferable. In 1988 the Association of Anaesthetists[9] advised that less than four beds or 200 admissions per year was not economic, and that the patient base was not large enough for staff to maintain the necessary skills.

In the UK there is a shortage of specialist pediatric intensive care beds, which means that many general units must also be proficient in the care of children.

A survey of intensive care in the United Kingdom

In 1988, the Medical Architecture Research Unit (MARU) published the results of a postal survey of all the ICUs and combined ICU/Coronary Care Units (CCU) in England.[4] This had been supplemented by visits to a small number of units to investigate specific planning and design issues highlighted in the survey. Two hundred and forty-six ICUs and ICU/CCUs were surveyed with an 80% response rate. The survey enquired about:

• background information – numbers of acute beds, operating theatres, accident departments, etc.;
• operational policies – admission policies, patients included/excluded, staff changing and gowning and catering;
• utilization – workload, bed utilization, referral patterns, use of cubicles;
• space provision – age of facilities, number of cubicles, number of beds in multi-bed bays, support space and its utilization;
• equipment and engineering services – storage, provision of medical gases, vacuum, electrical outlets, lighting and computing support;
• general comments including causes of dissatisfaction.

The survey provides an interesting snapshot of intensive care practice in the UK in the late 1980s.

Questions relating to background and policies showed that all the ICUs surveyed admitted patients with respiratory and postoperative insufficiency and that less than 10% excluded patients with coma, severe shock or multiple injuries. Less than half of ICUs admitted those suffering burns (44%) and only 18% admitted patients requiring renal dialysis. The burgeoning use of a variety of hemofiltration techniques is likely to have altered this figure.

Anesthesia and surgery were catered for in many units, 41% performing emergency tracheostomy. The advent of percutaneous tracheotomy may have modified this figure.

It was reported that in two-thirds of units nurses change into uniform at work and that this is supplemented with a plastic apron, although appropriate changing facilities were not always provided. The gowning of staff and visitors was uncommon. Staff generally eat meals on the unit and not in hospital dining facilities.

As to facilities, 55% of units responding were purpose-built, with an average age of 9.6 years. The average size of the units was 5.8 beds ranging from 1 to 13. Seventy-two per cent of units have four to six beds. MARU demonstrated minimal correlation between the numbers of acute hospital beds and the size of ICUs, including or excluding regional specialties. A similar conclusion was reached when the number of theaters or the presence of an Accident and Emergency Department were considered.

For the majority of units, the size was less than 2% of acute beds served, the average being 1%. Eighty per cent of ICUs had at least one single room, used in the main for source or protective isolation. No comment is made upon the influence of staff availability on the way such facilities are used.

The average length of stay was 4.4 days (range 1 to 21) with an occupancy of 62%; there was considerable variation, with those units admitting cardiac conditions having a greater throughput and shorter length of stay.

The analysis of major causes of dissatisfaction (Table 4.1) shows that over half the units were unhappy with

Table 4.1 Principal sources of dissatisfaction in 123 ICUs

Factor	Dissatisfied
Heating/ventilation/air conditioning	66
Lack of storage space	39
Layout	30
Lack of space	25
Lighting	14
Lack of daylight	13
Staff/visitors' facilities	12
Observation from nurse base	9
Lack of visitors' room	8

their heating, ventilation or air conditioning. Another significant source of discontent was the units (39%) who considered their storage space inadequate. Ventilators and mobile radiographic equipment provide the greatest problem (in 66% of units). Difficulties with supplies departments, and resulting over-ordering, had exacerbated shortages of storage space. The overall shortage of space was a recurring cause of dissatisfaction in the survey.

Twenty-five per cent of units were unhappy with inadequacies in the provision of windows, either in quantity or position. Sixty-three per cent had no space for teaching and 35% no relatives' overnight stay facilities.

This survey gives useful background against which to conduct a review of the facilities that a modern intensive care unit should provide.

Location

The Intensive Care Society publication *Standards for Intensive Care Units*[3] expanded on previous recommendations regarding the siting of an ICU in the hospital. While there are obvious advantages in being near operating rooms, not least because of the shared engineering services, there are other important considerations. The ICU should be accessible for clinical reasons to admissions/accident and emergency unit, recovery room, delivery unit, HDU/step-down unit, surgical and medical wards, and to the laboratories and imaging department.

A further recommendation was that coronary care and postoperative recovery patients should be kept in separate areas, although facilities and staff might be shared.

Accommodation

While requirements will vary with local needs, there are a number of functional areas that must be provided for any ICU (Table 4.2). In addition a reception area,

Table 4.2 Accommodation required in ICUs

Patient area
Management base
Storage
Offices – medical, nursing and secretarial
Staff lounge
Changing rooms including lavatories
Residents' bedroom
Laboratory area
Relatives' waiting room
Interview room
Kitchen
Cleaners' room
Seminar room
X-ray viewing area

workshop, computer room, treatment room, relatives' accommodation, X-ray dark room and satellite pharmacy should also be considered.

PATIENT AREA

A variety of shapes and sizes have been proposed for the patient area in intensive care units – open-plan and cubicle, square, rectangular and round. A circular intensive care unit of 12 beds was designed for the Methodist Hospital, Rochester, Minnesota.[10] The BMA Working Party on Intensive Care recommended that there should be one cubicle per two other open-plan beds, with each bed-space having an area of 200–300 sq ft (200 sq ft is $18.5\,m^2$). These broad conclusions have been repeated in subsequent reports including Hospital Building Note 27,[2] the ICS Standards,[3] and the Task Force on Guidelines of the Society of Critical Care Medicine (1988).[5] These define minimum dimensions, although they are often interpreted as 'ideal'.

The ICS report states that there should also be at least 2 m of unobstructed corridor space beyond the working area. Single rooms should be $30\,m^2$ in area and rectangular, not L-shaped, and accessible through doors large enough to allow easy passage of beds with traction and other equipment.

Standard 3 of the SCCM recommendations lays emphasis on the provision of a supportive environment that minimizes stress. The standard requires adequate windows citing the lesson learnt in Norwich, England,[11] about patients suffering hallucinations, delusions and depersonalization in a windowless ICU. Clocks, paintings and appropriate decor will all contribute to the reduction of stress for patients, and staff.

Further considerations are those of privacy and noise abatement. In the UK, nurse staffing constraints severely limit the use of individual rooms. Unless there are special requirements, such as barrier/reverse barrier nursing, most patients are treated in a large area that tends to be public and noisy. Floors have necessarily to be strong to support the weight of special equipment, and must be easy to clean. The result is often a surface that does not absorb sound, and a room that resonates to the multiplicity of alarms that are to be found in ICUs; standardization and modulation of these is urgently required.

Whether the beds are arranged in cubicles or in a large multi-bed area, they must be visible to nursing staff. In the UK there will generally be a nurse with each patient. As staff shortages and meal breaks will necessitate a 2 : 1 ratio at times, it is essential that patients can be easily observed from neighboring beds. Centralized monitoring is not an adequate substitute for direct observation.

Figure 4.1 is one of the floor plans for ICUs described in HBN 27 and shows many of the features that would be expected in a modern ICU. The basis for the unit is a large bay accommodating six bed-spaces; this is the model that has been used for recently built ICUs in the UK. A notable deficiency is in the provision for storage; the ICS recommends at least $12\,m^2$ per bed for consumables, equipment and linen.

The Nucleus hospital building programme in the UK uses a different design. These units have two three–bedded areas adjoining one another, one for intensive care, and one for coronary care (Fig. 4.2). There is one rather isolated cubicle for intensive care, and the available floor area is small.

Both designs contrast markedly with the ICU described by Piergeorge.[12] In 1978 the Baptist Hospital of Miami, a 515-bed Level II (community) hospital, decided that its existing ICU facility of 16 beds was inadequate. The hospital developed a 40-bed critical care facility of closed rooms in eight-bed modules, stocked identically (Fig. 4.3). Experiment, using movable plywood walls in a hospital warehouse, showed that a floor area of 225 sq ft as a 15 ft square was ideal; a change of shape conferred no advantage. Current thinking was confirmed.

The next decision related to the position of beds in the unit. Traditionally they are placed with their heads against the wall, and yet nurses spend up to 35% of their time at the patient's head, and respiratory therapists

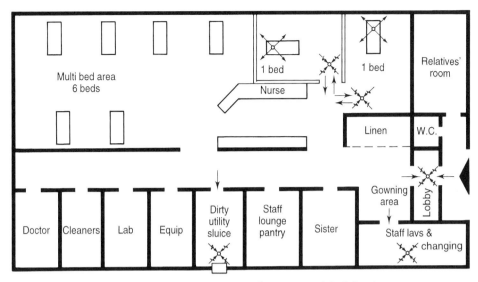

Fig. 4.1 Intensive care arrangement from Hospital Building Note 27.

50%. An arrangement was developed to improve bed head access which involved the provision of all services on a column at the bedside. This allowed access to the head of the patient at all times (Fig. 4.4). The principle is a further refinement of various stalactite, stalagmite or pendant systems developed elsewhere. As the bed is an island, it has to be fixed, and a toe-plate provided for one castor about which the whole can rotate.

Sliding glass partition doors, facing the nurses' central station, enable access (even with large pieces of equipment), minimize noise, and provide some privacy. Each room has a garden atrium to provide interest and natural light.

These contrasting styles reflect current thought in intensive care design, although all are now ten years out of date.

MANAGEMENT BASE

The ICU nursing philosophy in the UK is one of keeping the nurse at the bedside. This obviates the need for a 'central station', which may be regarded as more appropriate for coronary care. However, there is still the need for a primarily communications base from which the unit can be managed. This requires a console with at

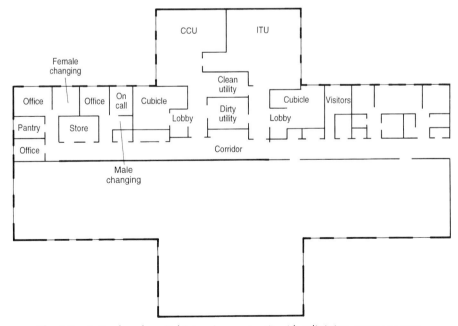

Fig. 4.2 A Nucleus hospital intensive care unit with adjoining coronary care.

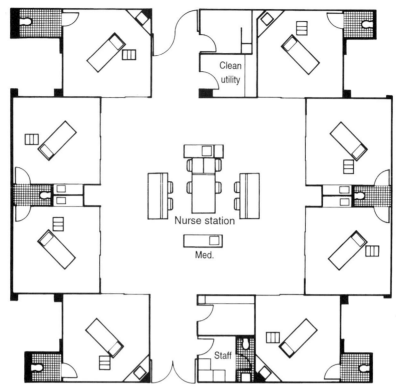

Fig. 4.3   Diagram of an eight-bed unit, Miami.

least two hospital telephone lines, a separate non-switchboard line, and where appropriate, an intercom. This will also accommodate a visual display unit (VDU) for a local or hospital computer system, and a printer (which should be quiet).

Nearby will be the unit drug store or pharmacy, storage for request forms, X-rays and other unit documentation. While patient records can be kept centrally, they are more readily accessible if kept on a chart desk near the bed. This also reduces the occasions

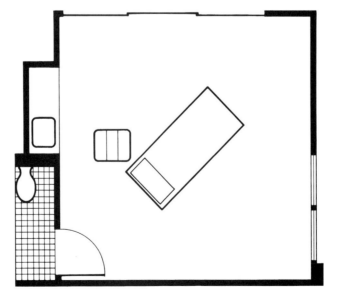

Fig. 4.4   Schematic diagram of a patient's room (Muse Organization, Miami–Denver, Architecture–Planning).

when nursing staff need to leave the patient. Drug/blood refrigerators, and emergency trolleys with a defibrillator, should also be stationed here.

STORAGE

In the light of comments in the MARU survey, the need for adequate storage space cannot be overstated. Storage for consumables must be near the patient, with at least 5 m^2 per bed being provided, half close to the patient, and half in a backup store. Storage for equipment must include provision for ventilators, portable X-ray machines, beds, trolleys, traction and many other smaller items. An additional 5 m^2 is required.

UTILITY ROOMS

A dirty utility room is required for bedpan storage, destruction and the disposal of contaminated dressings and linen. A clean utility room will allow the laying up of trolleys, etc.

LABORATORY

The MARU survey showed that 60% of units have a blood gas analyzer. It follows that there should be a small laboratory readily accessible from the unit to allow for the performance of blood gas analysis and blood glucose determination. The blood gas analyzer should incorporate a co-oximeter, for measurement of oxygen content in arterial and venous blood. Other near-patient testing (electrolytes, osmolality, lactate) can be performed depending upon local facilities, but all ought to be maintained by the clinical chemistry department. This should ensure regular service and calibration. An alternative arrangement might be the use of a vacuum tube system for rapid delivery of specimens and for timely, laboratory-based analysis.

WORKSHOP

For larger units a workshop providing a bench, electrical outlets, piped gases and scavenging, will enable local repair, adjustment, assembly and testing of equipment. However, the greater the complexity and range of equipment, the more use will be made of service contracts with suppliers and the need for such an area reduced.

PROCEDURES/TREATMENT ROOM

These have been used in the past for procedures such as tracheostomy and catheterization. However, increasing patient dependency, with greater dependence on support such as inotropes and hemofiltration, has made patient movement more hazardous. This, with the evolution of more percutaneous techniques such as tracheotomy, may be producing a decline in the use of such facilities.

SEMINAR ROOM

Teaching is a major activity in most large units and a seminar room has become an essential requirement for nurses, medical staff and other groups.

RECEPTION

A reception area and office are very desirable. A call bell to the unit from the reception area is very necessary.

RELATIVES' ROOMS

A waiting area of adequate size with radio and television, interview room and overnight stay facilities are all required. Separate facilities for smokers should also be provided.

CENTRAL SERVICES

The provision of central services, electricity, vacuum, medical gases, heating, lighting, etc. should all comply with the appropriate national standard (or higher).

Lighting should be without glare or flicker and compensated, to give a natural tint to flesh and assist in the recognition of cyanosis. Low-level lighting should be available to illuminate drains; all should be capable of flexible control to enable dimming at night and with illumination confined to selected patients. Emergency lights should be available and functioning, in case central supplies and standby generator fail (it can happen!).

Ventilation should be filtered and include an air conditioning system which will allow a choice of temperature and humidification. Single rooms should have 15 air changes each hour, and other patient areas at least three.

For hemodialysis a deionizer or reverse osmosis system may be needed in selected cubicles, and at strategic points in a larger patient area.

Fire safety

Standard hospital fire regulations will apply equally to ICUs. However rare they may be, it is important that plans for dealing with fire are regularly reviewed and that the fire officer's advice be sought, if changes are proposed, that may, for instance, obstruct access to fire escapes. Wiring is always ducted separately from piped gases, the latter always having good ventilation to wash out any leaking gas. Gas pipelines should not be used to earth electrical equipment.

Appropriate plans of the whole ICU area should be available for the fire department, and in case of fire, staff should know where shut-off valves for services are located.

Bedside services

These should be distributed to both sides of the bed and be easily accessible to short members of staff.

At least 16 mains electrical outlets are required for each bed, and an outlet for portable radiographic equipment should be easily accessible. Two suction outlets, tracheal and continuous low pressure, should be provided. Three oxygen and three air outlets are required, for flow meters, gas mixing devices, gas driven ventilators and other anesthetic machinery. If nitrous oxide or any other inhalational agent is provided, gas scavenging will be required.

Bedside storage may be provided on wall-railing or mobile 'dressers', which have shelving, cupboards, and drawers. Such furniture should not be so high as to obscure the view of the patient from adjoining beds. In addition, a chart board should be provided and easily accessible to nursing staff who are able to maintain sight of the patient.

Cross-infection

This is a particular hazard in such units although design considerations are relatively insignificant when compared with the risks from unwashed hands. A comparative study of nosocomial infection in an old intensive care ward and a new purpose-built unit, suggested that architectural design has little effect on the incidence of such infection.[13] The widespread use of disposable equipment is a major factor in the prevention of cross-infection, but the expense is such that use needs to be kept under continued review. A system of stock control is necessary because of the many items required; the involvement of nursing staff in the operation of the system should be minimized.

The gowning of staff and relatives has been largely abandoned in favor of protocols that aim to minimize cross-infection. Disposable aprons and gloves should be worn for patient contact and thrown away before moving between patients. Alcohol-based hand rubs should be available in every patient area and, to facilitate hand washing, scrub sinks should be readily accessible from each bed-space and within each cubicle. Self-sterilizing heated traps on sites are recommended.

Expired gases should be ducted from the unit to reduce the potential for cross-infection.

Equipment

Equipment must be inspected by a properly approved electrical and biomedical engineering (EBME) department before introduction into service, and appropriate arrangements made for regular in-house or contract servicing. This will normally cost about 10% per annum of the capital outlay. All electrical equipment should comply with appropriate electrical safety regulations.

Unfortunately few hospitals have planned replacement programs for medical and scientific equipment, for which 8–12 years to obsolescence is the norm; as a consequence funding is intermittent and often at short notice. Units should continually review the market for important equipment, so that they can make informed decisions at short notice when money becomes available. *Evaluation*, published by the Medical Devices Directorate of the Department of Health in the UK, is a useful source of regular information.

When choices are made the revenue consequences of this capital expenditure should be considered. 'Captive' disposables can be much more expensive than the generic equivalent, and the maintenance costs of similar apparatus can differ considerably. Other interested parties in the hospital need to be consulted: EBME departments and laboratories may be funding maintenance and need to know the costs. There may be servicing or supplies advantages in having equipment compatible with that used currently.

MEASUREMENT AND MONITORING

Monitoring needs will depend upon local requirements. However a *minimum* profile for each intensive care bed would be:

1. electrocardiograph
2. two pressure monitors
3. pulse oximetry
4. capnography
5. two temperature monitors.

All should be displayed by the bed, out of the line of sight of the patient, and have high and low visible and audible alarms. If thermodilution pulmonary flotation catheters are used, integrated cardiac output computation should be provided. It is hard to conceive of a modern ICU not requiring such a facility.

A data management system with facilities for trending variables, deriving hemodynamic data and printing the results is very advantageous. As much data management as possible should be performed at the bedside. This system should be distinguished from resource management and audit systems which handle, in the main, demographic, diagnostic and procedural data. Integration might be considered, to allow collation of diagnostic and physiological information.

Other monitoring to be considered includes transcutaneous O_2 and CO_2, mass spectrometry, electroencephalogram (EEG) and evoked potentials.

Although each patient will not require all the types of monitoring available, it is important that the facility to provide them is at every bed-space; it is a considerable inconvenience and danger to have to move patients to monitoring equipment. Modular monitors now make this more realizable. In determining equipment levels it is important to allow for the maximum potential requirement for a module; continually 'borrowing' from the next bed is not a good practice and discourages measurement.

A structural requirement for such monitoring is an appropriate conduit or trunking to each bed.

VENTILATORS

The choice of ventilators is always vexed. Some units will standardize on one (generally expensive) machine, while others have a selection with varying levels of sophistication. This latter approach, while providing a wide experience, increases training demands for doctors, nurses and engineers. The range of spares and ancillary equipment will also have to be greater. However, the needs of patients will vary and they can be matched with the most appropriate ventilator; the extra monitoring that is available on some machines may be helpful.

Whether or not disposable circuits are used, the ventilator should be easy to clean and have an autoclavable patient system.

While heat and moisture exchangers are now commonly used in ICUs for humidification, there are still patients who will need hot water bath humidifiers.

OTHER EQUIPMENT

Each bed will need an adequate provision of infusion and syringe pumps to enable pharmacological and fluid therapy. A heavily dependent patient who is septic and requiring sedation, hemodynamic and renal support, and receiving total parenteral nutrition will probably require 8–12 such devices.

Each bed-space should be provided with a full set of equipment for airway management.

Hemofiltration and renal dialysis machines should also be available, as should a fiberoptic bronchoscope for diagnosis and tracheobronchial toilet. Patient weighing scales are also required.

Medical records

The final common pathway for patient information is usually the ICU chart. These are generally large, completed daily, and provide a considerable storage problem, either within or without the medical record. There is a wide variety of such charts and little standardization. Important components are physiological data (cardiovascular, respiratory and renal), respiratory measurements, fluid balance, a record of results and drug/fluid prescription charts. Sedation and Glasgow Coma Scores may be included with other nursing notes.

Figure 4.5 shows the Birmingham Heartlands Hospital chart. In addition to the physiological data and provision of plenty of space for input/output and balances, there is space on the front of the chart for a detailed nursing record. On the rear is space for fluid prescription and a nursing model, on which a plan of management for the day can be clearly detailed. The human outline is used for noting the position of lines; dates of insertion are recorded so that a quick review of potential sites of sepsis is possible.

The advent of sophisticated 'electronic' records of intensive therapy should promote a review of the value of ICU data and the way in which it is stored. The costs of such systems are intimidating, even though significant cost/benefit realization is claimed to be possible.

Staffing

MEDICAL STAFF

Senior

Senior medical staff, known as consultants in the UK, should always be available for clinical advice and

McHENOL MODEL

Problem (Actual / Potential)	Plan	SHORT TERM GOAL	TIME	
1. RESPIRATION	a) C/O as per I.C.U. policy. Ventilator.			
(a) Requires mechanical ventilation.	b) Maintain the F1O2 at the correct/prescribed level. Top up water level in humidifier as necessary. Keep face/trachy mask, mini tracheostomy correctly in position.			
(b) Unable to maintain ABG's "within normal limits".				
(c) Requires an artificial airway.	c) Care of: Tracheostomy : E.T. tube : Minitrachy : Nasopharyngeal airway as per ICU policy.			
(d) Arterial line in situ.	d) Care of "A" line as per I.C.U. policy			
(e) Unable to cough and expectorate own secretions.	e) "Bag and Suck" as per I.C.U. policy _____ hrly. Thrice weekly sputums.			
2. CIRCULATION	a) Monitor heart rate continuously. Observe for irregularities. Report any changes. Obtain strips. Give drugs as prescribed.			
(a) Irregular pulse.	b) Monitor B/P via "A" line continuously. Give colloids/drugs as prescribed. Report any changes.			
(b) Unstable blood pressure (B/P/)	c) Titrate inotropes as required. Observe effects on monitor. Calibrate transducers. Ensure accuracy/settings of pump.			
(c) Inotropes in use.	d) Give drugs as prescribed. Record peripheral temp. Check colour and pulses of feet			
(d) Peripheral shutdown.	e) Warm using _____			
(e) Hypo/hyperthermia.	Cool using _____			
(f) Pulmonary artery catheter in situ.	Report significant gaps between peripheral and core temperatures.			
(g) C.V.P. line in situ.	f) Care of as per I.C.U. policy. g) Care of as per I.C.U. policy.			
3. NUTRITION, FLUIDS AND METABOLISM.	a) Check position of tube. Administer prescribed feeds. .Daily/Alt. daily weights.			
(a) Unable to eat so requires NG/OG feeding.	b) Free drainage. Aspirate _____ hrly. Chart accurately. Check PH. Give antacids as prescribed.			
(b) NG/.OG tube in situ. NG tube size	c) As per ICU policy. Infuse at prescribed rate. Monitor blood sugar. 24 hour urine collection.			
(c) Unable to tolerate NG feeds so requires parenteral nutrition.	d) Accurate recording of fluid intake/output hourly. Infuse fluids at prescribed rate. CVP monitoring as per ICU policy. Report if urine output below 0.5mls/kg/hr. Give prescribed drugs and review their effect.			
(d) Actual/potential disturbance of fluid balance/renal function.	e) Observe for signs of imbalance and report promptly. Administer fluids/ electrolytes at prescribed rate.			
(e) Disturbance of electrolyte balance.				
4. ELIMINATION	a) Daily urinalysis. Hourly output. Thrice weekly CSU. Change urimeter weekly/PRN. Clean catheter area PRN.			
(a) Urinary catheter in situ. Type _____ Size _____	b) Apply drainage bag carefully until drainage lessened. Shorten when required. Chart and describe drainage. Specimens twice weekly.			
(b) Wound drainage.	c) Monitor type, amount and frequency of bowel action. If diarrhoea occurs apply faecal drainage collector. Keep anal area clean and dry. Give drugs as required. If constipation occurs give laxatives/suppositories/ enema as prescribed.			
(c) Constipation/diarrhoea.				
5. REST/ACTIVITY	a) Change position _____ hourly. Use pressure relief aids. Active/passive movements. Daily bed bath. Mouth care _____ hourly. Eye care as per ICU policy.			
(a) Unable to move and care for self.	b) Set "self help" goals. Encourage change of position/sit out in chair. Stand up. Short walks.			
(b) Needs assistance and encouragement with mobility and care.	c) Minimise disturbances. Organise procedures to allow periods of rest. Dim lights at night. Orientate and re-orientate to time and place. Give analgesia as ordered/required and monitor effect.			
(c) Needs adequate rest and sleep.				
6. COMMUNICATIONS	a) Introduce yourself and others. Do not talk over patients. Use communication aids. Reassure and offer explanations to patients. Record information given.			
(a) Unable to communicate because of:- 1. Intubation 2. Tracheostomy 3. Language difficulty.				
7. Altered level of consciousness due to:-	To monitor neurological status and record observations _____ hrly.			
8. PSYCHOSOCIAL	a) Book hospital flat when available. Arrange room in Nurses rooms if needed. Inform relatives of canteen times & location. Inform rels. of nearest toilets.			
(a) Accomodation to relatives	b) Ensure frequent explanation of condition, treatment given by nursing & medical staff. Encourage family to ask questions. Re-inforce all information given. Keep documentation of all interviews and info. given.			
(b) Anxiety/Fear. Patients and Rels.	c) Nurse to be present at first interview with the admitting team. Keep complete record of all that is said at all interviews (to include names of those present).			
(c) Provide adequate information to rels.				
9 Wounds/Cross infection. State all wounds, drains etc present.	a) Write out in full. This must be individual to each patient. *note: All wounds should be assessed daily.			
10.	**10.**			
11.	**11.**			

FOOT NOTE: *Problems specific to patients/relatives should be identified by No. 10, 11, 12, etc I.E. No. 10 PAIN*

Fig. 4.5 The Birmingham Heartlands Hospital chart.

EVALUATION	SIG

ROUTE OR LINE	BOTTLE NO	FLUID	VOLUME	DRUG OR ELECTROLYTE AND DOSE TO BE ADDED	RATE	PRESCRIBER'S SIGNATURE	DRUG ADDITION		ADMINISTRATION		TIME BOTTLE STARTS	TIME BOTTLE FINISHES
							MADE BY	CHECK BY	GIVEN BY	CHECK BY		

PATHOLOGY REPORTS

TIME		TIME	
Hb		Urea	
Wbc		K +	
Platelets		Na +	
PcV		Creatinine	
PT		Glucose	
PTT		Calcium	
FDP		Albumin	
		Protein	

NUTRITION

PARENTAL
ENTERAL TYPE

TOTAL CALORIE

TOTAL NITROGEN

TOTAL POTASSIUM

TOTAL SODIUM

TOTAL VOLUME

CALCULATION OF INSENSIBLE LOSS

i) 0.5 mls/kg/Hour
ii) SUBTRACT HALF OF THIS VALUE IF PATIENT IS ON HEATED HUMIDIFIER.
iii) ADD 25% OF RESULTANT VALUE PEROC INCREASE IN TEMPERATURE > 37% OR SUBTRACT IF HYPOTHERMIC.

HOURLY SEDATION SCORE RECORD

4 = Unmanageable
3 = Actively breathing against ventilator
2 = Awake spontaneously, coughs, respiratory effort
1 = Rousable, coughs with tracheal suction
0 = Asleep, no response to tracheal suction
This scoring system is to be recorded on every patient in the unit

FLOW CHART

Flush Lines
N.G. giving sets
Catheter bag

SPECIMENS

Sputum
Urine C & S
24 hour urine
Blood cultures
U & E, s
Liver
Bone
Cardiac
Lipid
Creatinine
FBC
PT. PTT.

Chest X-ray
Ventilator tubing
Re-breathe bag
Nebuliser
Inspiron/bottle

Daily mouth tray
I/V giving sets
Wound dressing

** Flush lines to be changed as protocol.
  N/G giving sets to be changed daily.
  Catheter bags to be changed weekly/PRN.
  Wet and dry ventilator tubing to be changed as protocol.
  Nebulisers and inspirons to be labelled and changed as protocol.

CONSULTANT:

DATE ADMITTED:

DATE DISCHARGED:

DESTINATION:

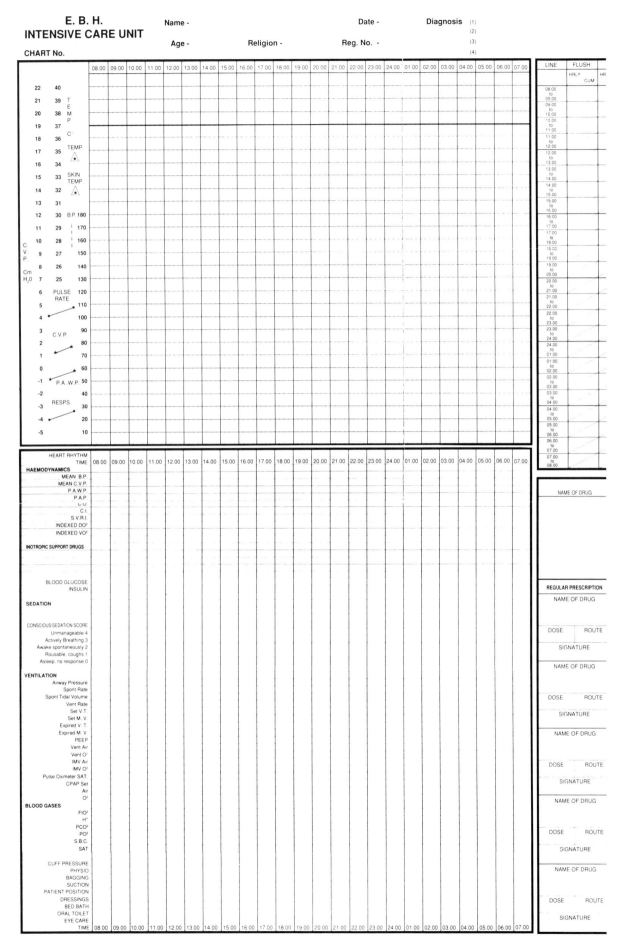

Fig. 4.5 *(cont.)* The Birmingham Heartlands Hospital chart.

Weight -   Tube/Trachy -   Days Intubated -   Admitting Cons -

Height -   Tube Size -   Days Ventilated -

B.S.A. -   INTAKE   Cut / Tied at -   OUTPUT   ALANCE

	HRLY	HRLY	HRLY	HRLY	HRLY	HRLY	TOTALS	HRLY	HRLY	HRLY	HRLY	HRLY	HRLY	HRLY	HRLY	TOTALS	PREVIOUS BALANCE	
CUM	CUM	CUM	CUM	CUM	CUM	CUM	CUM	CUM	CUM	CUM	CUM	CUM	CUM	CUM	CUM	CUM	PERIODIC	CUM

INSENS/LOSS   URINE   TOTALS

DRUG HYPERSENSITIVITIES   ASP TEST   TIME   RESULT   URINE ANALYSIS   TIME   RESULT

ONCE ONLY DRUGS

DOSE	ROUTE	TIME	DR'S SIG	TIME GIVEN	NURSE'S SIG

VARIABLE TIME DRUGS	TIME	SIG
NAME OF DRUG		
DOSE ROUTE		
SIGNATURE		

SPECIAL INSTRUCTIONS

TIME	INT	REGULAR PRESCRIPTION	TIME	INT
		NAME OF DRUG		
		DOSE ROUTE		
		SIGNATURE		

NAME OF DRUG		
DOSE ROUTE		
SIGNATURE		

NAME OF DRUG
DOSE   ROUTE
SIGNATURE

NAME OF DRUG
DOSE   ROUTE
SIGNATURE

Diary

TIME	EVENT	SIG	TIME	EVENT	SIG

NAME OF DRUG
DOSE   ROUTE
SIGNATURE

NAME OF DRUG
DOSE   ROUTE
SIGNATURE

NAME OF DRUG
DOSE   ROUTE
SIGNATURE

NAME OF DRUG
DOSE   ROUTE
SIGNATURE

NAME OF DRUG
DOSE   ROUTE
SIGNATURE

command an adequate sessional allocation for teaching and supervision during normal working hours. A senior doctor should also bear administrative responsibility for the unit, perhaps as director or clinical director. This role will include responsibility for resource provision and management.

The Kings Fund panel recommended that each ICU should have an individual or individuals responsible for:

- ensuring the unit has a clinical policy in the form of written guidelines;
- ensuring that the policy is implemented;
- collecting and evaluating data on clinical outcome and costs for the unit as a whole and for individual patients;
- coordinating the clinical care of individual patients.

In the UK the large majority of 'intensivists' are anesthetists,[7] with a few physicians and surgeons. In other parts of the world this varies, but again, anesthetists predominate.

The ICU should always be able to call on the services of the radiologist, clinical biochemist, hematologist, microbiologist, general surgeon, anesthetist and general physician. Chest physician, cardiologist, nephrologist, neurologist, cardiothoracic, orthopedic and neuro surgeons and otorhinolaryngologist will all make significant contributions.

Trainees

Intensive care units should have dedicated resident medical staff with responsibility extending throughout the day and night. This resident will be the final common pathway for all decisions about each patient, to ensure coordination of care from the disciplines involved.

While some residents may be career 'intensivists', a period of ICU training is valuable to many, if not all, trainees in hospital medicine; a 3-month attachment is probably a worthwhile minimum. If the resident has not been trained in anesthesia, a further tier of resident cover will have to be provided to ensure safe airway management.

Intensive care is not the province of the untrained. Even the most mundane practical skill can prove difficult and hazardous when performed on the critically ill. Nevertheless, intensive care provides an excellent forum for the teaching of therapeutics, resuscitation and monitoring. Dedicated training schemes for doctors wishing to specialize in intensive care have been available in North America and Australasia for some time and are just becoming available in the UK, where a scheme is available at senior registrar level. Lower in the training level the system is unstructured. As with

many subspecialty interests, there is no scheme for matching trainee numbers with available career posts.

NURSING STAFF

The generally accepted norm for the nurse staffing of intensive care is one trained nurse for each patient. This will equate to around six whole-time equivalent (wte) nurses per bed when working a 37.5-hour week. Allowance has to be made for patient 'dependency'. Some patients will not require a nurse at the bedside continuously, while others, e.g. unstable children, might require two. A method of scoring dependency, such as that advocated by the ICS,[3] gives a measure for assessing the demand in a unit (Table 4.3).

Table 4.3   Nurse dependency score

Dependency score	Patient type
C	Closed bed
0	Staffed but empty bed
0.5	Spontaneously breathing patient for simple monitoring perhaps postoperatively with opiate epidural or similar
1	Artificially ventilated patient
1.5	Ventilated patient receiving multiple infusions or requiring complex monitoring or needing very frequent endotracheal suction
2.0	As above but with very unstable cardiovascular system requiring frequent intervention; or
	As above but with the addition of dialysis, hemofiltration, plasma exchange or other extracorporeal circuitry

Additional problems may suggest a higher dependency score. A restless confused self-ventilating patient can require more nursing care than one who is stable and ventilated.

A senior nurse should be responsible for nursing care in the unit, and could have appropriate budgetary responsibility. In determining staffing levels, adequate allowance needs to be made for the other responsibilities of staff, such as teaching, ordering, restocking and training. With the rapid changes taking place in the specialty, the latter is of particular importance, enabling staff to keep up to date with new technology and techniques. Management development of senior nursing staff should be provided. Nurses undergoing postgraduate training in intensive care can make a significant service contribution and enhance the teaching environment. Student nurses should always be supernumerary.

OTHER STAFF

Secretarial and clerical support are often neglected when staffing of units is assessed; they have a vital contribution to make, allowing nursing and medical staff to devote as much of their time as possible to patients. The increasing information requirement within hospitals, for audit and management, and the need to enhance communications, make such a presence essential.

Cleaning should be performed by a person who is familiar with the unit and its procedures; who will not disconnect equipment inappropriately; who is aware of the need for patient confidentiality; and who has some knowledge of the problems of cross-infection.

Regular visits from a dietitian will provide advice about the feeding of patients, and will supplement the work of a nutrition team (see below).

Physiotherapy services, provided on a regular basis, are important to supplement and enhance the skills of the nursing staff. Nonrespiratory physiotherapy can easily be neglected in the critically ill and should not be forgotten.

Technical support, either from the EBME department or from a dedicated technician, is important. If this service is available on a 24 hour per day basis it will influence the equipment levels required for the unit. The less the availability of technical support, the greater the capital investment in equipment required.

Unit management

CLINICAL MANAGEMENT

There are two common patterns for clinical management in ICUs. The first, more common in Australia and North America, is where the intensive care medical staff take over complete responsibility for the patient on admission. The admitting team will then be consulted when required, as would any other discipline. The patient would then be discharged to the most appropriate team for continuing care; not necessarily that responsible for admission.

The second arrangement, which predominates in the UK, is where the patients remain under the care of the admitting consultant throughout their stay in the unit, and care is 'shared' with the ICU team. The balance of care will vary, with the clinical team involved and the admitting condition.

In both these circumstances, the final common

pathway for action and communication should be through the resident ICU medical staff.

SELECTION, ADMISSION AND DISCHARGE OF PATIENTS

Intensive care facilities are very expensive; such a resource should not be squandered on inappropriate admissions. One of the prime responsibilities of ICU staff (doctors, nurses and managers) is to define an admission and discharge policy which is 'owned' by the hospital's clinicians. This is a task not without its problems, particularly if ICU resources have always been stretched.

A policy detailing action to be taken if the ICU is full, is necessary under these circumstances. These policies should be reviewed on a regular basis. The Society of Critical Care Medicine[14] has published its recommendations on how this should be approached, as has the Kings Fund. The SCCM advocates a scheme of allocating patients to one of three priority groups and triaging on that basis. The second group includes those patients who only require monitoring and who could be nursed elsewhere, and the third group includes patients who have metastatic malignancy. It is apparent that a greater provision of intensive care beds in the USA allows a greater latitude for admission and triage than does that in the UK.

Admission criteria

General care units are expected to undertake the treatment of a broad spectrum of critically ill patients. Most will be adult medical and surgical patients who require ventilatory support. The management of acute ventilatory support on wards should not now take place! However, the need for ventilation should not be an exclusive determinant of admission to intensive care. The need to monitor therapy, fluid and pharmacological, may indicate admission.

The Kings Fund Panel proposed that intensive care should be given 'in the expectation of beneficial consequences *when such benefits can be achieved at acceptable cost*', and should not be given where possible harm outweighs the prospective gain. Likely outcome is therefore a major consideration, and the panel suggested the adoption of a simple scale:

1. expected to survive; potentially recoverable (a good chance);
2. prognosis uncertain;
3. death probable shortly, whatever is done;
4. death apparently imminent.

It recommends that intensive care should only be considered for the first two groups 'if the costs are not prohibitive'. While the scale is sensible, the ability of clinicians and relatives to segregate patients into these groups is limited. Public and professional expectation of survival is often unrealistic, while prediction of outcome is only appropriate to patient populations, and should not be applied to individuals,[15] some of whom succeed in confounding the medical soothsayer.

Having proposed this scale, the panel goes on to offer a number of qualifications that epitomize the dilemma faced by the practitioner of intensive care. It notes that patients whose death is probable may gain a temporary improvement in intensive care, allowing time for relatives and medical teams to come to terms with the inevitability of death: at the same time it questions this use of scarce resources! The panel also challenges the judgments made as to what constitutes benefit; is survival enough, is not quality of survival important, and who should assess that quality, doctors or the patient? Nevertheless, it is recommended that all ICUs have guidelines for admission to help staff determine priorities for treatment. Inevitability, particularly when managing emergencies, the presumption in favor of preservation of life will predominate.

Discharge criteria

The Kings Fund panel recognized four situations when discharge should be considered:

1. the patient is stable and has recovered;
2. the immediate threat to life has passed, but close observation is required;
3. the immediate threat has been alleviated, but death is expected shortly;
4. death is imminent, even with intensive therapy.

The first group will be discharged, as will the second if the hospital has suitable facilities elsewhere, e.g. an HDU. The last two groups provide difficult problems for those managing care. Many would wish to maintain support for these patients and their relatives at such a time, though there may be competing pressure for the resources. Withdrawal of support is always difficult; if the patient's views cannot be sought, the relatives should be fully involved with the decision; it should not be theirs to make, but rather theirs with which to agree. It is vital that throughout a period of intensive care, a realistic appraisal be given of a patient's condition and prognosis. It is all too easy in a 'multidisciplinary' environment, for such communication to be neglected or be misunderstood. Where large family groups are visiting key relatives should be identified, for discussion to take place, and information gained and given. Encouragement should be given to the adoption of objective criteria for the assessment of prognosis in the

critically ill, particularly when decisions are required about discontinuing or limiting intensive care. Here, again, recording of the duration of organ systems failure can be helpful, not just in clinical assessment, but in conveying the problem to relatives, who have to be involved in such decisions.

Issues that must be addressed include, who has final say about the admission of a patient, what arbitration mechanism might exist, and how decisions might be reviewed retrospectively if they are considered inappropriate.

The SCCM lists amongst patients who are least likely to benefit from continued treatment, those of advanced age with three or more organ system failures and who have not responded to intensive therapy; those with brain stem death; those with protracted respiratory failure who have not responded to aggressive efforts and who are also suffering from hematological malignancy; and a group with advanced cardiopulmonary disease or widespread carcinoma. Patients who are unlikely to require intensive care, because they are at low risk, are also included. There are patent difficulties in applying such criteria objectively.

Policies for the management of brain stem death and organ donation are also required.

TRANSFER OF PATIENTS

There will be many occasions when transfer of critically ill patients will be required, either within the hospital for operation/investigation, or to and from other hospitals. Appropriate management protocols and equipment should be provided.

Purdie *et al.*,[16] reviewing the early transfer of patients to a regional ICU, considered that this may decrease mortality in patients with complex critical illness and that more seriously ill patients may benefit from early referral. The mortality of patients transferred after 10 days was such as to make the benefit of further aggressive intensive care doubtful.

DATA COLLECTION

Any director of an ICU will quickly come to appreciate the wisdom of comprehensive data collection. Review of older papers about intensive care[16, 17] reveals the debate about length of stay. Average lengths of stay of 4.5 days, 7 days and 3 weeks, are all cited as the norm. The MARU survey demonstrates that little has changed. Case mix is also a factor, tetanus figuring highly in the debate and providing 6% of the admissions in Southampton in the 1960s – 75% survival was quoted.

Another statistic used is the proportion of patients

ventilated; however, the duration of ventilation (ventilated bed days) is more discriminating.

In 1990 the Intensive Care Society, recognizing the need for all ICUs to collect comparable data, issued guidance on how audit should be conducted in the UK.[19] They proposed a minimum data set, including demographic information, disease classification, severity of illness and outcome. To accompany this they suggest the collection of nurse staffing levels and workload (patient dependency).

The APACHE II system is widely used to assess sickness levels on admission, and may be scored daily. There are alternatives and developments such as the Riyadh Intensive Care Programme[20] and APACHE 3, both of which are available commercially.

Costing of therapeutic intervention is specifically excluded by the ICS because of data collection difficulties, although the use of a therapeutic intervention scoring system (TISS),[21] or a modification of the same, is recommended if this is to be done.

Diagnosis in the context of intensive care is very difficult. Various diagnostic coding systems are available but none are entirely satisfactory. The International Classification of Diseases Version 9 (ICD9) and ICD9-CM provide diagnoses; in 1994 ICD10 became available. The Office of Population Census and Studies Classification version 4 (OPCS4) gives a procedural classification, and various versions of Diagnostically Related Groups (DRGs) are available for costing. In the UK many groups are working with the Read Classification, which may well become the standard.

Outcome of treatment, in intensive care and in the hospital, should be collected, and, if possible, a year's follow up information obtained. Statistics on those patients refused admission/transferred elsewhere provide an invaluable tool for resource acquisition.

OTHER PROCEDURES AND POLICIES

Unit management should agree these with other relevant departments in the hospital. Pharmacy will be involved with therapeutic policies, and with the provision of total parenteral nutrition, perhaps through a nutrition team who visit the unit on a regular basis. It must be clear where prescribing responsibility lies; preferably it should be with the ICU resident.

Infection control is crucial; both nursing and medical staff should agree policies with regard to aseptic precautions, cleaning, and antibiotic use. A regular round reviewing these topics is very sound practice.

Investigational routines should be agreed with laboratories and radiology, to ensure that tests are timely and not excessive. Visits by the staff of those departments to ICU should be encouraged as a healthy dialogue can be encouraged and joint audit facilitated.

ROUNDS

Regular unit rounds form the core of patient review and teaching in any intensive care unit. An early morning round allows attendance of trainees and other disciplines, before the start of clinics and operating lists. Contractual allowance should be made for this. This can also coincide with staff handovers, ensuring full communication. A late afternoon or evening round can be briefer and anticipates overnight problems.

Conclusion

This review of general intensive care poses as many questions as answers; many remain unsolved despite years of consideration. The situation in the UK encapsulates problems that exist elsewhere, even in countries that devote far more of their gross national product to health care, a fact mirrored in their greater provision of intensive care.

In the UK the size and scale of intensive care provision fails to meet professional expectations. 'Intensivists' would argue that there are not enough intensive care beds and that they are often poorly supported. And yet it is probable that if the health care system provided the resources necessary to establish a level satisfying professional standards and requirements, this would considerably outstrip the funds available, or alternatively, divert support from other services. Professional groups are not alone in requiring these services. The expectations of patients (and their relatives) have been inflated such that demand may exceed the ability of the current service to provide care. Factors that in the past have assisted 'gate keeping' decisions are becoming of less import with increasing medical abilities. Chronological age is not regarded by patients, their relatives, or professionals, as a contraindication to major surgery. Biological age also becomes less relevant as medical advance enables the treatment of more extreme illness.

If health care systems are unwilling, for whatever reason, to provide adequate intensive care resources, politicians and the public at large will have to recognize the necessity of agreeing limitations in the use of such care. Emotive as it may be, some method of restricting demand will have to be agreed; for this the law is not the best medium!

It follows that, for patients, there must be equity, in distribution and access, to the care that is available. First come, first served, cannot be good enough when distributing a limited resource. Objective and clearly understood criteria for admission to and discharge from intensive care need to be agreed with the purchasers of health care, whether they be patients or their agents (health authorities or family doctors). This is not going to be an easy task.

In turn intensive care provision needs to be organized in an economic fashion. The debate about 'regionalization' of facilities needs to be pursued urgently, so that equipment and professional skills can be congregated in the most cost-effective fashion. This would result in the concentration of intensive care in a number of large units in each region; in turn not all district hospitals would have an ICU. The number of units would reduce, those left would be larger, and there would be an increased need for high dependency care.

Transport of the critically ill must, as a result, be better organized; there needs to be an increased willingness amongst clinicians to accept transfer of their patients to other hospitals and specialists. 'Regionalization' could improve equity as long as equality of access is maintained. Methods of funding such arrangements, including the necessary training overheads, must be found.

It follows that more ICUs should be modern and purpose-built. Careful consideration should be given to the views of the users in their design. Very few doctors or nurses working within ICUs have the opportunity to influence their design, let alone patients and relatives. When professional views are requested they are generally at very short notice with little opportunity to review the experience of others.

Proper training schemes with career progression should be provided for all staff; appropriate acknowledgment should be made of special skills and responsibility.

It is acknowledged that intensive care is a very expensive service benefitting a relatively small number of patients. The introduction into the hospital service of resource management, providing devolved budgets and more sophisticated costing systems, should enable accurate costs to be derived. If these are used to audit the outcomes of large numbers of intensive care patients, it should be possible to improve our knowledge of the effectiveness and cost-effectiveness of intensive care, and some of its components. We have yet to demonstrate that intensive care really is worthwhile!

Appendix
Definition of organ system failures

1. Cardiovascular failure
The presence of one or more of the following:
• vasoactive drugs used to support arterial pressure
• mean arterial BP <50 mm Hg
• episodes of ventricular fibrillation/tachycardia
• heart rate <40 bpm
• inadequate DO_2 causing base deficit >-10
• cardiac index <2.0 l/min/m^2

2. Respiratory failure
The presence of one or more of the following:
• respiratory rate >49/min
• $PaCO_2$ >6.65 kPa in the absence of opioid drugs
• $AaDO_2$ >47 kPa
  ($AaDO_2 = 95 \times FiO_2 - PaCO_2 - PaO_2$)
• dependence on mechanical ventilation for >3 days.
Mechanical ventilation *per se* does not constitute respiratory failure.

3. Renal failure
The presence of one or more of the following:
• urine output = <0.5 ml/kg/h for 24 h
• serum urea = >35 mmol/l
• serum creatinine = >300 μmol/l

4. Haematological failure
The presence of one or more of the following:
• WBC = <1000/mm^3
• platelets = <20 000/mm^3
• haematocrit = <20% in the absence of bleeding

5. Neurological failure
Best GCS = <8 in the absence of drugs

6. Hepatic failure
• encephalopathy
• Pugh score >3
• bilirubin >30μmol/l
• PT>1.5 in absence DIC

7. Metabolic failure
• uncompensated noncardiac base deficit >-10
• acute serum electrolyte shift requiring intravenous therapy

8. Gastrointestinal failure
• ileus/uncontrollable diarrhea
• hemorrhage
• pancreatitis

AaDO$_2$: Alveolar arterial oxygen difference
BP: blood pressure
bpm: beats per minute
DIC: Disseminated intravascular coagulation
DO$_2$: Oxygen delivery
FiO$_2$: inspired oxygen fraction
GCS: Glasgow coma score
PaCO$_2$: Arterial carbon dioxide partial pressure
PaO$_2$: Arterial oxygen partial pressure
PT: Prothrombin time
WBC: white blood cells.

References

1. British Medical Association Planning Unit. *Report of the Working Party on Intensive Care in the United Kingdom* London: BMA, 1967.
2. Hospital Building Note (HBN) 27. London: Department of Health and Social Security, Intensive Therapy Unit, 1970.
3. Intensive Care Society. *Standards for Intensive Care Units.* London: BioMedica Ltd.
4. Medical Architecture Research Unit (MARU). Intensive Therapy and Coronary Care Units: Postal Survey Report, 1988.
5. Society of Critical Care Medicine, Task Force on Guidelines. Recommendations for critical care unit design. *Crit Care Med* 1988; **16** (8): 796–811.
6. Intensive Care in the United Kingdom: Report from the Kings Fund Panel. *Anaesthesia* 1989; **44**: 428–31.
7. Cullen DJ. Results and costs of intensive care. *Anesthesiology* 1977;**47**: 203–16.
8. Intensive Care Society. *The Intensive Care Service in the UK.* London: The Intensive Care Society, 1990.
9. Association of Anaesthetists of Great Britain and Ireland. *Intensive Care Services – provision for the future.* London: Association of Anaesthetists of Great Britain and Ireland, 1988.
10. Wiklund PE. Intensive care units: design, location, staffing ancillary areas, equipment. *Anesthesiology* 1969; **31**: 122–36.
11. Keep P, James J, Inman M. Windows in the intensive therapy unit. *Aneasthesia* 1980; **35**: 257–62.
12. Piergeorge AR, Cesarano FL, Casanova DM. Designing the critical care unit: a multidisciplinary approach. *Crit Care Med* 1983; **11**: 541–5.
13. Huebner J, Frank U, Kappstein I *et al.* Influence of architectural design on nosocomial infections in intensive care units – a prospective 2-year analysis. *Intensive Care Med* 1989; **15**: 179–83.
14. Task Force on Guidelines, Society of Critical Care Medicine. Recommendations for intensive care unit admission and discharge criteria. *Crit Care Med* 1988; **16**(8): 807–8.
15. Knaus WA, Draper EA, Wagner DP, Zimmerman JE. APACHE II: a severity of disease classification system. *Crit Care Med* 1985; **13**: 818–29.
16. Purdie JAM, Ridley SA, Wallace PGM. Effective use of regional intensive therapy units. *Br Med J* 1990; **300**: 79–81.
17. Mason SA. Intensive care units. *Proc Roy Soc Med* 1966; **59**: 1293–6.
18. Burn JMB. Design and staffing of an intensive care unit. *Lancet* 1970; **i**: 1040–3.
19. Intensive Care Society. *Intensive Care Audit.* London: The Intensive Care Society, 1990.
20. Chang RWS, Jacobs S, Lee B, Pace N. Predicting deaths among intensive care unit patients. *Crit Care Med* 1988; **16**: 34–42.
21. Cullen DJ, Civetta JM, Briggs BA, Ferrara LC. Therapeutic Intervention Scoring System: a method for quantitative comparison of patient care. *Crit Care Med* 1974; **2**: 57–60.

CHAPTER 5

Specialist Care Units

MALCOLM WRIGHT———————————————————————

General principles for development of special care services   57
Integration of the SCU into the hospital   60
Types of specialist care units   61
Combined medical and surgical SCUs   64
Specialist surgical units   65
Medical special care units   66
Summary   68
References   68

This chapter will focus on the role of specialist care units (SCU) which offer some but not all of the range of services found in the general intensive care unit (GICU). It is neither feasible nor reasonable to admit to the GICU all patients requiring 'limited' intensive care. The development of general intensive care services in hospitals has recognized the value of aggregating patients with comparable levels of severity of illness regardless of the underlying pathology. Although the GICU is the locus of care for most critically ill patients in general hospitals, there are persuasive reasons for admitting certain categories of patient to SCUs dedicated to the provision of care for a narrow and easily recognized range of illnesses on the basis of pathology and clinical circumstances rather than severity of illness. Such SCUs provide specialized intensive care services directed at a narrower spectrum of diseases than would be found in the 'typical' GICU. In summary, the GICU tends to be severity-focused and the SCU tends to be pathology-focused.

In these units some or all of the elements of intensive care services may be provided, but therapy is focused on either a general problem occurring in a highly specialized category of patient or on a specialized single system problem occurring in a patient who may be relatively well. Organization of health services is one of the most sophisticated human social activities and at present it is clear that 'a wide range of organisational arrangements within hospitals determines where the ICU appears in an organisational chart . . .'.[1] The major differences in approach between the GICU and the SCU are summarized in Table 5.1.

This is neither a watertight nor an exhaustive differentiation, but it does serve to summarize some important points. These are that the GICU should have overall competence in managing multisystem disease whilst the SCU is largely selective in its admission policy. For example, the GICU in an adult general hospital might reasonably be expected to handle the problems of a burnt toddler for at least the first few hours until transfer to a special unit can be arranged. However, it is very unlikely that the pediatric burns unit would ever be expected to handle a case of adult renal failure. The GICU should be a generally safe venue from the point of view of early intervention in life-endangering emergencies in all comers, but in the SCU the major focus of medical and nursing attention is on the specific disease entity which has brought about admission to the SCU in the first place.

These important differences have implications for funding and staffing: SCUs frequently have regional, supraregional and even national responsibilities. A neonatal surgical unit may well serve several health authorities, all of which may refer work to the unit, but

Table 5.1 Comparison between the general intensive care unit (GICU) and the specialist care unit (SCU)

GICU	SCU
Patients admitted/accepted on basis of severity of illness	Severity not sole admission criterion; age, and pathology etc. also considered
Relatively nonselective admission criteria	Rigorous admission criteria
Wide range of therapies	Narrow specialized therapeutic repertoire
Most referrals from parent institution	Most referrals regional or supraregional
Easy establishment of outreach services	Inherent difficulties with outreach services
Relative ease of staffing and training of nurses and doctors	Often difficulties with recruitment and training of staff
Clinical research desirable	Clinical research essential

none of which may make a realistic contribution to the running costs of the unit. The need to liaise with large numbers of referring practitioners and institutions may create problems for the director of a major transregional unit who may experience substantial difficulty in establishing uniform referral and early treatment protocols because of the difficulties in imposing clinical discipline on other autonomous institutions and individuals. Although similar difficulties may beset the director of a GICU, over time the geographic and organizational integration of the GICU with a fairly large institution will lead to fairly standard lines of communication and patterns of prereferral management of patients.

In a GICU typically 75% or more of referrals will be from within the parent institution, but in a large SCU the proportion will be much lower. This means that relative to the size of the parent institution, the SCU may need to be substantially better funded and equipped than the GICU. This is particularly true in children's hospitals in which, wherever possible, inpatient care is avoided and so the proportion of pediatric ICU beds may be very high compared with the overall number of hospital beds.

The GICU in a large general hospital is invariably equipped to provide ventilatory support to all patients and usually has the capacity to carry out other system support maneuvers. This is not true of the SCU which may have a very limited capacity to support multiple organ failure and may need to recruit outside help should organ failure supervene.

The SCU may be inexorably tied to some other service. Thus a cardiovascular SCU may be part and parcel of the cardiac surgical service. A neonatal intensive care unit must of necessity be closely inte-

grated with the neonatal transport and retrieval service because management in transit is of the essence of neonatal critical care practice.

Finally, doctors are notorious empire builders. Much of the quality of present day critical care medicine is based upon the development of GICUs or SCUs which have been run as 'independent medical republics' within the broader hospital community. Whilst this model of care remains both attractive and successful, it is also highly addictive and expensive and hospital administrations are beset with submissions and plans for clinical units dealing with ever more circumscribed areas of medicine. Clearly limits need to be set, but the place and rigidity of those limits remains uncertain.

General principles for development of special care services

REPORTS FROM OFFICIAL BODIES

Recourse is frequently made to reports which attempt to quantify intensive care utilization or to estimate an ideal proportion of beds to be devoted to critical care facilities.[2–4] Unfortunately, such reports – often of impeccable pedigree and meticulously researched – are beset with a number of fundamental problems and should be interpreted with respectful skepticism for the following reasons.

Firstly they are inevitably couched in the cultural values of the community in which they are generated. A level of provision which would be seen as acceptable in one community might be regarded as disgracefully inadequate in another. Extrapolation from one country and culture to another is extremely hazardous.

Secondly, at all but the most clinically obvious level of organ failure there is no general agreement as to what constitutes an appropriate severity of illness to justify intensive care in either a GICU or a SCU and there is no general agreement on, or even a wholly effective measuring tool for, the level of intensive care to be made available. In other words, we all know what we mean by maximal severity and maximal therapy, but we do not agree on the lower cutoff points for defining either critical illness or intensive therapy. Attention was drawn to this issue as early as 1979 but the problem remains troublesome and unresolved.[5] This means that the level of severity at which this lower cutoff is set will determine the apparent demand for the service. Although enormous progress has been made in the sophistication and utilization of severity and therapy scoring systems, it would be unusual for prospectively gathered retrospective data of sufficiently high quality to be available at the time the decision to develop a new facility is made. Almost invariably, new units are developed on the basis of educated guesswork. At present, commercially available hospital management software remains disappointing in describing patient dependency or severity of illness.

Thirdly, regardless of the integrity of the committee or individual generating the report, such reports reflect the overall bias of their commissioners. If commissioned by government or other funding body, they tend to take a predictably rationalist approach to the provision of service. If generated by professionals in the field of critical care, there is a tendency for the report to err on the side of extravagance and become a Utopian wish-list rather than an achievable agenda. Where a 'needs assessment' is commissioned by a government this may be as a response to some 'scandalous' incident involving delay or mishandling of an individual case. Reports generated in a climate of indignation are not necessarily useful documents for achieving change and may run into difficulties in implementation.

Finally, no matter how worthy the reasoning behind a submission for a new or improved facility, if there is insufficient funding available, the plans will have to be revised and demands reduced to fit the available budget.

For these reasons policy statements, issues papers and pronouncements from relevant authorities should be used cautiously as guidelines for the provision of services in a specific community. Primarily they are useful for their qualitative value rather than their actual evaluations of ratios of beds to populations. It follows that any hospital wishing to develop a new service or enlarge an existing service should make every effort to gather data prospectively prior to the initiation of the service.

THERE SHOULD BE A DEMONSTRATED NEED FOR THE PROPOSED SERVICE

A SCU should occupy a unique niche and provide a service which is not and cannot readily be provided by referring hospitals or services and which is not already readily accessible. Whilst it is true to say that every general hospital should have certain core facilities such as operating suites and a GICU, it is quite wrong for specialized facilities to be duplicated on a 'me too' basis.

Ideally a prospective needs evaluation should be undertaken. For example a solid organ transplant service should be based upon documented evidence of the number of patients referred with or treated for end-stage organ failure. The options then are to either develop a local service or to continue to refer patients out to another facility.

A third option is frequently canvassed. This is to do neither and simply not offer a particular service. Although ethical arguments can be mounted which support this kind of rationing, in practice such a response tends to become a political issue very rapidly and ill-informed community pressure may precipitate inappropriate provision of advanced services for political expediency; this is often the costliest alternative in terms of both access and costs.

It should be borne in mind that there are significant costs in not providing an advanced clinical service. These include the costs of continuing to support a patient with worsening illness in a suboptimal environment. There are therefore potential savings to be made by the provision of curative care wherever possible. The classical example is the provision of kidney transplants as a cost-effective alternative to dialysis. There are also the substantial costs of escorted transport of critically ill patients to SCUs in another hospital. Transport of critically ill patients between health care institutions is potentially hazardous[6] and the sum of savings resulting from not providing a particular unit in a particular institution may be swallowed up in legal fees and settlements if a patient should come to harm in transit.

THE SERVICE SHOULD HAVE ACCESS TO SUFFICIENT NUMBERS OF PATIENTS

It is generally believed that there is a 'critical mass' of caseload where demanding technologies are concerned. Many studies have demonstrated a 'learning curve' illustrated by steadily improving outcomes during the early months or years of activity by clinical units. In blunt terms, this means that patients treated in a new and inexperienced facility have an increased risk of morbidity or death compared with those treated in an established and busy unit. It appears that extensive training of staff in an established facility can ameliorate but does not eliminate this problem.[7]

If access to high-technology medical care is to be widened, it is clear that new facilities must be brought on-line, but it is also clear that some risk to the first patients in a new facility is inevitable. A number of strategies can be employed to minimize this risk. These include prior training of key staff by attendance at a successful established unit, if necessary by residential attachment, workshops for support staff, graded start-up activities, 'dry run' and 'table-top' replication of the actual clinical situation, and tackling uncomplicated patients initially.

This last is often very hard to achieve as it is usual for any new clinical enterprise to be referred 'impossible' patients in the first instance. The result is that new units are frequently regarded as deathtraps and suffer from a loss of confidence and even ridicule from clinicians who have referred their patients too late for good results to be a realistic expectation.

IT SHOULD BE FULLY SUPPORTED BY RELEVANT GROUPS WITHIN THE HOSPITAL

There should be enthusiastic advocacy for the SCU, not only by those directly concerned, but by other members of the clinical and nursing staff. A SCU is unlikely to prosper if a number of influential stakeholders in the parent institution resent its establishment and feel that it is inappropriate, costly or a drain on other resources. Support must include a sufficiently generous allocation of staff of sufficient expertise for success to be a realistic expectation.

THERE SHOULD BE A POLICY FOR THE DEVELOPMENT OF SPECIFIC EXPERTISE WITHIN THE HOSPITAL

A team to operate the facility should be developed well before the unit is opened. A common mistake is to assume that a new clinical initiative can be managed by middle-grade medical staff according to a theoretical game plan devised by absentee consultants. Continuity of care is of the essence of all critical care and this continuity must be vested in consultants, not in the junior medical staff. Before clinical work begins, every member of the prospective team should be aware of their role in the organization.

Wherever possible individuals should be seconded to successful units for familiarization and training. These visits can be of enormous value in getting a new unit off to a successful start. In my experience the funding of such visits has proved a far more valuable use of 'soft' money from charities and public subscription than the subsidy of capital works or equipment purchases.

The purpose of such visits is two-fold. Firstly, they provide the opportunity to gain hands-on skills at an appropriate level. This cannot be done quickly. Experience is not readily gained by leaning over the shoulder of the expert. Every opportunity should be taken to actually do the job in question and become good at it under supervision. This is the opportunity for detailed note-taking about not only what is done, but exactly how it is done. Names of suppliers, catalogue numbers of equipment and costings can be obtained at these visits. It is important that nursing staff are included in this program of visits and that secondment should be of adequate duration. Hospital authorities tend to resent the salary implications of these secondments but the

money is well spent if the result is a thoroughly literate, confident and competent clinical team on commencement of a special service.

Secondly, the forging of links with centers of excellence elsewhere creates an invaluable resource backup. Sympathetic telephone assistance can be obtained at any hour of the day and night and both sides know who they are dealing with. The tendency to 'go it alone' must be resisted. Early failures and problems are almost inevitable but are much easier to cope with if problems have been discussed along the way with an established unit.

OPERATING PROTOCOLS SHOULD BE DEVELOPED PRIOR TO THE OPENING OF THE FACILITY

It is important to develop management protocols before the unit opens. These need not be detailed but should be based on orthodox and rational principles. Wherever possible existing skills should be incorporated into the operating procedures of a new unit. This means that standard techniques in use throughout the hospital need to be incorporated into management schedules. In addition to economizing on the time needed to develop new protocols, it permits easy transition from the known to the unknown and reduces the psychological threat inherent in any new venture. These protocols may need revision in the light of experience but to operate a new unit without a game plan is to court early failure. People must know what they are supposed to be doing and lines of communication must be drawn up for foreseeable emergencies. Nurses need to know their responsibilities and the limits of their roles and the nursing team should be involved in planning from the outset.

STAFF TRAINING AND FAMILIARIZATION SHOULD OCCUPY A MAJOR PART OF THE ACTIVITIES OF THE UNIT

Staff training should take place in three distinct phases. Firstly there should be the training initiatives required to develop new knowledge and skills. Secondly, when the unit has been in existence for a time it is important for all staff to pool their combined experiences and to make those protocol modifications which will be required for the future. Finally continuing education – targeted particularly at nursing staff – ensures that lessons learned are retained and that rational management plans do not degenerate into mere 'policy' but that all staff understand the clinical basis for their practice.

PROTOCOLS FOR REFERRAL AND CRITERIA FOR ACCEPTANCE OF PATIENTS SHOULD BE DEVELOPED

The purpose of these protocols is to ensure that referring clinicians understand the role and function of the unit and learn to identify those patients likely to do well with the new therapeutic initiative. It is likely that any new unit will have a cost structure which is higher than routine care within the hospital. Despite this, the admission policy should be fairly liberal at the outset in order that the unit can develop experience in assessing those likely to benefit from new therapies. In the light of experience firm and if necessary more restrictive admission criteria should be developed which will have widespread acceptance.

A PATIENT ASSESSMENT AND FAMILY SUPPORT TEAM MAY BE REQUIRED

For solid organ, chemotherapy and bone marrow transplantation units, it is usual for some form of comprehensive assessment to take place with the referring clinician making a case for the proposed intervention and the therapeutic team highlighting likely problem areas and recommending the necessary further treatment. This process provides an opportunity for the patient and family to become part of the therapeutic team rather than passive victims of the medical juggernaut. It is not clear whether such assessment really contributes to a good clinical outcome. It has also been suggested that the filtration process may tend to deny care to difficult cases in favor of straightforward ones. However, this process certainly provides for the patient and family a window into the therapeutic process and a more sympathetic mutual understanding between therapeutic team and patient.

The assessment team may comprise the relevant medical personnel, a senior member of the nursing team who will visit the patient and family prior to the treatment, a social worker and a liaison psychiatrist. For ongoing support in our own transplant unit we have relied heavily on the services of a former patient, herself a successful transplant recipient.

While the services of liaison groups and support persons may be invaluable, it is important to remember that the responsibility for medical and nursing decision making cannot be devolved either legally or ethically and that some patients may feel more comfortable disclosing their family intimacies only with core health care professionals. It should be clear from the outset that the support team are definitely helpers rather than executives and also that their role is no less confidential than that of the doctors and nurses involved in the actual care delivery.

CLINICAL AND FINANCIAL AUDIT SHOULD BE INCORPORATED FROM THE OUTSET

Money spent on data collection, curation and analysis is well spent. Although this is an unpopular chore at the outset, the benefits of well-founded decision making greatly outweigh the tedium of having to collect and analyze data. A climate of practice in which a clinical database is seen as fundamental as the oxygen supply must be maintained.

A database does not have to be complex and the services of a programmer although invaluable are by no means essential. Immense computing power is now available at minimal price using IBM or Macintosh computing systems. Small desktop computers running simple software packages are quite adequate to the task of collecting and organizing clinical data. Most standard database (e.g. dBase IV V2.0) and spreadsheet packages generate files which are readable and analyzable by major statistical programs such as SPSS/PC+,[9] thus enabling a wide range of statistical manipulations to be carried out. Regardless of research considerations, a sound clinical database has huge benefits for calculating workload, making future projections, computing costs and other important but tedious housekeeping tasks.

No matter how small or low-key the proposed SCU, it will provide opportunities for clinical research, evaluation and audit. There remains a huge shortage of information about the deployment and efficacy of critical care services and data from well-audited units remain the source for improvement in clinical management. Finally, SCUs however effective, become easy targets for cutbacks and bed closures because they are invariably costly relative to the usual beds in the unit. It is crucial for clinical and political reasons that resource utilization and outcome data be kept from the outset and that the database should be controlled by the medical and nursing directors of the unit.

Integration of the SCU into the hospital

COMBINED OR SEPARATE UNITS?

Should SCUs be integrated with the general intensive care services of the hospital or should they be separately administered?

A good case may be made out for the integration of all SCUs into a 'greater intensive care service'. Persuasive arguments may also be advanced for territorial divisions between SCUs to be maintained. The case for integration rests upon the familiar 'economies of scale' arguments together with the belief that there is sufficient overlap between the clinical scenarios likely to be encountered in each clinical grouping to justify a common medical and nursing approach.

The case for separation highlights the difficulties in training staff in all the care requirements of a particular clinical group. So it is claimed that, for example, the demands of burns patients differ so widely from those of GICU patients that it is logical to locate them separately and to have dedicated nursing staff.

In practice, it is usual for high-volume patients to be separately grouped. Therefore heart surgery patients are usually cared for separately from the GICU. However, SCUs with a lower volume of patients will need to rely heavily on the core GICU for provision of life-support technologies and the GICU will have to take responsibility for the necessity of developing and upgrading skills the SCU. For example, in our hospital, the renal dialysis and transplant service is operated separately from the main GICU, while the liver transplant service is operated utilizing the GICU extensively for pre- and post-operative care. This grouping reflects the large numbers of renal patients compared with the much smaller demand for liver transplantation, as well as the overall greater severity of illness in liver transplant patients.

What should be the criteria for combining or separating units?

It seems reasonable to use the likelihood or regularity of occurrence of organ failure as a criterion for self-sufficiency. Thus a cardiac surgical unit which regularly utilizes ventilatory support should clearly be self-sufficient in that regard and it would be quite usual for such a unit to make few demands on a GICU. On the other hand even a busy burns unit may only need to provide infrequent ventilatory support and would probably not seek to ventilate patients in the burns unit. Special problems relate to the development of SCUs in isolation or at outlying hospitals. By their nature, such units cannot offer a full range of GICU services and yet may treat some very sick patients with abundant potential for severe organ failure. Small or outlying hospitals may experience difficulty in providing a complete range of after-hours medical and diagnostic cover.

LOCATION OF SCUs IN THE HOSPITAL

The location of a SCU needs to be decided with attention to the ease of communication with and referral from feeder units. In general, complex units need to be situated near to major diagnostic and therapeutic services – in particular with easy access to operating rooms and imaging departments. An older generation of hospital buildings relied heavily on lifts for patient transfer and it is almost inevitable that some diagnostic or therapeutic service will be on another floor. It has been established[10] that movement of patients between special units and diagnostic services poses an additional risk, particularly if ventilatory support needs to be provided in transit. The time taken to make transfers between SCUs and other hospital services is not only a major inconvenience, but by tying up skilled staff it is an important contributor to costs. The notion of an intensive care floor or area of a hospital is attractive and workable. Different units each occupy their own area and may have differing management structures but are contiguous physically. These units may share a common pool of nurses and benefit from a shared after-hours junior medical service, shared radiology, and shared 'stat' laboratory services.

DEDICATED LABORATORY SERVICE

For over 30 years it has been assumed that an on-site laboratory ('stat-lab') is an essential feature of a GICU and for many SCUs and there is much commercial effort by the manufacturers of compact analysis equipment dedicated to reiterating this point to planners. Our experience has been that, provided that the on-site hospital laboratory offers a 24-hour service, then analysis of specimens transmitted from our intensive care floor to the main laboratory by air tube has resulted in rapid results with the added advantages of less blood-handling in the clinical area and also the automatic incorporation of the results into a national laboratory medicine quality assurance program. Although the concept of the 'stat-lab' is likely to survive for many years yet, the practice of junior medical staff analyzing blood in the clinical area divorced from any supervision or training by the chemical pathology service must be looked upon with increasing concern and our experience has shown that it can be phased out without detriment to the clinical service and with a reduction in capital outlay. Regardless of whether the actual analysis is carried out in a 'stat-lab' or in the main hospital laboratory, it is difficult to conceive of an intensive care service which could function without rapid access to high quality laboratory and radiology services. This should be a primary concern in the planning of new or expanded services.

Types of specialist care units

SCUs may be grouped in a number of ways. Table 5.2 shows just one convenient grouping. Some general

Table 5.2   Comparison of different types of special care unit

Type of unit	Typical nurse to patient ratio	Typical length of stay	Senior medical officer	Typical junior medical officer support	Additional support staff	Demand for family support	Environment (windows always essential)	Rehabilitation function
General intensive care unit	>1:1	4–6 days	Intensivist Anesthetist Physician	On ward 24-h	Scientist Research staff Therapist Dietitian	Moderate	Controlled climate	Minimal
Neonatal	>1:1	Weeks	Neonatologist	On ward 24-h	Scientist	Extreme	Highly controlled climate	Minimal
Step-down units	<1:1	Days	Intensivist (ideally)	On ward 24-h	Physiotherapist	Low	Routine hospital	Moderate
Pediatric	>1:1	Short as possible	Pediatrician or pediatric anesthetist	On ward 24-h	Scientist Research staff Therapist Teacher	High	Controlled climate	Some
Spinal injury	<1:1	Months	Rehabilitation team	In hospital	Physiotherapist Occupational therapist Assistance with lifting	High	Routine hospital	Dominant
Burns unit	1:1–4:4, depending on severity of burn	Weeks/months	Plastic surgeon	In hospital	Physiotherapist Occupational therapist Dietitian	High	Highly controlled climate	Prominent
Cardiac surgery	1:1	Hours/days	Cardiac surgeon or cardiologist	On ward 24-h	Physiotherapist Scientist	Moderate	Routine hospital	Low
Organ transplantation	Liver >1:1 Kidney <1:1	Variable	Variable	In hospital	Scientist Physiotherapist	High	Routine hospital	Low
Infectious disease	<1:1	Days/weeks	Infectious disease physician	In hospital	Ideally integrated with microbiology lab.	Moderate (high in AIDS patients)	Controlled climate Containment Isolation	Some
Marrow transplant/ oncology	>1:1	Days/weeks	Oncologist/ immunologist	From oncology team	Scientist Physiotherapist	High	Controlled climate Protective isolation	Low

Table 5.2 *Continued* Comparison of different types of special care unit

Type of unit	Typical nurse to patient ratio	Typical length of stay	Senior medical officer	Typical junior medical officer support	Additional support staff	Demand for family support	Environment (windows aways essential)	Rehabilitation function
Psychiatric	1 : 1	Brief	Psychiatry team	From psychiatry team	Psychologist Counsellor Toxicologist	Extreme	Routine hospital	Important
Geriatric	Variable	Days	Geriatrician	In hospital	Social worker Psychologist Therapist Assistance with lifting	High	Routine hospital	Fundamental
Renal and dialysis	<1 : 1	Brief but recurrent	Nephrologist	In hospital	Social worker Counsellor	Moderate but on-going	Routine hospital	Moderate
Coronary care	<1 : 1	Days	Cardiologist	In hospital	Social worker	Moderate	Routine hospital	Moderate
Poisoning	Variable	Hours	Pharmacologist/ anesthetist	In hospital	Social worker Psychologist Psychiatric liaison team	High	Routine hospital	Low

principles may be enunciated. Firstly, SCUs are not a substitute for a fully functional intensive care unit. Secondly, unless specific policies are laid down, SCUs can become 'independent warring republics'. It is important that the SCU does not become the 'alternative GICU' utilized by those clinician who for one reason or another do not like or cannot accept the policies of the GICU. These problems certainly bedevil critical care administration, but they should not be solved by diversion of patients to inappropriate clinical environments.

Combined medical and surgical SCUs

PEDIATRIC UNITS

There are persuasive arguments for separation of pediatric work from the mainstream of adult intensive care and within pediatric practice it is customary for neonates to be cared for separately from older children. Children have quite different care requirements from adults and if a child is sick enough to be in an intensive care unit he or she is sick enough to merit the care of a pediatrician skilled in the management of critical illness in children.

Access by parents and siblings is of crucial importance, not only to the families but also to the emotional well-being and development of the sick child, and this consideration constitutes a major subsidiary focus for care. Wherever possible children should be cared for in a dedicated pediatric unit, should be nursed out of sight of adult patients and as far as possible looked after by pediatrically trained nurses in association with their parents and siblings. As cancer therapy in children has become more commonplace there has been a recognition that the pediatric intensive care unit is a reasonable place for the care of children undergoing cancer therapy.[11] Nevertheless, these arrangements are not always feasible and Dawson *et al.* have reviewed their experience with almost 400 patients admitted to a predominantly adult GICU over a period of eight years. Their report makes the point that involvement of a pediatrician with the management was a crucial feature in the achievement of good outcomes.[12]

NEONATAL UNITS

The neonatal unit is a pivotal part of the interface between the pediatric service and the obstetric service. The main functions of such a unit are the care of babies with low birthweight and immature lungs and the care of babies with congenital deformities, especially in the

postoperative period. A recent report from the UK[13] highlights the problems of matching supply and demand for such a service. Neonatal units are usually situated in close proximity to a major maternity unit and are intimately integrated with both the pediatric and pediatric surgical and anesthetic services. No branch of medicine has generated greater controversy than neonatal intensive care. The issues are the high cost of care due mainly to the high staff ratios and the perceived poor results.

Smaller hospitals simply cannot afford to initiate or maintain a neonatal intensive care service and whatever the location of a neonatal service, a crucial feature is integration with the neonatal retrieval and transport team. In a compact country like the UK, this service may be predominantly by road ambulance, but in North America and Australia a large number of babies are transported to these units by the aeromedical service. Although the costs of such a service are usually borne by the referring institution, there is a need for the neonatal unit to be a resource base for education and training of nurses and doctors not only in the inpatient management of very small babies but in the prehospital care and aeromedical management.

SPINAL INJURY UNITS

Between 10 and 25% of all patients with spinal cord injury will be admitted initially to a GICU with a significant degree of respiratory failure. This is due to the combined effects of spinal cord injury and concomitant chest injury or other cause of respiratory failure.[14] Although most will recover sufficient respiratory function to lead an independent life outside hospital, the spinal injuries unit will require facilities for the continuation or resumption of ventilatory support. A small minority of patients will require ventilatory support either at night or permanently. This mandates the application of intensive respiratory care in a rehabilitation-focused environment. If long-term survival were to be the only goal, then round the clock ventilatory care in an intensive care environment would be ideal. Not only would this block an ICU bed indefinitely, but it would fail to capitalize on the limited but definite rehabilitation prospects available to the respiratory quadriplegic.

Accordingly, despite ventilator dependence around the clock, nursing levels for the long-term ventilator-dependent patient are limited, relatives may be recruited as assistants and novel options such as outings to parks and beaches are explored in the interests of mental rehabilitation. Here, overall well-being must be balanced against considerations of absolute safety. These aspects of overall care must be canvassed with the patient and relatives early in the course of disability in order to avoid the hospital being locked into an unsustainable commitment to care in a very high dependency environment.

All spinal injury patients are susceptible to infection. Lack of a powerful cough predisposes to chest infections and the need for catheterization predisposes to urinary infection. Skin breakdown is not common in a well-run unit, but this is at the expense of high levels of training and awareness amongst the patients and staff. Spinal injuries units are highly specialized care facilities where the skills of the GICU are practiced alongside the philosophies of rehabilitation medicine. Attempts to treat spinal cord injury outside a dedicated spinal injuries unit for more than a few days are doomed to disaster and should be vehemently discouraged. Where bed availability permits, spinal units are an ideal venue for the care of individuals with other paralyzing diseases following acute management, e.g. Guillain–Barre syndrome, because of the high degree of staff awareness of the hazards of skin breakdown.

STEP-DOWN AND HIGH DEPENDENCY UNITS

Following the development of GICUs in the 1960s there was a realization that there was a class of patients too sick for a general ward, but 'not sick enough for intensive care'. In the typical GICU there will be a ratio of at least one nurse per patient at all times. This is scarcely necessary for the routine care of many major postoperative cases, even though such patients may need to be nursed in a unit with a much higher level of care than a general ward. Applying the logic which led to the development of the early intensive care units, it is argued that some form of intermediate care area should be made available for these patients. The most usual solution to the problem is for a ward receiving patients immediately after discharge from the GICU to make a high dependency area with intense surveillance available – usually a cubicle under the direct supervision of a senior nurse. The next step is to argue that economies of scale will be achieved if all recently discharged patients can be grouped together in a 'step-down' unit.

There are difficulties with this approach which are not immediately apparent. The most important problem relates to the identification of an appropriate level of dependency to justify this intermediate level of care. As stated earlier, it is not difficult to identify patients who definitely need intensive care. It is much more difficult to identify the level of severity of illness which justifies high dependency but not 'intensive' care. There are also problems in deciding how much care is sufficient in an intermediate care area. Too little care and the unit becomes just another ward. Too much and we see another GICU. This is potentially dangerous because

the level of nursing and medical supervision in such an 'alternative' GICU may be inadequate to meet the clinical demands. The solution to this problem is to restrict admission to a step-down unit to only those patients who have been discharged from the GICU. There should be a policy which forbids direct admission from the wards or operating rooms directly to a step-down unit. The level of care given in a step-down unit is highly variable and ranges from simple pain relief and early mobilization on the one hand to all therapies and system support.

Many nonspecialist medical and surgical units will see merit in the establishment of a high dependency unit for their sickest patients. The facilities provided in such a unit must be unique to the clinical service. Many of these units work well, but they do have the capacity to delay the evaluation and admission to a GICU of severely ill patients.

Specialist surgical units

BURNS UNITS

Burns present an immense challenge to the surgical and intensive care services of any hospital. It is customary to regionalize the burns service in order to create a center of excellence with a substantial patient load. The burns patient mandates excellence in fluid management early in the illness followed by meticulous management of the burn wound and pain control throughout the later course. All this has to be achieved with meticulous control of sepsis. This creates a requirement for a closed unit with strict environmental controls. Ideally, burns units require a high degree of environmental cleanliness, control of temperature and humidity and laminar air flow ventilation. Utilization of special burn units is irregular because of the variable frequency of admissions. A strategy for maximizing the use of this intrinsically costly resource is to use the unit for other patients with similar clinical needs to thermal burns such as routine plastic surgery patients.[15] A novel suggestion which bears further examination has been the use of burns units as 'wound intensive care units'.[16]

POSTOPERATIVE CARDIAC UNITS

Modern cardiac surgical practice is dominated by large numbers of patients undergoing coronary artery bypass grafting (CABG). Typically a hospital undertaking this type of work will operate on at least one patient on each working day, i.e. 250 patients per year, and this is probably the lowest number that is worthwhile for a cost-effective unit. Although massive advances have been made in both preoperative work-up and in early postoperative care with impressively low mortalities, patients undergoing CABG surgery remain vulnerable to organ failure unless subjected to meticulous postoperative care. The aim of the postoperative cardiac unit is to operate a protocol-based management plan with the aim of getting patients stable and ambulant within 24 hours. Because of the enormous demand for cardiac surgery of this type, the limiting factor in cardiac surgical programs is often the availability of postoperative cardiac surgical beds and this means that patients must progress very rapidly through the unit. If patients are not able to be moved to a lower-dependency unit at the end of 24 hours, they are often moved to a different area such as the GICU. The reasons for this are two-fold. Firstly, this makes the bed available for scheduled cases and avoids bottlenecks. Secondly, the presence of a long-stay critically ill patient in a routine postoperative surgical unit constitutes a major environmental risk factor for the other patients. Infected or potentially infected patients should be transferred promptly to a GICU or infectious diseases unit.

ORGAN TRANSPLANTATION UNITS

Practice varies from hospital to hospital. Because of the degree of circulatory support which may be required, it is usual for patients undergoing heart or liver transplantation to be cared for in a high-level GICU or, in the case of a cardiac transplant, in a cardiac surgical unit. Kidney transplantation is a much less traumatic undertaking and typically such patients may be looked after in a medium dependency environment. It used to be thought that organ transplant recipients should be strictly isolated in order to reduce the likelihood of opportunistic infection. Experience has taught that nursing in isolation or otherwise has not been a major determinant of infective risk or of survival and many institutions are now abandoning or moderating their precautions.[17] In our own hospital our liver transplant patients are admitted to the general intensive therapy unit in the open area without any special precautions other than routine ward hygiene and cleanliness. Kidney transplant patients receive routine surgical ward care without additional precautions. In spite of this, our results seem comparable with other world centers.[18] Nevertheless, infection remains a major cause of death in organ transplant recipients and the issue of hospital-acquired infection cannot be treated lightly. Organ transplant units do have a place in the management of immunosuppression and the early detection of opportunistic infection.

Medical special care units

INFECTIOUS DISEASES UNITS

Florence Nightingale, writing in 1859, stated that 'No stronger condemnation of any hospital or ward could be pronounced than the simple fact that any zymotic disease has originated in it, or that such diseases have attacked other patients than those brought in with them.'[19] Over a century later, no satisfactory solution has been found to the problem of nosocomial infection first identified by this pioneer of hospital care (who, incidentally, did not believe in microorganisms!). Nevertheless, the infectious disease unit provides a partial solution to the problem.

Some illnesses mandate isolation in order to prevent the spread of infection either to the community or within the hospital. For example chickenpox is normally a trivial disease, but, occasionally, adults particularly can become extremely ill and need hospitalization. Diseases like chickenpox, infectious mononucleosis and mumps, although untreatable, are usually self-limited. Despite this, they can be devastating if they become epidemic amongst aged, disabled or immunocompromised patients and therefore it is usual to isolate such patients if they need to be admitted to hospital. Because such patients often present diagnostic problems – especially in the adult and even more so in the elderly – it is usual to group them under the care of an infectious disease physician. Such a physician will typically have charge of a unit capable of providing both protective and containment isolation. Theoretically, if barrier precautions are utilized correctly there should be little indication for quarantining patients because of the presence of hazardous organisms since most hospital pathogens are transmitted by contact. However, even the most effective precautions break down and although infective agents are readily transmitted in the inanimate environment, the addition of physical barriers between patients emphasizes the need to keep vulnerable and infected patients apart.

MARROW TRANSPLANT/ONCOLOGY UNITS

Patients receiving chemotherapy or radiotherapy as cancer treatment or in preparation for bone marrow transplantation are rendered profoundly susceptible to infection. Both radiotherapy and chemotherapy are capable of producing pulmonary damage which enhances the susceptibility to opportunistic infection. Typically these patients will be nursed in single accommodation using barrier gown techniques to reduce the numbers of potentially pathogenic organisms in proximity to the patient. Current practice is to use protective isolation with barrier nursing for patients receiving chemotherapy alone and to use more elaborate precautions including laminar-flow sterile air enclosures for patients undergoing total body irradiation in preparation for allogeneic marrow transplantation. Naturally, handwashing and avoidance of obvious sources of pathogens from visitors or foodstuffs (e.g. fresh salads) are enforced at the same time. Despite these precautions, oncology patients consistently become febrile and require extensive diagnostic workup. However bacteriological proof of the fever being caused by a specific bacterial infection is obtained in less than 50% of episodes.[20] Although reverse barrier nursing and protective isolation have been hallowed by practice for decades, their efficacy, such as it is, may be solely due to the necessary emphasis on handwashing as an essential part of the protocol. Since most pathogens encountered by the immunocompromised patient are either avoidable by handwashing, or endogenous to the patient from the outset, it is unlikely that elaborate (and costly) cleansing of the air and inanimate environment would make a large difference to infection and morbidity rates in susceptible patients. An unblinded study which compared standard care with simple protective isolation found no benefit to granulocytopenic patients.[21] The current situation seems to be that environmental control is probably effective in reducing the risk of infection in susceptible patients in the very short term, as in laminar-flow operating rooms. The techniques which are successful over hours are not extendable to days or weeks. Evidence showing a marked benefit from elaborate precautions is not available.

PSYCHIATRIC INTENSIVE CARE UNITS

A case has been made for the development of psychiatric SCUs. Several types of unit are described. The term has been used for an acute assessment unit with the aim of a high rate of discharge to the community in 48–72 hours.[22, 23] For the large numbers of violent, self-destructive or disruptive patients who present at major hospitals with acute psychiatric breakdown or other life-endangering complications of mental illness, admission to an acute therapeutic unit may be appropriate. Frequently the GICU is the only suitably staffed area for the care of these patients, which means that care necessarily focuses on sedation and restraint. Admission to the general ward means that sedation and restraint take place there also, but in a potentially hazardous setting. Recently the need for an acute therapeutic setting within the psychiatric department and supervised by the psychiatric unit has been recognized.[24] A Canadian psychiatric intensive care unit has demonstrated that most of its acute admissions were

either acutely psychotic or suffering from alcohol or other psychoactive substance abuse.[25] The criticism has been raised that the psychiatric unit is no place for a patient with a potential for life-endangering system failure. It can equally be argued that the GICU is no place for a hallucinating frightened schizophrenic. Obviously there is an imperative for multidisciplinary management using the hospital liaison psychiatry service and in this environment, the psychiatric intensive care unit fills a valuable role.

GERIATRIC INTENSIVE CARE UNITS

A recent report has focused on the generally unsatisfactory state of emergency care in the elderly.[26] With the increasing longevity of the population, and the increasing age of the hospital population, the extension of the concept of the geriatric assessment unit to a more interventive and intensive model for acute care is inevitable. There is the advantage that comprehensive assessment at an early stage by a team skilled in evaluation of the potential for rehabilitation may provide a strategy for deciding how much care is enough and how much is too much for a person at the natural end of his or her life. Patients are regularly transferred directly to the geriatric rehabilitation unit from our own general intensive care unit following major surgery or trauma. Recent work confirms the suspicions of many intensivists that age alone is a poor criterion for selecting patients for intensive care.[27]

RENAL AND DIALYSIS UNITS

The development of simple techniques for hemofiltration, hemodiafiltration and plasmapheresis using small filter cartridges running either on arterial pressure, or more commonly using a simple blood pump operating a veno-venous system, has made true hemodialysis in the intensive care unit a rare event. It is no longer necessary to transport critically ill patients to the renal unit for emergency dialysis. Similarly, the capacity for intensive care units to undertake emergency dialytic therapies has increased and sick renal patients are now typically cared for in the intensive care unit. For the chronic renal patient, the emphasis is increasingly on home dialysis, chronic ambulatory peritoneal dialysis (CAPD) and vigorous efforts to increase the renal transplant rate.

CORONARY CARE UNITS

Virtually synonymous in the lay mind with intensive care is the coronary care unit (CCU). The role of the CCU has changed dramatically in the past 30 years. The CCU was initially conceived as a venue for the early detection and prompt defibrillation of cardiac arrhythmia. The emphasis at this time was on resuscitation from life-endangering arrythmias. The concept of continuous monitoring for acute myocardial infarction was promoted following the acceptance that worthwhile survivals could be obtained following cardiopulmonary resuscitation.[28] The next phase of development was the emphasis on shock, but the treatment of cardiogenic shock has remained disappointing and it is now recognized that the major role of the CCU is in the management of acute cardiac symptoms due to unstable angina, acute dysrythmias and early myocardial infarction by prompt thrombolytic therapy, coronary vessel imaging and where appropriate by urgent coronary artery surgery.[29] In small or medium-sized hospitals, the CCU may have to be combined with the GICU in order to share space, beds, nurses and junior doctors. In larger hospitals, there are major divergences in role between the CCU and the GICU and these necessitate the establishment of separate units. Typically, the CCU is more like a general ward with facilities for patient privacy; life-support equipment tends to be less obtrusive than in the GICU. Central monitoring is very valuable as one nurse can observe the electrocardiogram (ECG) traces of several patients without hovering by the bedside. Indeed, it is possibly the only venue where central monitoring is truly valuable. Patients in the CCU may be partly ambulant and telemetric monitoring is used for these patients. The atmosphere of the ward must be conducive to reducing anxiety and alleviating boredom. Music and television are normally available. Ideally sitting rooms for visitors and convalescent patients are made available. If the CCU is integrated into a larger cardiology unit, facilities for angiography, catheterization and case conferences may need to be integral to the unit.

The ideal level of provision of coronary care beds remains unknown, as does the ideal length of stay. Because the chief benefits of CCU admission accrue to mainly 'healthy' patients with recent onset of symptoms, the benefits of the CCU facility can be maximized by a liberal admission policy with retention of those found to have actual infarction. An algorithm permitting accurate classification within 12 h has been devised.[30] This permits early re-use of CCU beds following discharge of low-risk patients.

Summary

1. The GICU should remain the treatment venue for critically ill patients. These patients are typically selected on the basis of perceived severity of illness.
2. The SCU provides care for subsets of patients with medical or surgical problems selected on the basis of presenting diagnosis.
3. The role of the SCU is to provide standardized treatment of a specific disease state. This role is particularly valuable if the patients are in large numbers, e.g. myocardial infarction.
4. There should be comprehensive backup of the SCU by a full GICU service. The SCU should not be allowed to become the 'alternative ICU'.
5. Management strategies for SCUs should incorporate proper data keeping and financial audit in order for the cost efficacy of the unit to be evaluated.

References

1. Groeger JS, Strosgerb MA, Halpern NA *et al*. Descriptive analysis of critical care units in the United States. *Crit Care Med* 1992; **20**: 846–63.
2. Task Force on Guidelines, Society of Critical Care Medicine. Recommendations for services and personnel for delivery of care in a critical care setting. *Crit Care Med* 1988; **16**: 809–11.
3. Field DJ, Hodges S, Mason E, Burton P, Yates J, Wale S. The demand for neonatal intensive care. *Br Med J* 1989; **299**: 1305–8.
4. Jacobs P, Noseworthy TW. National estimates of intensive care utilisation and costs: Canada and the United States. *Crit Care Med* 1990; **18**: 1282–6.
5. Knaus WA, Wagner DP, Draper EA *et al*. The range of intensive care services today. *J Am Med Assoc* 1981; **246**: 2711–16.
6. Ehrenwerth J, Sorbo, Hackel A. Transport of critically ill adults. *Crit Care Med* 1986; **14**: 543–7.
7. Laffel GL, Barness AI, Finkelstein S, Kaye MP. The relation between experience and outcome in heart transplantation. *New Engl J Med* 1992; **327**: 1220–5.
8. dBaseIV V1.5 [computer program]. Torrance CA: Ashton Tate, 1991.
9. SPSS/PC+ V2.0 [Computer program]. Chicago: SPSS Inc., 1990.
10. Link J, Krause H, Wagner W, Papadopoulos G. Intrahospital transport of critically ill patients. *Crit Care Med* 1990; **18**: 1427–9.
11. Woolery-Antill M. Development of a paediatric intensive care unit program for oncology patients. *J Assoc Paediatr Oncol Nurses* 1989; **6**: 33.
12. Dawson KP, Downward G, Mogridge RN. Children admitted to a general intensive care unit. *New Zealand Med J* 1989; **102**: 75–6.
13. British Association of Perinatal Medicine Working Group. Referrals for neonatal medical care in the United Kingdom over one year. *Br Med J* 1989; **298**: 169–72.
14. Davies WE. Spinal Cord Injuries. In: Jones ES (ed.) *Intensive Care*. Lancaster: MTP Press, 1982: 253–81.
15. Johnson KI, Meyer AA, Evans SK. Strategies to improve burn center utilisation. *J Burn Care Rehabil* 1988; **9**: 102–5.

16. Barillo DJ, Hallock GG, Mastropieri CJ, Troiani YM, Knowlton C. Utilisation of the burn unit for nonburn patients: the 'wound intensive care unit'. *Ann Plast Surg* 1989; **23**: 426–9.
17. Lange SS, Prevost S, Lewis P, Fadol A. Infection control practices in cardiac transplant recipients. *Heart and Lung* 1992 **21**: 101–5.
18. Opelz G. *Collaborative Liver Transplant Study Report.* Heidelberg: Ruprecht-Karls-Universität, May 1992.
19. Nightingale F. Sanitary conditions of hospitals. In: *Notes on Hospitals.* London: John W Parker and Son, 1859: 7.
20. Catovsky D, Hoffbrand AV. Acute leukaemia. In: Hoffbrrand AV, Lewis SM (eds) *Postgraduate Haematology.* Oxford: Heinemann Professional Publishing Ltd, 1989: 410–12.
21. Nauseef WM, Maki DG. A study of the value of simple protective isolation in patients with granulocytopenia. *New Engl J Med* 1981; **304**: 448–53.
22. Comstock BS. Psychiatric emergency intensive care. *Psychiatr Clin North Am* 1983; **6**: 305–15.
23. Basson JV, Woodside M. Assessment of a secure/intensive care/forensic ward. *Acta Psychiatr Scand* 1981; **64**: 132–41.
24. Goldney R, Bowes J, Spence N, Czechowicz A, Hurley R. The psychiatric intensive care unit. *Br J Psychiatr* 1985; **146**: 50–4.
25. Michalon M, Richman A. Factors affecting the length of stay in a psychiatric intensive care unit. *Gen Hosp Psychiatr* 1990; **12**: 303–8.
26. Sanders AB. Care of the elderly in emergency departments: conclusions and recommendations. *Ann Emergency Med* 1992; **21**: 830–4.
27. Chelluri L, Pinsky MR, Grenvik ANA. Outcome of intensive care of the 'oldest old' critically ill patients. *Crit Care Med* 1992 **20**: 757–61.
28. Julian DG, Valentine PA, Miller GG. Routine electrocardiographic monitoring in acute myocardial infarction. *Med J Austral* 1964; **1**: 433–6.
29. Julian DG. The history of coronary care units. *Br Heart J* 1987; **57**: 497–502.
30. Lee TH, Juarez G, Cook EF *et al.* Ruling out acute myocardial infarction. *New Engl J Med* 1991; **324**: 1239–46.

CHAPTER 6

Noninvasive Monitoring

ML PRICE

Cardiovascular monitoring   70
Respiratory monitoring   77
Conclusion   79
References   79

As intensive care medicine has developed, monitoring has advanced, leading to a better understanding of the physiology and pathology of disease processes. In the intensive care unit (ICU) monitoring has developed side by side with advances in technology. As technology has reduced in cost, increasingly complex monitoring has become more widespread. Initially technology allowed the measurement of pressure, flow and temperature; devices were developed to measure the most relevant physiological parameters using these variables, often by invasive means. Recent advances in electronics and computing have allowed faster and cheaper processing of electronic data. This in turn has allowed rapid processing of complex electronic signals which can be obtained from the patient using noninvasive methods. Information obtained in this way is being used increasingly to complement and replace data collected previously by invasive means.

Noninvasive monitoring in the ICU has many potential attractions. If noninvasive monitoring is to replace or supersede invasive monitoring, it should fulfill some if not all of the following criteria:

1. give a reliable measurement of the same variable if monitored invasively;
2. make the practicalities of monitoring easier so that it may be instituted by less experienced personnel;
3. have a similar response time to invasive monitoring;
4. produce results more rapidly than invasive monitoring;

5. limit risk of infection of staff by blood-borne disease;
6. give cost savings on disposable items;
7. give a continuous presentation of a variable where an intermittent one is available invasively;
8. measure different variables to those presently monitored, providing a different end point for treatment;
9. have lower complication rates than invasive monitoring.

The aim of this chapter is to concentrate on the more recent advances in noninvasive monitoring of the cardiovascular and respiratory systems, to compare their performance with invasive monitoring or evaluate their potential to complement data obtained from invasive monitoring in the ICU.

Cardiovascular monitoring

NONINVASIVE MEASUREMENT OF BLOOD PRESSURE

For continuous noninvasive blood pressure measurement to be practical in the ICU it must fulfill several criteria. These are as follows:

1. produce values for blood pressure which must be identical or at least consistently and predictably

70

different from those of direct arterial pressure monitoring;
2. work in all patients irrespective of vasoconstriction temperature or peripheral vascular diseases;
3. perform reliably throughout the entire range of blood pressures expected in an ICU setting;
4. not drift with time;
5. have a negligible response time;
6. not be prone to interference caused by patient movement.

Two basic principles are currently used to estimate systemic blood pressures, the photo-plethysmographic and tonometric methods. The Finapress (Ohmeda, Denver, CO, USA) uses a photo-plethysmographic method first described by Penaz[1] to estimate blood pressure from pulsation in the digital arteries of the fingers. A cuff is placed round a finger and inflated to a pressure that just causes the artery to collapse. It is maintained in this state by a servo pump mechanism attached to the cuff which is activated by changes in volume in the cuff, sensed by a photoelectric receiver. This servo mechanism means that the cuff pressure should always reflect arterial pressure. More recently the principle of arterial tonometry has been developed to a stage where it can be used in clinical practice. This differs from the Finapress in that the sensor flattens the artery rather than occluding it. This removes the effect of arterial wall tension produced by the curvature of the vessel. Pressure exerted on the sensor therefore reflects pressure in the artery.

The Finapress has been developed to a stage where it is now available commercially and many studies have been published to show its performance in clinical practice. Used intraoperatively in a variety of surgical patients, the overall correlation between invasive and noninvasive monitoring for systolic, diastolic and mean arterial pressures was poor ($r = 0.82, 0.68$ and 0.78, respectively).[2] The study of Stokes *et al.* also showed considerable interpatient variability with pressure with time. The recommendations of the American National Standards Institute suggest a mean difference of greater than ± 5 mm Hg and a standard deviation of more than 8 mm Hg between measured and actual pressure as the upper limits of error for noninvasive blood pressure monitoring.[3] Using these criteria, systolic, diastolic and mean blood pressures measured by the Finapress were only satisfactory in 11.9, 29.9 and 28.4% of patients, respectively, in this study. Considerable baseline drift of systolic, diastolic and mean pressures occurred averaging -7.8 mm Hg (range -12.5 to 15 mm Hg). In surgical procedures where profound systolic hypotension between 40–50 mm Hg was deliberately produced it has been shown that although there is good agreement with systolic, diastolic and mean pressures tend to overread with over 37% of readings overreading by 20% or more.[4] More recently an upgraded version of the Finapress 2300, the Finapress 2300E (Ohmeda, Denver, CO, USA), has been introduced. It has been shown that this is significantly more accurate than the Finapress 2300; however, it still demonstrates baseline drift and a tendency to overread mean and diastolic blood pressure. A study by Jones *et al.* concluded that, using the American National Standards Institute's recommendations, blood pressure readings obtained with the 2300E were still only acceptable in eight out of 15 patients.[5]

There are several potential sources of error using the Finapress, including the use of the correct cuff size and its accurate application.[6] In clinical practice the equipment may be prone to interference if it is disturbed. Vascular changes in the finger may also produce inaccuracies. Peripheral vasoconstriction has been shown to cause a reduction in arterial pressure in the fingers which is not matched to changes in systemic arterial pressures.[7] Changes in body temperature with consequent changes in peripheral perfusion may also cause problems. No studies have yet been published of its use in the ICU.

Arterial tonometry may offer greater potential for accurate continuous noninvasive measurement of arterial pressures in a wide age range of patients.[8] Differences in systolic, diastolic and mean arterial pressure showed negligible bias across the entire pressure range with limits of agreement of -12.2 to $+11.4$ mm Hg at the 95% confidence level. This would appear to be adequate for routine clinical use and falls within the guidelines from the American National Standards Institute, but again the practicality of use in the ICU has not been described and further studies are needed to assess this.

ASSESSMENT OF CARDIAC FUNCTION

Radionucleotide imaging

Noninvasive assessment of cardiac function until recently has involved the use of injected radioisotopes and the measurement of changes in emitted radiation throughout the cardiac cycle. In the past, measurement of emitted radiation has been difficult. The gamma camera is able to collect data and measure ejection fraction (EF) but its considerable cost, size, long acquisition time for information and need for an immobile patient during studies make its routine use in the ICU impractical.

A promising new device designed to measure emitted radiation and measure EF is the Cardioscint. The probe is hand held, light and can be positioned manually by an experienced operator aided by feedback from the computer. Signals are modified and information including EF and ventricular volumes can be presented on a beat to beat basis as the probe has a high temporal resolution. The Cardioscint has been shown to correlate well with EF measured by gamma camera.[9, 10] In the ICU it has been shown that the Cardioscint is a practical device able to monitor responses to therapy in a similar way to parameters derived from thermodilution catheters.[11]

Transesophageal echocardiography

Transesophageal echocardiography (TEE) is a technique that is becoming increasingly available for assessment of cardiac function. In the UK TEE is mainly used by cardiologists, but in the USA it is extensively used by anesthetists for assessment of cardiac function during anesthesia.

Transesophageal echocardiography has developed since the 1970s when transducers were attached to the end of flexible endoscopes. Their positional controls allow precise placement of the transducer relative to the posterior surface of the heart. Most endoscopes have transducers which allow imaging in the transverse axis. This allows assessment of the anatomy and size of the heart and movement of structures within the heart. These transducers usually have facilities to allow pulsed Doppler studies and colour flow mapping (CFM). These allow the assessment of direction and speed of blood flow within the heart. It is possible to use TEE in both adults and children.

The ability of TEE to measure both size and motion of the chambers of the heart allows the assessment of several aspects of cardiac function of interest in intensive care patients. It is possible to assess both global and regional ventricular function. Initially, direct observation was used to assess ventricular function. However practical automated systems are now becoming available which measure ventricular volumes and area fractional change on a beat to beat basis which correlates well with EF. Automation in this field is developing rapidly at present.

Transesophageal echocardiography is also able to assess regional ventricular function by visualizing wall motion abnormalities. Normal ventricle contracts during systole and relaxes during diastole. Ischemic or abnormal ventricle will contract less efficiently or not at all during systole, causing abnormal wall motion. The development of new wall motion abnormalities represents the onset of regional ischemia. It is also possible to assess cardiac contractility.[12]

Transesophageal echocardiography is also able to assess a wide variety of cardiac problems in the postoperative cardiac surgical patient. It is particularly useful for looking at valvular function, sources of embolism, endocarditis, thrombus and tumor. More general uses include the diagnosis of pericardial tamponade and intracardiac shunts.

Transesophageal echocardiography should not be used in patients with suspected esophageal pathology and if the airway is not protected the patient should be adequately starved. Like esophagoscopy, it is possible to use the technique in the sedated patient if needed. The overall complication rate is low but esophageal perforation has been reported as have a wide range of cardiac dysrhythmias, vocal cord paresis and dental damage. A recent review of 846 procedures[13] performed by cardiologists and anesthetists showed that 84.8% of two-dimensional and 79.7% of color flow studies were of good or excellent quality. As the technique becomes more widely available it is likely that the broad diagnostic scope of TEE will make it an essential item of equipment in the ICU.

MEASUREMENT OF PERFUSION

The concept that improving global oxygen delivery improves outcome was first proposed by Shoemaker.[14] The mechanisms of this 'global' approach in improving outcome were not fully understood at the time. It is not yet possible to measure global oxygen delivery noninvasively but it is possible to look at perfusion of specific organs and to relate this to global oxygen delivery. Recent interest in this has centered around the link between splanchnic perfusion and multisystem organ failure (MOF). Improved understanding of the possible mechanisms of MOF and 'sepsis syndrome' has pointed to the importance of relative ischemia of the gastrointestinal tract and consequent translocation of organisms and endotoxin across the gastrointestinal mucosal barrier.

There are two reasons why adequacy of splanchnic perfusion is theoretically a good measure of oxygen delivery. Firstly, it appears to compromise to a greater extent when oxygen delivery is low,[15] although redistribution of blood flow to the gut mucosa is altered to maintain mucosal blood flow during low flow states. Secondly, in sepsis, although mucosal blood flow is frequently maintained, intestinal oxygen consumption may be increased by as much as 100%. The altered balance between mucosal oxygen supply and demand explains the observation that superficial mucosa may become ischemic during sepsis. The majority of research published so far has taken gastric mucosal pH (pHim) as the measure of adequacy of oxygen delivery to the gut via the splanchnic circulation.

The principle of gastrointestinal mucosal tonometry may be applied to any fluid-filled viscus. Access to the mucosa of the gastrointestinal tract may be gained either by the oral or rectal route. Intramucosal pH measurements can then be taken from the stomach or sigmoid colon, respectively. The method most frequently used to do this is that of Fiddian-Green.[16] Carbon dioxide from the intestinal mucosa is allowed to equilibrate with a small fixed volume of normal saline in a silicone balloon at the end of a nasogastric tube. Equilibration of carbon dioxide between the gastric mucosa and normal saline is 95–98% complete in 1 hour. The partial pressure of carbon dioxide (CO_2) of the saline in the balloon is measured and arterial bicarbonate (HCO_3^-) is measured; this is assumed to represent the value of HCO_3^- found in the mucosa. Gastric intramucosal pH can then be calculated using the Henderson–Hasselbach equation:

$$pHim =$$
$$pK + \log \frac{\text{[arterial bicarbonate concentration]}}{F \times 0.03 \times PCO_2 \text{ of tonometer saline}}$$

where F is a correction factor that can be used to allow for equilibration for periods shorter than 1 hour and 0.03 is the solubility of CO_2 in plasma.

In animals a good correlation has been found between pHim measured by this method and directly measured intramucosal pH using microelectrodes.[17] The accuracy of measurements obtained can be affected by the clinical condition of the patient. The correlation is better in experimentally induced sepsis than in hypovolemic states.[17] In humans pHim correlates with hepatic venous PO_2, pH, mixed venous oxygen saturation and systemic oxygen delivery.[18]

Falsely low calculated values can arise for a variety of reasons. Hydrogen ions generated by the gastric mucosa can generate CO_2 when buffered by pancreatic bicarbonate, reducing calculated pHim. It has been suggested that in order to ensure reproducible measurements all patients should be treated with H_2 antagonists; however, there is evidence to suggest that normal values are similar in sedated patients whether they are receiving H_2 antagonists or not. Enteral feeding may cause a lowering of pH as it generates both hydrogen ions and HCO_3^- but this effect should be negated by the use of H_2 antagonists. Falsely high values for pHim are usually caused by failure to remove all the air from the balloon prior to filling with normal saline, but the recent systemic administration of bicarbonate will produce the same result. Sucralfate is not thought to have an effect on the accuracy of the tonometric measurement of pHim.

Clinically there is evidence that pHim is related to patient outcome, and that MOF and sepsis is greater in intensive care patients presenting with a low pHim [19,20] defined as a pHim of less than 7.35. It has been shown that therapy aimed at improving global oxygen delivery can improve patient outcome if pHim returns to normal values. Gastric intramucosal pH has been shown to be a predictor of patient mortality. Gastric intramucosal pH is 2.3 times more likely to predict death than any other variable.[20]

The measurement of pHim may be useful in predicting patient outcome, but its use as a goal to direct therapy is as yet unproven. Only one controlled study has shown an improvement in outcome by manipulating pHim. Gutierrez *et al.* showed no improvement in the mortality of patients presenting with a low pHim but demonstrated an improvement in mortality in patients in the group presenting with a normal pHim in whom there was a subsequent fall.[21] If a fall in pHim was detected, treatment was aimed at increasing global oxygen delivery. This is potentially a very important finding but needs to be confirmed by other studies.

Other parameters of peripheral perfusion have been shown to relate to both cardiac output and global oxygen delivery, although as yet no link between them and patient outcome has been demonstrated. Conjunctival oxygen tension (CjO_2) has been shown to correlate closely with mixed venous oxygen saturation and oxygen utilization in an animal model of septic shock.[22] Changes in CjO_2 precede changes in SvO_2. This method provides continuous information and is noninvasive. Conjunctival oxygen tension has also been shown to reflect cerebral blood flow in animals and humans. The normal range of CjO_2 is between 6.5 and 7.9 kPa. A target of greater than 0.5 kPa appears to confirm some advantage in overall survival in patients undergoing cardiopulmonary resuscitation.

The measurement of parameters of cutaneous perfusion on the assumption that they occur early in circulatory failure has not been promising. Toe temperature and transcutaneous oxygen tension correlate with oxygen transport and cardiac index in cardiogenic but not septic shock. In animals, hepatic hypoperfusion is paralleled by changes in subcutaneous PO_2, percutaneous PO_2 ($PctO_2$) and transconjunctival PO_2.[23] Interpatient variation of $PctO_2$ and variation of $PctO_2$ with other parameters such as and mean arterial pressure and PaO_2[24] means that it is unlikely that $PctO_2$ will be a reliable indicator of peripheral perfusion in the ICU.

NONINVASIVE MEASUREMENT OF CARDIAC OUTPUT

There are several potential methods available for the noninvasive measurement of cardiac output. The majority of recent publications concentrate on two methods, Doppler ultrasound and thoracic bioimpedance.

Doppler ultrasound

The principle of Doppler ultrasound in the measurement of cardiac output is simple. Velocity of blood flow can be measured in any vessel which carries the entire cardiac output. Blood velocity is calculated by measuring the Doppler frequency shift of sound reflected from red cells in the bloodstream. Blood velocity is calculated from the formula:

$$\text{Doppler frequency shift} = \frac{2FV \cos a}{c}$$

where c is the speed of sound in blood, α is the angle between blood velocity direction and the direction of incident pulse, V is the blood velocity and F is the transmitted frequency.

Measurement of blood velocity throughout the cardiac cycle allows the calculation of the flow velocity integral or stroke distance (SD). This represents the length of the column of blood ejected during a single cardiac cycle. The product of SD and the cross-sectional area of the vessel gives stroke volume (SV) and the product of SV and heart rate gives cardiac output (CO). Unfortunately, although the principle is simple in theory, inaccuracies can be introduced at several stages. To minimize errors caused by variability of SV throughout the respiratory cycle, it has been suggested that data from at least three cardiac cycles are pooled when calculating cardiac output.

Blood flow is assumed to be a square wave as this is the type of flow that is generally produced from a converging outflow tract. However, *in vivo* there may be variation in velocity of blood flow across the cross-section of the vessel. Blood velocity measurements taken from the periphery of the blood vessel may be substantially lower than those in the center. Blood flow from the pulmonary artery may conform to square wave flow better than aortic flow, making it a theoretically better artery to study. Unfortunately pulmonary artery flow does not take intracardiac shunts into account, which may again lead to errors.

Selection of the best signal is often left to the operator, creating the possibility of both interoperator and intraoperator variability. Both should be improved during the learning process. Reproducibility of results between operators in the clinical setting appears to be of the order of $\pm 5\%$, which is similar to thermodilution methods of measuring cardiac output.[25] It is possible that both types of variability may be improved by equipment with inbuilt expert systems which only process information from those signals which are assessed as acceptable by the software.

Calculation of aortic cross-sectional area presents a major problem when estimating cardiac output. Some systems allow the operator to enter an aortic diameter estimated from nomographic data from which the aortic cross-sectional area is calculated. Not only is there considerable interpatient variability in the aortic diameter, but aortic diameter also becomes more variable with increasing age. Nomographic data are therefore likely to be inaccurate. As the cross-sectional area is related to the square of the diameter, small inaccuracies in aortic diameter are magnified when cross-sectional area is calculated. Aortic cross-sectional area does not only differ between patients of the same age, height and weight, but also differs throughout the cardiac cycle, increasing by as much as 10% during systole and changing by as much as 12% with changes in systemic arterial pressure. Direct measurement of aortic cross-

sectional area using M-mode echocardiography is theoretically needed to overcome these problems. If it is used, all measurements should be taken in the long axis as vessels may be noncircular.

The angle at which the Doppler probe measures blood flow may introduce another error. In the suprasternal and esophageal approaches the angle of measurement is less than $25°$ to the long axis. As calculated blood velocity depends on the cosine of this angle, and at angles of less than $25°$ the cosine is greater than 0.9, the exact angle need not be measured. If the angle is greater than this then either a direct measurement or an estimate of the angle must be made and a correction factor introduced. The transtracheal Doppler system assumes that the angle between beam and aorta is $52°$. In practice the measured standard deviation (SD) of $\pm 3.8°$ means that an error of $\pm 14\%$ may be introduced at this stage.

Cardiac output can be measured by Doppler ultrasound using three approaches. The suprasternal approach is the only truly noninvasive method. The esophageal and transtracheal approaches are both minimally invasive but are potentially applicable in the ICU.

The suprasternal route is attractive as its ease of access allows measurement in fully conscious patients. The Doppler probe is positioned in the suprasternal notch and the beam angled behind the sternum. Clear signals are obtainable in approximately 90% of normal subjects. Factors making clear signals more difficult to obtain include obesity, short neck, tracheal intubation and tracheostomy, although the latter does not prevent signals being obtained. An air interface produced by mediastinal air following cardiac surgery can present problems in obtaining adequate signals whichever approach is used.

Transesophageal Doppler (TED) allows easy detection of ascending aortic blood flow. Probe sizes of 0.6 cm allow relatively atraumatic insertion of the probe. Advantages over the suprasternal approach are greater success in obtaining clear signals and the ability to monitor continuously following insertion of the probe. This is technically possible but clinically difficult with a suprasternal Doppler as it is difficult to fix the probe in a secure position.

Transtracheal Doppler (TTD) cardiac output (Applied Biometrics Incorporated, USA) uses a disposable tracheal tube with a transducer placed on the tip. The tracheal tube has a specially designed trapezoid cuff which approximates the transducer at a constant angle in close contact with the anterior wall of the trachea, providing good contact for a Doppler signal to be transduced. The tube is manipulated manually using visual and audio feedback until an optimal signal is obtained. The diameter of the proximal aorta is measured directly by the system, which in theory should give more accurate measurement of aortic cross-sectional area than estimates from a nomogram. Like esophageal Doppler, it is possible to obtain a continuous signal.

Several practical problems arise when using TTD. The signal may be lost on patient movement and the tube may need to be repositioned. Even in immobile patients in prolonged use the probe will need to be repositioned. Repositioning the tube requires cuff deflation which may lead to problems of hypoventilation and aspiration. One study has shown that the tube needed to be repositioned on average three times in an 8-hour period, the repositioning taking approximately 20–30 minutes during which time the cuff was deflated.[26] Aspiration was reported in two out of nine patients in this study. A further practical problem with TTD is that when correctly positioned to transduce a signal the tip of the probe has been shown to lie 2.7 cm (SD 1.3 cm) from the carina.[27] Endobronchial intubation is therefore a potential problem. These findings suggest that the system is unsuitable for general use in an ICU and if a continuous noninvasive system is required then the transesophageal system would seem safer.

Studies of cardiac output measured by Doppler ultrasound typify all studies of noninvasive monitoring in that initial optimism has been followed by studies showing poorer results. Published findings may be distorted by observer bias, poor study design and exclusion criteria and the greater likelihood of publication of studies with positive outcomes.

Studies comparing cardiac output measured by the thermodilution technique (COtd) and Doppler technique (COdopp) initially gave encouraging results with good correlation and regression coefficients.[28, 29] However, the evaluation of clinical studies comparing invasive and noninvasive monitoring techniques can be difficult.[30] Studies presenting results in the form of correlation and linear regression alone may be misleading. The more appropriate and now generally accepted statistical method for the comparison of two techniques which have inherent variability is that of Bland and Altman.[31] The average of the measurements of the two methods is plotted against the difference of each variable from the mean. This method calculates bias (any consistent difference between two techniques) and 95% confidence limits for the variable measured. Recent studies using this statistical approach have been less encouraging than earlier studies. In the largest study yet published (446 patients) Wong *et al.* showed a bias of −0.79 ± 1.95 l/min with limits of agreement of −4.6 to 3.11 l/min.[32] They also showed that agreement between COdopp and COtd was best in mechanically ventilated patients in sinus rhythm who had not undergone cardiac surgery. This study suggests that absolute values of cardiac output obtained from Doppler measurements should be viewed with some caution.

Studies looking at TED have shown similar results and have concluded that the technique is unreliable.

Hausen *et al.* could only detect adequate signals in 78% of patients and found the mean difference was 1.7 ± 1.67 l/min with limits of agreement of −1.56 to 4.99 l/min.[26] Siegel *et al.* showed a bias of 1.3 ± 1.1 l/min with limits of agreement of −3.6 to 3.11 l/min.[33] A comparison of cardiac output obtained by TTD and electromagnetic flowmeter (EMF) in animals suggested that there was no consistent bias which could be adjusted to improve agreement and that there was better agreement between thermodilution and EMF than between TTD and EMF. The mean difference between TTD and thermodilution was −0.3 ± 0.24 l/min, with limits of agreement of −0.5 and 0.4 l/min.[34] Overall results show a variable bias with a wide range of confidence limits and although the last study shows better results than the first two, all three studies concluded that TTD does not accurately measure cardiac output. Possible reasons for this have been mentioned. The complications and disadvantages described suggest that its routine use in the ICU in its present form is not indicated.

Cardiac output can be measured using transesophageal two-dimensional echocardiography. A study has shown that it was possible to image and measure the pulmonary artery in 76% of patients.[35] It also showed a mean bias of 0.03 l/min and the reported 95% confidence limit of 0.987 l/min was superior to that of the other studies mentioned. Considerable operator skill is needed to image the pulmonary artery but if transesophageal echo is already being used it may provide additional information with no extra morbidity.

Another potential use of Doppler in the assessment of the hemodynamic state of the patient is to derive other indices from the blood flow velocity waveform (Fig. 6.1). The initial rate of change in velocity of the waveform represents peak acceleration (PA). However, most equipment gives mean acceleration (MA) which represents the average rate of change of velocity with

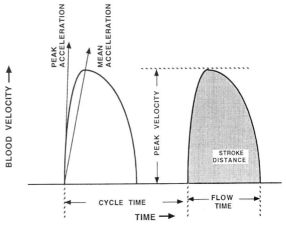

Fig. 6.1 Aortic velocity profile showing Doppler indices.

respect to the peak velocity of waveform. The peak velocity (PV) represents the maximum velocity that the blood reaches during a cardiac cycle. The flow time (FT) is measured as the length of time for which there is forward flow during a cardiac cycle. Flow time is influenced by heart rate as well as other hemodynamic changes. Changes in FT secondary to changes in heart rate can be corrected for by dividing the FT by the square root of the cycle time, giving corrected flow time (FTcorr).[36] The area under the flow velocity curve gives the stroke distance (SD). The product of SD and heart rate gives minute distance (MD).

Consistent changes in these indices have been shown to be produced by various hemodynamic maneuvers. Many studies have measured changes in various indices in response to such pharmacological and hemodynamic maneuvers. In assessing the results of these studies it is important to appreciate that in an intact subject changing just one variable is often impossible as homeostatic mechanisms will try to compensate for the variable changed. For example, the removal of 10% of a subject's blood volume will potentially lead to a compensatory tachycardia, peripheral vasoconstriction and perhaps a decrease in cardiac contractility by the Frank–Starling mechanism. Therefore no waveform change will represent a pure change of any one parameter. Results of these studies must therefore be interpreted, appreciating the way a normal (or abnormal) subject may respond to any pharmacological or hemodynamic manipulations.

Drugs affecting afterload have shown consistent changes in PV. Drugs increasing afterload will decrease the PV[37,38,40] in healthy volunteers. Drugs decreasing afterload will increase PV.[39–41] Changes in afterload also affect FT: decreases in afterload produce an increase in FT[38–41] and increases in afterload produce a decrease in FT.[38–40]

Stroke and minute distance are also affected, increases in afterload decreasing[38] and decreases in afterload increasing these indices.[38,41] Changes in preload produce changes in PV, FT and MA. Increasing preload (in normal or hypovolemic patients) increases PV, FT and FTcorr.[38–40] Decreasing preload decreases FTcorr.[38]

The effect of inotropes has also been studied. Positive inotropes increase PV[38,42] and negative inotropes decrease PV.[38,42] Peak acceleration and MA have been shown to correlate with invasive indices of contractility.[42] Peak acceleration and MA both increase when inotropes are administered. Peak acceleration is a more reliable index that MA as it correlates better with inotropic changes. Patients with cardiomyopathy have been shown to have lower values for PV, SD, MA and FT than normal subjects.[43] Unfortunately Doppler indices do not seem to be any better than conventional indices for defining inotropic state in a particular patient as 'normal ranges' of values are very variable.

Assessment of cardiac function using Doppler ultrasound has been shown to be useful in the clinical setting. In the ICU it has been shown to be useful in the optimization of positive end-expiratory pressure (PEEP)[44] and in the assessment of the response to vasodilators in heart failure.[45] The study of the use of these variables is still in its early stages but it is possible that Doppler indices may be more useful than measurements of cardiac output obtained by Doppler. They may provide us with a continuous dynamic method of assessing hemodynamic manipulation of the patient and be particularly useful in patients in whom the risk of complications of invasive monitoring is high.

Thoracic bioimpedance

Thoracic bioimpedance (TBIP) measures cardiac output by measuring changes in skin impedance to a small (2.5 mA) current applied across the thorax and neck. Eight electrodes, four sensing and four transmitting, are placed in fixed positions on the thorax and neck. Changes in thoracic impedance are caused by respiration, blood flow and thoracic water content. Changes in impedance are related to ventricular depolarization, which is detected by continuous ECG monitoring. In theory the change in impedance measured is caused by blood surges in the aorta and therefore can be related to cardiac output. A correction factor for height and weight is entered into the monitor and stroke volume is calculated on the principle described by Burnstein.[46]

Most studies looking at TBIP have found considerable problems with the technique. Many situations have been described which make measurements more difficult. The most widely reported group in whom significant problems arise is patients following cardiac surgery. There are many reasons proposed for this, some of which are specific to cardiac surgery, but some of which are more generally applicable. Wires in the chest may distort the thoracic electrical field and chest drains, bandages and internal jugular lines may affect positioning of electrodes, either physically or by obscuring landmarks such as the xiphoid process. A 2 cm error in placement of electrodes may result in a 20% error in estimation of stroke volume.[46] Specific cardiac conditions such as ventriculoseptal defect, valvular disease and large intrathoracic fluid shifts may also lead to inaccuracies in measurement. Other problems have been identified which may be seen in the general ICU as well as postoperative cardiac patients. Pacemakers which affect ECG timing, rapidly changing hematocrit, inotropes which produce changes in cutaneous blood flow, and patients who are outside the limits of average height for weight all cause problems. Dysrhythmias, particularly irregular dysrhythmias such as atrial fibrillation and ventricular ectopics (>10/min), may cause inaccuracy, as may tachycardia in a range between 120 and 150 beats per minute. Radiofrequency interference, particularly diathermy, can also interfere with signals. Most studies have shown no effect of intubation and ventilation on the agreement between cardiac output measured by thermodilution (COtd) and cardiac output measured by TBIP (CObip). The presence of sepsis also appears to have no effect on agreement. Studies have shown bias and limits of agreement of -1.5 ± 0.86 l/min and -3.2 to 0.22 l/min,[47] -0.4 ± 1.4 l/min and -3.2 to 2.4 l/min[48] and -0.7 ± 1.7 l/min and -4.1 to 2.7 l/min.[32] The major problem with TBIP is that it will give good results in some but not all patients. It is difficult to predict in which patients good results will be obtained without resorting to invasive measurements. It would appear to be better to avoid the use of TBIP in postoperative cardiac patients.

Respiratory monitoring

ARTERIAL OXYGEN SATURATION

The measurement of arterial oxygen saturation (SpO_2) by pulse oximetry represents a great advance in non-invasive respiratory monitoring. Its principle is based on the differential absorption of light of wavelengths of 660 nm and 940 nm by oxyhemoglobin and reduced hemoglobin. The ratio of pulsatile and baseline absorption of light at these two wavelengths differentiates between arterial and venous blood and filters out the variable absorption of light by bone and skin pigments.

Pulse oximetry is useful in the ICU as it gives a continuous estimation of SpO_2. As the response time is short early warning of impending hypoxemia is given before it is noticed clinically or by measurement of PaO_2 from arterial blood samples. It would therefore appear to be an ideal monitor in ICU where this sort of event is seen frequently.

There are several problems with pulse oximetry which may limit its use in the ICU. Hypothermia and poor peripheral perfusion are problems seen commonly in intensive care patients which can affect the accuracy of pulse oximetry. Hypothermia and hyperthermia can lead to problems by shifting the oxygen dissociation curve to the left or right, giving a false impression of PaO_2. Hypothermia, through its secondary effect of decreasing peripheral perfusion, can cause loss of pulsatile signals and failure to measure SpO_2. Hypothermia and vasoconstriction also increase the response time which may be as long as 6 min in severe hypotension. The ear lobe or forehead may be better monitoring sites than the finger when peripheral perfusion is low.

Dyshemoglobinemias are theoretically more common in the ICU and may produce inaccurate measurement of SpO_2. Carboxyhemoglobin and methemoglobin both reduce the total oxygen-carrying capacity of the blood, but as they are not measured by the pulse oximeter they can give falsely high estimates of SpO_2. In certain situations such as smoke inhalation, high carboxyhemoglobin levels may be anticipated and carboxyhemoglobin levels confirmed by co-oximetry. However endogenous carboxyhemoglobin is produced as a metabolic breakdown product of heme and hemolysis may also produce increasing levels of carboxyhemoglobin. Methemoglobin levels may be higher in ICU patients because many drugs used in the ICU will increase methemoglobin levels. Drugs that have been implicated include sodium nitroprusside, nitrates, sulfonamides, prilocaine, dapsone and metoclopramide. These sources of error have not yet been fully evaluated and studies into the importance of their effects in the ICU would be useful.

The site of the pulse oximeter probe may also influence the estimated SpO_2. There is generally a good correlation between SpO_2 at different sites in the same patient. However measurements from finger, toe, earlobe and forehead may vary in the same patient, leading to problems. Falsely low SpO_2 readings may lead to concern where none is needed. Limb position can also lead to false readings, increasing elevation producing lower measurements of SpO_2.[49] Partial occlusion of the vascular supply to the limb can lead to similar underestimates of SpO_2. Motion artifact and interference caused by ambient light may also give false readings of SpO_2. Venous pulsations can be mistaken for arterial pulsations by pulse oximeters, again leading to falsely low readings of SpO_2. This source of error is relatively rare but can be a problem in tricuspid regurgitation or occasionally when forehead probes are used.

The bias and precision of pulse oximeters in clinical practice above arterial saturations of 70% is approximately $\pm 3\%$. Pulse oximeters become increasingly inaccurate when SpO_2 is less than 70%. Once saturations reach 55% then bias increases from anything from $+1.58$ to -21.65%, depending on the manufacturer.[50] Anemia can lead to falsely low measurement of SpO_2. Instruments that are inaccurate at low SpO_2 will be more inaccurate in anemic patients.[51] Pulse oximeters made by different manufacturers have been shown to read consistently higher or lower than others,[52] but these differences are unlikely to be clinically significant.

Although it is clear that there are many sources of error associated with the use of pulse oximeters, they are widely used in the intensive care and high dependency settings. The obvious advantages of the continuous nature of the information they present along with their apparent accuracy in most situations means that their removal would be resisted by most physicians. In anesthesia, as in intensive care, the advantages of continuous monitoring of SpO_2 appear to be self-evident. Retrospective data from the USA on the use of pulse oximeters in anesthetic practice tend to support this. The rate of unforeseen events in an ICU is certainly higher than in anesthetized patients and therefore more likely to show benefit in terms of patient morbidity, but again the case is not proven. Any new technology introduced into the ICU must have the potential to improve outcome and aid nursing and medical care. All too frequently in the past new technology and therapy has been introduced on the assumption that it will improve patient outcome without any evidence to support this. Pulse oximetry falls into this category and a clinical study to confirm its benefits in the ICU is overdue.

PARTIAL PRESSURE OF ARTERIAL OXYGEN AND CARBON DIOXIDE

Percutaneous oxygen electrodes

Percutaneous oxygen electrodes are modified Clark electrodes which are designed to measure PaO_2 through 'arterialized' skin. Their main advantage over pulse oximetry is that they measure the arterial partial pressure of oxygen (PaO_2) rather than the saturation of hemoglobin. This is particularly important in the neonatal intensive care unit where high PaO_2 needs to be avoided. Percutaneous oxygen electrodes are attached to the skin which is heated to 43–45°C to 'arterialize' the blood. Heating the skin has several effects. It causes cutaneous vasodilation, producing increased diffusion of gases across the skin to the electrode. It also shifts the oxygen dissociation curve to the right, releasing oxygen from the hemoglobin. The resulting increase in partial pressure is balanced by an increase in tissue oxygen consumption at the higher temperature. When the system is set up an initial equilibrium period of 10–15 min is required. Response times of the probes vary but the 95% response time is approximately 30–60 seconds.

There are several practical problems with $PctO_2$ measurement which limit their use. Failure to exclude air when the probe is applied can lead to inaccuracy as can skin edema. Heating the skin can cause burns and blistering. This is more common in neonates than in adults but is also seen in states where peripheral perfusion is low. This means that the site of the probe must be changed frequently and the need for re-equilibration means that continuity of monitoring is lost.

Correlation between PaO_2 and $PctO_2$ is particularly good in neonates and children where skin thickness is small. In healthy cardiostable adults the correlation between PaO_2 and $PctO_2$ has also been shown to be good (>0.98).[53] The major problem with percutaneous oxygen monitoring is that values obtained depend not only on the oxygenation of cutaneous blood, but also on the cutaneous blood flow.[54] This depends on cardiac output and other factors that may cause cutaneous vasoconstriction such as exogenous or endogenous catecholamine levels. It has been demonstrated in both animal models of shock[54] and in humans[55] that there is significant linear correlation between cardiac output and $PctO_2$. The relationship between $PctO_2$ and cardiac output has led to the suggestion that $PctO_2$ may be used to assess the adequacy of cardiopulmonary resuscitation.[56] Alternations in $PctO_2$ with changes in cardiac output introduce a source of error which is probably more common in ICU patients than in normal subjects.

Subcutaneous oxygen tonometry

Subcutaneous oxygen tonometry has been proposed as a measure of oxygenation but its response time *in vitro* is approximately three times greater than $PctO_2$, and even longer *in vivo*. This presumably reflects a lag time in the response of tissue oxygenation to changes in arterial PaO_2. It would seem that these limitations make it of little use in clinical practice as a means of monitoring oxygenation, although it may be useful in measuring peripheral perfusion.

Percutaneous carbon dioxide electrodes

The complications and problems in the monitoring of percutaneous carbon dioxide ($PctCO_2$) are very similar to those of monitoring $PctO_2$. The measurement of $PctCO_2$ uses a modified heated Severinghaus electrode. Practical complications such as burns, response time and equilibration are similar to those encountered with percutaneous oxygen electrodes. Like $PctO_2$, $PctCO_2$ is affected by both cardiac output and $PaCO_2$; however, falling cardiac output causes a linear rise in $PctCO_2$.[56] In cardiostable patients $PctCO_2$ may be a better monitor of $PaCO_2$ than end-tidal carbon dioxide tension ($PetCO_2$) as it has been reported that the $PaCO_2$–$PctCO_2$ gradient is approximately 30% of, and less variable than, the $PaCO_2$–$PetCO_2$ gradient.

In the practical setting of the ICU, although there is still a significant correlation between the values of percutaneous and arterial measurement of oxygen and carbon dioxide, the considerable variability of the results produced means that $PctCO_2$ is likely to be a useful noninvasive monitor only in selected groups of patients. The values obtained will need to be regularly cross-checked with values obtained from arterial samples.

Capnography

The measurement of end-tidal carbon dioxide tension in exhaled breath can be achieved by one of three methods, mass spectrometry, infrared absorption spectrophotometry and Raman spectrophotometry. In theory the monitoring of PetCO$_2$ offers a continuous measurement of PaCO$_2$ by measuring alveolar partial pressure of carbon dioxide (PACO$_2$), which is in equilibrium with PaCO$_2$. Clinically the difference between PetCO$_2$ and PaCO$_2$ is found to be less than 1 kPa in normal subjects. This difference is explained by normal ventilation perfusion mismatch within the lungs. The difference increases as dead space ventilation increases.

Infrared absorption spectrophotometry is now the most commonly used method for measuring PetCO$_2$. Two methods of sampling PetCO$_2$ are currently used. The sidestream method draws gas samples from the breathing circuit and PetCO$_2$ is measured within the monitor. The mainstream analyzer uses a cuvette placed in the breathing circuit and a phototransducer is placed over the cuvette and heated to 40°C to prevent condensation forming. The mainstream analyzer has the advantage that results are instantaneous as no gas is withdrawn from the airway. Secretions and condensation are rarely a problem. However, the device is heavy and cumbersome, adds an additional 17–20 ml of dead space to the breathing circuit, and cannot be used in nonintubated patients. The sidestream analyzer is lighter, with a dead space as low as 3 ml. As the gas has to be aspirated to the monitor the response time is longer and will vary according to the length of tubing. Tubing may become blocked with condensation and secretions with consequent inaccuracies in results. One advantage of the sidestream analyzers is that the tube can be positioned to aspirate exhaled gases from the nose of spontaneously ventilating patients, allowing measurement of PetCO$_2$. However, mouth breathing may make results inaccurate. This method has been shown to produce a reasonable correlation between PetCO$_2$ and PaCO$_2$.[57]

Mass spectrometry has been used in the ICU and is able to measure CO$_2$ in many different patients, but sampling from each patient requires considerable lengths of tubing, thus delaying response time. Its expense and the limitation that only one sample can be processed at any one time means that the advantage of continuous estimation of PetCO$_2$ is lost.

Capnography is able to give useful information in the ICU patient but it must be interpreted correctly. Ideally the PetCO$_2$ would reflect the PaCO$_2$ at all times. Ventilation perfusion mismatch within the lungs means that this relationship does not always hold. Alterations in cardiac output and lung perfusion will significantly affect the PACO$_2$–PetCO$_2$ gradient. Pulmonary and gas emboli will decrease PetCO$_2$. Changes in cardiac output will also alter PetCO$_2$ and it has even been suggested that it may be used as an index for measuring cardiac output.[58] As ventilation perfusion relationships and changes in cardiac output are relatively frequent in ICU patients, PetCO$_2$ should not be used to estimate PaCO$_2$ unless the correlation is confirmed by frequent arterial

gas sampling. Conversely changes in the PACO$_2$–PetCO$_2$ gradient may be used to detect alteration in ventilation perfusion relationships within the patient.

There are several other uses of capnography within the ICU. Analysis of the capnogram can detect respiratory obstruction, bronchospasm, air trapping and rebreathing. It can also confirm placement of the tracheal tube and can act as an apnea alarm. Capnography may be useful in the assessment of effectiveness of cardiopulmonary resuscitation,[59] acting as a quantitative indicator of the volume of blood flow produced by external cardiac compression. It is possible both to ventilate and wean patients from ventilation in the short term, using capnography as the main indicator of adequacy of ventilation.[60]

Conclusion

The field of noninvasive monitoring is expanding rapidly at the moment. As new techniques become available they must be properly studied, not just to validate their accuracy but to assess their performance in the ICU setting, which may be very different from study conditions. Many new monitoring methods have been introduced over the years without this happening and we must resist the temptation to introduce new and usually costly equipment before it has been properly assessed.

References

1. Penaz J. Photoelectric measurement of blood pressure, volume and flow in the finger. In: Albert R (ed.) *Digest of the 10th International Conference on Medical Engineering*. Dresden: The International Federation for Medical/Biological Engineering, 1973: 104.
2. Stokes DN, Clutton-Brock T, Patil C, Thompson JM, Hutton P. Comparison of invasive and non invasive measurement of continuous arterial pressure using the Finapress. *Br J Anaesth* 1991; **67**: 26–35.
3. Association for the Advancement of Medical Instrumentation. *American National Standard for Electronic or Automated Sphygmomanometers*. Washington: American National Standards Inc., 1987: 313.
4. Aitken H, Todd JG, Kenny GNC. Comparison of the Finapress and direct arterial pressure monitoring during profound hypotensive anaesthesia. *Br J Anaesth* 1991; **67**: 36–40.
5. Jones RDM, Brown AG, Roulson CJ, Smith ID, Chan SC. The upgraded Finapress 2300E. *Anaesthesia* 1992; **47**: 701–5.
6. Gorback MS, Quill TJ, Lavine ML. The relative accu-

racies of two automated non invasive arterial pressure measurement devices. *J Clin Monitoring* 1991; **7**: 13–22.

7. Kurki T, Smith NT, Head N, DeSilver H, Quinn A. Non invasive continuous blood pressure measurements from the finger: optimal measurement conditions and factors affecting reliability. *J Clin Monitoring* 1987; **3**: 6–13.

8. Kemmotsu O, Ueda M, Otsuka H, Yamamura T, Winter D, Eckerle JS. Arterial tonometry for noninvasive blood pressure monitoring during anaesthesia. *Anesthesiology* 1991; **75**: 333–40.

9. Broadhurst P, Cashman P, Crawley J, Rafferty E, Lahiri A. Clinical validation of a miniature nuclear probe system for continuous on line monitoring of cardiac function of cardiac and ST segments. *J Nucl Med* 1991; **32**: 37–43.

10. Broadhurst P, Liu X, Cashman P, Rafferty E, Lahiri A. Spontaneous variability of left ventricular ejection fraction assessed with the Cardioscint. *J Nucl Med* 1992; **13**: 312–21.

11. Timmins AC, Giles M, Hinds CJ. Evaluation of a miniaturised nuclear detector for monitoring ejection fraction in critically ill patients. *Intensive Care Med* 1992; **18** (Suppl. 2): S176.

12. O'Kelly BF, Tubau JF, Knight A, London MJ, Verrier ED, Mangano DT and the Study of Perioperative Ischeamia (SPI) Research Group. Measurement of left venritcular contractility using transesophageal echocardiography in patients undergoing coronary artery bypass grafting. *Am Heart J* 1991; **122**: 1041–9.

13. Rafferty T, La Manita K, Davis E *et al*. Quality assurance for intraoperative transesophageal echocardiography monitoring: a report of 846 procedures. *Anesth Analg* 1993; **74**: 228–32.

14. Shoemaker WC, Appel PL, Kram HB, Waxman K, Lee TS. Prospective trial of supranormal values of survivors as therapeutic goals in high risk surgical patients. *Chest* 1988; **94**: 1176–86.

15. Shepherd A. Metabolic control of intestinal oxygenation and blood flow. *Fed Proc* 1982; **41**: 2084–98.

16. Fiddian-Green RG, Baker S. Predictive value of the stomach wall pH for complications after cardiac operations: comparison with other monitoring. *Crit Care Med* 1987; **15**: 153–6.

17. Antonsson JB, Boyle CC, Kruithoff KL. Validation of tonometric measurement of gut intarmural pH during endotoxemia and mesenteric occlusion in pigs. *Am J Physiol* 1990; **259**: G519–23.

18. Landow L, Phillips DA, Heard SO, Prevost D, Vandersalm TJ, Fink MP. Gastric tonometry and venous oximetry in cardiac surgical patients. *Crit Care Med* 1991; **19**: 1226–33.

19. Doglio G, Pusanjo J, Egurrola M *et al*. Gastric mucosal pH as a prognostic index of mortality in critical care patients. *Crit Care Med* 1988; **16**: 153–6.

20. Maynard N, Bihari D, Beale R *et al*. Assessment of splanchnic oxygenation by gastric tonometry in patients with acute circulatory failure. *J Am Med Assoc* 1993; **270**: 1203–10.

21. Gutierrez G, Palizas F, Doglio G *et al*. Gastric intramucosal pH as a therapeutic index of tissue oxygenation in critically ill patients. *Lancet* 1992; **339**: 195–9.

22. Van der Linden J, Modig J, Wilklund L. Conjunctival oxygen tension in experimental septic shock. *Int J Clin Monitoring* 1989; **6**: 37–43.

23. Soini HO, Takala J, Nordin AJ, Makisalo HJ, Hockerstedt KA. Peripheral and liver oxygen tensions in haemorrhagic shock. *Crit Care Med* 1992; **20**: 1330–40.

24. Hasibeder W, Haisjakl M, Sparr H, Klaunzer S, Horman C, Salak N, Germann NR, Stronegger WJ, Hackl M. Factors influencing transcutaneous oxygen and carbon dioxide measurements in adult intensive care patients. *Intensive Care Med* 1991; **17**: 272–5.

25. Gardin JM, Dabestani A, Matin K. Reproducibility of Doppler aortic flow measurements: studies on intraobserver, inter-observer and day to day variability in normal subjects. *Am J Cardiol* 1984; **54**: 1092–5.

26. Hausen B, Sfers HJ, Rhode R, Haverich A. Clinical evaluation of transtracheal Doppler for continuous cardiac output estimation. *Anesth Analg* 1992; **74**: 800–4.

27. Perrino AC, Luther M, Ehrenwerth T. Transtracheal Doppler: a safe technique? *Anesth Analg* 1992; **74**: S236.

28. Huntsman LL, Stewart DK, Barnes SR, Colocousis JS, Hessel EA. Noninvasive Doppler determination of cardiac output in man. *Circulation* 1983; **67**: 593–602.

29. Chandaratna PA, Nanna M, McKay C, Nimalasuriya A, Swinn R, Elkayam U, Rahimtoola SH. Determination of cardiac output by transcutaneous continuous wave ultrasonic Doppler computer. *Am J Cardiol* 1984; **53**: 234–7.

30. La Mantia KR, O'Connor T, Barash PG. Comparing methods of measurement: an alternative approach. *Anesthesiology* 1990; **72**: 781–3.

31. Bland JM, Altman DG. Statistical methods for assessing agreement between two methods of clinical measurement. *Lancet* 1986; **i**: 307–10.

32. Wong DH, Tremper KK, Stemmer EA *et al*. Noninvasive cardiac output: simultaneous comparison of two different methods with thermodilution. *Anesthesiology* 1990; **72**: 784–92.

33. Seigel LC, Fitzgerald DC, Engstrom RH. Simultaneous intraoperative measurement of cardiac output by thermodilution and transtracheal Doppler. *Anesthesiology* 1991; **74**: 664–9.

34. Gregoretti S, Henderson CT, Bradley EL. Simultaneous cardiac output measurements by transtracheal Doppler, electromagnetic flowmeter and thermodilution during various haemodynamic states in pigs. *Anesth Analg* 1991; **73**: 455–9.

35. Savino JS, Troianos CA, Aukburg S, Weiss R, Reichek N. Measurement of pulmonary blood flow with transesophageal two-dimensional echocardiography. *Anesthesiology* 1991; **75**: 445–51.

36. Bazett MC. An analysis of the time relationships of electrocardiograms. *Heart* 1920; **7**: 353–6.

37. Harrison M, Clifton G, Berk M, De Maria A. Effect of blood pressure and afterload on Doppler echocardiographic measurements of left ventricular function in normal subjects. *Am J Cardiol* 1989; **64**: 905–8.

38. Singer M, Allen MJ, Webb AR, Bennett ED. Effects of alterations in left ventricular filling, contractility, and systemic vascular resistance on the ascending aortic velocity waveform of normal subjects. *Crit Care Med* 1991; **19**: 1138–45.

39. Singer M, Clarke J, Bennett ED. Continuous haemodynamic monitoring by oesophageal Doppler. *Crit Care Med* 1989; **17**: 447–52.
40. Bedotto J, Eichhorn E, Greyburn P. Effects of left ventricular preload and afterload on ascending aortic blood velocity and acceleration in coronary artery disease. *Am J Cardiol* 1989; **64**: 856–9.
41. Elkyam U, Gardin JM, Berkley R, Hughes C, Henry W. The use of Doppler flow velocity measurement to assess the haemodynamic response to vasodilators in patients with heart failure. *Circulation* 1983; **67**: 337–83.
42. Wallmeyer K, Wann S, Sagar K, Kalbfleisch J, Kloppfensten S. The influence of preload and heart rate on Doppler echocardiographic indexes of left ventricular performance: comparison with invasive indexes in an experimental preparation. *Circulation* 1986; **74**: 181–6.
43. Gardin JM, Iseri LT, Elkayam U. Evaluation of cardiomyopathy by pulsed Doppler echocardiography. *Am Heart J* 1983; **106**: 1057–61.
44. Singer M, Bennett D. Optimization of positive end expiratory pressure for maximal oxygen delivery to the tissues using oesophageal Doppler ultrasonography. *Br Med J* 1989; **298**: 1350–3.
45. Elkayam U, Gardin JM, Berkley R. The use of Doppler flow measurements in patients with heart failure. *Circulation* 1983; **67**: 377–83.
46. Burnstein DP. A new stroke volume equation for calculating thoracic electrical bioimpedance: theory and rationale. *Crit Care Med* 1986; **14**: 902–4.
47. Saladin V, Zussa C, Risica G *et al*. Comparison of cardiac output estimation by thoracic electrical bioimpedance, thermodilution and Fick method. *Crit Care Med* 1988; **16**: 1157–9.
48. Seigel LC, Schafer SL, Martinez GM, Ream AK, Scott JC. Simultaneous measurements of cardiac output by thermodilution, esophageal Doppler and electrical impedance in anesthetised patients. *J Cardiothoracic Anesth* 1988; **2**: 590–5.
49. Vegfors M, Lindberg L, Lenmarken C. The influence of changes in blood flow on the accuracy of pulse oximetry in humans. *Acta Anaesthesiol Scand* 1992; **122**: 1672–5.
50. Severinghaus JW, Naifeh KH, Koh SH. Errors during profound hypoxia in 14 pulse oximeters. *J Clin Monitoring* 1989; **5**: 72–81.
51. Severinghaus JW, Koh SO. Effect of anaemia on pulse oximeter accuracy at low saturation. *J Clin Monitoring* 1990; **6**: 85–88.
52. Taylor MB, Whitwam JG. The accuracy of pulse oximeters: a comparative clinical evaluation of five pulse oximeters. *Anaesthesia* 1988; **43**: 229–32.
53. Rooth G, Hedstrand U, Tyden H, Ogren C. The validity of the transcutaneous oxygen tension method in adults. *Crit Care Med* 1976; **4**: 162–5.
54. Tremper K, Waxman K, Shoemaker WC. Effects of hypoxia and shock on transcutaneous PO_2 values in dogs. *Crit Care Med* 1979; **7**: 526–31.
55. Tremper K, Waxman K, Bowman R, Shoemaker WC. Continuous transcutaneous oxygen monitoring during respiratory failure, cardiac decompensation, cardiac arrest and CPR. *Crit Care Med* 1980; **8**: 377–81.
56. Tremper K, Shoemaker WC. Continuous CPR monitoring with transcutaneous oxygen and carbon dioxide sensors. *Crit Care Med* 1981; **9**: 417–18.
57. Liu S, Lee T, Bongard F. Accuracy of capnography in non intubated patients. *Chest* 1992; **102**: 1512–15.
58. Isserles S, Breen P. Can changes in end tidal pCO_2 measure cardiac output? *Anesth Analges* 1991; **73**: 808–14.
59. Falk JL, Rackow EC, Marx HW. End tidal carbon dioxide concentration during cardiopulmonary resuscitation. *New Engl J Med* 1988; **318**: 607–11.
60. Withington DE, Ramsay JG, Saoud T, Bilodeau J. Weaning from ventilation after cardiopulmonary bypass: evaluation of a new technique. *Can J Anaesth* 1991; **38**: 15–19.

CHAPTER 7

Invasive Hemodynamic Monitoring

RINALDO BELLOMO, MICHAEL R PINSKY

Introduction   82
Usefulness of invasive monitoring   84
Does an invasive hemodynamic monitoring technique benefit the patient?   85
Three fantasies of hemodynamic monitoring   86
Types of invasive hemodynamic monitoring   92
Proven indications for hemodynamic monitoring   97
Probably appropriate (but not proven) indications for hemodynamic monitoring   97
Unproven indications for hemodynamic monitoring   99
Recommendations for clinical practice   100
Recommendations for future research   101
References   101

Introduction

RATIONALE FOR INVASIVE HEMODYNAMIC MONITORING IN THE CARE OF THE CRITICALLY ILL

Critical care medicine is a technology intensive field of medicine. The intensive care unit (ICU) is one of the primary sites within the hospital where novel monitoring devices and treatments are tried initially, before their widespread acceptance or rejection by the medical community, and before their usefulness has been documented in the scientific literature. Because advances in technology related to the diagnosis and treatment of disease progress quickly and because critical care medicine often utilizes technological developments and novel therapies from disparate sources within medicine, it is often not possible to determine which new therapies or diagnostic procedures will ultimately be effective and which will either not improve care or actually worsen the probability of a good outcome. This nihilistic argument has often been used as defense for the compassionate use of unproven therapies or diagnostic techniques in the critically ill. In the ICU risk/benefit ratios are hard to define and may vary for reasons not easily quantified. Still, one needs to approach new therapies and diagnostic procedures based on the assumption that if they are to be used in critically ill patients, there must be some rationale which can be easily articulated to the patient, the patient's family, other health care providers, and other interested parties.

In this regard, a logical progression of ethical arguments can be developed by which specific therapies or diagnostic procedures are defended. The first level of defense comes from historical controls, wherein prior experience using similar therapies have been shown to be beneficial. Using this level of defense, the mechanism by which the benefit is achieved need not be understood or even postulated. Few therapies commonly used in the ICU still fall into this category. The next level of understanding and defense comes from a greater appreciation of the pathophysiology of the process being treated and the presumed mechanism by which the treatment improves outcome. The most common arguments for the use of hemodynamic monitoring lie at this level, and here also lie the greatest number of flaws in such arguments. The assumption is that if one knows how a disease process creates its effect, preventing the process from altering measured bodily functions should prevent the disease process from progressing. The final level of defense comes from clear documentation that a given therapy or diagnostic procedure, by directing therapy in otherwise unexpected ways, improves outcome in terms of survival and quality of life. Few ICU therapies or even the 'package deal' of global ICU care have been shown to improve survival. The one often quoted exception comes from the data demonstrating that intubated and ventilated patients not treated in an ICU setting have a greater likelihood of untoward events and mortality related to complications of mechanical ventilation than they would if cared for in a GICU.[1] Unfortunately, few other conditions can boast such documented benefits from ICU care. In this instance the main benefit comes from the rapid identification of acute airway obstruction from secretions, inadvertent airway disconnections and/or self-extubation.

NEW TECHNOLOGIES AND THE ICU

Perhaps no therapy or procedure has impacted more on the diagnostic approaches or therapies utilized in the care of the critically ill than invasive hemodynamic monitoring.[2] Within this context, we define invasive hemodynamic monitoring to include arterial,[3] central venous, and pulmonary arterial catheterization.[4] The assumption is commonly made that, by measuring specific hemodynamic variables and based on our knowledge of cardiopulmonary physiology, specific patterns can be identified in the derived cardiopulmonary data which correspond to specific pathophysiological processes. Furthermore, these newly diagnosed processes could not have been readily or reliably diagnosed without these data. The argument continues that patients so diagnosed will respond selectively to specific therapies which would otherwise be detrimental in other critically ill patients with similar overt clinical signs. In the following section we will explore the physiological basis for some of the hemodynamic data defining decision making in the ICU and will underscore some of the major problems inherent in this approach.

IS THERE A DEFINABLE RATIONALE FOR THE CARE OF THE CRITICALLY ILL?

Our understanding of the pathophysiology of many critical illnesses is rudimentary at best. As we discover new disease processes which are operative in common

diseases and/or cause common diseases to develop in uncommon ways, we begin to realize that some aspects of diagnosis and therapy which we previously considered unimportant are central to survival, whereas others thought central to the disease process are merely epiphenomena of a larger and more malignant process, totally ignored by us in the past. It should not be surprising, therefore, to learn that our ability to cure patients with either acute lung injury presenting with the adult respiratory distress syndrome (ARDS)[5] or acute renal failure,[6] of any cause, has not improved in over 25 years.[7] Clearly, over the past 25 years we have been missing some basic problems present in these patients while making major advances in other areas of medical science and technology.

The commonly reported observation of the minimal effect that critical care medicine has on mortality in many types of critical illness flies in the face of the very logic for which critical care medicine in general, and the ICU in particular, were developed. Critical care medicine espouses to treat patients with titrated care to maintain or recover normal physiological variables while arresting or reversing any underlying pathological process. Supportive resuscitative efforts, it is hoped, will allow those critically ill patients who can recover to do so with a minimal amount of suffering. At present, however, it is not clear how effective we have been at attaining this goal, even in a partial way. Why is this so?

How can it be that the intensivist, the critical care nurse and the respiratory therapist, with all their efforts and successes to their credit, with all their new advanced machines and monitoring systems, their weaning and resuscitation protocols and textbooks explaining in clear terms the mechanisms by which disease is supposed to work, have not been more successful in curing their patients? The answer to this question may have two parts. Firstly, we probably see patients now who are more ill in terms of basal organ system function.[7] Critically ill patients are older, thus the average age for a myocardial infarction in 1993 is more than 10 years older than in 1963. We are also more aggressive in how we treat the chronically ill prior to the onset of acute decompensation. We are better at preventing the less sick patient receiving nonintensive care from deteriorating quickly in response to the same level of insult. For example, we push intravascular fluids and give empiric antibiotic therapy in septic patients prior to the onset of hypotension or the return of positive blood cultures. We restrict potassium and free water in patients with decreasing renal function[6] or we restrict fluids, give oxygen, bronchodilators and other forms of therapies to patients with impending respiratory failure. Secondly, all our supportive therapies do only that: support. They do not cure or eradicate disease. Positive pressure ventilation, with or without positive end-expiratory pressure (PEEP), does not treat acute lung injury. It merely maintains a certain degree of alveolar ventilation allowing gas exchange to be adequate for the other metabolic functions. Similarly, dialysis techniques (hemodialysis, peritoneal dialysis, continuous hemofiltration with dialysis, etc.) merely maintain a more physiologic internal milieu but do not treat directly the cause of the renal failure. Furthermore, organ-supportive therapies may make the function of the very organ system they are attempting to support or replace deteriorate. They may also worsen the function of remote organ systems.[8]

Thus, if hemodynamic monitoring is to improve patient survival, we need to better understand the complex pathophysiology of the diseases we treat, the role of diagnostic procedures in establishing prognosis and guiding therapy, and the impact that novel or established therapies based on such procedures will have. To the extent that information on critically ill patients derived from hemodynamic monitoring can stabilize physiology and allow more definitive therapies to work or prevent deterioration of organ systems, then such monitoring may have a place in the management of the critically ill. To the extent that such monitoring only confirms what is known and does not alter care, its inherent morbidity will only decrease the efficacy of intensive care.

Usefulness of invasive monitoring

Invasive hemodynamic monitoring, by the percutaneous insertion of catheters into a vascular space and transducing of pressures sensed at their distal ends, allows for the continuous display of the complex waveforms that are present within these vascular spaces. Much information relevant to the physiological basis for the patient's cardiovascular status is present in this data.[9] Unfortunately, little of this information is actually used clinically or in a physiologically relevant fashion.[10,11] Other information besides distal pressure can be ascertained from indwelling intravascular catheters. Blood from the distal ports can be sampled to measure oxygen content, pH, gas tensions, and various chemistries. Using the principle of indicator dilution, one can intermittently measure pulmonary blood flow as an estimate of cardiac output by either thermodilution or dye dilution methods.[12] Furthermore, especially adapted pulmonary arterial catheters allow for the continuous measurement of mixed venous oxygen saturation[13] and, now, pulmonary arterial blood flow. In combination with continuous arterial blood sampling techniques one can also intermittently measure thoracic blood volume and lung water. Finally, using a rapid response thermistor to sense temperature change from the thermal bolus, one can also estimate right ven-

Table 7.1   Physiological variables derived from invasive monitoring

Unitary measures

Arterial pressure
Mean arterial pressure (MAP)
  Organ perfusion inflow pressure
Arterial pulse pressure and its variation during ventilation
  Left ventricular stroke volume changes and pulsus paradoxes
Arterial pressure waveform
  Aortic valvulopathy, input impedance and arterial resistance

Central venous pressure (CVP)
Mean central venous pressure
  If elevated, that effective circulating blood volume is not reduced
Central venous pressure variations during ventilation
  Tricuspid insufficiency, tamponade physiology

Pulmonary arterial pressure (Ppa)
Mean Ppa
  Pulmonary inflow pressure
Pulmonary artery pulse pressure and its variations during ventilation
  Right ventricular stroke volume, pulmonary vascular resistance changes during ventilation, and the degree of change in intrathoracic pressure

Pulmonary artery occlusion pressure (Ppao)
Mean Ppao
  Left atrial and left ventricular intralumenal pressure and by inference, left ventricular preload
Ppao waveform and its variation during occlusion and ventilation
  Mitral valvulopathy, atrial or ventricular etiology of an arrhythmia, accuracy of mean Ppao to measure intralumenal LV pressure, and pulmonary capillary pressure (Ppc)

Calculated measures
Calculated measures using multiple measured variables including cardiac output by thermodilution (COtd), arterial and mixed venous blood gases (ABG and VBG, respectively)

Vascular resistances
Total peripheral resistance = MAP/COtd
Systemic vascular resistance = (MAP − CVP)/COtd
Pulmonary arterial resistance = (mean Ppa − Ppc)/COtd
Pulmonary venous resistance = (Ppc − Ppao)/COtd
Pulmonary vascular resistance = (mean Ppa − Ppao)/COtd

Ventricular pump function
Left ventricular stroke volume (SVlv) = COtd/HR
Left ventricular stroke work (SWlv) = (MAP − Ppao)/SVlv
Preload-recruitable stroke work = SWlv/Ppao

Oxygen transport and metabolism
Global oxygen transport or delivery (DO_2) = CaO_2/COtd
Global oxygen uptake (VO_2) = $(CaO_2 − CvO_2)$/COtd
Venous admixture
Ratio of dead space to total tidal volume (Vd/Vt) = $PaCO_2$/$(PaCO_2 − PetCO_2)$

Right ventricular function using RV ejection fraction (EFrv) catheter-derived data
Right ventricular end-diastolic volume (EDVrv) = SV/EFrv
Right ventricular end-systolic volume (ESVrv) = EDVrv − SV

Key: HR: heart rate.
$PaCO_2$: arterial carbon dioxide tension.
$PetCO_2$: end-tidal carbon dioxide tension.
Other abbreviations are explained in the table.

tricular (RV) ejection fraction, and, by calculation, RV volumes.[14,15] Using these measures of cardiovascular function the intensivist can now assess numerous aspects of cardiopulmonary function at the bedside. Data derived from measures of cardiac output, heart rate, vascular pressures and specific blood gas components can be used to solve simple algebraic equations whose solution gives estimates of vascular resistance, muscular pump function, gas exchange and oxygen metabolism.[16] The list of most of the potential variables that can be estimated from invasive monitoring is impressive. A partial list of such derived variables and their implications by technique is included in Table 7.1. The accuracy to which these measures can be made, the effects of ventilation and PEEP on the accuracy of these measures, and the limitations of present technologies have all been debated before; numerous studies, chapters in textbooks and monographs have addressed these issues in detail.

What is not often discussed, however, is the efficacy that this new information lends to the overall management of the patient. We propose a list of four tests that may be useful in answering the question: Does an invasive hemodynamic monitoring technique benefit the patient? Following this list of tests we will discuss the practical limitations in the application of each and the specifics of three types of invasive hemodynamic monitoring used at present: arterial, central venous and pulmonary arterial catheterization.

Does an invasive hemodynamic monitoring technique benefit the patient?

Tests for documentation of effectiveness of invasive monitoring

1. Information received from invasive monitoring cannot be acquired from less invasive and less risky monitoring systems.
2. Information received from invasive monitoring improves the accuracy of diagnosis, prognosis, and/or treatment based on known physiological principles.
3. The changes in diagnosis and/or treatment result in improved patient outcome (morbidity and mortality).
4. The changes in diagnosis and/or treatment result in more effective use of health care resources.

Based on these four tests, there are very few situations in which invasive monitoring has a proven role.[10] However, application of these stringent tests to other noninvasive diagnostic procedures routinely accepted clinically as useful, are also lacking. For example, the use of cardiac catheterization for the diagnosis of clinically significant coronary artery disease as the initial diagnostic procedure has never been documented and may be inferior to less invasive nuclear and echocardiographic studies.

Having said that few definitive data support the use of cardiovascular monitoring in the large picture of improved patient outcome and cost-effectiveness, it is still the overall perception of critical care providers that information derived from invasive hemodynamic monitoring has greatly improved our ability to diagnose the immediate cause of cardiopulmonary insufficiency, titrate resuscitative measures which would otherwise be potentially dangerous to the patient, and prognosticate as to the chance of survival of the critically ill patient.[17,18] How then is it that these technologies now assumed to be useful appear not to have induced the rewards of improved patient survival and decreased morbidity? One obvious superficial answer to this question is that these techniques have probably played a major role in reducing morbidity and mortality in many specific groups of patients, such as acute postoperative cardiac or trauma patients,[18] and other numerous acute reversible situations in which the underlying state of the host is normal and the insult short-lived. However, for many other patients, this answer may not be correct.

Other answers to this question are not known, but may relate to inherent errors in our perception of the pathophysiology of critical illness. First of all, we often use hemodynamic data derived from invasive monitoring incorrectly by assuming that the measures reflect in an analog fashion measures of more relevant physiologic variables. Secondly, our inability to analyze more than one or two independent variables at one time, despite the fact that numerous variables interact to determine the final physiologic picture, means that we simplify the data, often to the detriment of understanding the operative underlying process, their natural course, and their response to therapy. Finally, although we may correctly diagnose the operative pathophysiologic process and give the most appropriate therapy available to reverse or minimize its effects, if the therapy does little to minimize the etiology of the dysfunction, then it should not be assumed to reduce patient morbidity and mortality. Three examples of common misunderstandings in the application of physiologic principles to the assessment of cardiovascular status follow.

Three fantasies of hemodynamic monitoring

PULMONARY ARTERY OCCLUSION PRESSURE IS SYNONYMOUS WITH LEFT VENTRICULAR PRELOAD

Much of the theory and practice of applying hemodynamic monitoring in the assessment of cardiovascular instability relates to applications of data derived from such monitoring to infer the status of filling of the left ventricle.[4] Whether the left ventricle is underfilled, overfilled, impaired in its ability to contract or hypercontractile are all important bits of information one needs to know to select the most physiologically sound resuscitative efforts. Clearly, our ability to diagnose the etiology of cardiovascular instability and acutely correct it is one of the major accomplishments which can be claimed by intensivists in their defense of critical care medicine. As will be discussed later, it is not clear, however, if these acute stabilization maneuvers actually reduce long-term mortality and costs for the majority of critically ill.

Our understanding of the determinants of cardiac pump function has developed greatly since the initial studies of Frank and Starling around the end of the nineteenth century and the beginning of the twentieth century. Frank noted that cardiac muscle strips, unlike skeletal muscle strips, increased their force of contraction when stretched above their resting length. Starling expanded this observation to show that this increased force of contraction was related to end-diastolic volume, presumably because the way end-diastolic volume increases is to increase end-diastolic fiber length. For a similar increase in end-diastolic volume, a more effective ventricle will develop a greater stroke work than a less effective ventricle (Fig. 7.1). This concept is central to most diagnostic and therapeutic protocols used to assess cardiac function.[19] Now, however, we understand that the Frank–Starling relationship of preload-dependent force of contraction is a unidimensional description of the mechanical quality of ventricular ejection as described by time-varying elastance.[20] Time-varying elastance describes the contractile history of the left ventricle through systole in the pressure–volume domain. Time-varying elastance is the relative stiffness of the ventricle over time as mechanical systole develops from end-diastole. It can be calculated experimentally as a plot of the slopes of the isochronic pressure–volume relations during ejection as end-diastolic volume is rapidly varied (Fig. 7.2). The slopes of these sequential pressure–volume lines reflect the obligatory pressure–volume domain that the left ventricle (LV) must be in after the initiation of systole. Since

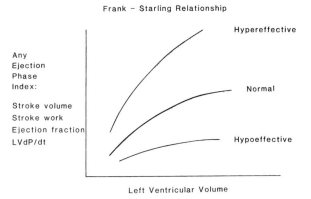

Fig. 7.1 Schematic representation of the contractile behavior of three idealized hearts demonstrating the relation between changes in left ventricular end-diastolic volume on the *x*-axis and systolic functional parameters on the *y*-axis. Note that under all conditions, increases in end-diastolic volume are associated with directionally similar changes in ejection phase indices. What categorizes the ventricular response as being 'hypereffective, normal or hypoeffective' is the *relative change* in ejection phase index for change in end-diastolic volume.

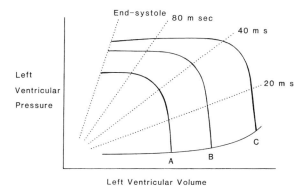

Fig. 7.2 Schematic representation of the systolic phase of the cardiac cycle for three idealized hearts, A, B and C, with identical diastolic compliance and contractility, but with progressively increasing end-diastolic volumes. The dotted lines reflect isochronic lines following the initiation of systole. These lines define for all three beats what the left ventricular pressure and volume data pairs must be at each specific time interval following systole. This increasing slope of these isochronic line reflects increasing stiffness (elastance) of the left ventricle over time, hence the name time-varying elastance, used to describe this phenomena. Note that all ejection phase indices, such as ejection fraction, stroke volume, stroke work and $(dP/dt)_{max}$ increase as left ventricular end-diastolic volume increases. However, load-dependent indices, such as time-varying elastance, are unaffected by these changes.

elastance increases its slope during both the isometric and ejections phase of systole, the slope of the elastance curve after the initiation of contraction will be steeper than the slope for LV diastolic compliance immediately preceding it. This fact underlies the physical basis for the Frank–Starling relationship. Using a real example of time-varying elastance from a patient to illustrate this point (Fig. 7.2), it can be seen that end-diastolic volume must have a profound effect on ejection phase indices. Conceptually, time-varying elastance, as shown in Fig. 7.2, can be seen to approximate the ribs of a fan with its hinge near the origin of the pressure volume axis. The lowest rib at the border of the fan lying near the *x*-axis (volume axis) describes the relation between LV pressures and volume during diastole, whereas the uppermost rib of the fan, being the maximal stiffness of the ventricle near end-systole, describes end-systolic elastance (end-systolic pressure–volume relations or ESPVR). Each rib then reflects the pressure–volume domain at a given time following the initiation of systole. It can be seen from this analogy that if the ventricle were to start ejecting at a larger end-diastolic volume, then it would be starting further from the hinge of the fan. Since each rib represents a fixed point in time during systole, the larger the end-diastolic volume, the further up the pressure axis it must travel to keep its appointed relation between pressure and volume by the next time point. Thus, increasing end-diastolic volume will increase all measures of ejection phase indices, such as stroke volume, stroke work, LV rate of change of pressure (d*P*/d*t*), velocity of circumferential fiber shortening (Vcf), and LV ejection fraction. This dependence of ejection phase indices on preload makes their use to assess cardiac function with a changing preload dubious at best. Still, one may effectively argue that if LV end-diastolic volume is above some minimum value and measures of ventricular function are still depressed relative to normal values, then the ventricle has impaired performance. If such a patient also has evidence of hemodynamic instability, then it is logical to conclude that a component of that instability can be ascribed to impaired ventricular pump function and measures directed at reversing or minimizing this dysfunction should be undertaken. Which measures should be taken is a subject for another forum.

It should be obvious from the above discussion that intensivists consider the preload-dependent nature of left ventricular performance to be central in the understanding of cardiac physiology. In fact, demonstrating that preload, i.e. LV end-diastolic volume, is above some minimum value, whereas cardiac output and stroke work are depressed, is essential for the diagnosis of cardiac pump dysfunction.[16,18,21] Similarly, demonstrating that preload is reduced in the setting of hemodynamic instability presumes the diagnosis of inadequate preload as the most likely cause of the hemodynamic instability. Furthermore, such documentation of reduced preload implies that therapeutic maneuvers aimed at increasing LV preload are indicated. Based on these concepts and the fundamental truth that the heart can only pump out that which it receives, intensivists focus their initial resuscitative energies on optimizing LV preload prior to considering the use of other therapies in the acutely hemodynamically unstable patient. Although this overall conceptual framework is valid and relevant to the management of the critically ill, problems arise when one attempts to apply it at the bedside using data derived from hemodynamic monitoring.

The problem with the above constructs is that they require that one measure LV end-diastolic volume. Furthermore, substituting LV and diastolic pressure for end-diastolic volume as an approximation of preload still requires LV catheterization. Such catheterizations are not easy to perform and cannot be routinely sustained for long periods of time because of the risks of arterial embolization and hemorrhage. The introduction of a bedside insertion of a pressure-guided balloon flotation pulmonary arterial catheter with the subsequent ability from the pulmonary artery occlusion pressure to directly reflect LV filling pressure has revolutionized our diagnostic approaches to the care of the hemodynamically unstable patient.[4] In fact, pulmonary artery occlusion pressure, or 'wedge' pressure, as it is often incorrectly called, is often used synonymously with the concept of 'preload'. The first fantasy in hemodynamic monitoring is the assumption that a specific pulmonary artery occlusion pressure (Ppao) or wedge pressure reflects a specific LV preload. Furthermore, Ppao can be elevated to values in excess of 20 mm Hg with markedly reduced LV preload, and can be as low as 5 mm Hg in patients with adequate preloads.[22–24] If these statements are true, and they are, what are the logical constructs which allow or inhibit one from using Ppao as an estimate of LV preload? The following discussion follows the logic from the physiologically correct LV end-diastolic volume to the clinically expedient Ppao.

If one assumes that LV preload is synonymous with LV end-diastolic volume, then to accurately assess LV preload one should measure LV end-diastolic volume. Although this can be attempted at the bedside indirectly using nuclear stethoscopes and radiolabeled blood markers or echocardiography, these measures are not universally available, have their own significant inaccuracies, costs, risks and limitations and cannot easily be done at a moment's notice. As a first approximation of LV end-diastolic volume one can measure LV end-diastolic pressure. This is routinely done in the cardiac catheterization laboratory during LV catheterization. Unfortunately, the relation between LV end-diastolic pressure and end-diastolic volume, which is the final point on the LV diastolic compliance curve, is not linear but curvilinear. It is convex to the pressure axis, being markedly so as LV volumes exceed normal limits due to the combined effects of myocardial distension and pericardial volume restraint.[24] Furthermore, LV diastolic compliance can be reduced (made stiffer) by several common clinical events, such as ischemia,[25] tachycardia,[26] and hypothermia[27] (Table 7.2). Similarly,

Table 7.2 Conditions characterized by variations in the relation between left ventricular end-diastolic pressure and end-diastolic volume

Acute decreases in left ventricular diastolic compliance
1. Acute myocardial ischemia
2. Hypothermia
3. Tachycardia (HR >120 beats/min)
4. Acute right ventricular dilation (acute cor pulmonale)
5. Increased pericardial pressure secondary to pulmonary hyperinflation and tamponade

Chronic decreases in left ventricular diastolic compliance
1. Infiltrative diseases of the myocardium
2. Pericardial fibrosis and constriction
3. Myocardial hypertrophy (left- or right-sided)

Acute increases in left ventricular diastolic compliance
1. Acute resolution of cor pulmonale
2. Acute resolution of myocardial ischemia prior to stunning (<5 minutes total ischemic time)
3. Vasodilating drug infusion (may be due to causes 1 and 2 above)

Chronic increases in left ventricular diastolic compliance
1. Dilated cardiomyopathies

HR: heart rate.

LV diastolic compliance can be increased (made more compliant) by other common clinical conditions, such as resolution of acute cor pulmonale or ischemia and the infusion of vasodilators, such as nitroprusside[28] (Table 7.2). Finally, the position of the diastolic compliance curve can be shifted in a parallel fashion to the pressure axis by the presence or absence of the pericardium, and by pericardial disease (effusions and constriction).[29] Therefore, LV end-diastolic pressure may reflect LV preload but may also misrepresent changes in LV preload when any of the above conditions occur or resolve. However, if these complicating forces are held constant, changes in end-diastolic pressure should directly reflect changes in end-diastolic volume. Thus, maneuvers which increase LV end-diastolic pressure should be expected to improve ejection phase indices to the degree that the LV is responsive to changes in LV preload. Still, measurement of LV end-diastolic pressure using left heart catheterization carries high risks of arterial embolization, hemorrhage and arrhythmias.[17,30–33].

Measures of left atrial pressure (Pla) are easier and are associated with fewer incidences of arrhythmias and hemorrhage than measures of LV pressure, but cannot be easily made except in some patients after cardiac or

thoracic surgery in whom direct access to the left atrium through a pulmonary vein can be achieved. Still, Pla is often used to reflect LV preload in both experimental studies and clinically.[34,35] However, Pla measures share all the same limitations of LV end-diastolic pressure measures in assessing LV end-diastolic volume with the added limitation of not accurately reflecting LV end-diastolic pressure, but rather mean LV diastolic pressure. Thus, under conditions in which atrial contraction materially increases LV end-diastolic pressure, such as in exercise and tachycardia, measures of Pla may underestimate LV end-diastolic pressure. Finally, if obstruction exists between the left atrium and the left ventricle or if the mitral valve is incompetent, measures of Pla may grossly overestimate LV filling pressures while still accurately reflecting the back-pressure to pulmonary venous blood flow. In practice, however, neither measures of LV pressure nor Pla are feasible in the routine monitoring of critically ill patients. Hence, the great excitement when a simple bedside method for the estimation of mean Pla was introduced.

Pulmonary artery occlusion pressure is the pressure at the distal tip of a pulmonary artery catheter once the balloon at the tip of the catheter has been inflated enough to allow the balloon to advance and occlude a medium sized (6–8 mm diameter) pulmonary artery. This results in a stoppage of blood flow from this point in the downstream pulmonary circulation until the first point of anastomosis between this vascular bed and the remaining pulmonary vasculature. The pulmonary vasculature, unlike the systemic vasculature, has little cross blood flow from one arterial bed to another. Thus, the next point in the pulmonary circulation where blood flow occurs in the medium sized pulmonary veins (the J-1 point) is approximately 2–5 cm from the left atrium. If a continuous column of blood exists in the occluded vessels downstream from the occlusion site, then the pressure at the distal tip will reflect a dampened pressure signal from this J-1 point or from the site of final vascular obstruction, whichever comes first. With a patent pulmonary vasculature, the pressure at the site of initial flow in the medium sized pulmonary veins is almost identical to that at the left atrium. Thus, Ppao is a common clinical estimate of Pla.[23] Furthermore, under the most clinical conditions, total obstruction of the pulmonary vascular bed downstream from the site of balloon occlusion is uncommon. Exceptions to this rule include hypotension and hypoperfusion following the initial insertion of the flow-directed pulmonary artery catheter, or markedly increased mean or end-expiratory airway pressure with occlusion of the pulmonary vasculature as it passes through the alveoli, the so-called West zone 1 and 2 conditions. However, one can readily determine at the bedside whether the measured Ppao reflects a pulmonary venous pressure or alveolar pressure. This is accomplished by observing the behavior of the Ppa pressure signal during a positive pressure breath both prior to and following balloon occlusion. Since in the nonoccluded state some blood flow must occur through the pulmonary circulation for the patient to be alive, Ppa changes during ventilation must reflect proportional changes in intrathoracic pressure. Furthermore, since alveolar pressure increases more than intrathoracic pressure during inspiration, owing to the obligatory increase in transpulmonary pressure, if Ppao reflects a patent vasculature then it will vary by no more than Ppa does during ventilation. If Ppao reflects the pressure within an obstructed pulmonary vessel (i.e. alveolar pressure), then it will increase more during inspiration than did either systolic or diastolic Ppa measures taken just a moment before. Thus, one should be readily able to identify in which patients Ppao measures can be taken to reflect Pla by their behavior during positive pressure ventilation.[36]

Given that one has an accurate measure of Ppao which reflects a dampened Pla signal, can we use this as a measure reflecting LV end-diastolic volume? Pulmonary artery occlusion pressure, like Pla and LV pressures, is influenced by its surrounding pressure: intrathoracic pressure (Table 7.3). Intrathoracic pres-

Table 7.3 Conditions associated with a varying relation between pulmonary artery occlusion pressure (Ppao) and left ventricular end-diastolic pressure (Plv_ed), such that Ppao overestimates Plv_ed

Pulmonary hyperinflation
1. Catheter tip in Zone I or I conditions (alveolar pressure > pulmonary venous pressure)
2. 'Overwedging' of the balloon in the pulmonary arterial lumen (includes eccentric balloon inflation)
3. Positive-pressure ventilation
4. Sustained positive end-expiratory pressure: PEEP, CPAP, auto-PEEP (dynamic hyperinflation), and air trapping

Primary vascular obstruction
1. Mitral valvular disease (stenosis and insufficiency)
2. Left atrial myxoma or thrombus
3. Pulmonary venous pathology (pulmonary veno-occlusive disease, fibrosis, tumor, *in situ* thrombosis)

Other vascular and pulmonary abnormalities
1. Intracardiac shunt (ASD or VSD)
2. Aortic regurgitation
3. Tachycardia
4. Pneumonectomy

CPAP: continuous positive airways pressure.

sure varies widely during ventilation. Since measures of any of these vascular pressures are made relative to a neutral atmospheric pressure background, changes in intrathoracic pressure will directly alter the measured vascular pressure in a straightforward algebraic sum relation. If intrathoracic pressure increases, as occurs during positive pressure inspiration, then these pres-

sures will appear to increase as well. To minimize this problem, often referred to as the 'respiratory artifact', measures of all intrathoracic pressures are usually made at end-expiration when intrathoracic pressure is assumed to be both minimal and constant over time.[22] However, end-expiratory Ppao measures may still overestimate Pla if mitral regurgitation or tachycardia develop, because the increased retrograde pressure waves created by left atrial contraction will add with the mean Ppao values to give a 'standing wave' increase in the baseline pressure. Furthermore, if hyperinflation exists, either due to the addition of positive end-expiratory pressure (PEEP) or air trapping, then intrathoracic pressure will remain elevated above its normal level even at end expiration. The external PEEP effect on Ppao measures can be easily removed by briefly disconnecting the patient from the ventilator at end expiration and observing the 'nadir' Ppao that occurs within 1 to 2 seconds following disconnection. If Ppao does not change, then on-PEEP values of Ppao will reflect off-PEEP Pla. If nadir Ppao values are less than on-PEEP Ppao, then the on-PEEP Ppao values overestimate Pla and one must use this nadir Ppao technique or other methods to assess Pla in that patient.[3]

Based on the above discussion, Ppao is not synonymous with LV preload and may change in the opposite direction to the actual changes in LV preload under conditions often seen in the ICU. For example, during an acute ischemic event or following cardiopulmonary bypass for cardiac surgery, LV diastolic compliance decreases, such that for the same LV end-diastolic volume (preload) a greater Ppao is required. However, once that end-diastolic volume is achieved, there may be little evidence of grossly impaired systolic pump function. Thus, it is often difficult to use Ppao measures alone to define the hemodynamic determinants of a given clinical condition when changes in LV diastolic compliance are also occurring.

Having said all this, is there reason not to adopt a nihilistic approach to the use of Ppao to reflect LV end-diastolic volume? The answer is most definitely yes. Firstly, patients with low Ppao (<5 mm Hg) cannot be assumed to have an expanded LV preload, although they may have an adequate LV end-diastolic volume for their condition. Secondly, if changes in Ppao directionally track changes in ventricular pump function, cardiac output, and the development or resolution of pulmonary edema, then this trending is valuable for the moment-to-moment fluid and inotropic management of these patients. Furthermore, in many patients the above confounding events do not occur during the brief time interval of the therapeutic trail, making the use of directional changes in Ppao reasonable in the assessment of response to therapy. These points are repeated again in the section below on indications for hemodynamic monitoring.

OXYGEN DELIVERY AND OXYGEN CONSUMPTION MEASURES DESCRIBE THE METABOLIC STATUS OF THE PATIENT

The metabolic determinants of global oxygen metabolism are complex. The primary goal of the cardiorespiratory system is to maintain from moment to moment adequate amounts of oxygen to meet the metabolic demands of the tissues. Under most circumstances, the body's metabolic demands vary as needed and global oxygen delivery follows to meet these demands. In other words, the 'independent variable' in the oxygen supply–demand relation is demand, not supply. It follows that under almost all conditions oxygen supply and demand must covary as a normal and expected aspect of homeostasis. Oxygen supply is often varied externally through therapeutic interventions which increase the oxygen content of blood (transfusion and enriched inspired oxygen) and the flow of blood (fluid resuscitation and the use of vasoactive and inotropic drug therapies). Furthermore, oxygen supply also may vary as a consequence of disease, as manifest by hemodynamic instability. Under conditions in which hemodynamic instability occurs, tissue hypoperfusion can develop, limiting oxygen delivery to the tissues to levels below which they can still function normally.[18,37] These conditions are collectively referred to as shock. Clear examples of tissue hypoperfusion shock include severe hemorrhage, tamponade, acute massive myocardial infarction, and massive pulmonary embolism inducing acute cor pulmonale. Unless the initiating processes can be rapidly reversed and the patient's circulation supported, these processes are uniformly fatal. Profound hypoxemia and anemia can also induce organ system dysfunction and death via similar mechanisms, but surprisingly different presentations. Apparently blood flow and arterial oxygen content alter tissue function differently, with flow being the more critical factor.[38] The reasons for this are still unclear, but may relate to the effect that high flow has on wash out of anaerobic metabolic products. However, in all cases of cardiovascular insufficiency with oxygen delivery to the tissues reduced to levels below which organ system function can be maintained, primary therapy is directed at increasing oxygen delivery while reversing the initiating process. In that regard, physicians often utilize data derived from invasive monitoring to assess the adequacy of oxygen delivery and its response to specific therapeutic interventions by how changes in oxygen delivery affect oxygen consumption.

Much confusion exists in the literature and among field workers in the field around the analysis of oxygen supply–demand relations in the critically ill.[39] Much attention has focused in recent years on the concept of 'pathological oxygen supply-dependence'.[40] This entity describes a tissue oxygen consumption which varies as oxygen delivery varies, but without evidence of varying tissue oxygen demand. In other words, the tissues appear to use as much oxygen as they can be given. Does such a circumstance exist in critically ill man? If it does, then measures of oxygen consumption will be more dependent on delivery than on tissue metabolic needs and may not be useful in the management of patients.

Many possible mechanisms could explain 'pathological' oxygen supply dependency. Firstly, the covariance seen could be nonpathological covariance of consumption and delivery as seen in normal conditions. Basal oxygen consumption of critically ill patients is not constant but varies over time. Muscular activities, such as moving in bed or being turned, 'fighting the ventilator', and breathing spontaneously can easily double resting oxygen consumption. In the patient with an intact and functioning cardiopulmonary apparatus, this will translate into an increase in both oxygen delivery and consumption. In support of this observation, most studies examining these relations in critically ill patients do not alter oxygen delivery while preventing consumption from muscular work from varying, they merely observe how changes in delivery and consumption interact as some nonspecific intervention alters oxygen delivery.[41–45] Furthermore, when patients are sedated and paralyzed, it is difficult to demonstrate oxygen delivery–consumption covariance.[46–47] Secondly, the covariance could reflect an artifact of the method of measuring delivery and consumption using invasive hemodynamic monitoring. Measures of oxygen delivery and consumption based on data derived from pulmonary arterial and arterial catheters share two of the three variables which derive both, namely cardiac output and arterial oxygen content.[48] Thus, mathematical coupling of errors must make calculated delivery and consumption covary. In support of this concern, when oxygen uptake at the mouth is used to estimate consumption, little covariance of oxygen delivery and consumption can be demonstrated. Thirdly, there could be actual subcellular dysfunction, such that damaged tissues have altered mitochondrial metabolism with uncoupled oxidative phosphorylation. Under these conditions, which include calcium poisoning of the cell, mitochondria metabolize oxygen to carbon dioxide but do not produce high-energy phosphates. This is analogous to cyanide poisoning. Although documented to occur in certain types of reperfusion injury following prolonged ischemia, this phenomenon has not been demonstrated in tissues in association with moderate hemorrhage or sepsis.[49] Finally, the apparent covariance could reflect the 'payback' by the circulation of an 'oxygen debt' incurred during the initial hypoperfusion state.[50] This is analogous to the persistent elevated oxygen delivery and consumption seen following the termination of vigorous exercise. Tissue anaerobic metabolism, which supported metabolic function over the short run when oxygen delivery was inadequate to maintain such activity on a purely aerobic fashion, is now being 'recharged' by subsequent oxygen delivery. Although this scenario often occurs in exercise and with the initial resuscitation from acute hypoperfusion states, it cannot explain the continued covariance of oxygen consumption to delivery. One caveat in this argument remains. If blood flow distribution is deranged, then blood flow may not go to specific tissues which need it the most. Thus, some tissues may be chronically dysoxic and when given more oxygen, they will increase their consumption. Still, this theoretical argument cannot explain the large increases in oxygen consumption which are normally attributed to supply dependency described in clinical studies. Furthermore, only at the very limits of tissue survival do we see evidence that oxygen uptake is primarily dependent on oxygen delivery. Experimentally, when tissues have their oxygen delivery reduced so much that consumption falls, they acutely become dysfunctional.[37, 51] If this hypoperfusion state persists, then permanent cell damage occurs.

In conclusion, neither measures of oxygen delivery or consumption, if above some threshold value, can be used to define inadequate global blood flow. Furthermore, increases in delivery may naturally be associated with increases in consumption. Thus, demonstrating that consumption increases in response to a therapeutic maneuver is not proof of prior tissue hypoperfusion.

Finally, measures of global oxygen delivery and consumption may bear little relation to actual oxygen demands, delivery and uptake in different regional tissue beds.[38, 52] It is a fundamental assumption of medicine that the body autoregulates the distribution of blood flow among and within organs to meet specific metabolic demands. Tissues increase their oxygen uptake primarily by increasing both their local blood flow, through vasodilation, and the amount of oxygen their extract per unit of flow.[52] Accordingly, global measures of arterio-venous oxygen content differences (extraction ratio) should reflect the limits to which this delivery is being stretched. If the extraction ratio increases too much, the tissues may be unable to receive enough oxygen to meet their metabolic requirements and tissue metabolism will be limited. This is the metabolic basis for the observed maximal level of exercise seen in healthy individuals. Unfortunately, regional tissue oxygen demands may have little relevance to remote tissue oxygen requirements. Any voluntary skeletal muscle contraction can be considered exercise for the critically ill and will be associated with an increased oxygen requirement. Spontaneous ventilation, 'fighting the ventilator', restlessness, seizures, and moving in bed all constitute exercise and all are associated with an increase in regional oxygen requirements. Thus, the common finding of a covariance of oxygen delivery and consumption in many critically ill patients, despite little evidence of increase metabolic demand of specific organs such as the gut, heart and brain, should not be surprising. Such covariance is both normal and what would be seen in noncritically ill patients if measurements were taken. Still, if a patient is sedated and paralyzed, changes in global oxygen consumption may reflect either oxygen 'supply dependence' or varying intrinsic metabolic rates due to fever, catabolism, anabolism or inflammation.

Thus, to use oxygen delivery–consumption data for most critically ill patients based on either single data pairs in time or even multiple points in time without attention to extraneous factors which could also alter oxygen metabolism, would be like trying to describe a hockey game without a single photograph! This 'snapshot' approach to defining global and regional oxygen metabolism and overall tissue wellness is inadequate for the task and often leads to erroneous conclusions, from which patient care may not benefit. Measures of oxygen delivery and extraction are probably more clinically relevant than those of consumption because they reflect the tissue extraction reserve. If the extraction ratio of blood is high, then the tissues are incapable of removing more oxygen from the blood.[53] In these conditions either increasing oxygen delivery or decreasing oxygen requirements seems appropriate. However, the detailed use of these relations in clinical practice is fraught with far too many inaccuracies and confounding variables to allow it to be a primary tool in assessing the adequacy of resuscitative efforts.

MEAN ARTERIAL PRESSURE REFLECTS CARDIOVASCULAR STABILITY

As essential aspect of hemodynamic monitoring is the identification of cardiovascular instability. Documentation of how cardiovascular status changes over time in response to disease progression and therapeutic interventions represents one of the most basic aspects of the clinical application of hemodynamic monitoring. Central to this monitoring is the measure and continuous display of arterial pressure and the display of mean arterial pressure (MAP) as the electrically averaged arterial pressure per heart beat. Numerous therapeutic protocols and alarm systems use decreases in MAP below some nadir value to trigger concern and the institution of new or more aggressive therapies. In that regard, it has become commonplace in the ICU to equate a MAP above some minimum value as hemodynamic stability. The assumption is that since MAP is the major central determinant of organ perfusion pressure, if MAP exceeds some minimum value, organ perfusion is adequate. This assumption is often false.

Several errors exist in this logic which make the routine application of this rule dangerous to the care of the critically ill patient. Firstly, although MAP is a major determinant of organ perfusion, intraorgan vascular resistance and venous outflow pressure are the two other determinants. Neither of these necessarily varies in the same direction as MAP nor stays constant when MAP is constant. Secondly, normal homeostatic mechanisms functioning through carotid body baroreceptors vary arterial vascular tone in such a fashion as to maintain MAP relatively constant despite varying cardiac output. For example, in animal models and in patients with hemorrhagic shock, blood pressure is usually well maintained until a considerable amount of intravascular volume is lost.[52] Furthermore, when MAP does start to decrease, severe hypotension usually occurs rapidly. Thus, MAP is remarkably stable and relatively insensitive as a marker of cardiovascular instability. Indeed, indirect measures of sympathetic tone, such as heart rate, respiratory rate, and peripheral capillary filling and peripheral cyanosis, probably reflect better estimates of cardiovascular status than does MAP. If this is true, and it is, why then the extreme focus on MAP clinically? The answers to this question are multiple.

First of all, MAP is the input pressure for organ blood flow. Increases in MAP, all else being equal, will increase organ perfusion. In disease states associated with a decreasing cardiac output, MAP may decrease. Baroreceptor reflexes induce an increase peripheral sympathetic vasomotor tone which tend to maintain MAP. Although vasoconstriction of nonvital peripheral organs occurs in response to decreases in cardiac output, cerebral and coronary blood flows do not decrease and may actually increase. Presumably this occurs because the cerebral and coronary vessels have few alpha adrengeroc receptors. Thus, systemic hypoperfusion primarily decreases blood flow to nonvital organs. The gut, kidneys, muscles and skin demonstrate a marked reduction in blood flow in response to marked sympathetic stimulation. Accordingly, short-term survival is ultimately linked to MAP through the maintenance of cerebral and coronary blood flows. This logic supports the extreme concern intensivists have for patients who develop acute hypotension and the aggressive efforts made to reverse it.[54] If profound hypotension persists for even a brief period of time, irreversible cerebral and cardiac damage can occur.

However, one cannot take this crisis level management approach to cardiovascular control for prolonged periods of time because the remaining nonvital visceral organs will also become ischemic and fail.[55] Blood flow to organ systems, not MAP, is the primary factor determining long-term viability of those organ systems. Thus, in the resuscitation phase of cardiovascular insufficiency, care must be taken to balance concerns about vital organ perfusion via MAP and nonvital visceral organ viability.[50] If, for example, the method by which

MAP is maintained in a patient with cardiovascular instability due to volume loss and manifested by hypotension and hypoperfusion is to increase peripheral vasomotor tone, then MAP may increase, but nonvital organ perfusion will decrease further. If such a patient also presents with a falling urine output, then the artificially increased peripheral vasomotor tone induced by vasopressor infusion may increase MAP, but would be unlikely to increase either renal perfusion or urine output. The fear here is that if one were to measure cardiac output in such a hypovolemic patient before and after initiation of vasopressor therapy, one may readily document a transient increase in cardiac output, due to increased peripheral vasomotor tone. However, blood flow to nonvital visceral organs may well be compromised. Accordingly, measures of organ system function, rather than cardiac output and MAP, represent the most logical methods to define adequacy of resuscitation efforts.

On the opposite end of the organ system balance, MAP is not only the perfusion pressure for coronary blood flow but also the pressure load against which the left ventricle must eject.[20] Increases in MAP increase LV afterload, increasing LV stroke work and myocardial oxygen consumption, whereas decreases in MAP reduce LV afterload, minimizing LV stroke work and myocardial oxygen consumption. In patients with cardiac dysfunction or in whom MAP is labile due to pain, hypovolemia, recovery from general anesthesia, and other disorders of sympathetic tone, measures which tend to maintain MAP constant will minimize the workload on the left ventricle and simplify the intravascular fluid management of the patient. As a corollary to this point, increases in MAP and the rate of rise of the arterial pulse pressure induce a lateral stress of vascular suture lines. Keeping MAP and the pulse pressure below some specific values, by whatever means (beta adrenergic blockage, sedation), is clearly indicated in these patients.[54,55]

Thus, MAP does not reflect hemodynamic stability when it is normal, but often represents shock states once it is depressed. If one waited for MAP to fall below some nadir value prior to initiating therapy for cardiovascular instability, then many a patient would be at risk for nonvital organ damage and increased morbidity and mortality.

Types of invasive hemodynamic monitoring

ARTERIAL CATHETERIZATION

Arterial catherization is an extremely common invasive procedure in the ICU. A small gauge catheter is inserted, usually by Seldinger technique or, occasionally, by surgical cut-down, typically, either in the radial or femoral artery. Other less common sites include the dorsalis pedis, brachial and axillary arteries. The procedure is performed in critically ill patients for the monitoring of arterial blood pressure and the sampling of arterial blood for the measurement of arterial blood gases (Table 7.4). Arterial lines may also be used to

Table 7.4 Arterial catheterization

Indications for arterial catheterization
1. As guide to synchronization of intra-aortic balloon counterpulsation

Probable indications for arterial catheterization
1. Guide to management of potent vasodilator drug infusions to prevent systemic hypotension
2. Guide to management of potent vasopressor drug infusions to maintain a target MAP
3. As a port for the rapid and repetitive sampling of arterial blood in patients in whom multiple arterial blood samples are indicated
4. As a monitor of cardiovascular deterioration in patients at risk for cardiovascular instability

Useful applications of arterial pressure monitoring:
Diagnosis of cardiovascular insufficiency
1. Differentiating cardiac tamponade (pulsus paradoxus) from respiration-induced swings in systolic arterial pressure
   Tamponade reduces the pulse pressure but keeps diastolic pressure constant. Respiration reduces systolic and diastolic pressures equally, such that pulse pressure is constant

2. Differentiating hypovolemia from cardiac dysfunction as the cause of hemodynamic instability
   Systolic arterial pressure decreases more following a positive pressure breath as compared to an apneic baseline during hypovolemia. Systolic arterial pressure increases more during positive pressure inspiration when LV contractility is reduced

obtain peripheral blood without resorting to repeated venepuncture. Cannulation is performed in adults with either an 18- or a 20-gauge catheter. If the radial artery is used, physicians often check the status of the collateral circulation using an Allen's test, the logic being that the hand has two end arteries supplying the digits. If the radial artery becomes occluded because of radial arterial catheterization, collateral blood flow from the ulnar artery will be the only blood supply to the hand. Allen's test is performed by occluding the radial and the ulnar arteries by pressure at the wrist with two separate fingers. After the hand has become pale and cool, the finger depressing the ulnar artery is released and the time it takes to restore color to the hand is noted.

Although Allen's test suggests the presence of an adequate collateral circulation, one prospective study of radial artery insertion demonstrated that the incidence of distal ischemia was identical under conditions in which the test demonstrated the presence or absence of collateral flow. Thus, it is not clear if lack of clinical evidence of collateral circulation in the hand precludes the insertion of a radial artery catheter in that hand. The method of catheter insertion can be either by transfixion (with deliberate puncture of the posterior wall of the vessel) or by the direct threading technique.[56]

Like other invasive procedures, arterial catheterization is associated with a number of complications. A prospective study performed in the late 1970s[57] found a 4% incidence of catheter-related septicemia and an 18% incidence of significant colonization of the catheter tip (semiquantitative method). A more recent study,[58] however, showed that, with the use of continuous flushing and of a blood sampling stopcock, catheter-related bacteremia could be reduced to less than 1%. Clinically important thrombosis or distal embolism is equally uncommon, with large series reporting incidences of 0.6%[59] or less.[60] A number of risk factors for infection (use of a surgical cut-down, inflammation of the catheter site, prolonged cannulation) and thrombosis (small vessel, repeated cannulation attempts, prolonged cannulation, large catheter size) are known and should be used as an indication to remove the catheter.[3,61] The routine practice of changing arterial catheters at fixed intervals, however, is not recommended because the potential complications of reinsertion probably exceed the risk of infection or thrombosis in an otherwise normally functioning and appearing arterial catheter.

CENTRAL VENOUS CATHETERIZATION

Percutaneous catheterization of the central veins allows the measurement of central venous pressure (CVP), the administration of fluids, of parenteral nutrition and of certain drugs, which owing to the direct tissue toxicity cannot be given via a peripheral route. Central venous catheterization also allows the sampling of venous blood without resorting to repeated venepuncture. While its usefulness in the acute and chronic administration of hypertonic fluids is undisputed, it is unclear what the clinical usefulness of monitoring CVP may be.[18] Clearly, CVP is a useful variable as its value falls in the extremes. In a hypotensive patient, a CVP of 0 mm Hg would provide useful information concerning the need for fluid administration. In such a situation, the etiology of hypotension is most unlikely to be acute ventricular failure, since cardiac failure should be associated with some increases in CVP. It is less clear what a CVP of 12 mm Hg means in a mechanically ventilated patient with sepsis and hypotension. Similarly, in a hypotensive patient, a CVP of greater than 20 mm Hg implies more than adequate intravascular volume, such that further fluid administration may be of little benefit and possibly some detriment. Many questions about CVP as it relates to ventricular function remain unanswered for individual patients. For example, it is not clear how CVP correlates with RV end-diastolic volumes, or how it relates to LV end-diastolic volume. Ultimately, it is not clear if there is a definable relation between CVP and cardiac output. In many situations a great deal of guesswork is required. A recent study[62] of critically ill patients in whom the RV end-diastolic volume index was obtained by means of a modified pulmonary artery catheter equipped with a fast response thermistor, showed that there was no correlation between CVP and RV end-diastolic volume. In some patients with modest CVP, the RV end-diastolic volume index was, in fact, markedly elevated and fluid administration resulted in a fall in cardiac index. In this common clinical situation, such patients would have received fluids in the unproven and often mistaken hope that cardiac output would rise. Despite these caveats in the critically ill, the CVP can provide a relatively accurate estimate of left atrial pressure when there is no right ventricular dysfunction or pulmonary vascular disease. Therefore, CVP can be used as a 'poor man's' measure of LV end-diastolic pressure in patients with preserved cardiopulmonary function.[22] Unfortunately, such patients are a minority in modern ICUs when one addresses the specific issue of who requires invasive monitoring. Furthermore, the measure of CVP comes at a risk of complications which is similar to that of the pulmonary artery catheter[63] with the exception of problems related to intracardiac transit and injury related to the balloon or the tip. It is important, therefore, to carefully consider and understand the value and limitations of the hemodynamic information to be obtained before inserting a central venous line for the sole purpose of cardiovascular monitoring.

Having dismissed the measure of mean or end-expiratory CVP as misleading and of limited value, there are still specific instances in which its measure may be useful. First of all, if a central venous access catheter is inserted for the infusion of drugs, such that a central venous port is available for monitoring, then no increased risk is associated with that monitoring. In this scenario, the demonstration of a markedly elevated or low CVP supports the diagnosis of a relative expanded or reduced intravascular volume, respectively. Furthermore, respiration-induced variations in CVP are classically used to demonstrate acute tricuspid regurgitation, tamponade and atrial fibrillation. However, it is not clear if one would insert a central venous catheter specifically to make such diagnoses. Finally, Madger *et al.*[64] suggested an interesting and novel application of the analysis of the CVP waveform during spontaneous

ventilation. Using the principle that decreases in intrathoracic pressure will decrease CVP only if the right ventricle is not on the 'flat part' of its Starling curve, based on the teaching of Guyton, they reasoned that, if CVP did not decrease during inspiration, the right ventricle was relatively overfilled and therefore not volume responsive. However, if CVP decreased during inspiration, further fluid administration would increase cardiac output. They demonstrated that in markedly fluid-overloaded patients in heart failure, CVP did not decrease during inspiration, while in the remainder of 'volume responsive' patients CVP decreased.

PULMONARY ARTERY CATHETERIZATION

The percutaneous catheterization of the pulmonary artery using a balloon-tipped, blood flow-directed flotation catheter was first described in 1970.[4] Since its initial description, the pulmonary artery catheter has become a well established part of the critical care physician's armamentarium and its insertion is now a common procedure in the operating room and the ICU. From a monitoring point of view, the pulmonary artery catheter allows the direct and continuous measurement of the CVP and pulmonary artery pressures (Ppa), and the intermittent measurement of the pulmonary artery occlusion pressure (Ppao) and cardiac output (by the thermodilution technique). Furthermore, with a catheter sampling port in the pulmonary artery, measures of mixed venous blood gases and arterial oxygen content can be made. Specially equipped catheters are available which, through fiberoptic sensors, can measure mixed venous oxygen saturation continuously, and through a rapid response thermistor, RV ejection fraction with each measure of cardiac output. Knowledge of these variables and of other invasively or noninvasively obtained information (heart rate, body surface area, arterial pressure, etc.) permits the measurement of a plethora of additional calculated hemodynamic variables (systemic vascular resistance, oxygen delivery index, oxygen extraction, left ventricular stroke work index, coronary perfusion pressure, etc.) which may be of use in the management of critically ill patients (Table 7.1). As discussed in the first sections of this chapter, few of these measures or derived variables have, by themselves, led to measurable improvement in the treatment of the critically ill. The possible exception to this statement is the study by Shoemaker *et al.*,[65] which provides documentation that surgical patients at risk for developing multiple organ failure whose hemodynamic status was driven by the goal of attaining a target level of global oxygen delivery, had a reduced mortality, length of stay, and cost of hospitalization when compared to similarly treated patients in whom no specific target value for oxygen delivery was set. Despite the results of this optimistic clinical trial, the current major uses of the pulmonary arterial catheter are primarily in the determination and monitoring of cardiac output and Ppao.

Cardiac output is measured by the thermodilution method and the averaging of multiple determinations. This method is reproducible, simple to perform and has been shown to correlate well with either the Fick or the dye dilution method.[12,66] There are a number of caveats which one needs to be aware of in relation to the thermodilution method of measuring cardiac output. These include the presence of tricuspid incompetence and of an intracardiac shunt, the effect of variations in intrathoracic pressure associated with normal respiration and intermittent positive pressure ventilation and that of high levels of PEEP.[67] It appears that the averaging of three consecutive measurements performed at random during the respiratory cycle will sufficiently even out the impact of the above factors.[67,68] The present dogma states that the normal variation in cardiac output measures by thermodilution which can occur within the range of noise of the system is ±15–20%.[66] This level of inherent variation in measured cardiac output reflects some errors in the measuring systems, to be sure, but most of the error comes from inherent noise in the system which is not an artifact but actual flow variation. The thermodilution technique does not measure aortic blood flow – it measures pulmonary arterial blood flow. Pulmonary arterial blood flow varies markedly during ventilation, as respiration-associated changes in intrathoracic pressure vary RV filling by phasically varying the pressure gradient for venous return. Although taking the average of three or more thermal injection-derived cardiac output measures to reflect mean cardiac output represents a reasonable approach to this inherent variability in the measures signal, Jansen *et al.*[67] demonstrated that if the variation was systematically incorporated into the measuring technique, by injecting at evenly partitioned points within the ventilatory cycle when the cycle was regular from one breath to the next, the derived mean cardiac output had a variability of less than 5% of the simultaneously measured mean cardiac output using either the Fick technique or cardiac green dye dilution curves. However, the technique of respiration-partitioned measures of cardiac output is cumbersome, requiring a computer-driven mechanical thermal injector timed off by the airway pressure signal. It also requires a fixed ventilatory rate throughout the entire time needed to collect the four or five measures of cardiac output (approximately 4 minutes).

Pulmonary artery occlusion pressure is obtained when the inflated balloon at the tip of the catheter allows distal migration and occlusion of a pulmonary artery segment (wedging). This transient obstruction to blood flow should allow rapid equilibration of pressure between this distal occluded segment of pulmonary artery and the remainder of the downstream pulmonary vasculature to a point near the left atrium. This having occurred, the pressure tracing from the orifice of the catheter tip should reflect, under normal conditions, the left atrial pressure. As a point of reference, occlusion pressure is not true wedge pressure. Wedge pressure, if measured, is often slightly lower than Ppao. Wedge pressure connotes that pressure sensed when a small catheter in the pulmonary artery is advanced until it fully occludes its vessel's lumen, or wedges into the vessel. Obviously, this can only occur once the catheter has traveled into a very distal small pulmonary artery. The measure of Ppao, on the other hand, reflects the measure within a medium sized pulmonary artery once its lumen has been occluded by a fairly large sized balloon (diameter 6–9 mm). The capacitance of the occluded pulmonary artery downstream from the balloon and the real potential for sensing collateral blood flow from other pulmonary arteries and the bronchial circulation make the measure of mean Ppao slightly greater than pulmonary artery wedge pressure, but the change in pressure during ventilation less. Still, it seems that the term 'wedge' is so ingrained into our vocabulary that its excision is nearly impossible.

The simplicity of Ppao concepts belies the complexity of factors that play a clinically important role in determining the actual correctness of the obtained numerical value and the accuracy with which it reflects pulmonary capillary pressure and left atrial pressure. Firstly, the tip of the catheter must be in the correct position (true wedge). A number of criteria can be used to establish this: the mean Ppao should be lower than or equal to the diastolic Ppa, a typical though dampened left atrial pressure waveform should be seen, and blood gas analysis from blood taken from the occluded tip should reveal a high degree of oxygen saturation and a PCO_2 less than arterial blood. Secondly, the pressure measurement system should be free of sources of potential errors. This requires the presence of appropriate tubing, the absence of air bubbles from the tubing, correct positioning of the transducer at the zero point (the phlebostatic axis), avoidance of tubing movement and correct interpretation of respiratory artifacts. Even so, errors persist.[69] Once these potential sources of error have been eliminated, there still remains a myriad of situations in which the Ppao may not reflect the left ventricular end diastolic pressure (Table 7.2). Furthermore, in many commonly encountered clinical situations, even though the Ppao may correctly reflect the LV end-diastolic pressure, the relationship of that pressure and LV end-diastolic volume or preload cannot be predicted (Table 7.3). For all of these reasons, the use of the Ppao as a measure of LV preload in critically ill patients is fraught with a high probability of error. More recently, the development of optic fibers and of accurate reflection spectrophotometry has led to the additional ability to continuously measure the oxygen saturation of mixed venous blood (SvO_2). This innovation offers the potential for an early detection of global tissue hypoxia, with a fall in oxygen saturation indicating the absence of an adequate supply of oxygen to the periphery.[13] The logic of this measure is that since oxygen extraction in the periphery is the final limiting step prior to tissue hypoxia, if SvO_2 falls, then extraction processes of the capillary beds are being stressed and may reach or exceed their limits to supply adequate amounts of oxygen to their metabolically active cells. The argument continues that if SvO_2 is above some threshold value, for example 60%, then most tissues can still extract additional oxygen from the blood. If, however, the SvO_2 falls to lower levels, then some tissues must be at or below that level of oxygen extraction necessary to maintain tissue well-being. Finally, if global oxygen consumption is constant and arterial oxygen content constant, then SvO_2 reflects directly cardiac output. This last argument falls short of being correct too many times to be clinically useful. However, changes in SvO_2 are useful clinical monitoring techniques to assess the adequacy of neuromuscular paralysis, sedation, and inotropic support in an otherwise controlled critically ill patient. Perhaps the most common use of this system for these last few purposes is in the routine ICU management of the postoperative cardiac surgery patient. Like other measurements obtained by means of a pulmonary artery catheter, this further piece of information requires attention to errors of measurement and errors of interpretation. The measurement of SvO_2 can be influenced by blood pH, blood flow velocity and erythrocyte shape. It can also be altered by the infusion of lipid emulsions,[70] vessel wall artifacts, incorrect positioning of the catheter, the presence of methemoglobinemia and the administration of methylene blue.[71]

The interpretation of SvO_2 measurements requires consideration of and the integration of multiple clinical and hemodynamic data. A fall in SvO_2 may just as likely indicate an increase in oxygen demand by nonvital organs (shivering) with maintained and adequate oxygen delivery to vital structures as it may mean that occult hemorrhage is progressing and becoming significant enough to limit cardiac output. As a global measure of tissue oxygenation, it fails to provide information about regional oxygenation. For example SvO_2 data provide little useful information about the adequacy of renal or gastrointestinal oxygenation. Furthermore, in sepsis, where the problem appears to be blood flow distribution and tissue oxygen utilization, SvO_2 may be >60% even though obvious signs of hypoxic organ system dysfunction and lactic acidosis are present.[72] In patients with significant peripheral shunts (liver disease) SvO_2 may be >80% despite clinically obvious evidence of global tissue hypoxia. It

appears, therefore, that, while a fall in SvO_2 provides a relatively sensitive index of global tissue hypoxia in most patients, its specificity is limited and the therapeutic impact of the measurement over and above other indices of global tissue oxygenation yet undetermined.

Another refinement in the area of pulmonary artery catheterization, has been the provision of a rapid-response thermistor and the development of computer algorithms that allow the simultaneous measurement of cardiac output and right ventricular (RV) ejection fraction.[14, 15, 73] The computer-driven mathematical model uses a single exponential wash out curve which reduces variability to 7–8%. By measuring RV ejection fraction and cardiac output by two independent methods from the same thermal injection, one can further calculate RV end-diastolic volume as the ratio of stroke volume to RV ejection fraction. The measure of RV ejection fraction, like the measurement of other hemodynamic variables, has a number of limitations that must be kept in mind when interpreting it. Severe tachycardia (>120 beats/min), arrhythmias, tricuspid regurgitation or intracardiac shunts will significantly reduce the accuracy of estimating RV ejection fraction. Furthermore, RV ejection fraction changes significantly during the respiratory cycle, so that randomized measurements can show large differences. Correct catheter positioning is particularly important. Nonetheless, derived calculations of RV end-diastolic volumes may be a clinically useful guide to fluid administration[62, 74, 75] and to the effect of inotropic agents.[76] Our understanding of the determinants of RV function is just now emerging, and it is appearing more and more as if the rules defining RV function are unique to the right ventricle. Therefore, it may be premature to apply knowledge derived from LV physiology to define or predict RV behavior.

Though generally safe, the pulmonary artery catheter, like other types of invasive hemodynamic monitoring, carries with it the risk of complications. These relate to central venous cannulation, catheter floating and catheter presence. Central venous cannulation is associated with the induction of pneumothorax,[63] arterial puncture, bleeding and hematoma formation. Floating of the catheter can cause ventricular arrhythmias and knotting may develop.[30] Finally, long-term catheterization can lead to venous thrombosis and septicemia,[17, 77] as well as distal catheter tip migration with pulmonary infarction and pulmonary artery rupture with major hemorrhage.[31] The frequency of all these complications depends on the experience of the physician inserting the catheter and can vary from 1 to 10%.[32, 63] These risks make it mandatory to carefully assess the risk/benefit ratio of catheter insertion in any patient considered a potential candidate for this type of invasive hemodynamic monitoring.

Proven indications for hemodynamic monitoring

ARTERIAL CATHETERIZATION

The only proven indication for arterial catheterization is for the synchronization of an intra-aortic balloon counterpulsation device.[21, 78] Table 7.4 lists some of the proven and probable indications for the insertion of an arterial catheter in the critically ill patient. It is important to note, however, that even though this device may be useful in the management of a number of critically ill patients, there is no proven indication for its use.[79]

CENTRAL VENOUS CATHETERIZATION

There is no proven indication for the use of central venous catheter for the sole purpose of hemodynamic monitoring. Central venous catheterization is clearly indicated for the infusion of hypertonic substances or drugs which, if infused peripherally, would induce thrombophlebitis, vasospasm, or might trigger hemolysis.

PULMONARY ARTERY CATHETERIZATION

There is no proven indication for the insertion of the pulmonary artery catheter[10] and, to our knowledge, there is no ongoing randomized controlled study seeking to establish a scientifically proven indication for its use.

Probably appropriate (but not proven) indications for hemodynamic monitoring

ARTERIAL CATHETERIZATION

There are a number of clinical situations in which collected experience and international consensus strongly suggest that the benefits of arterial catheterization and the information obtained from it significantly outweigh the risks. Catheterization appears indicated when infusion of a potent vasodilator agent (nitroprusside/nitroglycerine) becomes necessary for the control

of severe hypertension or to reduce myocardial afterload in acute cardiac failure. It is probably also indicated when infusion of a potent vasopressor agent (norepinephrine, dopamine, phenylephrine) becomes necessary as part of a controlled hypertension protocol for the treatment of vasospasm associated with intracranial hemorrhage. Equally, a number of critically ill patients will display a clinically important degree of hemodynamic instability in association with severe sepsis. In these patients the administration of potent vasoactive and inotropic drugs and the presence of major vasomotor instability often result in rapid (over seconds) and unpredictable fluctuations in blood pressure. These patients may also derive benefit from monitoring via an intra-arterial catheter.

The guidelines described above refer mainly to patients in the intensive care setting. However, similar principles should govern arterial catheterization in the operating room and probably apply not only to patients in whom hemodynamic instability has already developed but also to those in whom it can be reasonably anticipated that it will (coronary grafting in patients with impaired ventricular function, major organ transplantation, cases requiring emergency surgery following trauma, leaking aortic aneurysms, etc.).

Arterial catheterization is probably indicated when multiple arterial blood gas samples need to be collected[16] over a short period of time to assess ventilatory status and gas exchange[8] during acute respiratory failure. This probable indication for arterial catheterization is being progressively eroded by the developments of noninvasive respiratory monitoring techniques. The development of pulse oximetry,[80, 81] in particular, poses a major challenge to the need for repeated blood gas measurements. This is particularly so when one considers the present availability of continuous capnography by measurement of expired carbon dioxide.[82] This noninvasive approach allows a continuous approximate, but clinically adequate, assessment of the patient's arterial carbon dioxide tension in the majority of cases. In patients with severe pulmonary disease, in whom the correlation with arterial carbon dioxide tension would be less predictable, trends in end-tidal CO_2 may still provide sufficient information for satisfactory clinical monitoring. Finally, the gradient between end-tidal CO_2 and arterial CO_2 may also provide additional, clinically useful and presently unavailable information, as it correlates well with the dead space/tidal volume ratio[83] in patients with pre-existing pulmonary disease. More recently, the numerical value of this gradient has been reported to be of utility in the management of patients with respiratory failure.[84]

Furthermore, even in the absence of capnography, measurement of venous blood gases provides a limited but often perfectly adequate degree of approximation for the assessment of a patient's arterial carbon dioxide tension and pH. In the light of the above observations, it is unclear whether there is any role at all for arterial catheterization for the sole purpose of frequent arterial blood gas analysis in the presence of a reliable pulse oximeter and of venous access.

CENTRAL VENOUS CATHETERIZATION

It is particularly difficult to define the probable indications for central venous catheterization for the sole purpose of hemodynamic monitoring. It may be indicated in otherwise healthy patients experiencing hypovolemia secondary to major fluid loss (diarrhea, vomiting, polyuria, etc.) or to hemorrhage. In these cases the central venous pressure probably provides sufficient information on the state of intravascular filling to appropriately guide fluid therapy. In more complex patients with sepsis or cardiac dysfunction, pulmonary artery catheterization is preferable. The one possible use of CVP measures in hemodynamic monitoring may be in the patient with a mechanical heart valve in the tricuspid or pulmonary positions, since in these specific conditions it is impossible to measure pulmonary arterial pressures with a balloon flotation catheter.

PULMONARY ARTERIAL CATHETERIZATION

The probable indications for pulmonary artery catheterization pertain to the need to assess cardiac function and global oxygen delivery, the need to assess the patient's intravascular volume status, the need to measure pressures in the pulmonary vasculature, and the ability to diagnose intracardiac shunts by sequential measurement of oxygen tension in the right side of the heart. Table 7.5 lists some of the probable indications and possible uses of pulmonary arterial catheterization. The scientific data to support these indications are incomplete and the subject of much controversy.[23, 24, 33, 65, 85–87]

The reason for the divergent views expressed in the literature was addressed in the initial sections of this chapter but also stems from the absence of well-conducted, prospective, randomized and controlled studies evaluating the clinical utility of the pulmonary artery catheter in very specific and well-defined patient populations. This is not surprising. By the time the need for such studies became apparent, the use of the catheter had become widely entrenched in clinical practice. If a study were performed to analyze the impact of pulmonary arterial catheterization in patients with a common and uniform critical illness such as myocardial infarc-

Table 7.5   Probable indications for pulmonary arterial catheterization

Data necessary for diagnosis
1. Distinguishing primary (non-cardiogenic) from secondary (cardiogenic) pulmonary edema
2. Diagnosis of acute ventricular septal defect
3. Diagnosis of acute cardiac tamponade

Data necessary for management
1. Vasoactive drug therapy for cardiogenic shock with or without acute mitral regurgitation
2. Cardiac dysfunction with ischemia requiring intra-aortic balloon counter-pulsation
3. Balancing fluid and vasoactive therapy in acute lung injury states (ARDS)
4. Assessing pulmonary pathology and response to ventilator therapy in acute lung injury states
5. To assess global cardiac output and systemic oxygen delivery
6. To direct vasodilator therapy in the management of pulmonary hypertension associated with acute cor pulmonale
7. To continuously monitor mixed venous oxygen saturation as an estimate of the adequacy of oxygen delivery to oxygen requirements in hemodynamically unstable patients

tion, it is likely that no statistically significant results would be achieved if mortality was the end point. In fact, such a study was done in a large group of affiliated hospitals.[85] The authors found that the presence of a pulmonary artery catheter did not reduce mortality in patients with acute myocardial infarction. A probable reason for this finding is simple. Thousands of patients would have to be recruited to demonstrate even a 25% decrease in mortality even if such improvement existed. Based on the Worchester study[85] there is no case for hemodynamic monitoring in uncomplicated myocardial infarction. In patients with cardiogenic shock the major determinant of survival is not the use of sophisticated hemodynamic monitoring but the extent of myocardial damage. It is probable, therefore, that if such a study was ever completed in the most critically ill patients following myocardial infarction, it would show that the use of the pulmonary artery catheter does not alter outcomes in myocardial infarction. Such findings would not help the clinician in making a decision as they would tell him little, for instance, about the usefulness of the catheter in complicated cases who fall short of the definition of cardiogenic shock. The same principles apply to other large groups of patients. Many coronary artery bypass patients would probably do well without the pulmonary artery catheter. Large patient numbers would be needed to demonstrate any clinical utility for its use. Whatever the results of such a study, the physician would still have to make individual decisions in high-risk patients on the basis of his/her experience and the information in the literature. Even assuming that large studies could be performed or that appropriate 'high-risk' patients could be selected in a multicenter investigation, it would not be sufficient to simply randomize patients to receive or not to receive the catheter. A clear picture of how the catheter was used for patient management must be made available (i.e. no use can be demonstrated for a map, no matter how accurate, if the user does not know how to navigate, does not know how to read the map and does not know where he or she wants to go). Unfortunately, there is plenty of evidence that physicians may either not use the information obtained by the pulmonary artery catheter optimally[9] or that they may not have adequate knowledge to do so.[2,11] This appears to be an international problem.[88] Information on how the catheter was utilized will still be insufficient for an adequate assessment of the overall usefulness of the catheter in the absence of evidence that the hemodynamic goals initially set for a given pathophysiological derangement were actually achieved and that they were achieved within a reasonable period of time. From the above preliminary considerations, it is clear that a scientific appraisal of the indications for pulmonary catheter use is highly desirable but will require a complex and very careful study structure.

Unproven indications for hemodynamic monitoring

ARTERIAL CATHETERIZATION

The arterial catheter is often 'routinely' inserted in patients admitted to the ICU, even when there is no evidence of hemodynamic instability. In this setting, it is used for 'routine' monitoring of blood pressure and 'routine' measurement of arterial blood gases. There is no evidence in favor of this type of clinical practice and it probably represents an inappropriate form of invasive monitoring from the point of view of cost, patient comfort and morbidity.

Arterial catheterization allows for the continuous display of the arterial waveform. This beat-to-beat display of the systolic to diastolic pressure allows one to examine in detail many interactions induced by ventilation. Although not *per se* an indication for arterial catheterization, these data are extremely valuable in specific situations in assessing the determinants of cardiovascular instability. Respiratory-induced changes in systolic arterial pressure of greater than 12 mm Hg is defined as pulsus paradoxus. More interesting from a physiologic perspective, however, is the effect of spontaneous ventilation on not only systolic arterial pressure but pulse pressure as well. Pulse pressure,

which is the pressure difference between systolic and diastolic pressures, is not readily measured indirectly using a sphygnomanometer, since the two measures must be made on the same heart beat and must also be differentiated in time with regard to inspiration. Two important clinical conditions induce pulsus paradoxus: pericardial disease and airflow obstruction. Tamponade, by limiting absolute biventricular volumes, decreases LV end-diastolic volume during spontaneous inspiration as the increased venous blood flow expands the right ventricle, decreasing LV diastolic compliance. The result of this interaction is an inspiration-associated decrease in stroke volume without a change in mean arterial tone. Thus, systolic pressure decreases along with pulse pressure but diastolic pressure is relatively constant. This is in contrast to airflow obstruction, which by markedly decreasing intrathoracic pressure without changing lung volume very much primarily decreases both systolic and diastolic pressures with minimal decreases in stroke volume or pulse pressure.[89] Thus, by examining the arterial pulse pressure waveform during spontaneous ventilation one can readily separate tamponade from bronchospasm and upper airway obstruction. Since these disease processes have different prognoses and treatment, such a differentiation is important clinically.

Another use of the arterial pressure waveform was suggested by Perel *et al.*[90] They demonstrated that positive pressure ventilation was associated with phasic decreases in systolic arterial pressure as compared to an apneic (end-expiratory) baseline. This fall in systolic arterial pressure decreases in hemorrhagic states, is minimized with fluid resuscitation, and can be reversed to become an increase in systolic pressure in fluid-resuscitated heart failure states. Although the exact mechanism by which this process occurs is still not defined, it appears to track fluid requirements, as documented in one clinical study. This example is given not merely to suggest that changes in arterial pressure may be useful in directing fluid therapy, but also to underscore the vast amount of potentially useful information available for hemodynamic monitoring which routinely is ignored.

CENTRAL VENOUS CATHETERIZATION

A central venous catheter is sometimes inserted for the sole purpose of monitoring ventricular preload. The limitations inherent to this approach to hemodynamic monitoring have been previously discussed and, in the opinion of the authors, this represents a potentially misleading way of obtaining hemodynamic information. The risk/benefit ratio of the procedure is probably unfavorable. This argument also applies to the use of the central venous catheter for sampling of central venous blood gases.

PULMONARY ARTERIAL CATHETERIZATION

As previously discussed, much debate surrounds the possible indications for the insertion of the pulmonary artery catheter. Predictably, it is not clear what are 'unproven' or 'inappropriate' indications for its use. Nonetheless, in the opinion of the authors, there are a number of clinical situations where the use of the pulmonary artery catheter appears to have a particularly low degree of support, either in the literature or in clinical practice. Use of the catheter for the monitoring of cardiac output as an indicator of cardiovascular stability or routinely in the setting of uncomplicated myocardial infarction appears of unproven benefit. Equally, the use of the SvO_2 number as the sole form of assessment of changes in cardiac output or of its adequacy is not only of unproven value but may lead to incorrect clinical decisions.

As discussed above under the 'Three fantasies of hemodynamic monitoring', oxygen delivery/consumption measures may not reflect tissue oxygenation nor response of the body to therapeutic maneuvers aimed to improve tissue oxygenation. A number of studies have emphasized the concept that, in some critically ill patients, oxygen consumption may be pathologically dependent on oxygen delivery.[41-45,53] The findings of these investigations, although controversial,[46,47] have led a number of physicians to the use of the pulmonary artery catheter as a means of monitoring oxygen delivery and consumption. The information obtained is then used to guide hemodynamic manipulations aimed at providing oxygen delivery levels that meet even dramatically supranormal pulmonary artery-calculated levels of global oxygen consumption. The protagonists of this approach believe that this style of hemodynamic management results in increased survival.[48,50,91] A contrary view is that covariation of oxygen consumption and oxygen delivery does not represent 'oxygen supply dependency' but simply 'oxygen demand dependency' and that, therefore, it does not indicate dysoxia.[92,94] Furthermore, from the strict point of view of pulmonary artery-derived data, there is great concern that the oxygen consumption–delivery covariation seen in some critically ill patients may simply by artifactual and related to a 'mathematical coupling' effect.[93,95] Finally, the achievement of high cardiac outputs in critically ill patients who ultimately achieve a lower mortality may simply reflect an otherwise unmeasured difference in illness severity that is, independent of hemodynamic manipulations, associated with an inherently favorable outcome. Whatever the correct interpretation may turn out to be, there is presently no proven evidence for the use of the catheter for the sole purpose of monitoring oxygen delivery and consumption.

The availability of catheters with rapid-response thermistors makes it now possible to measure RV ejection fraction and end-diastolic volume. Such catheters can also be combined with continuous mixed venous oxygen saturation measurement.[96] This technology, although available and validated, has yet to be adequately studied clinically and there presently are no proven indications for its use.

Recommendations for clinical practice

It is difficult to offer specific recommendations for clinical practice in the absence of sufficient scientific data to guide them. It is clear, however, that a nihilistic approach to invasive hemodynamic monitoring, while possibly scientifically orthodox, ignores the vast amount of work that is available and falls short of a thoughtful, reasonable, and pragmatic assessment of the situation. It would seem prudent, at this stage, to use invasive hemodynamic monitoring for proven or probably appropriate indications as outlined above. Furthermore, the insertion of invasive monitoring devices should be performed either by adequately trained physicians or under their close supervision since the risks of catheter insertion fall markedly with the experience of the operator. Equally, the interpretation of the information collected and the management of the subsequent hemodynamic manipulations are also best carried out either by trained physicians or under their close supervision with attention paid to the interaction of multiple variables in the overall clinical picture, rather than to one specific variable. An invasively monitored patient should be cared for in an ICU where trained nursing, paramedical and medical staff are available 24 hours a day. It is unacceptable practice to make therapeutic decisions on the basis of a single set of invasively acquired hemodynamic data and then return 12 hours later to see the results of their delegated and medically unsupervised application. This sort of behavior, common when medical staff are not routinely caring for the patients in the ICU, cannot be defended for the majority of hemodynamically unstable patients being treated today. If personnel and equipment are not available within one hospital for the care of a critically ill patient, then provisions should be made for the safe and expedient transfer of that patient to another medical setting in which such facilities exist. Finally, it is vital that in every patient who is a potential candidate for invasive hemodynamic monitoring, an assessment be made of the individual risk/benefit ratio of any planned invasive procedure so that, even in the absence of hard and fast scientific data, current 'best clinical practice' is adhered to.

Recommendations for future research

There is a clear need for prospective controlled randomized studies in the area of invasive hemodynamic monitoring, particularly in relation to the use of the pulmonary artery catheter.[97] Any study, however, that does not define beforehand the specific information from the invasive monitoring to be acquired, how it will be interpreted and how it will modify or direct therapy, and what end points will be deemed unsuccessful, will be of limited clinical value. These future studies must focus on specific patient groups likely to require close hemodynamic monitoring and therapeutic manipulations. Furthermore, such groups need, by necessity, to have potentially curable diseases or potentially effective treatment, otherwise even the most accurate of hemodynamic monitoring and the best of supportive therapies will only postpone death without minimizing morbidity or mortality. Predefined hemodynamic variables must be collected in a standardized way. These data must also be interpreted in a consensual way by appropriately trained medical personnel. Predefined hemodynamic goals for given clinical situations and associated cardiovascular states must be the consensual object of therapy. This consensual therapy applied to a given hemodynamic state must then be shown to have altered it and to have achieved the preset target within an acceptable time-frame. If future studies ignore the need for such sophisticated study designs we may never know whether the more than a million pulmonary artery catheters inserted in the USA every year represent an excess or whether the meager 6000 to 8000 used in the UK (40 times less than in the USA) represent substandard patient care. Furthermore, and perhaps more importantly, good science will succumb to technology.

The above recommendations for future studies must also be seen within the wider context of our presently limited understanding of the pathophysiology of many of the conditions we treat. We do not yet know whether 'correcting deranged physiology' is sufficient to alter outcome for most critical illnesses. We do not know what the target of such corrections should be. We do not know how global hemodynamics and oxygen delivery data relate to specific organs and their oxygen supply. We do not understand the pathogenesis of septic multiple organ failure. Neither do we understand the mechanisms that lead to its resolution. Much presently unmonitored data may well drive the processes that we measure and our therapies may, in large part, be randomly useful. Until more basic research allows us to gain insight into the pathophysiologic basis of what we think we monitor and manipulate, our efforts are likely to meet with limited success.

In conclusion, invasive hemodynamic monitoring must come of age in order to survive the fast approaching challenge of both increasingly sophisticated and accurate noninvasive alternatives and cost containment policies of medical care. It can only do so if firm foundations for its use are established objectively. This requires not only prospective, controlled and randomized studies, but further advances in our understanding of pathophysiologic processes, better definitions of therapeutic goals, and a better understanding of how and what aspects of the disease process need to be treated.

References

1. Rogers RM, Weiler C, Ruppenthal B. Impact of the respiratory intensive care unit on survival of patients with acute respiratory failure. *Chest* 1972; **62**: 94–7.
2. Bone R [editorial]. High-tech predicament: pulmonary artery catheter. *J Am Med Assoc* 1990; **264**: 2933.
3. Davis FM, Stewart JM. Radial artery cannulation. *Br J Anaesth* 1980; **52**: 41–7.
4. Swan HJC, Ganz W, Forrester JS, Marcus H, Diamond G, Channette D. Catheterization of the heart in man with the use of a flow-directed balloon tipped catheter. *New Engl J Med* 1970; **283**: 447–51.
5. Montgomery AB, Stager MA, Carrico CJ *et al*. Causes of mortality in patients with the adult respiratory distress syndrome. *Am Rev Respir Dis* 1985; **132**: 485–9.
6. Abreo K, Moorthy V, Osborn M. Changing pattern and outcome of acute renal failure requiring hemodialysis. *Arch Intern Med* 1986; **146**: 1338–41.
7. Pinsky MR. Multiple systems organ failure: malignant intravascular inflammation. In: Pinsky MR, Matuschak GM (eds) *Multiple Systems Organ Failure. Crit Care Clin* 1989; **562**: 195–8.
8. Matuschak GM, Rinaldo JE. Organ interactions in the adult respiratory distress syndrome during sepsis, role of liver in host defense. *Chest* 1988; **94**: 400–6.
9. Connors AF, Dawson NV, McCaffrey DR, Gay BA, Siciliano CJ. Assessing hemodynamic status in critically ill patients: do physicians use clinical information optimally? *J Crit Care* 1987; **2**: 174–80.
10. Robin ED. The cult of the Swan–Ganz catheter. Overuse and abuse of pulmonary flow catheters. *Ann Intern Med* 1985; **103**: 445–9.
11. Iberti TJ, Fischer EP, Leibowitz AB *et al*. A multicenter study of physician knowledge of the pulmonary artery catheter. *J Am Med Assoc* 1990; **264**: 2928–32.
12. Levett JM, Replogle RL. Thermodilution cardiac output: a critical analysis and review of the literature. *J Surg Res* 1979; **27**: 392–404.

13. Kandel G, Aberman A. Mixed venous oxygen saturation. Its role in the assessment of the critically ill patient. *Arch Intern Med* 1983; **143**: 1400–2.

14. Dhainaut JF, Brunet F, Monsallier JF *et al.* Bedside evaluation of right ventricular performance using a rapid computerized thermodilution method *Crit Care Med* 1987; **15**: 148–52.

15. Vincent JL, Thirion M, Brimioulle S, Lejeune P, Kahn RJ. Thermodilution measurement of right ventricular ejection fraction with a modified pulmonary artery catheter. *Intensive Care Med* 1986; **12**: 33–8.

16. Wiedemann HP, Matthay MA, Matthay RA. Cardiovascular-pulmonary monitoring in the intensive care unit (Part 1). *Chest* 1984; **85**: 537–49.

17. Davis MJ, Cronin KD, Domanique E. Pulmonary artery catheterization. An assessment of risks and benefits in 220 surgical patients. *Anesth Intensive Care* 1982; **10**: 9–14.

18. Shoemaker WC, Kram HB, Appel PL, Fleming AW. The efficacy of central venous and pulmonary artery catheters and therapy based upon them in reducing mortality and morbidity. *Arch Surg* 1990; **125**: 1332–8.

19. Ross J Jr, Peterson KL. On the assessment of cardiac inotropic state. *Circulation* 1973; **47**: 435–8.

20. Suga H, Sagawa K. Instantaneous pressure–volume relationships and their ratio in the excised supported canine left ventricle. *Circ Res* 1983; **53**: 306–18.

21. Sturm JT, McGee MG, Fuhrman TM *et al.* Treatment of postoperative low output syndrome with intraaortic balloon pumping: experience with 419 patients. *Am J Cardiol* 1980; **45**: 1033–6.

22. Rajacich N, Burchard KW, Hasan FM, Singh AK. Central venous pressure and pulmonary capillary wedge pressure as estimate of left atrial pressure: effects of positive end-expiratory pressure and catheter tip malposition. *Crit Care Med* 1989; **17**: 7–11.

23. Raper R, Sibbald WJ. Misled by the wedge? The Swan–Ganz catheter and left ventricular preload. *Chest* 1986; **89**: 427–34.

24. Fein AM, Goldberg SK, Walkenstein MD, Dershaw B, Braitman L, Lippman ML. Is pulmonary artery catheterization necessary for the diagnosis of pulmonary edema? *Am Rev Respir Dis* 1984; **129**: 1006–9.

25. Pirzada FA, Ekong EA, Vokonas PS *et al.* Experimental myocardial infarction. XVIII Sequential changes in left ventricular pressure–length relationships in the acute phase. *Circulation* 1976; **53**: 970–5.

26. Bourdillon PD, Lorell BH, Mirsky I *et al.* Increased regional myocardial stiffness of the left ventricle during pacing-induced angina in man. *Circulation* 1983; **67**: 316–23.

27. Courtois MR, Kurnik PB, Ludbrook PA. The sensitivity of isovolumic relaxation to hypothermia during myocardial infarction. *J Am Coll Cardiol* 1988; **11**: 201–6.

28. Brodie BR, Grossman W, Mann T *et al.* Effects of sodium nitroprusside on left ventricular diastole pressure–volume relations. *J Clin Invest* 1977; **59**: 59–68.

29. Grossman W, McLaurin LP. Diastolic properties of the left ventricle. *Ann Intern Med* 1976; **84**: 316–26.

30. Sprung CL, Marical CH, Garcia AA, Sequeira RF, Pozen RG. Prophylactic use of lidocaine to prevent advanced ventricular arrhythmias during pulmonary artery catheterization: prospective, double-blind study. *Am J Med* 1983; **75**: 906–10.

31. Barash PG, Nardi D, Hammond G *et al.* Catheter-induced pulmonary artery perforation, mechanisms, management and modifications. *J Thorac Cardiovasc Surg* 1981; **82**: 5–12.

32. Shah KB, Rao TK, Laughlin S *et al.* A review of pulmonary artery catheterization in 6245 patients. *Anesthesiology* 1984; **61**: 271–5.

33. Robin ED [editorial]. Death by pulmonary-artery flow-directed catheter. *Chest* 1987; **92**: 727–31.

34. Pinsky MR, Guimond JG. The effects of positive end-expiratory pressure on heart–lung interactions. *J Crit Care* 1991; **6**: 1–15.

35. Pinsky MR, Vincent JL, DeSmet JM. Estimating left ventricular filling pressure during positive end-expiratory pressure in humans. *Am Rev Respir Dis* 1991; **143**: 25–31.

36. Teboul JL, Besbes M, Andrivet P *et al.* A bedside index assessing the reliability of pulmonary artery occlusion pressure measurements during mechanical ventilation with positive end-expiratory pressure. *J Crit Care* 1992; **7**: 22–9.

37. Gutierrez G, Lund N, Bryan-Brown CW. Cellular oxygen utilization during multiple organ failure. In: Pinsky MR, Matuschak GM (eds) *Multiple Systems Organ Failure. Crit Care Clin* 1989; **5**: 271–87.

38. Fink MP, Kaups KL, Wang H *et al.* Maintenance of superior mesenteric arterial perfusion prevents increased intestinal mucosal permeability in endotoxic pigs. *Surgery* 1991; **110**: 154–61.

39. Bartlett RH, Dechert RE [editorial]. Oxygen kinetics: pitfalls in clinical research. *J Crit Care* 1990; **5**: 77–80.

40. Nelson DP, Beyer C, Samsel RW *et al.* Pathological supply dependence of O_2 uptake during bacteremia in dogs. *J Appl Physiol* 1987; **63**: 1487–92.

41. Powers SR, Mannal R, Neclerio M *et al.* Physiologic consequences of positive end-expiratory pressure ventilation. *Ann Surg* 1973; **178**: 265–72.

42. Danek SJ, Lynch JP, Weg JG *et al.* The dependence of oxygen uptake on oxygen delivery in the adult respiratory distress syndrome. *Am Rev Respir Dis* 1980; **122**: 387–95.

43. Mohsenifar Z, Goldbach P, Tashkin DP, Campisi DJ. Relationship between O_2 delivery and O_2 consumption in the adult respiratory distress syndrome *Chest* 1983; **84**: 267–71.

44. Bihari D, Smithies M, Gimson A, Tinker J. The effects of vasodilatation with prostacyclin on oxygen delivery and uptake in critically ill patients. *New Engl J Med* 1987; **317**: 397–403.

45. Clarke C, Edwards JD, Nightingale P, Mortimer AJ, Morris J. Persistence of supply dependency of oxygen uptake at high levels of delivery in adult respiratory distress syndrome *Crit Care Med* 1991; **19**: 497–502.

46. Annat G, Viale JP, Percival C *et al.* Oxygen uptake and delivery in the adult respiratory distress syndrome. *Am Rev Respir Dis* 1986; **133**: 999–1004.

47. Pepe PE, Culver BH. Independently measured oxygen consumption during reduction of oxygen delivery by positive end-expiratory pressure. *Am Rev Respir Dis* 1985; **132**: 788–93.

48. Russell JA, Ronco JJ, Lockhart D, Belzberg A, Kiess M, Dodek PM. Oxygen delivery and consumption and ventricular preload are greater in survivors than in nonsurvivors of the adult respiratory distress syndrome. *Am Rev Respir Dis* 1990; **141**: 659–65.
49. Hotchkiss RS, Karl IE. Reevaluation of the role of cellular hypoxia and bioenergetic failure in sepsis. *J Am Med Assoc* 1992; **267**: 1503–10.
50. Shoemaker WC, Appel PL, Kram HB. Tissue oxygen debt as a determinant of lethal and nonlethal post-operative organ failure. *Crit Care Med* 1988; **16**: 1117–21.
51. Kobayashi S, Clemens MG. Kupffer cell exacerbation of hepatocyte hypoxia/reoxygenation injury. *Circ Shock* 1992; **37**: 245–52.
52. Schlichtig R, Kramer D, Pinsky MR. Flow redistribution during progressive hemorrhage is a determinant of critical O_2 delivery. *J Appl Physiol* 1991; **70**: 169–78.
53. Kariman K, Burns SR. Regulation of tissue oxygen extraction is disturbed in adult respiratory distress syndrome. *Am Rev Respir Dis* 1985; **132**: 109–14.
54. Macho JR, Luce JM. Rational approach to the management of multiple system organ failure. In: Pinsky MR, Matuschak GM (eds) *Multiple Systems Organ Failure. Crit Care Clin* 1989; **5**: 379–92.
55. Vincent JL, DeBacker D. Initial management of circulatory shock as prevention of MSOF. In: Pinsky MR, Matuschak GM (eds) *Multiple Systems Organ Failure. Crit Care Clin* 1989; **5**: 369–78.
56. Jones RM, Hill AB, Nahrwold ML, Bolles RE. The effect of method of radial artery cannulation on post cannulation blood flow and thrombus formation. *Anesthesiology* 1981; **55**: 76–8.
57. Band JD, Maki DG. Infections caused by arterial catheters used for hemodynamic monitoring. *Am J Med* 1979; **79**: 735–41.
58. Shinozaki T, Deane R, Mazuzan JE, Hamel AJ, Hazelton D. Bacterial contamination of arterial lines: a prospective study. *J Am Med Assoc* 1983; **249**: 223–5.
59. Gardner RM, Schwartz R, Wong HC, Burke JP. Percutaneous indwelling radial artery catheters for monitoring cardiovascular function. *New Engl J Med* 1974; **290**: 1227–31.
60. Shapiro BA. Monitoring gas exchange in acute respiratory failure. *Respir Care* 1983; **28**: 605–7.
61. Bedford RF. Long-term radial artery cannulation: effects on subsequent vessel function. *Crit Care Med* 1978; **6**: 64–7.
62. Reuse C, Vincent JL, Pinsky MR. Measurement of right ventricular volumes during fluid challenge. *Chest* 1990; **98**: 1450–4.
63. Cobb DK, High KP, Sawyer RG et al. A controlled trial of scheduled replacement of central venous and pulmonary artery catheters. *New Engl J Med* 1992; **327**: 1062–8.
64. Magder S, Georgiadis G, Cheong T. Respiratory variations in right atrial pressure predict the response to fluid challenge. *J Crit Care* 1992; **7**: 76–85.
65. Shoemaker WC, Appel PL, Kram HB, Waxman K, Lee TS. Prospective trial of supranormal values of survivors as therapeutic goals in high-risk surgical patients. *Chest* 1988; **94**: 1176–86.
66. Stetz CW, Miller RG, Kelly GE, Raffin TA. Reliability of the thermodilution method in the determination of cardiac output in clinical practice. *Am Rev Respir Dis* 1982; **126**: 1001–4.
67. Jansen JRC, Schreuder JJ, Bogaard JM, van Rooyen W, Versprille A. Thermodilution technique for measurement of cardiac output during artificial ventilation. *J Appl Physiol* 1981; **51**: 84–91.
68. Snyder JV, Powner DJ. Effects of mechanical ventilation on the measurement of cardiac output by thermodilution. *Crit Care Med* 1982; **10**: 677–82.
69. Morris AH, Chapman RH, Gardner RM. Frequency of wedge pressure errors in the ICU. *Crit Care Med* 1985; **13**: 705–8.
70. Seghal LR, Seghal HL, Rosen AL, Gould SA, Moss GS. Effects of intralipid on measurement of total hemoglobin and oxyhemoglobin in whole blood. *Crit Care Med* 1984; **12**: 907–9.
71. Varon AJ, Anderson HB, Civetta JM. Desaturation noted by pulmonary artery oximeter after methylene blue injection. *Anesthesiology* 1989; **71**: 791–4.
72. Miller MJ, Cook W, Mithoefer J. Limitations of the use of mixed venous pO_2 as an indicator of tissue hypoxia. *Clin Res* 1979; **27**: 401A.
73. Kay HR, Afshary M, Barash B et al. Measurement of ejection fraction by thermodilution techniques. *J Surg Res* 1983; **34**: 337–46.
74. Boldt J, Kling D, Moosdorf R, Hempelman G. Influence of acute volume loading on right ventricular function after cardiopulmonary bypass. *Crit Care Med* 1989; **17**: 518–22.
75. Eddy AC, Rise CL. The right ventricle: an emerging concern in the multiple injured patient. *J Crit Care* 1989; **4**: 58–66.
76. Vincent JL, Reuse C, Kahn RJ. Effects on right ventricular function of a change from dopamine to dobutamine in critically ill patients. *Crit Care Med* 1988; **16**: 659–62.
77. Rowley KM, Clubb KS, Smith GJW, Cabin HS. Right sided infective endocarditis as a consequence of flow-directed pulmonary artery catheterization. A clinical study of 55 autopsied patients. *New Engl J Med* 1984; **311**: 1152–6.
78. Lefemine AA, Kosowsky B, Madoff I, Black H, Lewis M. Results and complications of intraaortic balloon pumping in surgical and medical patients. *Am J Cardiol* 1977; **40**: 416–20.
79. Bolooki H. Current status of circulatory support with an intra-aortic balloon pump. *Cardiol Clin* 1985; **3**: 123–33.
80. Taylor MB, Whitwam JG. The current status of pulse oxymetry: clinical value of continuous non-invasive oxygen saturation monitoring. *Anaesthesia* 1986; **41**: 943–9.
81. Yelderman M, Newa W Jr. Evaluation of pulse oxymetry. *Anaesthesiology* 1983; **59**: 349–52.
82. Tobin MJ. Respiratory monitoring in the intensive care unit. *Am Rev Respir Dis* 1988; **138**: 1625–42.
83. Yamanaka MK, Sue DY. Comparison of arterial end-tidal PCO_2 difference and dead space/tidal volume ratio in respiratory failure. *Chest* 1987; **92**: 832–5.
84. Murray IP, Modell JH, Gallagher TJ, Banner MJ. Titra-

tion of PEEP by arterial minus end-tidal carbon dioxide gradient. *Chest* 1984; **85**: 100–4.

85. Gore JH, Goldberg RJ, Spodick DH, Alpert JS, Dalen JE. A community-wide assessment of the use of pulmonary artery catheters in patients with acute myocardial infarction. *Chest* 1987; **92**: 721–7.

86. Tuman KJ, McCarthy RJ, Spiess BD *et al*. Effect of pulmonary artery catheterization on outcome in patients undergoing coronary artery surgery. *Anesthesiology* 1989; **70**: 199–206.

87. Rao TLK, Jacobs KH, El-Etr AA. Reinfarction following anesthesia in patients with myocardial infarction. *Anesthesiology* 1983; **59**: 499–505.

88. Singer M, Bennett ED. Hemodynamic monitoring in the United Kingdom. Enough or too little? *Chest* 1989; **95**: 623–6.

89. Rebuck AS, Read J. Assessment and management of severe asthma. *Am J Med* 1971; **51**: 788–98.

90. Perel A, Pirov R, Cotev S. Systolic blood pressure variation is a sensitive indicator of hypovolemia in ventilated dogs subjected to graded hemorrhage. *Anesthesiology* 1987; **67**: 498–502.

91. Siegel JH, Farrell EJ, Miller M *et al*. Cardiorespiratory interaction as determinant of survival and the need for respiratory support in human septic states. *J Trauma* 1973; **13**: 602–7.

92. Quinn TJ, Weissman C, Kemper M. Continual trending of Fick variables in the critically ill patient. *Chest* 1991; **99**: 703–7.

93. Vermeij CJ, Feenstra BWA, Bruining HA. Oxygen delivery and oxygen uptake in post operative and septic patients. *Chest* 1990; **98**: 415–20.

94. Weissman C, Kemper BA, Elwyn DH, Askanazy J, Hyman AI, Kinney JM. The energy expenditure of the mechanically ventilated critically ill patient. *Chest* 1986; **89**: 254–9.

95. Stratton HH, Feustel PJ, Newell JC. Regression of calculated variables in the presence of shared measurement error. *J Appl Physiol* 1987; **62**: 2083–93.

96. Dorman HB, Spinale FG, Kratz JM, Alpert CC, Ford M. Use of a combined right ventricular ejection fraction-oximetry catheter system for coronary bypass surgery. *Crit Care Med* 1992; **20**: 1650–6.

97. Bennett D, Boldt J, Brochard L *et al*. Expert panel: the use of the pulmonary artery catheter. *Intensive Care Med* 1991; **7**: 1–8.

CHAPTER 8

Imaging

D J TAWN, S N JONES

Introduction   105
Equipment   105
Pathological processes   109
Conclusion   121
References   121

Introduction

There have been rapid advances in imaging technology over the last two decades. Critically ill patients present the clinician with complex diagnostic challenges, and a close liaison between clinician and radiologist is essential to determine the appropriate sequence of imaging tests. Techniques available include routine radiography, contrast investigations, ultrasound, computed tomography (CT), nuclear medicine and magnetic resonance imaging (MRI). Before requesting an investigation, the following points should be considered:[1]

1. The anatomical site to be imaged.
2. Which investigation will yield the most information?
3. What information must be obtained from the test?
4. Can the patient be moved safely?

If it is not possible to move a patient from the intensive care unit (ICU), then only radiography using a mobile unit and ultrasound will be possible; a few hospitals have a mobile gamma camera for bedside nuclear medicine studies. Therefore, there are considerable advantages if the patient's condition can be stabilized to allow safe transport to the radiology department, but each case needs to be decided on its merits.[2] Full resuscitation facilities must be readily available in the radiology department, and a doctor must be in attendance.

Equipment

PLAIN FILM RADIOGRAPHY

Most plain films performed on ICU patients are produced using mobile X-ray equipment, with the patient in a standard hospital bed.[3] Occasionally, if the condition of the patient permits, radiography can be performed in the radiology department. Patients who have sustained severe trauma are usually radiographed in the casualty X-ray room, prior to any transfer.

MOBILE X-RAY UNITS

Films produced using mobile X-ray units are often suboptimal for a number of reasons:[2]

1. Mobile generators are not capable of producing the large exposure factors that fixed generators can give. The exposures are adequate for chest radiographs, but inadequate for diagnostic abdominal or spinal films.
2. The distance between the X-ray tube anode and film (the focus–film distance, FFD) is reduced, and an

antero-posterior (AP) projection used, which leads to increased magnification and difficulties in standardization, which is necessary when comparing a series of films.

3. Often the patient is radiographed in the supine, rather than the erect, position. This can lead to difficulties in interpretation. However, a well penetrated supine film is preferable to an attempted erect film with the patient slumped and rotated.

4. In many cases, the clinical condition of the patient will preclude cooperation with respiratory instructions; blurring due to respiratory movement may thus be a problem. This problem is exacerbated if long exposure times are necessary.

Despite these problems, the modern mobile X-ray machine is capable of producing high-quality chest films, although exposures may not be sufficient to produce diagnostic abdominal films. Lateral decubitus films can be attempted to show large quantities of free intraperitoneal gas in cases of suspected bowel perforation.

Two main types of mobile X-ray machine are in common use; both are independent of fluctuations in mains electricity supply during the exposure. They are the capacitor discharge unit and the battery-operated mobile unit.[4]

Capacitor discharge unit

Here, a high-voltage capacitor is used as a reservoir of electrical energy for the exposure. The capacitor is charged at a relatively slow rate to the kilovoltage (kV) selected by the radiographer. When the exposure is made, charge flows across the X-ray tube at a rate determined by the filament temperature. As charge from the capacitor is used, so the charge on the capacitor falls, and the voltage reduces as well.

The X-ray exposure is started and finished by means of cathode-biased switching (grid-controlled tube). An additional lead shutter is closed when the tube is not exposing, to avoid leakage currents producing radiation when the machine is not making an exposure. These machines must be stored in an uncharged state to avoid leakage radiation.

Capacitor discharge units are easy to use, independent of the mains supply during exposure, and very short exposure times are possible with low-power exposures, which is ideal for chest radiography. However, they tend to be large and cumbersome and have to be charged before each exposure, although this only takes 10–12 seconds. The machine must, therefore, be used within a cable length of an electrical socket. The exposure must be made immediately following the charging, or charge will leak away from the capacitor. There is no indication of the exposure time used.

Battery-operated mobile unit

This type of machine is often referred to as the 'cordless mobile', as it is used entirely independently of the mains electrical supply. Power is supplied by batteries, usually three nickel–cadmium cells giving 40 V each, or two 12 V car batteries.

The direct current (DC) electrical supply is converted to alternating current (AC) in a multiphase, high-frequency form. A high-tension transformer is used to boost the voltage to the required level, and the supply is rectified before being applied to the X-ray tube.

The batteries are rechargeable from the mains electrical supply, although many exposures (in the hundreds) of average values are possible on one charge.

Technique

There is no consensus among radiologists between high- and low-kilovoltage techniques for chest radiography.[5] Some prefer a high-kilovoltage technique for departmental films, in the range 130–150 kV. This technique has the advantage of very short exposure times, minimizing respiratory blur in uncooperative patients. Contrast is reduced, so there is a more uniform appearance across the film, providing good penetration of the mediastinum and good visualization of the pulmonary markings. Calcifications, bony structures and some monitoring devices are not so well shown. The use of an antiscatter grid, or air gap technique, is essential to prevent image degradation from scattered radiation.

Using a low-kilovoltage technique, high-contrast films are obtained. However, good penetration of the mediastinum requires either a longer exposure time, or higher tube current. This increase in exposure may result in overpenetration of the lungs. This technique uses voltages in the range 60–70 kV.

For departmental films, in order to obtain minimal magnification of organs within the chest and to minimize distortion of the relative size of structural detail at differing distances from the film, focus–film distances (FFD) of 150 cm and 180 cm are in general use. For high-kilovoltage films using an air gap technique, the FFD may be increased to 200 cm. At these distances, in conjunction with the use of small focal spot X-ray tubes (0.3 and 0.6 mm) and high-definition screens, maximum sharpness is obtained.

The situation is slightly different with mobile units. Such units are not capable of delivering 150 kV, but very satisfactory results can be obtained in the range 110–125 kV. An antiscatter grid must be used, which is often incorporated into a grid cassette. Grid lines will therefore appear on the film. There is no problem in producing voltages in the range 60–70 kV, and with suitable intensifying screens, exposure times will be in the millisecond range. A grid cassette is not necessary.

Mobile films are nearly always produced using an AP projection, and hence there will be cardiac magnification. A FFD of 150 cm should be used where possible, and the FFD should never be less than 120 cm.

Recently, computed radiography has been used for mobile chest radiography, with very encouraging results.[6] In this technique, a reusable photostimulable phosphor plate is used in place of the conventional cassette and film. The phosphor plate is constructed with a thin coating of europium-doped barium fluorobromide. The plate is housed in a cassette, which is exposed in the same manner as a conventional film cassette. The latent image, stored on the phosphor plate, is scanned by a helium–neon laser, which stimulates luminescence. The signal is detected by a photomultiplier and subsequently digitized. The digital information is processed and recorded by laser printer onto film. Such imaging plates have wide dynamic range, so retakes due to incorrect exposure are rare. In addition, high-quality images can be obtained with a reduction in radiation dose to the patient as compared with conventional radiographs. Digital acquisition of the image allows postprocessing such as contrast manipulation and edge enhancement. The theoretical disadvantage of computed radiographic systems is reduced spatial resolution. Conventional film/screen combinations achieve a resolution of 10 line pairs/mm or better; computed systems have a resolution of 5 line pairs/mm at best in adult chest radiography. However, as long as the pixel size used is less than 0.4 mm, accurate detection of subtle abnormalties such as septal lines or small pneumothoraces is possible. Computed radiography has been shown to be at least as good as, if not superior to, conventional radiography in the demonstration of drainage tubes and central venous catheters.

Radiation protection

There are strict regulations governing the protection of patients, staff and the general public against ionizing radiation in the radiology department.[7] In the UK, the reader is referred to the Ionising Radiation Regulations of 1985 and 1988.[8] However, it is necessary to be particularly careful when using mobile X-ray equipment. A temporary controlled area in the vicinity of operating mobile equipment should be set up. In our hospital this is defined as:

> ... all points which are within the primary beam before it strikes a suitable beam stop (patient, wall, floor, etc.), or which lie within two metres of the X-ray tube, or where the primary beam strikes the patient, shall be the Controlled Area.

Access to the controlled area is limited to radiographic staff and other staff who may be required to support the patient. When the radiographic exposure is being made, staff must stand as far away from the patient as possible (at least 2 m) and wear protective lead rubber aprons. If anyone is required to support the patient during the exposure, that person must wear protective apron and gloves, and avoid the direct beam by standing to one side and away from the X-ray tube. A record must be kept of his/her name, the date, the number of exposures and the radiographic technique used. The same member of staff should not be used for this help too frequently. The radiographer must wear a dosemeter under the protective body apron. A verbal warning must be given prior to the exposure, to allow other members of staff to withdraw as far as possible.

CONTRAST ENHANCED RADIOGRAPHY

The place of contrast-enhanced radiography is limited in the critically ill patient, since these techniques require that the patient is moved to the radiology department. Mobile image intensifiers are available for use in the operating theatre, and for the insertion of pacemaker electrodes, but all other fluoroscopic procedures should be performed in the main radiology department.

Excretion urography (IVU)

The main equipment requirement for excretion urography is the capability to perform tomography. Critically ill patients undergoing urography may have impaired renal function, and will not have been dehydrated, so that concentration of contrast medium by the kidneys is likely to be poor. Such patients are also likely to have copious bowel gas overlying the kidneys, impairing visualization, hence, tomography is essential. Nonionic contrast media should be used, as these are less nephrotoxic.[1]

Real-time ultrasonography and computed tomography have significantly decreased the demand for excretion urography and the main indications now are renal trauma and suspected renal colic.

General fluoroscopy

General fluoroscopy equipment comprises an X-ray tube, an image intensifier with television chain and a movable, tilting tabletop.

Permanent images can be produced using conventional film cassettes or 100 mm camera, and dynamic studies can be recorded onto video tape. Digital fluoroscopy is a recent development. The image from the intensifier is digitized and displayed on a monitor, where postprocessing of the image is possible, e.g. edge enhancement and contrast manipulation. The digital information is processed and recorded onto film by a laser imager. Rapid sequences of up to eight images a second can be recorded and displayed in a cine-loop.

Angiography

Arteriography is best performed in a dedicated room. Digital vascular imaging (DVI) or digital subtraction angiography (DSA) produce images of the contrast-filled artery lumen, with the background bones and soft tissues subtracted out. A series of small injections of contrast medium are made into the vessel, with the image intensifier positioned over the region of interest, and digital images are acquired as the bolus of contrast medium passes through the vessel. Direct injection into the arterial system through a catheter introduced via the common femoral artery is the usual method, and produces the best images. Intravenous DSA is possible, using a catheter in the superior vena cava or right atrium. However, a much larger volume of contrast medium is necessary and image quality is not as good.

ULTRASOUND

Ultrasonography was first introduced into medicine in the early 1950s, but initial development was slow and practical imaging equipment was not available until the late 1960s. Early gray scale imaging used analog signal processing and storage, but this has been supplanted by digital technology.[9]

Although modern ultrasound equipment is very complex, the machines are not large and are mobile. The main difficulty with the critically ill patient is the presence of dressings and monitoring devices, which may limit access for the transducer. If there is excessive bowel gas, especially in patients with an ileus, image quality will be impaired. However, even with these limitations, ultrasound is a most valuable tool in the investigation of abdominal pathology in the critically ill patient.

COMPUTED TOMOGRAPHY

Computed tomography employs a tightly collimated fan beam of X-rays, which is transmitted through the patient, in a sequence of narrow layers, or slices.[10] Modern scanners are of three main types:

1. Third generation – an array of detectors is mounted opposite the X-ray tube and rotates with it.
2. Fourth generation – the X-ray tube rotates within a fixed ring of detectors.
3. Helical scanners – the X-ray tube rotation is com-

bined with movement of the patient table, which allows acquisition of true volume metric data.

Scan times are now in the range of 2–4 seconds per slice for conventional scanning, but can be reduced still further for sequential or dynamic scanning.

The main use for CT in the critically ill patient is the investigation of acute cerebral events, and also in the investigation of possible aortic dissection. It has a role in the investigation of intra-abdominal pathology, where it is complementary to ultrasound.

MAGNETIC RESONANCE IMAGING

Magnetic resonance imaging (MRI) is a new and exciting addition to the radiologist's armory.[11] The physics of MRI is complex, but uses the principle that certain atomic nuclei possess magnetic moment, i.e. they can be likened to tiny bar magnets. When such nuclei are subjected to a strong magnetic field, they will align along the lines of force of the magnetic field. They can align either parallel to the field (low-energy state), or antiparallel to the field (higher-energy state). A small excess of nuclei will align in the lower-energy state. If energy, in the form of a radiofrequency pulse at a critical frequency (the resonance frequency), is applied to these nuclei perpendicular to the magnetic field, they will excite or flip to a higher-energy state. As soon as the radiofrequency terminates, the nuclei will return to the lower-energy state, releasing the absorbed energy as the MR signal. Protons, being the most abundant magnetic nuclei in the human body, are used as the nuclei for study.

Acquisition times for MR imaging are quite long compared with those for CT. As the patient is confined within a tube for a long period of time (up to an hour), it is very difficult to monitor critically ill patients. Also, as the patient is in a strong magnetic field, any monitoring and ventilation equipment must be contructed using nonmagnetic materials, both in order to function properly and not to cause image degradation. For these reasons, the uses of MRI for imaging the critically ill patient are limited.

NUCLEAR MEDICINE

Nuclear medicine techniques depend upon the detection of the distribution of radioactivity within the body. In the majority of nuclear studies a radioactive tracer is administered, usually by intravenous injection.[12] The biological property of the radiopharmaceutical used must be matched to the physiology under investigation. Commonly used radiopharmaceuticals are listed in Table 8.1. The detection device most commonly used is a gamma camera and the image produced is a map of the

Table 8.1 Radiopharmaceuticals commonly used in nuclear medicine

Radiopharmaceutical	Uses
[99m]Tc albumin macroaggragates	Lung perfusion
Krypton 81m or xenon 133	Lung ventilation
Thallium 201	Myocardial perfusion
[99m]Tc diethylene-triamine pentaacetic acid (DTPA)	Renography
[99m]Tc albumin or red blood cells	Left ventricular function/ bleed

distribution of radioactivity within the patient. Sequential images can be acquired, allowing regional changes in radioactivity to be studied. Gamma cameras are easily linked to computer systems, can perform studies rapidly with relative ease of patient positioning, and can perform tomographic images.

Pathological processes

THE THORAX

The lung

Collapse and consolidation

Loss of volume

Collapse of the left lower lobe is not infrequent in postoperative patients, especially following cardiac surgery.[2] Complete left lower lobe collapse causes a triangular opacity behind the heart outline, with blurring of the medial portion of the left hemidiaphragm. The left hilum is drawn downwards and there is compensatory expansion of the upper lobe, with splaying of the pulmonary vessels. Partial collapse of a lobe is more difficult to diagnose and compensatory expansion of the unaffected pulmonary segments is a useful sign. Right upper lobe segmental or subsegmental collapse may occur if following general anesthesia the endotracheal tube has been advanced inadvertently into the ostium of the right main bronchus. This can obstruct the upper lobe bronchus. If the tip of the endotracheal tube is advanced well into the right main bronchus, it will obstruct the left main bronchus, causing collapse of the left lung.

Pneumonia

Patients in an ICU are subject to a wide variety of infectious agents, but there are certain radiographic features that can be helpful in suggesting the nature of the causative organism.[13] Inflammatory infiltrates do not cause collapse, but they may cause an increase in volume of the affected segment. An 'air bronchogram' may be present, indicating that while the alveoli are filled with inflammatory material, the more centrally placed bronchi remain patent.

Cavitation within the area of consolidation suggests an infection with either staphylococci or klebsiella.

Diffuse reticulonodular and alveolar infiltrates, with a predominantly perihilar distribution, in an immuno-comprised host, suggest a *Pneumocystis carinii* pneumonia. A similar type of shadowing, but predominantly affecting the periphery of the middle and lower lobes, also in immunocompromised patients, is characteristic of cytomegalovirus infection.

In practice, these infections cannot be differentiated radiographically with any degree of reliability, and often occur together in the same patient. Mycoplasma and viral pneumonias can also cause a diffuse reticular pattern, with superimposed alveolar infiltrates.

It must be remembered that steroid therapy will change both the appearance and course of inflammatory processes in the lung, possibly masking the usual radiographic appearances entirely. If the steroid treatment is discontinued during antibiotic therapy, it is possible for the radiographic appearance to deteriorate while the clinical condition improves.

Pulmonary emboli

Pulmonary embolism and infarct occur postoperatively, following abdominal or pelvic surgery or hip replacement, classically 10 days after the operation.[12] The plain chest film is often within normal limits in pulmonary embolism without infarction. Enlarged central (hilar) pulmonary arteries, with abrupt tapering and peripheral oligemia in the affected segment, is the classical finding – the 'Westermark' sign.[14] Local arterial dilatation can also be seen – the 'knuckle' sign.[15]

Segmental parenchymal consolidation without an air bronchogram, associated with line shadows and possibly pleural effusions, occurs in pulmonary embolism with infarction. Similar appearances can be seen in pneumonias and septic emboli associated with subacute bacterial endocarditis (SBE) and intravenous drug abusers. Cavitation due to necrosis can occur in large pulmonary infarcts.

Ventilation and perfusion (VQ) lung scintigraphy can provide the definitive diagnosis in patients without underlying chronic airways disease. In elderly patients with airways disease, radionuclide scans may suggest the diagnosis but are not usually definitive.[16] For patients who are at risk of developing pulmonary emboli, but are a poor risk for pulmonary arteriography, there may be a case for performing a preoperative VQ scan, to provide a baseline study.

Pulmonary arteriography will provide the definitive diagnosis in equivocal scintigraphic cases, and can be performed with a relatively small contrast burden if facilities for digital angiography are available.

Aspiration

In the severely ill patient, when an area of consolidation appears in the lung, aspiration must be considered. Changes of aspiration tend to be seen in the upper lobes of the supine patient, but because the aspirate is highly irritant, changes may be widespread. Indeed, the widespread changes can mimic pulmonary edema owing to increased pulmonary capillary permeability. Normal heart size and the absence of signs of pulmonary venous hypertension will help to differentiate this from cardiogenic pulmonary edema. Resolution usually occurs within 5 days in survivors, though 25% of patients will suffer a secondary infection.[17]

Near drowning and inhalation of smoke or noxious gases can result in similar widespread pulmonary opacities, which usually resolve in 5 days or so.

Diffuse alveolar shadowing

There are very many causes for this appearance in the lung; only those likely to be encountered in the ICU are described.

Cardiogenic pulmonary edema

The classical presentation is that of bilateral, symmetrical interstitial and confluent alveolar shadowing. This may be preceded by a predominantly interstitial phase, with linear densities radiating from the hila (Kerley A lines), and short linear densities in the costophrenic angles and above (Kerley B lines). Pulmonary venous hypertension with prominence of the upper lobe vessels is almost invariably present, though this sign can only be elicited on an erect chest film. Cardiomegaly is usually present when the pulmonary edema is due to left heart failure. Heart size is more difficult to assess on mobile chest radiographs, though it has been shown that if the cardiac diameter is more than 55% of maximum thoracic diameter, the heart is likely to be enlarged.[18] The onset of radiographic changes coincides with the onset of symptoms and resolution is rapid following appropriate diuretic therapy (within minutes or hours).

Patients with chronic airways disease may exhibit asymmetrical alveolar shadowing, with sparing of emphysematous areas of lung. Asymmetry may also be due to the immobility of patients in the ICU. For example, unilateral edema may occur if the patient has been lying on one side for some time, the dependant lung being affected. Unilateral pulmonary edema also occurs following the too rapid re-expansion of a pneumothorax. The presence of a chest drain on the affected side is a clue in this situation.

Overtransfusion or fluid overload will give a similar picture of widespread pulmonary edema, which clears rapidly with appropriate therapy.

Neurogenic pulmonary edema

A number of intracranial conditions can be associated with the development of pulmonary edema including epileptic seizures, cranial trauma and surgery, intracranial hemorrhage and cerebral tumors. The edema is abrupt in onset, and may be asymmetrical. It usually clears within 1 or 2 days, sometimes spontaneously, or following the surgical relief of raised intracranial pressure. The mechanism for the development of pulmonary edema is not clear.

Renal failure

Uremia is associated with the development of bilateral, symmetrical pulmonary shadowing, similar to cardiogenic pulmonary edema. Occasionally, the radiographic density of these infiltrates appears greater than usual. This is due to the fibrinous nature of the edema, with hemorrhage, cellular infiltration and organization.

Fat embolism

Fat embolism following trauma is common, but most cases go unrecognized because of mild clinical symptoms and minimal radiographic changes. The chest radiograph shows bilateral, peripheral alveolar infiltrates, predominantly in the middle and lower lobes. These changes appear 1 or 2 days following the trauma and resolution can take up to a week or more.

The fat embolism syndrome may progress into fully developed adult respiratory distress syndrome.[19]

Adult respiratory distress syndrome (Fig. 8.1)

The adult respiratory distress syndrome (ARDS) is a condition of unknown cause, in which altered pulmonary capillary permeability to fluid allows the accumulation of proteinaceous fluid in the interstitial tissues and alveoli of the lung. Conditions associated with ARDS are legion.[20]

Four distinct phases of ARDS have been described.[21] In the first phase, lasting some 24 hours following the pulmonary insult, there is deterioration in the patient's clinical condition, but no changes are evident on the chest radiograph. The development of interstitial pulmonary edema heralds the second phase, which is rapidly followed by alveolar edema. All this occurs between 24 and 36 hours after the onset. During phase three, between 36 and 72 hours, the patient's condition continues to deteriorate, without further change in the chest radiograph. If the patient survives, the final phase is slow resolution of the radiograph from 72 hours to 6 weeks.

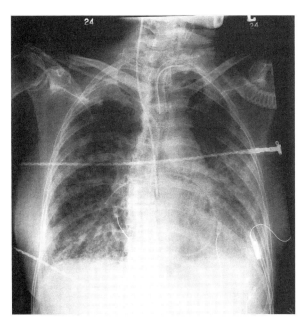

Fig. 8.1 Adult respiratory distress syndrome (ARDS). There is marked bilateral alveolar shadowing. There is an internal jugular central venous line and a Swan–Ganz catheter, which has been inserted via the right subclavian vein.

Prognosis in ARDS is poor, but there is little or no long-term morbidity in survivors and radiographic resolution is usually complete.

Interstitial emphysema, pneumomediastinum and pneumothorax can complicate ARDS, probably an indication of the increased airway pressure required to maintain ventilation.

Pulmonary contusion and hemorrhage

Traumatic hemorrhages in the lung cause asymmetrical alveolar opacities, with greater involvement on the side of maximum impact, which may be evident by rib fractures. These hemorrhages are the most common complication of the blunt chest trauma and are invariably evident within 6 hours of the injury, unlike fat embolism. Resolution is rapid, within 1 week.

Nontraumatic pulmonary hemorrhage causes bilateral alveolar shadowing, which clears within 2 or 3 days following a single bleeding episode. Reticular changes may persist for several more days in affected areas.

Pulmonary interstitial emphysema

Pulmonary interstitial emphysema is the earliest sign of barotrauma, a complication of positive pressure ventilation. It is due to rupture of the airway, probably at alveolar level, which allows air to enter the interstitial tissues of the lung and to dissect along the peribronchial and perivascular connective tissue, causing edema and

hemorrhage. There is reduction of lung compliance and compression of small vessels. Hence, both pulmonary ventilation and circulation are compromised. Air may dissect centrally into the mediastinum, or peripherally, where rupture of the pleura will give a pneumothorax. Air may track from the mediastinum into the soft tissues of the neck, resulting in subcutaneous emphysema.

Radiographically, pulmonary interstitial emphysema can be identified as perivascular gas collections, giving a 'bubbly' appearance to the lung.[22] This early stage is seldom seen in isolation (except in infants), as it is more common to see the secondary effects of pneumomediastinum and pneumothorax.

The mediastinum

Widening of the mediastinum

Even with AP mobile radiographs of the chest it is possible to assess the mediastinum for widening. A medistinal width of 8 cm or more above the carina, or if the mediastinum forms more than 25% of the width of the chest at this level, indicates that there is significant widening of the mediastinum.[23]

Postsurgical hemorrhage

Widening of the mediastinum is almost invariably present following mediastinal or cardiac surgery. A preoperative AP chest film should be performed to aid postoperative assessment.[24] The mediastinum will progressively decrease in width from the second or third postoperative day. If there are any clinical signs of active hemorrhage, chest radiographs should be performed at hourly or 2 hourly intervals, to determine any progressive increase in the width of the mediastinum. If this is the case, it indicates arterial hemorrhage in the postoperative patient. CT is very sensitive in demonstrating a mediastinal hematoma, even in the absence of the findings on a plain film, but the combination of a progressively widening mediastinum with clinical features of hemorrhage warrants further surgical exploration, and the delay necessary to obtain a CT scan not justified.

Trauma to the aorta and great vessels

A major deceleration trauma can cause a shearing injury to the aorta, usually just distal to the origin of the left subclavian artery. This region is a transition zone between the relatively mobile aortic arch and the tethered descending aorta. In 80–90% of cases the aortic transection is complete and the patient will succumb immediately.[19] In a small group of patients the transection is not complete, and the advential tissues preserve the integrity of the aorta for a short time. At least 50% of this group of lesions will rupture in the next 24 hours, and most of the remainder will do so in the subsequent few weeks. Only 2% of patients will survive, with the formation of a pseudoaneurysm.[24]

On the supine chest film, the following features may be present:

1. Widening of the mediastinum.
2. Blurring of the contours of the aortic arch.
3. An apical pleural cap, usually on the left.
4. Deviation of the trachea or nasogastric tube to the right.[25]
5. Depression of the left main bronchus.
6. Widening of the right paratracheal stripe and the paraspinal lines.

All these signs indicate a mediastinal hematoma, and are not diagnostic of aortic rupture. Such a hematoma can also occur with injury to the trachea or main bronchi, or with spinal injury. While CT will be more sensitive in demonstrating the hematoma, and may even demonstrate the aortic rupture, aortography should be performed next, as this will both demonstrate the rupture and provide the surgeon with all the necessary anatomical information prior to immediate surgery. There will inevitably be a high proportion of normal aortograms. However, if CT is being performed in a patient with multiple injuries (e.g. head or abdomen), it may be worthwhile performing a few sections through the mediastinum at the same time. This would add only a few minutes to the examination, and may detect some of the minority of cases of aortic damage that present without plain film abnormalities.[26]

Dissection of the aorta

Hypertension is the main predisposing factor; the dissection usually starts near the aortic root and extends distally. The De Bakey classification outlines three types:

• Type I: commences in ascending aorta, and extends around the arch into the descending or abdominal aorta.
• Type II: also commences in the ascending aorta, but is confined to it.
• Type III: commences distal to the origin of the left subclavian artery and extends distally.

From a surgical point of view, a better classification combines all cases involving the ascending aorta (De Bakey Types I and II) into Type A, and the remainder (De Bakey Type III) are called Type B. Type A dissections require surgical intervention, but Type B dissections are better treated conservatively.

The chest radiograph findings consist of widening of the mediastinum and localized dilatation of the thoracic aorta, involving the aortic knuckle. If there is an associated hematoma, the appearance is similar to that in aortic trauma.

In suspected cases of aortic dissection, a combination of echocardiography and contrast-enhanced CT provides the best noninvasive approach to imaging.[27] Ultrasound will identify the intimal flap within the aortic root and will also demonstrate any associated pericardial effusion. Contrast-enhanced CT will also show a flap in the aortic arch, and will show the extent of the dissection down the aorta. MRI scanning is developing a place in the imaging of aortic dissection and may supplant other modalities.

Aortography, using the transfemoral root, will demonstrate the true and false lumens in the majority of cases, and is usually performed preoperatively. It is not required in cases that are being managed conservatively.

Pneumomediastinum

Pneumomediastinum occurs most frequently following positive pressure ventilation of the lung. As such, it is one of the effects of barotrauma. Other causes of pneumomediastinum include tracheal damage during intubation, rupture of the esophagus (during endoscopy or traumatic nasogastric intubation), closed chest trauma (including cardiopulmonary resuscitation), paroxysmal coughing, or following surgery to the neck or abdomen. Air in the mediastinum can track up into the neck or downwards into the retroperitoneum. Infection can also pass with the air, leading to a retroperitoneal or subphrenic abscess.[2]

Radiographic signs of a pneumomediastinum are a line shadow parallel to the cardiac border, representing the displaced mediastinal pleura. The diaphragmatic outline extends across the midline (continuous diaphragm sign) and the cardiac border is unusually sharply defined. Secondary signs include pneumothorax, soft tissues emphysema of the neck and thorax, and a pneumoperitoneum.

The heart

Cardiac enlargement may be chronic due to ischemic heart disease or a congenital anomaly. Comparison with any previous films will be helpful. Cardiac enlargement may also be due to a pericardial effusion. If there is clinical evidence of cardiac tamponade, a pericardial effusion can be demonstrated by echocardiography. Ultrasound can also be used to guide the drainage of such an effusion.

In patients with a fractured sternum, enlargement of the cardiac outline may signify a developing hemopericardium. Again, this can be confirmed by echo-cardiography.

The pleura

Pleural effusion

Pleural effusions can be difficult to diagnose on the mobile chest film, especially if the patient is not in the erect position. When the patient is supine, the fluid layers lie posteriorly, giving a uniform 'hazy' appearance to one or both lungs. Apical capping is an important sign, and with a unilateral effusion the overall increased radiodensity of the lung will be obvious when compared with the normal side. If there is any doubt about the diagnosis a lateral projection should be performed. Ultrasound will demonstrate an effusion and is useful in guiding the drainage of a loculated effusion.

A subpulmonary pleural effusion must be remembered in the differential diagnosis of apparent elevation of the diaphragm. It can usually be demonstrated by taking a lateral decubitus film, with the patient lying on the affected side.

Pneumothorax

A pneumothorax occurs when air enters the potential space between the visceral and parietal pleura, causing collapse of the underlying lung away from the chest wall. When air can enter this space during inspiration, but cannot leave it during expiration, a tension pneumothorax develops, with shift of the mediastinum away from the affected side. This is a potentially life-threatening condition.

Causes of a pneumothorax include spontaneous (due to rupture of a pleural bleb), positive pressure ventilation (barotrauma), asthma, chest trauma (both blunt and penetrating) and iatrogenic (postsurgical or puncture during attempted subclavian venous catheterization).

A pneumothorax may be difficult to diagnose on supine or semierect mobile chest radiographs, as the air accumulates anteriorly and can be quite difficult to see, even when quite large.[28] A film taken in expiration, or a lateral decubitus film with the affected side raised, can aid in identification. The subtle signs of a pneumothorax on the supine frontal film are unusual clarity of the contours of the mediastinum on the affected side, with depression of the diaphragm anteriorly. In a recent study, supine chest radiographs detected only 40% of pneumothoraces, compared with 100% for CT.[29] In cases of chest trauma, there may be an associated hemothorax and rib fractures may be present. Mediastinal shift away from the side of the pneumothorax indicates developing tension and the need for immediate decompression and drainage.

The diaphragm

Elevation of the diaphragm

The diaphragm appears higher on supine films than on erect films, so allowance must be made for the patient's position during the radiograph. However, a marked discrepancy between the two domes of the diaphragm must be viewed with suspicion. Apparent elevation of the diaphragm may be due to a subpulmonary effusion (see above), a phrenic nerve palsy, or a subphrenic fluid collection, e.g. abscess or hemorrhage.

Fluoroscopy will reveal paralysis of the diaphragm, with or without paradoxical movement of the affected side.

An increased distance between the fundal gas bubble of the stomach and the lung base may alert the clinician to either a subpulmonary effusion or a subphrenic collection on the left. Ultrasound can be used to determine whether the fluid is above or below the diaphragm, and can estimate the size of a subphrenic abscess.[30]

Rupture of the diaphragm

Rupture of the diaphragm can occur following a severe deceleration trauma, such as a road traffic accident. The mortality rate in this condition may be as high as 20–25%, which is an indication of the severity of the trauma. Rupture of the diaphragm can only be diagnosed from the plain film when there is herniation of abdominal viscera into the chest, or when fluid or air is seen to traverse the diaphragm. Seventy per cent of ruptures are on the left side,[31] and the stomach will herniate upwards. The diagnosis of herniation of the stomach can be facilitated by the passage of a nasogastric tube. Herniation of solid abdominal organs can be confirmed by ultrasound or CT. The diaphragm is readily identifiable by ultrasound, and herniation of the liver, spleen or bowel can be demonstrated through a rupture. CT will demonstrate the herniation of abdominal organs, but will not show the site of the rupture.

The chest wall

Rib fractures

Multiple rib fractures do not usually cause any diagnostic problems. A 'flail' segment may be identified, necessitating artificial ventilation. Fractures of the first three pairs of ribs indicate severe trauma, and there may be associated spinal or vascular injury. If there are clinical signs of hemorrhage and mediastinal widening, then aortography should be performed. Fractures of the lower three pairs of ribs may be associated with rupture of the liver or spleen, or with renal trauma.

Sternal fractures

Fractures of the sternum are often overlooked on frontal or oblique chest films, as they are almost or completely invisible. A lateral film of the sternum is required to make the diagnosis. Sternal fractures are usually the result of steering wheel trauma, and are of little significance of themselves, but they do indicate a significant impact. They should alert the clinician to possible mediastinal, cardiac or thoracic spinal injury.

Dehiscence of the sternum is a complication of a median sternotomy for cardiac surgery and occurs in 4–5% of cases. On the radiograph, there may be a radiolucent stripe down the center of the sternum, which represents air in the dehisced incision, and is present in approximately 36% of cases.[32]

Iatrogenic devices

Radiography provides a quick and simple method for verifying the correct positioning of various catheters, drains and leads.

Central venous catheters

Ideally, the tip of the catheter should be in the superior vena cava, above the level of its entry into the right atrium, to avoid interference with the cardiac conduction system. Central venous pressure (CVP) lines may be inserted via an antecubital, subclavian or external jugular vein. Not infrequently, the line will have been inadvertently directed into the neck from the subclavian vein, and will require repositioning.[2] This can sometimes be achieved with a brisk injection of normal saline. Subclavian venous puncture carries the risk of pneumothorax or mediastinal hematoma. Rarely, fluid may collect in the pleura. All catheters may coil, knot or fracture, leading to embolism.

Swan–Ganz catheters

The tip of the catheter should be maintained 6–8 cm beyond the bifurcation of the main pulmonary artery, in either the left or right pulmonary artery. When the wedge pressure is to be measured, a balloon at the catheter tip is inflated, and the flow of blood carries the tip peripherally until it wedges into a smaller pulmonary artery branch. Once the measurement has been made, the balloon is deflated, and the catheter returns to a more central location. Catheters of this type have a tendency to migrate peripherally into the lung, and may cause peripheral emboli and enfarction.[2] The balloon is radiolucent, and must be kept deflated to avoid the risk of thrombus formation. The position of these catheters must be monitored carefully to minimize these risks. If there is clinical suspicion of a peripheral embolus, a selective angiogram can be performed through the catheter.

Nasogastric tubes

The course of a nasogastric (NG) tube should be demonstrated to its most distal point. NG tubes may not reach the stomach, or may coil in the pharynx or esophagus. Occasionally, the tube may be inserted into the tracheobronchial tree, though usually this provokes severe reflex coughing. However, no substance should be introduced via the NG tube until correct position has been confirmed.

Endotracheal tubes

Endotracheal (ET) tubes are inserted into the trachea to access the airway for ventilation and management of secretions. There is an inflatable cuff at the tip of the tube. The chest radiograph is important in assessing the position of the tip of the ET tube, which may move on flexion and extension of the neck by up to 5 cm. The tip of the tube should ideally be 5 cm above the carina with the neck in the neutral position. If the ET tube is inserted too far, it tends to pass into the right main bronchus and hence obstruct the left main bronchus, causing collapse of the left lung (Fig. 8.2). Ischemia of the tracheal mucosa is a risk, if the inflated cuff dilates the trachea, with tracheostenosis as a late complication.

Tracheostomy tubes

Tracheostomy tubes are inserted when long-term artificial ventilation is required. The tube tip should be placed centrally in the airway at the T3 level. Complications of tracheostomy include pneumothorax, pneumomediastinum and subcutaneous emphysema.

Chest drains

Chest drainage tubes are used to treat both large pleural effusions and pneumathoraces. If the patient is supine, the tip of the tube should be placed anteriorly and superiorly to treat a pneumothorax, but posteriorly and inferiorly for a pleural effusion. If both fluid and air are present in the pleural cavity, two drainage tubes may be necessary.[2] A radio-opaque line usually runs along pleural tubes to aid identification on the chest film. This line is interrupted where there are side holes. It is important to confirm that all the side holes are within the thorax.

Failure of re-expansion of the lung, with increasing air drainage through the chest drain, indicates the likelihood of a bronchopleural fistula. The location of such a fistula can be demonstrated by injecting a water-soluble nonionic contrast medium into the drainage tube.

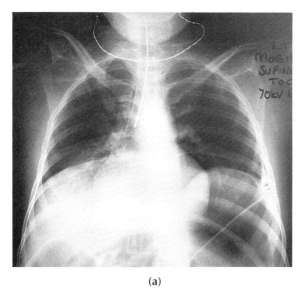
(a)

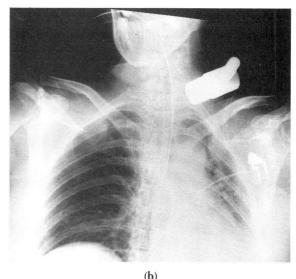
(b)

Fig. 8.2 (a) The endotracheal tube has been inserted too far and enters the right main bronchus. (b) If not corrected, this can lead to collapse of the left lung.

Pacemaker electrodes

Temporary epicardial wires may be inserted during cardiac surgery, and these are evident as thin, metallic opacities overlying the heart. Transvenous pacing electrodes are usually inserted via the subclavian route, and insertion should be performed under fluoroscopic guidance using a mobile image intensifier. The tip of the electrode should be in the region of the apex of the right ventricle, and fluorscopic guidance should avoid inadvertent placement of the electrode into the coronary vein or right ventricular outflow tract. Full assessment of the position of a pacemaker electrode requires both frontal and lateral chest films. If the patient is not pacing properly, the chest film may indicate an incorrect or unstable position of the electrode tip, or a fracture of the wire.[33]

Intra-aortic balloon pumps

Intra-aortic balloon pumps are used in patients suffering from cardiogenic shock, usually following cardiac surgery. The pump consists of a catheter, the end of which is enveloped by a long, inflatable balloon. It is inserted via the femoral artery and the balloon is positioned in the thoracic aorta. The tip of the catheter should be just distal to the origin of the left subclavian artery. If the catheter is advanced too far, the balloon will occlude the left subclavian artery. If it is not advanced far enough, branches of the abdominal aorta may be occluded. The principle of these pumps is that the timing of inflation and deflation of the balloon increases coronary perfusion during diastole, and also reduces left ventricular afterload.

THE ABDOMEN

Plain films of the abdomen are of limited use when performed using mobile equipment. Departmental films are essential when assessing the patient with an acute abdomen. Ultrasound equipment is freely mobile, and can be of great assistance for assessing abdominal problems in patients who cannot be moved from ICU. CT is also a very useful technique for assessing intra-abdominal pathology, when the patient can be moved safely. As yet, MRI is limited for abdominal work.

The acute abdomen

Bowel perforation

Departmental plain film radiography remains the mainstay for diagnosing perforation of the bowel. The essential films are a supine abdominal film and an erect chest film, which best visualizes free gas beneath the diaphragm. If the patient is too ill for an erect chest radiograph, then a film taken using a horizontal beam with the patient lying on his/her left side (left lateral decubitus) should be performed. With the patient in this position, free gas tracks between the liver and the diaphragm. The patient needs to be in the erect or decubitus position for at least 10 minutes before the film is taken, to allow small quantities of gas to accumulate. Signs of free intraperitoneal gas on the supine abdominal film include seeing both sides of the bowel wall (Wriggler's sign) and visualizing the falciform ligament of the liver (Fig. 8.3).

A water-soluble contrast agent can be given orally if perforation of the stomach or duodenum is suspected, and a water-soluble contrast enema will demonstrate a

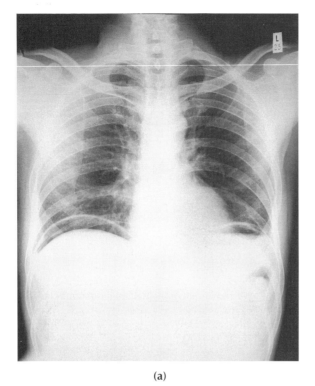

(a)

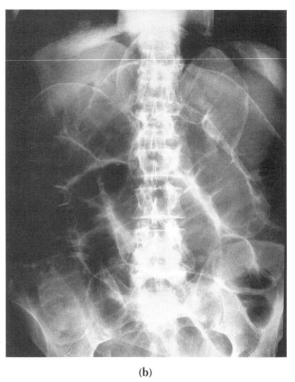

(b)

Fig. 8.3 Intestinal perforation. (a) Erect chest film. Free gas is apparent beneath the diaphragm. (b) Supine abdominal film. There is marked dilatation of small bowel, and both sides of the bowel wall are evident – Wriggler's sign.

colonic perforation. However, most patients proceed direct to laparotomy.

CT will demonstrate much smaller volumes of free peritoneal gas than does plain film radiography, but is seldom used for this. Ultrasound has little to offer.

Bowel obstruction

It has been demonstrated that the erect abdominal film does not contribute greatly in the assessment of intestinal obstruction, but does provide increased sensitivity in some cases.[34] The problem arises in deciding which patients would benefit from the erect film. In practice, some clinicians find the erect film easier to interpret than the supine film (as multiple fluid levels will be visualized) when looking for obstruction. A supine film should be performed initially, and if this is equivocal radiographically, an erect film should then be performed. The supine film only is used to follow up cases of proven obstruction.

Ultrasound examination will demonstrate dilated, fluid-filled loops of bowel throughout the abdomen. However, this technique is not the primary method of diagnosis.

Choledocholithiasis (Fig. 8.4)

Dilated bile ducts, both intra- and extra-hepatic, are easily demonstrated by ultrasound examination. With

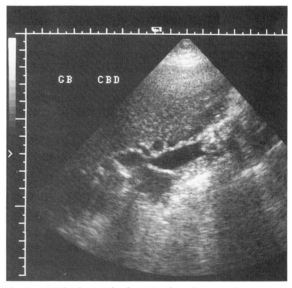

Fig. 8.4 Bile duct calculus. On this ultrasound examination of the upper abdomen, a calculus is seen within the common bile duct. Note the acoustic shadowing beyond the calculus.

newer equipment, it is usually possible to predict both the level of obstruction and its cause. A common cause of biliary obstruction, especially in the acutely symptomatic patient, is a calculus in the bile duct. The detection rate of bile duct calculi is currently in the range 75–80%.[35] The common bile duct is usually dilated, and can be traced down to the pancreatic head. A calculus will appear as an echogenic focus with acoustic shadowing. Only in about 10% of patients will the calculus be located in the proximal duct. Intra-hepatic calculi are rare, but characteristic in patients with recurrent pyogenic hepatitis.

Intra-abdominal sepsis

Acute cholecystitis/empyema

Approximately 33% of individuals with gallstones will develop acute cholecystitis. Persistant impaction of a calculus in the neck of the gallbladder or the cystic duct is the cause. The clinical manifestations of acute cholecystitis can be confusing, and the differential diagnosis includes such diverse conditions as peptic ulcer, acute appendicitis and acute pancreatitis. An ultrasound examination is the investigation of choice. Calculi will be present in the gallbladder, in association with local tenderness (the sonographic Murphy's sign).[36] The gallbladder wall may be thickened and adjacent fluid may be evident. Intraluminal echoes may be present, either as, 'sludge' or dispersed, indicating an empyema. An empyema can be drained percutaneously, using a pigtail drain, inserted under ultrasound guidance. Emphysematous cholecystitis can be demonstrated with intramural or intraluminal gas. The full extent of the gas may not be appreciated with ultrasound, so a CT scan is usually performed for confirmation. Gangrenous cholecystitis and gallbladder perforation can both be demonstrated by ultrasound.

Acalculus cholecystitis occurs in 5–10% of patients with acute cholecystitis. Sonographic detection of this condition is hampered by the lack of gallstones, but the other signs of acute cholecystitis will be present. Cholescintigraphy is of limited value. It has a high sensitivity for diagnosing acalculus cholecystitis (90–95%), but an unacceptably low specificity (38%).[37]

Intra-abdominal abscesses

Subphrenic abscesses usually occur in the postoperative patient, as a result of intraoperative sepsis. Occasionally, they can occur as a complication of a traumatic pneumomediastinum. Pelvic abscesses can occur postoperatively, or following pelvic inflammatory disease. Abscesses also occur as a complication of diverticular disease of the colon.

Abscess cavities appear as echo-poor or echo-free mass lesions on ultrasound, displacing adjacent structures. Abscesses can be drained percutaneously using ultrasound to guide the placement of a pigtail drainage catheter.

Occasionally, gas within an abscess can be recognized on a plain abdominal radiograph, although this is often retrospectively.

CT is a very sensitive technique for demonstrating abscess cavities within the abdomen and pelvis, and the image is not degraded by bowel gas, which can be a problem with ultrasound.

Acute appendicitis

In the overwhelming majority of normal individuals the appendix is not visible on ultrasound examination. The demonstration of an inflamed appendix may therefore aid the diagnosis in equivocal cases. The inflamed appendix has a target-like appearance in cross-section, and a serpiginous appearance in longitudinal section. An appendix abscess or periappendiceal phlegmon is easily visualized, though CT is superior in distinguishing between them. Both CT and ultrasound can be used to guide percutaneous drainage techniques.

Ultrasound may also identify an alternative pathology to appendicitis, e.g. pelvic inflammatory disease, endometriosis, ectopic pregnancy or ovarian cyst.[38]

Acute gastrointestinal hemorrhage

Finding the source of bleeding from the gastrointestinal tract can be a difficult and time-consuming task. Investigation of upper gastrointestinal hemorrhage is usually endoscopy or barium study, though scintigraphy may be useful. For a lower gastrointestinal hemorrhage, investigations may include colonoscopy, angiography and nuclear medicine studies. The endoscopist's view may be impaired by active hemorrhage, but this is necessary for scintigraphy or angiography. Angiography is usually reserved for situations in which active bleeding has been confirmed, and interventional procedures (e.g. embolization) may be of benefit in controlling the hemorrhage.[39]

Renal disease

Many patients in the ICU will have some impairment of renal function. It is important to distinguish obstructive uropathy from renal parenchymal disease. Ultrasound examination will readily identify a hydronephrosis, and can be used to guide the placement of a nephostomy tube. Injection of contrast medium into the nephrostomy tube (nephrostogram) can be performed to identify the site, and possibly the cause, of the obstruction. Renal parenchymal disease may cause increased echogenicity of the renal cortex and loss of corticomedullary differentiation. The Doppler signal from the renal artery changes in character with renal parenchymal disease, but it can be very difficult to obtain a satisfactory signal from the renal artery. Duplex scanning is very useful in assessing the transplant kidney, because of easier access.

Acute renal artery embolism is a surgically correctable cause of acute renal failure. While ultrasound may identify cortical infarcts within the kidney, isotope renography will demonstrate the lack of perfusion more readily.[39]

Aortic aneurysm

Rupture of an abdominal aortic aneurysm carries a very high mortality, as the patient succumbs before medical treatment is available. However, some aneurysms will leak into the retroperitoneum, giving a localized hematoma, at least for a while. Occasionally, the hematoma will wall off, giving a pseudoaneurysm. The patient will present with abdominal pain and shock. Sonography will demonstrate aortic aneurysms with ease, and in most cases the position relative to the renal artery origins. A retroperitoneal hemorrhage or hematoma will also be shown. Contrast-enhanced CT will also demonstrate the aneurysm, and may show the extent of hemorrhage more accurately (Fig. 8.5). However, if a

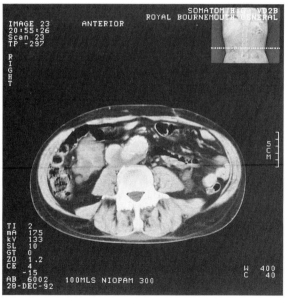

Fig. 8.5 Ruptured aortic aneurysm. Contrast-enhanced CT scan of abdomen. Contrast-enhanced blood is seen to extravaste from the aortic lumen, causing a retroperitoneal hematoma, which displaces the IVC to the right.

leaking aortic aneurysm has been demonstrated sonographically, performing a CT scan, with its consequent delay, cannot be justified.

Blunt abdominal trauma

Both ultrasound examination and CT scanning have a place in the assessment of the patient who has suffered blunt abdominal trauma. Most trauma victims with abdominal injuries only will survive long enough to receive medical care. These patients may die as a result of inadequate intravascular volume replacement or unrecognized abdominal injuries. Ultrasound is quick and mobile, so can be used in the resuscitation room if required. Its main disadvantage is the problem of bowel gas, which may be copious in trauma patients, since this may limit the visualization of some internal organs. CT can identify injuries to all abdominal organs, evaluate the retroperitoneum and identify fractures of the spine or pelvis. However, serious injuries can have subtle manifestations on the CT examination, so meticulous technique and attention to detail are essential.

The spleen is the most commonly injured organ in blunt abdominal trauma.[40] Ultrasound can readily identify a splenic rupture and associated hemorrhage (Fig. 8.6). CT is also very accurate in diagnosing splenic

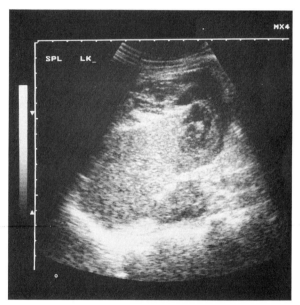

Fig. 8.6 Ruptured spleen. This ultrasound examination demonstrates a laceration in the tip of the spleen, with a surrounding hematoma.

injury, with sensitivities and specificities above 95%. The liver is the next most frequently injured organ. Lacerations can be hard to identify on both ultrasound and CT. Subcapsular and intrahepatic hematomas are much easier to identify. Renal injuries occur in approximately 10% of patients with blunt abdominal trauma. CT is more sensitive than excretion urography in the detection of renal injuries, and is superior in assessing the extent and geometry of the injury.[41] CT is also superior in identifying associated injuries to adjacent structures, as occurs in 10–20% of cases. Bladder injuries are usually assessed using retrograde cystography, but if abdominal CT is being performed for other injuries, the bladder can be adequately examined also.

THE HEAD

The development of CT in the past decades has had a great impact on the evaluation of acute cerebral episodes and head trauma. MRI is gaining ground in many areas, but CT maintains its pre-eminent position for evaluating acute head injury because of the difficulty in monitoring the acutely and severely injured patient during an MRI scan. However, CT underestimates the severity of many types of cerebral trauma, especially brain stem injury, nonhemorrhagic cortical contusions and diffuse axonal injury.[42]

Head injury

Skull fracture

Good plain film radiography of the skull will identify the vast majority of cranial vault fractures. Basal skull fractures are more difficult to identify, and fluid levels in the paranasal sinuses or opacification of the mastoid air cells may be the only signs visible on plain films. The standard skull series consists of three views, the frontal, the Towne's and the lateral. More than 90% of vault fractures will be visible on the lateral film, so this is the most important film to obtain if there is difficulty. The presence of a skull fracture may indicate a more severe intracranial injury, and such patients should be admitted for observation. However, if neurological symptoms or signs develop, a CT scan is indicated, whether or not a skull fracture is present.

Extradural hematoma

An extradural hematoma is a collection of blood in the potential space between the inner table of the skull and the dura. Such hematomas are usually lenticular (biconvex) in shape and have a high attenuation value on CT. They may be associated with cerebral contusion and subdural collections.[43] The middle meningeal artery is usually the source of hemorrhage. The mass effect caused by an extradural hematoma in the posterior fossa can be rapidly life-threatening.

Subdural hematoma

Subdural hematomas arise in the space between the dura and arachnoid membranes. These hematomas are usually crescentic in shape, though other configurations can occur if adhesions are present. In the elderly, subdural hematomas can occur after a trivial injury. Subdural collections may cause a marked mass effect.

On CT scans, acute subdurals appear hyperdense, but chronic subdurals are hypodense. At a critical time in their evolution, subdural collections will be isodense with the adjacent brain, and evident only by their mass effect. Not surprisingly, bilateral isodense subdurals are easily overlooked. The appearance of subdural collections on MRI depends not only on the stage of evolution, but also on the pulse sequence used.

Intracerebral hematoma

Intraparenchymal hematomas may be isolated, or associated with other injuries. On CT, these hematomas are high-attenuation, rounded or irregular collections of blood within the brain, sometimes with surrounding, low-attenuation edema. The hematoma may enlarge in the immediate post-traumatic period and liquefaction may occur. Hematomas usually appear as high-signal lesions on T2-weighted MR images.

Contusions

Contusions are parenchymal lacerations, with associated hemorrhage. Lesions are usually cortical, or near the gray-white matter junction. Bland contusions appear as ill-defined low-attenuation areas on CT, but these lesions may become hemorrhagic at a later stage, with areas of high attenuation appearing. MRI is more sensitive at detecting hemorrhage within an area of contusion.[42]

Cerebral edema

Cerebral edema is invariably present in traumatic brain injury. On CT, there is loss of normal differentiation between gray and white matter, and the attenuation is lower than that of normal brain. There may also be cerebral swelling, with loss of the cortical sulci and compression, and possibly obliteration, of the ventricles and subarachnoid cisterns.

Diffuse axonal injury

After severe head trauma, patients may present in a comatose state, despite a relatively benign-appearing CT examination. Close examination of the scan may reveal diffuse cerebral swelling with small petechial hemorrhages in the white matter. This is the appearance of diffuse axonal or shear injury, usually due to rapid acceleration–deceleration forces. MRI is much more sensitive in the detection of diffuse axonal injury, and is better for assessing its extent.[42] Lesions are small, located entirely within the white matter and of high signal on T2-weighted images. MR imaging should be performed when there is a significant disparity between the patient's clinical state and the CT examination.

Brain stem injuries

Brain stem trauma can be difficult to visualize on CT scans due to the bone artefact that occurs in the posterior fossa. MR images are far superior in assessing the brain stem, especially as the majority of injuries are diffuse axonal injuries.

Subarachnoid hemorrhage (Fig. 8.7)

Cranial trauma is the most common cause of sub-arachnoid hemorrhage, and subarachnoid blood is invariably present following significant head trauma, though it may not be a prominent feature on the CT

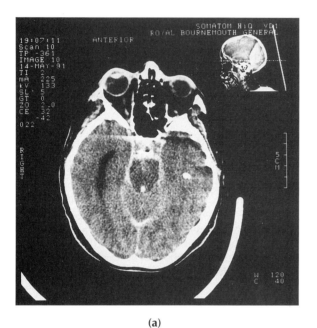

(a)

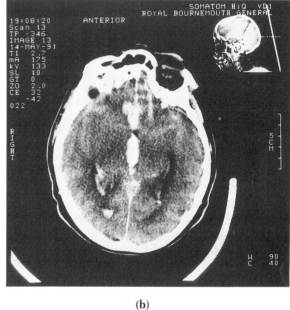

(b)

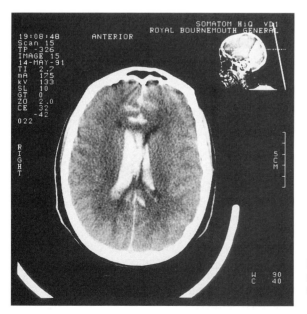

(c)

Fig. 8.7 Subarachnoid hemorrhage. CT scan of brain (three levels). High-attenuation (white) blood is present around the brain stem (a), in the third ventricle (b) and in the lateral ventricles (c).

images.[44] However, a significant number of subarachnoid hemorrhages occur spontaneously, often following rupture of an aneurysm. Blood appears as high-attenuation material within the cerebrospinal fluid spaces, and layering may occur. The distribution of blood may give a clue to the site of the aneurysm. Intravenous contrast enhancement to try to visualize the aneurysm is not indicated, as the patient should be transferred to a neurosurgical center for carotid and vertebral arteriography.

In demonstrating an acute subarachnoid hemorrhage, MRI is nowhere near as sensitive as CT.

Cerebral infarction

Cerebral infarction results from the disturbance of blood supply to a region of brain. Most infarcts are spontaneous, due to pre-existing vascular disease, but infarcts may also be the result of trauma (including neurosurgery). They may be either hemorrhagic or nonhemorrhagic in nature. Hemorrhagic infarcts result from spontaneous hemorrhage from an intracranial vessel. The resulting hematoma will appear on CT as a high-attenuation collection of blood, surrounded by low-attenuation edema. Nonhemorrhagic infarcts are due to thrombotic or embolic phenomena and appear as low-attenuation areas in the distribution of the affected artery. Occasionally it can be difficult to differentiate between a resolving hemorrhagic infarct and a neoplastic lesion on a plain CT scan. Neoplastic lesions are likely to enhance to a much greater extent than infarcts, but intravenous contrast medium can extend an infarct in the acute phase, so the contrast-enhanced scan should be delayed into the recovery phase.

Small lacunar infarcts imply embolic episodes, for which a cause should be sought. If carotid artery disease is suspected, a duplex ultrasound scan of these vessels should be performed.

Conclusion

The advances in imaging technology over the past two decades have resulted in a vast improvement in the investigations available to assess the critically ill patient. In the first section of this chapter, we have outlined the equipment and investigations now available. In the second section, we have tried to show which examinations are appropriate for investigating the various conditions which may be encountered. Many of the technologies are complex, so close collaboration is required between the clinician in charge of the patient and the radiologist to ensure appropriate use of the facilities available.

References

1. Kumar AB, Frisby JR. Imaging techniques in intensive care. In: Oh TE (ed.) *Intensive Care Manual*, 3rd edn. Sydney: Butterworths, 1990: 594–608.
2. Ovenfors CO, Hedgcock MW. Intensive care unit radiology. *Radiol Clin North Am* 1978; **16**: 407–39.
3. Underwood GH, Newell JD. Pulmonary radiology in the intensive care unit. *Med Clin North Am* 1983; **67**: 1305–24.
4. Forster E. Equipment for mobile, dental, accident and skull radiography. In: *Equipment for Diagnostic Radiography*. Lancaster: MTP Press Limited, 1985: 118–29.
5. Clark KC. Respiratory system. In: *Positioning in Radiography*, 9th edn. London: William Heinemann Ltd, 1973: 344–70.
6. Jennings P, Padley SPG, Hansell DM. Portable chest radiography in intensive care: a comparison of computed and conventional radiography. *Br J Radiol* 1992; **65**: 852–6.
7. *Guidance Notes for the Protection of Persons against Ionising Radiations arising from Medical and Dental Use*. Oxford: National Radiation Protection Board, 1988.
8. *The Ionising Radiation (Protection of Persons Undergoing Medical Examination or Treatment) Regulations*. London: Her Majesty's Stationery Office, 1985 and 1988.
9. Lees WR. Ultrasound. In: Sutton D (ed.) *A Textbook of Radiology and Imaging, 4th edn.* London: Churchill Livingstone, 1987: 1773–1809.
10. Isherwood I, Forbes WStC, Griffin JF. CT scanning: the body. In: Sutton D (ed.) *A Textbook of Radiology and Imaging, 4th edn*. London: Churchill Livingstone, 1987: 1691–1737.
11. Isherwood I, Jenkins JPR. MRI: technical aspects – CNS and spine. In: Sutton D (ed.) *A Textbook of Radiology and Imaging, 4th edn*. London: Churchill Livingstone, 1987: 1654–90.
12. Donaldson RM. Nuclear imaging. In: Tinker J, Rapin M (eds) *Care of the Critically Ill Patient*. Berlin: Springer-Verlag, 1983: 985–1004.
13. Scanlon GT, Unger JD. The radiology of bacterial and viral pneumonias. *Radiol Clin North Am* 1973; **11**: 317–37.
14. Westermark N. On the Roentgen diagnosis of lung embolism. *Acta Radiol* 1938; **19**: 357–72.
15. Williams JRK, Wilcock WC. Pulmonary embolism: Roentgenographic and angiographic considerations. *Am J Roentgenol* 1963; **89**: 333–42.
16. Secker-Walker RH. Nuclear medicine in lung disease. In: *Special Procedures in Chest Radiology*. Philadelphia: WB Saunders, 1976.
17. Bynum LJ, Pierce AK. Pulmonary aspiration of gastric contents. *Am Rev Respir Dis* 1976; **114**: 1129–36.

18. Kabala J, Wilde P. Unpublished data.
19. Dee PM. The radiology of chest trauma. *Radiol Clin North Am* 1992; **30**: 291–306.
20. Hudson LD. Causes of adult respiratory distress syndrome – clinical recognition. *Clini Chest Med* 1982; **3**: 195–212.
21. Putman CE, Ravin CE. Adult respiratory distress syndrome. In: Goodman LR, Putman CE (eds) *Intensive Care Radiology*. 1978.
22. Ovenfors CO. Pulmonary interstitial emphysema. *Acta Radiol* 1964; **224** (Suppl.).
23. Gundry SR, Burney RE, MacKenzie JR *et al*. Assessment of mediastinal widening associated with traumatic rupture of the aorta. *J Trauma* 1983; **23**: 293–9.
24. Gundry SR, Burney RE, MacKenzie JR *et al*. Traumatic pseudoaneurysms of the thoracic aorta. *Arch Surg* 1984; **119**: 1055–60.
25. Tisnado J, Tsai FY, Ais A *et al*. A new radiographic sign of acute traumatic rupture of the thoracic aorta: displacement of the nasogastric tube to the right. *Radiology* 1977; **125**: 603–8.
26. Richardson P, Mirvis S, Scorpio R *et al*. Value of CT in determining the need for angiography when findings of mediastinal hemorrhage are equivocal. *Am J Roentgenol* 1991; **156**: 273–9.
27. Tottle AJ, Wilde P, Hartnell GG, Wisheart JD. Diagnosis of acute thoracic aortic dissection using combined echocardiography and computed tomography. *Clin Radiol* 1992; **45**: 104–8.
28. Rhea JT, Van Sommerberg E, McLoud TC. Basilar pneumothorax in the supine adult. *Radiology* 1979; **133**: 593–5.
29. McGonigal MD, Schwab CW, Kauder DR *et al*. Supplemented emergent chest computed tomography in the management of blunt torso trauma. *J Trauma* 1990; **30**: 1431–5.
30. Landry M, Harless W. Ultrasonic differentiation of right pleural effusion from subphrenic fluid on longitudinal scans of the right upper quadrant: importance of recognising the diaphragm. *Radiology* 1977; **123**: 155–8.
31. Arendrup HC, Jensen BS. Traumatic rupture of the diaphragm. *Surg Gynaecol Obstet* 1982; **154**: 526–30.
32. Berkow AE, Demos TC. The midsternal stripe and its relationship to postoperative sternal dehiscence. *Radiology* 1976; **125**: 525.
33. Grier D, Cook PG, Hartnell GG. Chest radiographs after permanent pacing. Are they really necessary? *Clin Radiol* 1990; **42**: 244–9.
34. Field S, Guy PJ, Upsdell SM, Scourfield AE. The erect abdominal radiograph in the acute abdomen: should its routine use be abandoned? *Br Med J* 1985; **290**: 1934–6.
35. Dong B, Chen M. Improved sonographic visualisation of choledocholithiasis. *J Clin Ultrasound* 1987; **15**: 185–90.
36. Ralls PW, Colletti PM, Lapin SA *et al*. Real time sonography in suspected acute cholecystitis. *Radiology* 1985; **155**: 767–71.
37. Mirvis SE, Vainright JR, Nelson AW *et al*. The diagnosis of acute acalculus cholecystitis: a comparison of sonography, scintigraphy and computed tomography. *Am J Roentgenol* 1986; **147**: 1171–5.
38. Laing FC. Ultrasonography of the acute abdomen. *Radiol Clin North Am* 1992; **30**: 389–404.
39. Parekh JS, Teates CD. Emergency nuclear medicine. *Radiol Clin North Am* 1992; **30**: 455–74.
40. Rosoff L, Cohen JL, Telfer N *et al*. Injuries of the spleen. *Surg Clin North Am* 1972; **52**: 667–85.
41. Gay SB, Sistrom CL. Computed tomographic evaluation of blunt abdominal trauma. *Radiol Clin North Am* 1992; **30**: 367–88.
42. Sklar EML, Quencer RM, Bowen BC *et al*. Magnetic resonance applications in cerebral injury. *Radiol Clin North Am* 1992; **30**: 353–66.
43. Tapiero B, Richer E, Laurent F *et al*. Post-traumatic extradural hematomas. *J Neuroradiol* 1984; **11**: 213–26.
44. Johnson MH, Lee SH. Computed tomography of acute cerebral trauma. *Radiol Clin North Am* 1992; **30**: 325–52.

CHAPTER 9

Intensive Care Laboratory

ROHINI NAIDOO, DOMINIC JA COX

Summary   123
Does the unit need its own laboratory facilities?   123
Staffing   124
Standards   124
Quality assurance and control   126
Equipment   128
Conclusion   131
References   132

Summary

The advances in technology which have enabled ventilators to become lung function laboratories and ECG monitors to diagnose cardiac disarrythmias, have also made complex clinical pathology testing possible at the bedside of the critically ill patient. This change has been brought about by the development of solid phase chemistry, electronics, microprocessors, enzyme and ion selective electrodes, biosensors and the simplification and miniaturization of the components making up the instruments. Most tests require less than 0.5 ml of whole blood and a minimum of technical expertise on the part of the operator. However, just because a test is easier to perform, this does not necessarily mean that it is either clinically justified, more useful, more accurate or more easily interpreted.

The more technically unskilled the personnel who use the equipment, the more rigorous the quality control and assurance has to be. It is the purpose of this chapter to recognize that 'near patient testing' or 'bedside biochemistry' is here to stay and is a very real step forward in the treatment of the critically ill. However, it requires careful planning and an almost obsessional attention to detail by those providing the service.[1] There are certain minimum standards which must be followed by the intensive care laboratory if it is to become a viable reality. It is recommended that when ever possible, compliance with standards established by national accrediting agencies must be met.

Does the unit need its own laboratory facilities?

Any evaluation of intensive care utilization, be it staffing costs or numbers of Swan–Ganz catheters used, must review cost benefit analysis (CBA) and cost-effectiveness analysis (CEA). Quality is not always the opposite of efficiency. An intensive care unit which captures economies of scale may render high-quality services at lower cost. Furthermore, doing things correctly the first time is cheaper than doing things incorrectly or unnecessarily.[2] The objective of CBA is to maximize net benefits, i.e. costs discounted over time. The objective of CEA is to place in order the preferred alternatives for reaching a goal. Thus CEA can only indicate which of the alternatives is the more cost-effective; it cannot determine whether the benefit is worth the cost.

The purpose of intensive care has been defined as 'the

reduction of avoidable mortality and morbidity in those who are critically ill.'[2] The quicker the laboratory results are obtained, the nearer to 'real-time' monitoring and thus treatment of biochemical or haematological variables can be. If, by reducing the 'turn around time' of samples, there is a concurrent reduction in avoidable morbidity or mortality, then a cost benefit analysis would justify setting up a 'stat' laboratory in intensive care.

'Turn around time' must not be confused with analytical laboratory time, which may well be only a matter of minutes for urgent specimens. The turn around time is the time from a sample being obtained from the patient to the moment when the resulting information from that sample is acted upon clinically. Zaloga[3] recently reported a typical therapeutic turn around time of greater than 3 hours for sodium and potassium in a university hospital intensive care unit (ICU), the laboratory component of which was 7 minutes. The therapeutic turn around time for the same tests in our own intensive care laboratory is approximately 2 minutes, with the added benefit of a significantly smaller sample size and thus a reduction in iatrogenic anaemia.[4]

Having established a need for the 'on site' 'stat' or 'satellite' laboratory in the ICU (known from now on as the 'intensive care laboratory'), four main issues should be addressed. These are:

1. staffing
2. standards
3. quality assurance and control
4. equipment and tests required

Staffing

One of the fundamental reasons for siting the laboratory as near to the patient as possible is the need for urgent results in acute or emergency situations. For this reason the results are inevitably going to be used clinically, without being subjected to the scrutiny and validation normally carried out by clinical laboratories before results are released to clinicians. However, someone has to take the responsibility for subsequently scrutinizing and validating the results of these tests. This person must be skilled in analytical procedures and interpretation in order to highlight problems with the test procedures at an early stage. Depending upon the workload of the intensive care unit, this person could be co-opted as a 'visiting expert' from the main pathology laboratory or could be permanently on the intensive care unit staff. UK accreditation standards demand that this person be a medical consultant (qualified in pathology) or clinical scientist of equivalent status.[5]

Current practice in the UK is to allow medical and nursing staff direct access to the very carefully chosen analytical devices on the intensive care unit, thus the tests are carried out by the clinical staff who are directly involved with the care of the patient. In other European countries, for instance France, this would be illegal. The role of the clinical scientist or responsible clinical pathologist is to train these technically unskilled users in terms of safe practice and to educate them regarding quality control and assurance. He/she must also be available to troubleshoot any technical problems which arise and also take responsibility for running both the internal and external quality assurance schemes. On our own unit the clinical scientists are responsible for the choice of equipment, the training of medical and nursing staff, and the overall laboratory performance, safety and quality control. They are also responsible for other aspects of medical technology applied to the critically ill, including monitoring and ventilation technology, audit, research and education. The laboratory component of their work would typically take up about a third of their workload.

It is essential that whoever is employed is qualified to the appropriate level and has the authority to intervene and shut down the facilities if standards cannot be maintained.

Standards

This type of laboratory is not going to be used by fully trained and qualified analysts most of the time, and so it is particularly important that it meets the standards required by routine pathology laboratories for accreditation by the relevant supervising body (Clinical Pathology Accreditation in the UK, Clinical Laboratory Clinical Amendments of 1988, Joint Commission on Accreditation of Health Care Organization, College of American Pathologists in USA).[6,7] The standards can be subdivided as follows:

ORGANIZATION AND ADMINISTRATION

1. There should be a laboratory handbook documenting procedures and use of instrumentation. This need not be overlong or complicated. Some explanation of laboratory philosophy should be included stressing importance of quality control to nonexpert analysts. Each member of staff allowed access to the laboratory should be given a copy of the booklet at the end of their introductory training.
2. There should be a documented line of managerial and scientific responsibility for the laboratory.
3. There should be formal arrangements for meetings

between senior laboratory staff (or responsible person) and institutional management.

4. There should be at least an annual review of the service, including future objectives and audit, and budget requirements.

STAFFING AND DIRECTION

1. The laboratory should be professionally directed by a suitably qualified medical consultant or clinical scientist of equivalent status.
2. There should be orientation and induction of new staff (medical, nursing, and domestic) regarding health and safety and Control of Substances Hazardous to Health (COSHH), or other relevant requirements.
3. Regular minuted meetings which may be part of the routine intensive care staff meetings should be held to reinforce health and safety and discuss problems.
4. Fire drills should be carried out.

FACILITIES AND EQUIPMENT

1. Appropriate office and laboratory space should be provided. Wherever possible the office should be separate from the laboratory area. Food and drink must never be taken into the laboratory area. The laboratory space must be consistent with safe working practices for the services offered.
2. Preventive maintenance programs must be carried out for all instruments to meet the manufacturers' requirements. Preventive maintenance is not just a biannual service visit by the service engineer. It is a requirement under the Consumer Protection Act 1988 in the UK.[8]
3. There should be appropriate facilities for data storage and retrieval. If this data is held on computer then the laboratory must be registered under the Data Protection Act (UK only). There should be adequate facilities for communication of results, e.g. telephone, intercom, etc.
4. There should be appropriate, properly maintained scientific equipment to meet the demands of the service. This includes the provision of relevantly trained staff for any specialist equipment. All equipment should conform to current health and safety requirements, and there should be a planned replacement programme.[9] Manufacturer's user manuals should be available.
5. Lighting, heating, wipe-clean lab tops, and facilities for the proper disposal of specimens should be to an approved standard.
6. There should be adequate storage space for reagents and records. Acids, caustics and corrosives will all need to be kept and where necessary will need to be stored in accordance with local regulations (COSHH in UK). Refrigerators and freezers should be dedicated to the laboratory and not used for anything else.
7. All staff should be required to wear gloves, and these should be provided in various sizes close to each analyzer. All should wear disposable plastic aprons or an approved alternative and where necessary should wear protective goggles. Most intensive care nurses will be experienced in handling patient specimens and body fluids and protecting themselves by the sensible application of 'universal precautions.' Medical staff may need more encouragement regarding the rudiments of laboratory safety. Instructions on action to take upon blood spillage and decontamination of the area should be available, as should the appropriate disinfectant/decontaminant. Needles should NEVER be brought into the lab area on the end of syringes (or any other way). 'Sharps boxes' should be provided for safe disposal of specimens and syringes.

POLICIES AND PROCEDURES

As mentioned earlier, all members of staff who are authorized to use the laboratory will have been given a handbook in which the policies and procedures should address the following issues:

1. If the laboratory is required to analyze samples from outside the ICU then the system of labelling the samples, requests for procedures, identifying the doctor requesting the test, etc. should conform to that of the main laboratory.
2. Reports of results should include adequate patient identification, time and date, and when relevant a validation record. Most instruments will have a printer with all this information generated automatically (except patient ID).
3. There should be written policies relating to specimen collection, handling and disposal. These should concur with the requirements of the 'universal precautions' policy of the unit. The advice of the infection control team in the hospital may be helpful in this context.
4. If the hospital is a major accident reception center the policy and procedure document should be easily accessible.
5. There should be a written record of all reagents, calibration and quality control materials.
6. There should be a written protocol for the performance of each test. When appropriate this should include the preparation of the equipment and sample, specify the reagents used, outline any calculations required for the interpretation of the results, and an interpretation of the internal quality

control procedures. All test procedures should be carried out according to the manufacturer's instructions. Failure to comply with this could mean that the instrument warranty is invalidated.

7. There should be a written procedure for the reporting of results of each test. There should also be a written document of validation, procedures and reference ranges. Additionally data on potential pitfalls or interferences with test results should be available.

8. There should be written procedures for the regular maintenance of equipment, identifying the member of staff responsible if necessary.

9. There should be a written procedure for the decontamination of all items of equipment and the working space.

10. The whole point of having a laboratory, or laboratory equipment, in the ICU is that it should be available for use 24 hours a day. There should be a written policy describing the procedure for dealing with breakdowns at times when the responsible person in charge of the equipment is not on duty.

STAFF DEVELOPMENT AND EDUCATION

1. There should be a written program of training for all members for staff (medical, nursing, technical, and scientific) to include:

   ● Health and safety matters related to specimens, equipment, and reagents.
   ● Aspects of patient confidentiality.
   ● The use of individual pieces of equipment, the performance of analytical procedures and the relevance of results to the patient's clinical condition.

2. There should be an appropriate site for training and continuing education – this would normally be part of the staff facilities of the unit generally.

3. There should be opportunities for staff responsible for the laboratory to attend seminars, meetings and conferences, as part of a continuing education program.

4. There should be an established staff appraisal scheme.

EVALUATION

1. The unit laboratory should take part in a national external quality control scheme (NEQAS).

2. There should be a formal review of NEQAS and internal quality control results. Nurses and medical staff must be included in this review.

3. There should be a formal clinical audit of the service. Turn round times should be monitored, clinical users

should be asked about their understanding of results and their impression of the laboratory service should be sought.

4. The intensive care laboratory staff should help and participate in audit of other clinical specialities where appropriate.

Quality assurance and control

Quality assurance (QA) is the name given to a wide range of practices which allow a laboratory to achieve predefined analytical goals. It involves identifying and minimizing errors in each step of the analytical process from patient preparation before taking a sample through to result interpretation. *Quality control* (QC) is the term which describes the day-to-day techniques and practices that are used to monitor how well a particular method for measuring a blood analyte is performing.

In order for a QA policy to work in ICU laboratories it is necessary to have adequate financial resources and facilities in addition to trained staff who are technically competent and able to deal with any problems that may arise. In addition, QA procedures need to be in constant use and practiced by all staff members.[10]

QUALITY ASSURANCE PROCEDURES

Errors can be introduced at any stage of the analytical process and so there has to be some means of controlling these possible sources of error.

Control of pre-analytical variables

Pre-analytical variables include the following:

1. Correct patient identification and preparation
2. Adequate flushing of arterial lines prior to sampling
3. Adequate specimen collection into an appropriate container with the correct preservative or anticoagulant.
4. Correct specimen identification
5. Turn around time.

In smaller ICU laboratories these are not significant problems as the nursing and medical staff analyze blood samples as and when appropriate, but an emphasis has to be placed on adequate and thorough training of all staff members with respect to sample collection and analysis. In addition, there has to be a standard protocol concerning volumes of sample to be collected, volumes of liquid anticoagulant used, timing, etc. In larger laboratories staffed by a number of technical staff, pre-analytical errors are a more important consideration and should be controlled by the use of sample labelling, worksheets and log books.

Control of analytical variables

Method selection and evaluation

The most important factor in achieving quality control is the selection and evaluation of the analytical method to be used. An analytical method needs to be assessed for:

1. Accuracy or bias, which is the agreement between the best estimate of a quantity and its true value.
2. Precision (expressed as coefficient of variation, %CV), which means how well replicate measurements agree. It highlights random errors, since it measures how much scatter there is between results.
3. Specificity, which is the ability of a method to measure only the analyte that it is supposed to measure and not other substances.
4. Sensitivity, which is the smallest result distinguishable from a blank sample with 95% probability. At this point the measurement is possible but it may be inaccurate.[11,12]

In addition to these, the speed of analysis, the sample volume required, the cost of the technical skill required for an analysis and how robust a method is, also need to be considered.

Control materials

In order to check whether an analytical method is performing well and providing correct results, a control material is used. This is a specimen which has known concentrations of the analytes being measured and it is analyzed in the same way as patient samples using the selected instruments and methods. The observed value obtained for that control sample is then compared to an expected value, this being either a range of acceptable values or upper and lower limits for the control material (control limits).

An ideal control material would have the properties listed below:

1. stable over long periods of time
2. available in aliquots or vials that can be analyzed periodically
3. little vial to vial variation
4. same matrix as the test specimen
5. concentration of analytes should cover normal and abnormal ranges.

In the case of blood gas analysis it is not possible to achieve these properties with serum samples and so manufacturers of blood gas machines provide vials of aqueous quality control materials for their equipment, which cover the acidotic, normal and alkalotic ranges seen clinically. Other analytes, such as electrolytes and enzymes, require a quality control material which is serum based. There are a number of commercial companies that supply lyophilized quality control sera, which the user makes up into a liquid form with an accurately measured volume of deionized or sterile water. The quality control material is analyzed daily in the case of blood gases and in the case of other analytes, should ideally be analyzed with each sample or batch of ten samples.

Quality control charts

A quality control chart is an easy way of comparing the observed values obtained for quality control materials with the expected values. It consists of a graph of the observed value plotted against time, with the upper and lower control limits for a control material clearly indicated. When the method is performing well, the observed values lie within the control limits, but as soon as the values fall outside these control limits, it serves as an indication to a possible problem with the method, which should then be identified and corrected. To prepare a control chart, the control material is analyzed at least 20 times. The control limits are determined by calculating the standard deviation (SD) using the equation:

$$SD = \sqrt{\left(\frac{\sum x_i^2 - [(\sum x_i)^2/n]}{n - 1}\right)}$$

where x_i is the individual measurement and n is the number of measurements made.

The control limits are most commonly set to include either 95 or 99% of the control sample measurements, i.e. 2SD or 3SD respectively, assuming that the distribution of error of the control values follow a normal Gaussian pattern. Each time the control sample is analyzed (daily or with each batch), the value obtained or a statistic derived from the value, depending on the type of chart used, is plotted. There are a variety of chart types but for ICU purposes the easiest to use are the Levey–Jennings control chart and the cumulative sum control chart.

Levey–Jennings control chart

The individual control values are plotted against time for each analyte. The control limits are set at ±3SD if there are two or more control observations and ±2SD if there is only one control observation. With this chart, if a value falls outside the control limits it indicates a possible problem with a method.[13]

Cumulative sum control chart (CUSUM)

The difference between the observed value and the expected value is calculated for the control sample and this difference is added to the cusum of the previous day, and the product is plotted. The chart is interpreted by looking at the angle of the cusum line. The steeper the angle, the more out of control the method, thus systematic errors are detected.[14]

External quality assurance

In addition to the day-to-day analysis of control materials to check that methods are working well, an intensive care laboratory should also participate in a regional or national external quality assurance scheme (EQAS) if it measures analytes such as electrolytes, liver and cardiac enzymes and drug levels. The reason for this is that internal quality control detects and distinguishes between daily systematic and random errors, but does not assess the laboratory performance, which EQA does. The way an EQA scheme works is outlined below.

Identical specimens are distributed once or twice monthly by the scheme organizers to participating laboratories, who then analyze the specimens for the various analytes using their routine methods and handling them in the same way they do patient samples. The results are then returned to the scheme organizers who statistically analyze the results together with results from other laboratories in the country using the same methods and equipment. Finally the EQAS organizers return a summary report to the individual laboratory with results expressed in a number of ways:

1. Histograms showing the distribution of results.
2. Levey–Jennings charts for each analyte showing deviations from the mean.
3. Mean values for all methods combined, each method group and the individuals method.
4. SD or coefficient of variation (CV) for all methods combined, each method group and the individuals method. This allows the performance of individual laboratories to be seen in relation to others.
5. Variance index score (VIS). This acts as a monitor of bias or systematic error from the method mean in addition to imprecision; however, the degree to which each of these contribute to the error is not known.
6. Mean running variance index score (MRVIS). This is the VIS for the last ten results which can be plotted graphically. This score monitors changes in performance with time but it is insensitive to single poor results.

In addition to monitoring laboratory performance, the EQA scheme should also act as an advisory body to the participating laboratories with respect to improving their performance and hence the quality of results.[15]

Control of postanalytical variables

Once a sample has been analyzed there is still room for error in terms of result reporting and interpretation. When looking at patient results the user of the intensive care laboratory should be aware of the variety of factors that influence the result. These are summarized below:

1. Age and sex of the patient.
2. Nutritional status and temperature.
3. The method and time of sampling.
4. Interference from drugs, either due to the pharmacological action of a drug or drug metabolite on a test component or as a result of chemical interference of a drug or drug metabolite with the actual method for measuring that test component.[16,17]
5. Hemolysis. Since whole blood samples are nearly always analyzed, this factor is an important and often overlooked source of error. The color of hemoglobin can interfere with photometric measurements and therefore affect the precision of a test. Furthermore during hemolysis, hemoglobin and other substances are released, which can affect specific chemical reactions in tests, e.g. free hemoglobin interferes with the diazotization procedure in the bilirubin assay. Other substances such as potassium, aspartate transaminase and lactate dehydrogenase are also released and thus produce erroneously raised levels.[18,19]

Equipment

Since the intensive care laboratory is required to analyze whole blood samples taken from the patient only moments beforehand, the most cost-effective piece of equipment required is a supply of preheparinized syringes at each bedside. These will contain a fixed amount of balanced heparin (preferably lithium heparin),[20,21] thus avoiding both dilutional errors due to aspirating an arbitrary amount of liquid heparin into a conventional syringe and analytical errors in Na^+ and Ca^{2+} measurements that arise when using sodium heparin. If the samples need to be stored on ice for any length of time the use of syringes with air vents should be avoided, since the melting ice will mix with the sample unless great care is taken.

It is not the intention of this review of standards to single out any particular instrument or manufacturer. The choice of analyzer is dependent on the local requirements. Whenever appropriate the advice of the main pathology laboratory should be sought when deciding upon a method, analyzer or supplier. It should be remembered, however, that the intensive care laboratory is a potentially more hostile environment in which to house delicate instruments than is the main laboratory. It is recommended that other ICUs are consulted regarding the performance of a proposed instrument.

Although good maintenance and planning can prevent analyzer breakdowns, the inevitable will happen. It is important to check that the nearest service engineer/technician is based within a reasonable distance and that the service contract, that comes with the analyzer, specifies a maximum 'down time' from the call to the suppliers of the instrument.

Different analyzers measuring different analyses may be deployed in intensive care unit laboratories, depending on the specialist slant of the hospital or unit. Irrespective of the type of equipment used for whole blood analysis, there are a few golden rules to be followed if it is to be safely and effectively operated by staff with limited technical and analytical expertise:

1. It should be self-calibrating.
2. It should only give results if it is calibrated.
3. The sample path should be easily inspected for blockages and *all* parts of it should be accessible, so that clots (which will occur even on the best run unit) can be easily and quickly removed without resorting to the use of bent needles and other unsatisfactory methods.
4. The waste bottle should be sealed and cause no environmental or health hazard to the users. It is also desirable that the instrument shuts itself down when the waste container is full and cannot be restarted until it has been emptied.
5. There should be full documented compliance with all local and governmental electrical safety requirements.

There are differences of design philosophy between manufacturers of equipment, and the choice of which path to follow when equipping an intensive care laboratory will be dependent to some extent on the number and type of patients treated on the unit or monitored by the laboratory. Large multichannel analyzers which measure everything at once are marginally quicker and almost always cheaper in terms of running costs. However, if they go wrong for any reason the whole of the laboratory analytical capability is lost. A small ICU with a limited throughput of samples per day may find it more efficient to have discrete analyzers for blood gases, electrolytes, glucose, etc. A larger, busier unit will require a faster 'all in one' type of analyzer and back-up analyzers which can be used to avoid queuing and delays during normal down times, due to maintenance of the main analyzer.

The instruments described below are regarded as essential to the intensive care laboratory.

BLOOD GAS ANALYZER

A blood gas analyzer is required for measuring pH, PCO_2, PO_2, calculating HCO_3, base excess/deficit, O_2 content, and alveolar-arterial oxygen gradient ($AaDO_2$). Most of the modern gas analyzers on the market allow the user to carry out extensive calculations regarding oxygen uptake by the lungs, oxygen transport by the blood and, if a mixed venous sample is analyzed, oxygen release by the hemoglobin to the tissues. Often a co-oximeter is interfaced to the analyzer, enabling among other things more accurate hemoglobin measurements to be undertaken. Again, most of these modern instruments either have an in-built program for recall and storage of service and maintenance records and quality control procedures, or can be linked to a computer which will store the information directly.

ELECTROLYTE ANALYZER

Analyzers incorporating potentiometric ion-selective membrane electrodes are by far the most suitable. Whole blood samples can be measured directly, thus eliminating the need for centrifugation and dilution (necessary for flame photometers). However, it should be realized that the analyzer will be set up and calibrated to measure ionic activity at and around the normal levels in blood. If urine electrolytes are required, then the samples will need to be accurately diluted and the analyzer recalibrated. If urine analysis is to be a routine part of the laboratory activity then it would probably be better to invest in a separate analyzer.

The most commonly analyzed electrolytes are Na^+, K^+ and Ca^{2+}, with Mg^{2+} being introduced in the latest generation of instruments. Some analyzers include a pH electrode and will 'correct' the result back to a pH of 7.4. This is usually unnecessary in an ICU since the vast majority of samples will have been taken from the arterial circulation, and the activity at the actual arterial pH will be more clinically relevant. Although all ion-selective electrode analyzers measure direct ion *activity* in the blood, most manufacturers provide a 'fudge factor' offset to enable the results to be reported as *concentrations* similar to the results by classic flame photometry. It is important that the person responsible for the laboratory liaises closely with the senior chemical pathologist in the main laboratory to ensure consistency of results throughout the hospital. Calcium results can also cause a problem since most biochemistry departments will report total calcium results rather than ionized and the clinicians receiving the results must be made aware of the difference.

BLOOD GLUCOSE ANALYZER

The most common method of measuring blood glucose in intensive care units is by using dry reagent strips. The glucose in the blood reacts with the reagent for a set period of time, causing a color change which the doctor or nurse then compares to a color chart or reads using a reflectance meter. The accuracy of such tests is affected by hematocrit but more importantly by operator error and at best should only be used as an indicator of high or low blood glucose levels.[22]

There are various alternative methods for determining blood glucose levels more accurately in the intensive care laboratory area or at the bedside. The technique is made more accurate by eliminating operator responsibility. The most accurate methods involve an analyzer sampling a preset amount of blood from a syringe and are usually based on an enzymatic reaction within the analyzer. Although the initial outlay for the analyzer may be quite high the running costs per test may well be less than inaccurate hourly glucose strip tests. A recently introduced method involves using a precise amount of blood drawn into a microcuvette by capillary action, therefore independent of the operator. The microcuvette, which contains a mixture of dry chemicals, is then inserted into a dedicated photometer and after a suitable time for an enzymatic reaction to take place a blood glucose reading is given.[23] This method has the advantage of not being affected by hematocrit, but it is a more expensive test. A variant on the bedside glucose strip method is a combined amperometric and enzymatic method.[24] This method has the advantage of being fast (results in 30 seconds) and does not require timing or wiping of blood from the reagent strip, but accuracy does rely on the size of the blood sample on the end of the strip. In addition, the method involves a glucose oxidase reaction which is dependent on oxygen content and so the blood PO_2 of ventilated patients may produce higher results.

HEMOGLOBIN ANALYZER

Most ICUs need to have a fast and accurate method of measuring hemoglobin, but some will make do with hematocrit (Hct). Hand-held battery operated microcentrifuges are available which measure Hct at the bedside, however they are not recommended for general intensive care use since they can easily generate an aerosol of blood. Some blood gas and electrolyte analyzers will measure whole blood conductivity and interpret the results as a hematocrit reading. The most successful discrete hemoglobin analyzer works on

similar principles to the microcuvette outlined above for glucose. This time the reagent in the microcuvette hemolyzes the blood and the subsequent free hemoglobin is analyzed, absorbance measurements being taken at the isobestic points on the visible spectrum (570 and 880 nm). Co-oximetry remains the most accurate method of determining hemoglobin by absorbance measurements; it also has many advantages from a clinical point of view, giving additional quantitative information about the hemoglobin types measured.

LACTATE ANALYZER

Lactate concentrations are easily measured in whole blood using technology where blood lactate reacts with an immobilized enzyme contained within a membrane, to produce a current.[25] Some methods involve pipetting of samples for analysis and so are unsuitable for intensive care laboratories if unskilled personnel are to carry out the analyses.

ADDITIONAL ASSAYS

In addition to these pieces of equipment, an intensive care laboratory may also measure other analytes such as proteins, enzymes, drugs and some hematology assays if it is thought that these measurements would benefit patient treatment and be more cost-effective than having the same tests performed by the pathology laboratories. However, the methods available usually require serum or plasma samples, so a means of centrifuging blood samples would be a necessity. The equipment used can also be more sophisticated and involve more complicated techniques, therefore one requires a detailed knowledge of the actual methodologies in order to interpret results, as many factors influence these results.

PROTEIN AND ENZYME ANALYZERS

Instrumentation ranges from large multichannel analyzers, which carry out many tests on large batches of samples, down to smaller dry chemistry analyzers that can be used for smaller numbers of samples. All of these use methods where the reaction causes a change of color of one of the components, which can be detected using absorbance measurements.

DRUG ANALYZERS

Drug levels can be determined using a wider variety of methods including wet and dry reagent colorimetric methods, immunoassay, gas–liquid chromatography (GLC) and high-performance liquid chromatography (HPLC). The majority of these require specialist training in both the techniques and result interpretation.

HEMATOLOGY ANALYSIS

Most ICUs will not need to monitor more than total hemoglobin and/or hematocrit. However, relatively simple bedside analyzers for measuring prothrombin time (PT), activated partial thromboplastin time (APTT) and international normalized ratio (INR) are available. For these tests a disposable cartridge is inserted into the analyzer and one drop (approx. 45 μl) of fresh whole blood is drawn by capillary action through the cartridge. The distance it travels after being activated is tracked by a laser within the analyzer. The analyzers have proved to be extremely reliable when used by nonexpert analysts in the emergency operating room and the ICU. At present the only drawback is the cost of the cartridge.[26] Automated coagulation analyzers are available which can give detailed analysis of all clotting factors, D-dimers and heparin and antibody levels, etc. These analyzers are really beyond the technical skills of the ordinary users of the intensive care laboratory.[27]

Thromboelastography is undergoing a renaissance as a means of assessing coagulation and fibrinolysis in fresh whole blood samples (350 μl). The basic technique is simple and on our ICU is routinely carried out by junior medical staff, contributing to a more rational use of blood and blood products in the identification and treatment of coagulopathies.[28]

PERCUTANEOUS/EXTRACORPOREAL AND IN VIVO ANALYZERS

Continuous measurements of all the various biochemical and hematological variables currently measured by laboratory instruments in the intensive care laboratory will be the next major leap forward in intensive care monitoring. The biggest problem so far with all the current methods available is one of calibration and verification (QC) of the results which the instrument is showing.

Transcutaneous methods of monitoring PO_2 and PCO_2 are based on the same electrode technology as those in the blood gas analyzer. Recent advances in design have seen these encased in tough ceramic surrounds, but they still require frequent membrane changes and calibration checks.[29] In the adult intensive care patient the transcutaneous measurements may not correlate with blood gas results but this does not necessarily mean that they are wrong – local variations in tissue perfusion can be highlighted by this technique,

first pointed out by Rithalia *et al.*,[30] leading to the now famous quotation from Shoemaker and Vidyasagar that 'the instruments were giving us the right answers but we were asking the wrong questions'.[31]

In-line/on-line extracorporeal devices can measure blood gases and electrolytes by either removing a blood sample automatically from an extracorporeal blood pathway such as a continuous hemofiltration or extracorporeal membrane oxygenation circuit, or by fluorescence-based optical sensors, placed 'in-line' on the circuit. *In vivo* blood gas analysis can now be performed using optical fibers placed in the bloodstream with chemical sensors on the tip of the fiber bundle. The devices have been shown to give reasonable trend results over a short period; however, two-point calibrations are impossible and so sensitivity cannot be adjusted or checked.

Conclusion

In this chapter we have deliberately not provided a shopping list of specific manufacturers' equipment needed to set up an intensive care laboratory. The choice must be made locally in consultation with experienced laboratory staff and other ICUs. We have attempted to present a philosophy, namely the elimination of errors by organization, education and a relentless attention to detail by those responsible for the laboratory and those using it.

Under the Consumer Protection Act in the UK and similar legislation in Europe and the USA, the manufacturer of an instrument may be held liable if a patient is harmed as a result of erroneous laboratory analysis. In order not to share liability the hospital would have to prove that the intensive care laboratory procedures were carried out as meticulously as if the test had been done in the main laboratory. This means that documented evidence of QC, service records, evidence of staff training, etc. will have to be available. If the manufacturer can show any fault on the part of the hospital then the costs of the claim would have to be met by the hospital or health authority. The same standards that apply for laboratory instrumentation also apply to instruments attached to the patient which give *in vivo* data. The drawbacks regarding calibration and drift have been mentioned earlier, but if a therapeutic maneuver is instigated, stopped or changed as a result of data obtained from an 'in-line' potassium or blood gas analyzer, then the same documented evidence of maintenance records, calibration and QC would have to be available.

Close cooperation with the main pathology laboratories is vital for safety and improvement to patient treatment. Whilst it is undesirable for an ICU to 'go its own way' and start up a mini-pathology service of its own without consultation, it is equally unrealistic of directors of pathology services to insist that every single blood test required by an intensive care unit has to come down to the main laboratory.

The purpose of the on-site intensive care laboratory is to be part of the patient monitoring process. Frequent observations (analyses) are made in almost real-time, enabling trend analysis of biochemical and hematological data to be made in conjunction with the hemodynamic, respiratory and fluid balance data which are already being recorded. The 'art' of intensive care lies in pulling all the strands of information together and making a complete picture, the 'science' is simple – just make sure the information obtained is correct. There are no half measures when it comes to providing an intensive care laboratory service; with proper planning it can be cost-effective, of cost benefit and safe.

References

1. Eastaugh SR. In: Daver MA (ed) *Financing Health Care Economic Efficiency and Equity*. Westport, CN: Auburn House Publishing Company, 1987.
2. Jennet B. *High Technology Medicine Benefits and Burdens*. Oxford and New York: Oxford University Press, 1986.
3. Zaloga GP. Evaluation of bedside testing options for the critical care unit. *Chest* 1990; **97**(Suppl.): 5.
4. Smoller BR, Kruskall MS. Phlebotomy for diagnostic tests in adults – pattern of use and effect on transfusion requirements. *New Eng J Med* 1986; **3**: 1233–5.
5. HN (90) 18 *Scientific and Technical Services*. London: Department of Health and Social Security, 1990.
6. The CPA Accreditation Handbook. Sheffield, UK: Clinical Pathology Accreditation (UK) Ltd.
7. Clinical Laboratory Clinical Amendments 1988. HCFA – Transmittal 217: Appendix A. Washington: Department of Health and Human Services (DHHS), USA, 1988.
8. Consumer Protection Act 1988. London: HMSO, 1988.
9. Health Equipment Information HE1(98) 1982. London: NHS Procurement Directorate, 1982.
10. Westgard JO, Klee GG. Quality assurance. In: Teitz NW (ed.) *Textbook of Clinical Chemistry*. Philadelphia: WB Saunders: 424–54, 1986.
11. Westgard JO, Carey RN, Wold S. Criteria for judging precision and accuracy in method development and evaluation; *Clin Chem* 1974; **20**: 825–33.
12. Westgard JO, Hunt MR. Use and interpretation of common statistical tests in method–comparison studies. *Clin Chem* 1973; **19**: 149–57.
13. Levey S, Jennings ER. The use of control charts in the clinical laboratory. *Am J Clin Path* 1950; **20**: 1059–66.
14. Westgard JO, Groth T, Aronsson T *et al*. Combined Shewhart–cusum control chart for improved quality control in clinical chemistry. *Clin Chem* 1977; **23**: 1881–7.
15. Broughton PMG. Quality assurance. In: Williams DL, Marks V (eds) *Principles of Clinical Biochemistry – Scientific Foundations*. Oxford: Heinemann, 1988.
16. Young DS, Pestaner LC, Gibberman V. Effect of drugs on clinical laboratory tests. *Clin Chem* 1975; **21**: 1D–432D.
17. Salway JG. Drug interference causing misinterpretation of laboratory results. *Ann Clin Biochem* 1975; **15**: 44–8.
18. Van der Woerd-de Lange JA, Guder WG, Schleicher E *et al*. Studies on the interference by haemoglobin in the determination of bilirubin. *J Clin Chem Clin Biochem* 1983; **21**: 437–43.
19. Frank JJ, Bermes EW, Bickel MJ *et al*. Effect of in-vitro haemolysis on chemical value of serum. *Clin Chem* 1978; **24**: 1966–70.
20. Sachs C, Raboume PH, Chaneac M, Kindermans C, Dechaux M, Falch-Christiansen T. Preanalytical errors in ionised calcium measurements induced by the use of liquid heparin. *Ann Clin Biochem* 1991; **28**: 167–73.
21. O'Leary TD, Langton SR. Effect on biochemical parameters of blood collected into heparinised syringes. *Ann Clin Biochem* 1989; **26**: 106–7.
22. Ashworth L, Gibb I, Alberti KG. Hemocue: Evaluation of portable photometric system for determining glucose in whole blood. *Clin Chem* 1992; **38**: 1479–82.
23. Weiner K. An assessment of the effect of haematocrit on the Hemocue blood glucose analyser. *Ann Clin Biochem* 1993; **30**: 90–3.
24. Matthews DR, Burton SF, Bown E *et al*. Capillary and venous blood glucose measurements using a direct glucose sensing meter. *Diabetic Med* 1991; **8**: 875–80.
25. Foxdal P, Nergquist Y, Eckerbom S. Improving lactate analysis with the YSI 2300 GL: haemolysing samples makes results comparable with those for deproteinised whole blood. *Clin Chem* 1992; **38**: 2110–14.
26. Ansell J, Tiarks C, Hirsh J, McGehee W, Adler D, Weibert R. Measurement of the activated partial thromboplastin time from a capillary (fingerstick) sample of whole blood. A new method for monitoring heparin therapy. *Am J Clin Path* 1991; **95**: 222–7.
27. Castillo JB, Farag AM, Mammen EF, Sachs RJ. Prothrombin times and clottable fibrinogen determination on an automated coagulation laboratory (ACL-810). *Thrombosis Res* 1989; **55**: 213–19.
28. Mallett SV, Cox DJA. Thromboelastography. *Br J Anaesth* 1992; **69**: 307–13.
29. Rithalia SV. Developments in transcutaneous blood gas monitoring: a review. *J Med Eng Techn* 1991; **15**: 143–53.
30. Rithalia SVS, George RJD, Tinker J. Continuous tissue pH and transcutaneous pO_2 measurement as an index of tissue perfusion in critically ill patients. *Resuscitation* 1981; **9**: 67–74.
31. Shoemaker WK, Vidyasagar D. Physiological and clinical significance of Ptc O_2 and Ptc CO_2 measurements. *Crit Care Med* 1981; **9**: 689–90.

CHAPTER 10

Respiratory Support

WILLIAM T PERUZZI, BARRY A. SHAPIRO────────────────────────────

Introduction   133
Nonventilatory respiratory support   133
Positive airway pressure therapy   138
Extrapulmonary gas exchange   151
Conclusions   152
References   152

Introduction

The respiratory support of critically ill patients entails several different modalities. Appropriate and timely attention to nonmechanical ventilatory support will often preclude the need for more intensive care at a later time. Additionally, attention to these factors will often shorten the time course of mechanical ventilation and intensive care unit care as well. The various types of nonventilatory respiratory support, such as oxygen therapy and bronchial hygiene, will be discussed.

The provision of mechanical ventilatory support has become more complex as our clinical sophistication and technologic capabilities have expanded. Decisions concerning the type of ventilatory support that should be provided have become more complex as well. This chapter will provide information concerning the various options that are available for the provision of mechanical ventilatory support and some basic information about their clinical applications.

Another factor to consider is that, as our technologic capabilities have expanded, the pulmonary disease processes that we are faced with supporting have become more complex. In fact, at times parenchymal lung disease can become so severe and complex as to render most forms of mechanical ventilatory support inadequate. In this light other options for support of respiratory function have been devised, such as extra-corporeal and intracorporeal gas exchange devices. The usefulness and limitations of these techniques will be considered as well.

Nonventilatory respiratory support

OXYGEN THERAPY

When dealing with lung pathology potentially amenable to oxygen administration, the indications for oxygen therapy and the available methods of oxygen administration must be considered. In order to understand the indications for oxygen therapy, the physiologic responses to hypoxemia and/or hypoxia must be appreciated. First, there is an increase in minute ventilation which increases alveolar ventilation and the work of breathing. Second, there is an increase in cardiac output. This maintains oxygen delivery in the face of a decrease in oxygen content and increases the stress placed on the cardiovascular system. Therefore, the goals of oxygen therapy are to improve oxygen content and subsequently decrease the work of breathing and myocardial stress.

Oxygen content is determined by the concentration of hemoglobin (Hb) in the blood, the percentage of the Hb that is saturated with oxygen, and the amount of oxygen dissolved in the plasma (Equation 1).

$$CaO_2 = [Hb] \times \%SaO_2 \times 1.34 + PaO_2 \times 0.003$$
$$(Eqn\ 1)$$

It should be obvious that the primary determinant of oxygen content is the Hb concentration (g/dl) and the degree of hemoglobin saturation (expressed as a decimal). At atmospheric pressure the amount of oxygen dissolved in the plasma ($PaO_2 \times 0.003$) is usually negligible.

Oxygen delivery systems

There are three basic types of gas delivery systems: rebreathing systems, nonrebreathing systems, and partial rebreathing systems. *Rebreathing systems* collect exhaled gases into a reservoir on the expiratory limb of the system which contains a carbon dioxide absorber. This permits the re-entry of expiratory gases into the inspiratory gas flow without rebreathing of carbon dioxide. This system has been used primarily in the delivery of anesthetic gases in order to conserve expensive volatile anesthetics.

Most oxygen delivery systems are *nonrebreathing systems* in that all expiratory gases are vented in such a fashion that exhaled carbon dioxide is not rebreathed during subsequent breaths. This is often accomplished with one-way valves to prevent mixing of inspired and expired gases.

A *partial rebreathing system* is one in which the initial portion of the expired gases, consisting mainly of gas from the anatomic dead space, is expired into a reservoir, while the latter portions of the expiratory gases are vented to the atmosphere through one-way valves. The expiratory gases from the anatomic dead space contain very little carbon dioxide and, therefore, can be rebreathed without significant consequences. The reservoir also receives fresh inspiratory gas flow; thus, the patient breathes both expiratory gas, containing little carbon dioxide, and fresh inspiratory gas. Hence, the term partial rebreathing system.

Nonrebreathing systems are further divided into high-flow (fixed performance) and low-flow (variable performance) systems. A high-flow system means that the inspiratory gas flow rate delivered by the system is sufficient to meet the peak inspiratory flow demands of the patient. Thus, all inspiratory gas is supplied by the oxygen delivery system and the inspired oxygen concentration (FiO_2) is both known and stable. In order to accomplish this the inspiratory gas flows must be three to four times the measured minute ventilation.[1,2] High-flow oxygen delivery systems are indicated whenever there is a need for a consistent and predictable FiO_2, especially in patients with unstable ventilatory patterns. Conversely, a low flow system delivers a fixed amount of oxygen to the patient and entrainment of room air is necessary in order to meet the patient's peak inspiratory flow rates. In this circumstance the FiO_2 is variable and unpredictable if the patient has an abnormal or changing pattern of ventilation. If the patient has a stable, normal pattern of ventilation, however, low-flow oxygen delivery systems can deliver a predictable and consistent FiO_2 (Table 10.1).

Table 10.1 Low-flow oxygen delivery devices, flow rates and FiO_2. Predicted FiO_2 values for low-flow systems assume a normal and stable pattern of ventilation

Low-flow system	Oxygen flow rates (l/min)	FiO_2
Nasal cannula	1	0.24
	2	0.28
	3	0.32
	4	0.36
	5	0.40
	6	0.44
Simple face mask	5–6	0.40
	6–7	0.50
	7–8	0.60
Partial rebreathing mask	6	0.60
	7	0.70
	8	0.80
	9	0.80+
	10	0.80+
Nonrebreathing mask	10	0.80+
	15	0.90+

It must be understood that use of a low-flow oxygen delivery system does not imply delivery of low oxygen concentrations. For example, it is possible to calculate the FiO_2 for a low-flow system, such as a nasal cannula, if certain assumptions are made as follows:

1. the anatomic reservoir (nose, nasopharynx and oropharynx) comprises approximately $\frac{1}{3}$ of the anatomic dead space ($\approx 150\,cm^3$) and is approximately $50\,cm^3$;
2. the oxygen flow rate is 6 l/min (100 ml/s) via the nasal cannulae;
3. the patient's respiratory rate of 20 breaths/minute results in a 1-second inspiratory phase and a 2-second expiratory phase;
4. there is negligible gas flow during the terminal 0.5 second of the expiratory phase, thus allowing the anatomic reservoir to completely fill with oxygen.

Using the above assumptions the FiO_2 can be calculated for variable tidal volumes (V_t) as outlined in Table 10.2. This variability in FiO_2 at 6 l/min oxygen flow clearly demonstrates the effects of a changing ventilatory pattern on FiO_2. In general, the larger the V_t or the faster the respiratory rate, the lower the FiO_2. The smaller the V_t or lower the respiratory rate, the higher the FiO_2. With a stable, unchanging ventilatory pattern and

Table 10.2 Variability in FiO_2 with low-flow oxygen delivery systems and variable patterns of ventilation

	$Vt = 500 cm^3$	$Vt = 250 cm^3$
Anatomic reservoir	$50 cm^3 O_2$	$50 cm^3 O_2$
Inspiratory phase (1 s)	$100 cm^3 O_2$	$100 cm^3 O_2$
Entrained room air	$350 cm^3 O_2$	$100 cm^3$
Oxygen from entrained room air (21% O_2)	$70 cm^3 O_2$	$20 cm^3 O_2$
Total volume O_2/V_t	$220 cm^3/500 cm^3$	$170 cm^3/250 cm^3$
FiO_2	0.44	0.68

oxygen flow rate, low-flow systems can deliver a relatively consistent FiO_2.

Low-flow systems

Low-flow oxygen devices are the most commonly employed oxygen delivery systems because of their simplicity, ease of use, familiarity, economics, and patient acceptance. In most clinical situations these systems are acceptable and are the preferred choice.

Nasal cannula

The nasal cannula is the most frequently used oxygen delivery device because of its simplicity, ease of use, and comfort. To be effective the nasal passages must be patent in order to allow filling of the anatomic reservoir; however, the patient does not need to breath through the nose. Oxygen will be entrained from the anatomic reservoir even in the presence of mouth breathing. If the oxygen flow rate exceeds 4 l/min, the gases should be humidified to prevent drying of the nasal mucosa.[3] Flows >6 l/min will not significantly increase FiO_2 > 0.44 and are often poorly tolerated by the patient.

Simple face mask

A simple face mask consists of a mask with two side ports. The mask provides an additional 100–200 cm^3 oxygen reservoir and will provide a higher FiO_2 than a nasal cannula. There are open side ports in the sides of the mask to allow entrainment of room air and venting of exhaled gases. A minimum flow of 5 l/min is necessary to prevent carbon dioxide accumulation and rebreathing. Flow rates greater than 8 l/min will not increase the FiO_2 significantly >0.6.

Partial rebreathing mask

A partial rebreathing mask is similar in construction to the simple face mask, but it also incorporates a 600–1000 ml reservoir bag into which fresh gas flows. The first third of the patient's exhaled gas fills the reservoir bag. Since this gas is primarily from anatomic

dead space, it contains very little carbon dioxide. With the next breath, the patient inhales a mixture of the exhaled gas and fresh gas. If the fresh gas flows are ⩾8 l/min and the reservoir bag remains inflated throughout the entire respiratory cycle, adequate carbon dioxide evacuation and the highest possible FiO_2 should occur. The rebreathing capacity of this system allows some degree of oxygen conservation which may be useful during transportation with portable oxygen supplies.

Nonrebreathing mask

A nonrebreathing mask is similar to a partial rebreathing mask but with the addition of three unidirectional valves. Two of the valves are located on opposite sides of the mask. They permit venting of exhaled gas and prevent entrainment of room air. The remaining unidirectional valve is located between the mask and the reservoir bag and prevents exhaled gases from entering the fresh gas reservoir. As with the partial rebreathing mask, the reservoir bag should be inflated throughout the entire ventilatory cycle in order to ensure adequate carbon dioxide clearance from the system and the highest possible FiO_2.

To avoid air entrainment around the mask and dilution of the delivered FiO_2, masks should fit snugly on the face, but should avoid excessive pressure. If the mask is fitted properly, the reservoir bag should respond to the patient's inspiratory efforts. Unfortunately, if fresh gas flows and the volume of the reservoir bag are insufficient to meet inspiratory demands, the patient could be compromised. Therefore, masks may be fitted with a spring loaded tension valve that will open and allow entrainment of room air as needed to meet inspiratory demands. If such a valve is not present another option is to remove one of the unidirectional valves that prevent room air entrainment. If the total ventilatory needs of the patient are met by the non-rebreathing system, then it functions as a high-flow system. If room air entrainment occurs, then a low-flow system is operating.

Tracheostomy collars

Tracheostomy collars primarily are used to deliver humidity to patients with artificial airways. Oxygen may be delivered with these devices; but, similar to other low-flow systems, the FiO_2 is unpredictable, inconsistent, and depends upon the ventilatory pattern.

High-flow systems

Although high-flow systems are more complex, more labor-intensive to initiate and maintain, and more expensive, clinical situations in which it is important to deliver a precise FiO₂ require their availability and use.

Venturi mask

These masks entrain air using the Bernoulli principle and constant pressure-jet mixing.[4] This physical phenomenon is based on a rapid velocity of gas (e.g. oxygen) moving through a restricted orifice. This produces viscous shearing forces which create a sub-atmospheric pressure gradient downstream relative to the surrounding gases. This pressure gradient causes room air to be entrained until the pressures are equalized. In this manner, flows high enough to meet peak inspiratory demands of the patient can be generated. As the desired FiO₂ increases, the air/oxygen entrainment ratio decreases with a net reduction in total gas flow. Therefore, the probability of the patient's needs exceeding the total flow capabilities of the device increases with higher FiO₂ settings. Occlusion of or impingement on the exhalation ports of the mask can cause back-pressure and alter gas flow ('Venturi stall'). In addition, the oxygen injector port can become clogged, especially with water droplets. Therefore, aerosol devices should not be used with these devices; if humidity is necessary, a vapor-type humidifier (see 'Humidification' below) should be used.

There are two basic types of Venturi systems:

1. a fixed FiO₂ model which requires specific inspiratory attachments that are color-coded and have labelled jets which produce a known FiO₂ with a given flow; and
2. a variable FiO₂ model which has graded adjustments of the air entrainment port which can be set to allow variation in delivered FiO₂.

Aerosol mask and T-piece

An FiO₂ greater than 0.40 with a high flow system is best provided with a large volume nebulizer and wide-bore tubing. Aerosol masks, in conjunction with air entrainment nebulizers or air/oxygen blenders, can deliver a consistent and predictable FiO₂ regardless of the patient's ventilatory pattern. A T-piece is used in place of an aerosol mask for patients with an endotracheal or tracheostomy tube.

An air entrainment nebulizer can deliver an FiO₂ of 0.35–1.0, produce an aerosol, and generate flow rates of 14–16 l/min. As with Venturi masks, a higher FiO₂ results in less room air entrainment and lower flow rates. Should a greater total flow be required, two nebulizers can feed a single mask and increase the total flow.

Air/oxygen blenders can deliver a consistent FiO₂ in the range of 0.21–1.0 with flows up to 100 l/min. These devices are usually used in conjunction with humidifiers.

HUMIDIFICATION

The administration of dry oxygen lowers the water content of the inspired air. The use of an artificial airway bypasses the nasopharynx and oropharynx, where a significant amount of warming and humidification of inspired gases takes place. As a result, oxygen administration and the use of artificial airways increase the demand on the lung to humidify the inspired gases. This ultimately leads to drying of the tracheal and bronchial mucosa, decreased mucocilliary clearance and inspissated secretions. To prevent these complications, a humidifier or nebulizer should be used to increase the water content of the inspired gases.

A humidifier increases the water vapor in a gas. This can be accomplished by passing gas over heated water (heated passover humidifier); by fractionating gas into tiny bubbles as gas passes through water (bubble humidifiers); by allowing gas to pass through a chamber which contains a heated, water saturated wick (heated wick humidifier); or by vaporizing water and selectively allowing the vapor to mix with the inspired gases (vapor phase humidifier).

A nebulizer increases the water content of the inspired gas by generating aerosols (small droplets of particulate water) of uniform size which become incorporated into the delivered gas stream and then evaporate into the inspired gas as it is warmed in the respiratory tract. There are two basic types of nebulizers. Pneumatic nebulizers operate from a pressurized gas source and are either jet or hydronomic. Electric nebulizers are powered by an electrical source and are referred to as 'ultrasonic.' There are several varieties of the above nebulizers which are more dependent on design differences than on the power source.

BRONCHIAL HYGIENE

Bronchial hygiene is useful and effective when the patient is carefully evaluated, the goals of therapy are clearly defined, and the appropriate modalities are applied.

Prophylactic vs therapeutic

Prophylactic bronchial hygiene therapy is administered to patients who are essentially free of acute pulmonary pathology with the intention of preventing inadequate bronchial hygiene. Therapeutic bronchial hygiene therapy is aimed at the reversal of pre-existing inadequate bronchial hygiene; specifically, the mobilization of retained secretions and the reinflation of atelectatic lung regions.

Incentive spirometry

The incentive spirometer is an effective and inexpensive prophylactic bronchial hygiene tool. This device provides a visual goal or 'incentive' for the patient to achieve and sustain a maximal inspiratory effort. When performed on an hourly basis, this modality provides optimal lung inflation, distribution of ventilation, and an improved cough. Thus, atelectasis and the retention of bronchial secretions are prevented. Incentive spirometry can also be helpful in the diagnosis of acute pulmonary pathology in that a sudden decrease in the ability of a patient to perform at a previously established level may herald the onset of severe atelectasis, pneumonia, or other pulmonary pathology. For incentive spirometry to be effective the patient must be cooperative, motivated and well instructed in the technique (by the respiratory therapist, nurse or physician); a vital capacity >14 ml/kg or an inspiratory capacity >12 ml/kg should be obtainable; and the patient should not be tachypneic or on a high FiO_2.

Suctioning

Removal of bronchial secretions via suction is a commonly employed bronchial hygiene technique. Performed appropriately this procedure is safe and effective. Performed without appropriate caution, it can result in significant complications or death.

Airway suctioning can be accomplished safely in patients with artificial airways (endotracheal or tracheostomy tubes) in place. In this circumstance, the patient should be ventilated with a manual resuscitation bag providing a high FiO_2 ('preoxygenation'). This will minimize the hypoxemia induced by removal of the patient from an oxygen source and the application of suction to the airways. A sterile suction catheter should then be placed into the airway and advanced, without the application of a vacuum, beyond the tip of the artificial airway until it can no longer be easily advanced. The catheter should then be withdrawn slightly before suction is applied. Suctioning is then accomplished by the intermittent application of a vacuum and the gradual withdrawal of the catheter in a rotating fashion. The duration of the entire procedure should not exceed 20 seconds. Following completion of suctioning the patient should be manually ventilated with an oxygen-enriched atmosphere to ensure adequate lung re-expansion and oxygenation. The patients should be monitored for signs of distress, bronchospasm, hemodynamic instability or arrhythmias throughout the entire procedure.

Suctioning of the tracheobronchial tree without an artificial airway in place (i.e. nasotracheal suctioning) carries several risks. Since the patient cannot be manually ventilated and 'preoxygenated' prior to the procedure, hypoxemia and hemodynamically significant arrhythmias can occur.[5,6] In addition, passing the suction catheter through the vocal cords can result in laryngospasm or vocal cord injury with subsequent airway obstruction. Because of these concerns, suctioning of the tracheobronchial tree in the absence of an artificial airway cannot be recommended.

Suctioning of the tracheobronchial tree should only be undertaken in the presence of appropriate indications. The primary indication is the presence of bronchial secretions that can be identified visually or on auscultation. Rising airway pressures in mechanically ventilated patients may also indicate the presence of retained bronchial secretions. Mucosal irritation, trauma and bleeding can be precipitated by frequent and aggressive suctioning in the absence of bronchial secretions. 'Routine' suctioning of the airway should be discouraged except in neonates, where small airway diameters can be acutely obstructed by a small accumulation of secretions.

Humidification

Air inspired through the nose is warmed and nearly 90% humidified by the time that it passes through the pharynx. This humidification process is bypassed in patients with artificial airways in place. If adequate humidification of inspired gases is not provided prior to gas entry into the trachea, the deficit of humidity is provided by moisture from the mucous blanket of the tracheobronchial tree. This results in drying of the tracheobronchial tree, ciliary dysfunction, impairment of mucus transport, inflammation and necrosis of the ciliated pulmonary epithelium, retention of dried secretions, atelectasis, bacterial infiltration of the pulmonary mucosa and pneumonia. Humidification of inspired gases must always be provided to patients with artificial airways in place.

Aerosol therapy

An aerosol is a suspension of fine particles of a liquid in a gas. Aerosols have three basic applications in respiratory care. They are used as an aid to bronchial hygiene, to humidify inspiratory gases and to deliver medications. When dealing with medical aerosols for inhalation, the particle size is very important. Particle size should be 3 μm or less in order for gravitational effects to be sufficiently small to permit deposition in the pulmonary tree.

When used as an aid to bronchial hygiene, water is one of the most important physically active agents. Aerosol therapy can be very useful in the hydration of dried, retained secretions and the restoration and maintenance of the mucous blanket. This, in conjunction with appropriate cough mechanisms and other bronchial hygiene techniques, will permit the mobilization of retained secretions. Care must be taken, however, because aerosols used for these purposes can result in clinical deterioration due to either increased airway resistance (bronchospasm) or swelling and expansion of dried secretions followed by worsening hypoxemia. These detrimental effects can be ameliorated by the administration of a bronchodilator and/or techniques to mobilize the expanding secretions.

There is controversy about whether 'bland aerosol' therapy is of significant therapeutic value. While some studies may indicate improvement with this therapy, there are many variables which are difficult, if not impossible, to control (i.e. cough, bronchial drainage, other therapy, other disease states, etc.). The etiology of clinical improvement is difficult to determine. Therefore, the usefulness of bland aerosol therapy has been called into question.[7]

The delivery of medications for the reversal and prevention of bronchoconstriction is an important application of aerosol therapy. Table 10.3 lists the names, dosages, mechanisms of action, etc. for the most commonly used aerosolized pharmacologic agents.

Chest physical therapy

Chest physical therapy (CPT) techniques can be classified into those which promote bronchial hygiene, improve breathing efficiency, or promote physical reconditioning. The CPT techniques considered here will be those concerned with bronchial hygiene.

Postural drainage

Postural drainage is a technique that utilizes different body positions to facilitate gravitational drainage of mucus from various lung segments. Diseases that are amenable to postural drainage therapy include cystic fibrosis, bronchiectasis, chronic obstructive pulmonary disease, acute atelectasis, lung abscess and others. In hospitalized patients the basilar lung regions can often benefit from postural drainage because most hospital bed positions do not permit adequate drainage of these segments. When dealing with postural drainage of unilateral lung disease, it is best to follow with drainage of the contralateral lung. The reason for this is that cross-contamination of the nondiseased lung is always a possibility. It is important to avoid inappropriate positioning during postural drainage. Patients with increased intracranial pressure or congestive heart failure may not tolerate head down positioning to facilitate drainage of the basilar lung segments. Also, it is important to avoid direct pressure on sites of injury, surgery or burns.

Chest percussion and vibration

These techniques are used to loosen and mobilize secretions that are adherent to bronchial walls.[8] When used in conjunction with appropriate postural drainage and coughing techniques they can facilitate bronchial hygiene efforts significantly. Chest percussion is performed by rhythmic 'clapping' with cupped hands over the lung areas in question. This generates a mechanical energy wave that is transmitted through the chest wall to the lung tissue and loosens adherent mucus. Chest vibration is accomplished by placing the hands on the chest wall and generating a rapid vibratory motion in the arms, from the shoulders, and gently compressing the chest wall in the direction that the ribs normally move during exhalation.[9] This is most effective when performed during exhalation. Relative contraindications to these techniques include fractured ribs, 'fragile bones' (i.e. osteoporosis), coagulopathies, and undrained empyema.

Intermittent positive pressure breathing

Intermittent positive pressure breathing (IPPB) is the application of inspiratory positive pressure to the airway in order to provide a significantly larger tidal volume, with a physiologically advantageous inspiratory to expiratory pattern, than the patient can produce spontaneously. It should not be confused with positive pressure ventilation delivered with a mechanical ventilator that is intended to provide ventilatory support. IPPB is useful in disease states in which the patient's depth of breathing is limited. This type of therapy is very expensive; therefore, for this mode of therapy to be indicated the patient's vital capacity should be less than $15 \, cm^3/kg$ and the IPPB treatment should augment this by at least 100%.

Positive airway pressure therapy

POSITIVE PRESSURE VENTILATION (PPV)

Indications

The need for mechanical ventilatory support arises when the cardiopulmonary reserves of the patient are overwhelmed or compromised by a pathologic situation. In these circumstances either the ventilatory mechanism is rendered ineffectual or the work of breathing (WOB) becomes *detrimental*[10] to the patient's physiologic homeostasis and respiratory muscle fatigue develops. In either event, mechanical ventilatory support is a modality that permits the clinician to support the patient while the underlying pathologic process is being reversed.

Table 10.3 Aerosolized bronchodilators and antiasthmatic drugs

Drug	Method	Dosages[a]	Frequency	Duration of action (h)	Effects	Mechanism
Sympathomimetics						
Isoetharine hydrochloride 1% (Bronkosol)	Nebulized MDI[b]	0.25–0.50 ml in 4.0 cm³ 2 puffs (10 mg/puff)	q2–4h	1.5–3.0	Bronchodilation, tachycardia	β_2-Agonist increase in cAMP
Metaproterenol sulfate 5% (Alupent)	Nebulized MDI[b] Rotocaps[c]	0.3 ml in 4.0 cm³ 2 puffs (0.65 mg/puff) 1–2 capsules (200 µg/cap)	q4–6h or qid	≤5	Bronchodilation	β_2-Agonist increase in cAMP
Albuterol (Ventolin, Proventil)	MDI[b] Nebulized	2 puffs (90 µg/puff) 2.5–5.0 mg in 4 cm³	q4–6h or qid	≤6	Bronchodilation	β_2-Agonist increase in cAMP
Racemic epinephrine 2.25%	Nebulized	0.5 ml in 3.5 cm³	q1h, prn	<1	Mucosal decongestion	Weak β_2 and mild α mucosal vasoconstrictor
Isoproterenol (0.5%)	Nebulized	0.25–0.50 mg in 3.5 ml	q2–4h	1.5–2.0	Bronchodilation, tachycardia, vasodilation, flushing	Prototype β-agonist; significant β_1 side effects
Anticholinergic drugs						
Ipratroprium bromide (Atrovent)	MDI[b]	2 puffs (18 µg/puff)	q4h or qid	3–4	Bronchodilation	Cholinergic blocker increasing β stimulation
Antiallergy agents						
Cromolyn sodium 1% (Intel)	Nebulized MDI[b] Spinhaler[c]	20 mg in 2–4 cm³ 2–4 puffs (800 µg/puff) 1 capsule (20 µg/cap)	q6h or qid	6	Stabilization of mast cell membranes	Suppression of mast cell response to Ag-Ab reactions; used prophylactically
Beclomethasone acetonide (Vanceril, Beclovent)	MDI[b]	2 puffs (42 µg/puff)	q6h or qid	6	Anti-inflammatory	Anti-inflammatory; inhibits leukocyte migration; potentiates effects of β-agonists
Flunisolide (Aerobid)	MDI[b]	2–4 puffs (250 µg/puff)	bid		Anti-inflammatory	Anti-inflammatory; inhibits leukocyte migration; potentiates effects of β-agonists
Triamcinolone (Azmacort)	MDI[b]	2 puffs (100 µg/puff) 4 puffs (100 µg/puff)	tid–qid bid		Anti-inflammatory	Anti-inflammatory; inhibits leukocyte migration; potentiates effects of β-agonists
Dexamethasone sodium phosphate (Decadron)	Nebulized	0.25 ml (1 mg) in 2.5 cm³	q6h	6	Anti-inflammatory	Anti-inflammatory; inhibits leukocyte migration; potentiates effects of β-agonists

[a] Dosages may vary. References to specific drug inserts are recommended.
[b] MDI = metered dose inhaler.
[c] Rotocaps and Spinhaler = inhaled powder.
[d] Ag-Ab = antigen–antibody.

q: every
qid: four times daily
bid: twice daily
tid: three times daily
prn: as required

There are four basic clinical indications for mechanical ventilatory support:

1. apnea;
2. acute ventilatory failure;
3. impending ventilatory failure; and
4. hyperventilation for intracranial pressure (ICP) control.

Apnea is a circumstance that can occur in a variety of clinical situations. It is often related to prescribed or illicit drug administration, such as narcotics or neuromuscular blocking agents. It can also occur with certain types of central nervous system (CNS) injury or profound cardiovascular instability.

Acute ventilatory failure (respiratory acidosis) is a diagnosis based upon arterial blood gas (ABG) analysis demonstrating an acute rise in $PaCO_2$ and an acute fall in pH.[11] This circumstance indicates that, for whatever reason, the patient is incapable of spontaneously maintaining normal carbon dioxide homeostasis. If the situation is not corrected and/or the patient is not appropriately supported, the process can be expected to progress eventually to death.

Impending ventilatory failure is a clinical diagnosis made independent of ABG analysis. In this circumstance the clinician is making the assessment that the patient's clinical presentation is consistent with significant WOB which exceeds their cardiopulmonary reserves and is *detrimental* to their physiologic homeostasis. Therefore, if left unabated, this condition will eventually progress to respiratory muscle fatigue and acute ventilatory failure. Clinical signs of detrimental WOB include tachypnea, dyspnea, intercostal retractions, use of accessory muscles of ventilation, tachycardia, hypertension, diaphoresis, etc.

Hyperventilation for ICP control is included here because, although many patients with CNS injuries will hyperventilate spontaneously, mechanical ventilation is the only way to assure the consistent maintenance of a desired $PaCO_2$.

Initiation of mechanical ventilation

First, *establish the airway and manually support ventilation* with a manual resuscitation bag. Manual ventilation allows the clinician to gradually take over ventilation and vary the pattern in conjunction with patient efforts. During the early stages of mechanical ventilation, this will permit a smooth transition to positive pressure ventilation. Second, *establish hemodynamic stability*. It is not uncommon for patients to demonstrate cardiovascular instability during this process. Often delays in establishing the airway, stress of intubation, sedative drugs and inappropriate support are blamed for this occurrence. However, such instability

often occurs in the absence of any of the above mentioned factors and is actually due to:

1. a decrease in catecholamine levels, with subsequent vasodilatation and decreased cardiac output, related to the relief of respiratory distress;
2. decreased venous return related to PPV; or
3. a combination thereof.

Third, if not already in place, *establish appropriate monitors and support*, such as intravenous and intraarterial catheters, electrocardiographic monitor, etc. Fourth, *establish the ventilatory pattern* by manually supporting the patient until they relax and adopt the slow deep pattern of PPV. If the patient will not tolerate the anticipated ventilatory pattern, appropriate sedation should be applied until they are comfortable, stable and in synchrony with ventilatory support. Finally, connect the patient to the ventilator for maintenance of PPV.

Full vs partial ventilatory support

Full and partial ventilatory support are discussed here in terms of conventional, volume preset mechanical ventilatory techniques. Full and partial ventilatory support with pressure preset/volume variable modes will be discussed under individual sections relating to these techniques.

Full ventilatory support

When initiating mechanical ventilatory support during an acute episode of ventilatory failure, it is imperative that the patient be adequately supported. In this context the concept of full ventilatory support is important. Full ventilatory support means that the ventilator provides all of the work that is required to maintain carbon dioxide excretion. This can be accomplished with ventilator rates of 8–10 breaths/min and tidal volumes of 12–15 cm^3/kg. In patients who are stable hemodynamically, this will usually result in a $PaCO_2$ <45 mm Hg. Patients with a significantly decreased cardiac output or severe pulmonary pathology may demonstrate high dead space ventilation (high V/Q) and the $PaCO_2$ may be higher.

Partial ventilatory support

Spontaneous ventilation carries some benefits (e.g. improved V/Q matching, improved venous return, etc.) which are negated by mechanical ventilatory support. Following the acute deterioration, when patients are more stable, rested, and therapy has been in place, they may be able to tolerate a portion of the WOB, but not all of it. In this circumstance it is possible to allow the ventilator to perform that WOB which is detrimental to the patient's cardiopulmonary homeostasis while allowing the patient to perform that amount of work that produces beneficial effects. This concept has been termed partial ventilatory support and is usually accomplished with the same tidal volumes as outlined for full ventilatory support, but with slower rates (<6 breaths/min).

Modes of positive pressure ventilation

There are various modes by which positive pressure ventilation may be applied. There are an equal or greater number of viewpoints concerning which mode is most appropriate for any given clinical situation. Suffice it to say that all of the methods are equally effective when applied correctly in an appropriate circumstance. The ensuing discussion will concentrate on the technical and clinical considerations concerning the available modes of mechanical ventilatory support. The nomenclature pertaining to mechanical ventilation is controversial. The nomenclature used here will be chosen to provide clarity of concepts, but every attempt has been made to incorporate the most current and generally accepted terminology.[12] Certain terms must be defined in order to describe clearly how mechanical breaths are delivered. The term *trigger* indicates that which begins the inspiratory cycle; *limit* describes that variable which cannot be exceeded during the inspiratory phase; and *cycle* is used to indicate those variables which end the inspiratory phase. Table 10.4 summarizes the various modes of mechanical ventilatory support and the factors that control their ventilatory cycles.

Table 10.4 Modes of mechanical ventilation and the factors controlling the ventilatory cycle

Ventilator mode	Initiated	Limited	Cycled
CMV	Time	Volume	Volume/time
A/CMV	Pressure	Volume	Volume/time
IMV	Time	Volume	Volume/time
SIMV	Pressure	Volume	Volume/time
Pressure support	Pressure	Pressure	Flow
Pressure control	Time	Pressure	Time
APRV	Time	Pressure	Time

Volume preset (pressure variable)

Control mode ventilation (CMV)

In this mode the ventilator essentially ignores the efforts of the patient and delivers a breath at a preset time, with a preset volume, and is limited by flow or pressure. This mode of ventilation is most effectively used in anesthetized or heavily sedated and/or paralyzed patients. Patients who are awake and cognizant tolerate this

mode poorly because it prevents spontaneous breathing or effective interaction with the ventilator and, thus, is very uncomfortable and psychologically distressing to patients. This is the primary reason that this mode of mechanical ventilatory support has been relegated to use in the operating room with anesthetized patients.

Assist/control (A/C)

Assist/control ventilation is an adaptation of the CMV mode that permits patient participation in the ventilatory cycle. In the assist/control mode the patient's spontaneous inspiratory effort triggers a positive pressure breath to be delivered by the ventilator. A 'backup' rate is set as a safety measure and insures that, should the patient become apneic or otherwise unable to trigger a breath, an adequate minute ventilation is maintained. Since in this mode each attempt at a spontaneous breath results in the delivery of a full volume positive pressure breath, assist/control can only be used effectively for delivery of full ventilatory support. Because the patient generally initiates the positive pressure breath with inspiratory muscle activity, energy expenditure is necessary at the beginning of the breath and continues throughout the entire cycle.[13,14] The amount of energy expended may be significant and, in patients with extremely limited cardiopulmonary reserves, it has been suggested that the 'backup' rate be set above the patient's spontaneous rate in order to suppress the spontaneous ventilatory efforts.[15]

Intermittent mandatory ventilation (IMV) and synchronized intermittent mandatory ventilation (SIMV)

IMV provides a continuous flow of fresh inspiratory gas past the airway that permits the patient to breathe spontaneously between intermittently delivered positive pressure breaths. This mode of ventilation has been demonstrated to result in less hyperventilation and alkalosis, and greater hemodynamic stability in infants and adults. In addition to these advantages, the advent of IMV permitted gradual withdrawal of mechanical ventilatory support rather then the 'all or nothing' level of support associated with the CMV or A/C modes. Thus, with IMV the patient can be allowed to assume the work of breathing in a step-wise fashion and the level of support can be titrated to the patient's needs. This mode was the first to allow provision of partial ventilatory support. SIMV was developed because the IMV breaths were delivered without regard to the phase of the spontaneous respiratory cycle and some investigators felt that this led to detrimental effects on the hemodynamic status of the patient. Synchronization of the breath delivery has not proven to be of significant benefit, but it remains the prevalent mode of ventilation provided on most mechanical ventilators because of technical advantages.

IMV/SIMV vs A/C controversy

Since the inception of IMV/SIMV a tremendous debate has raged over the advantages and disadvantages of these modes as compared with the A/C mode of mechanical ventilatory support. The proposed advantages of IMV/SIMV include a decreased risk of respiratory alkalosis, a decreased need for sedation, lower mean airway pressure, an improved distribution of ventilation, a more rapid withdrawal of ventilatory support, a decreased risk of respiratory muscle atrophy, and less interference with cardiovascular function; whereas, the purported disadvantages of IMV/SIMV include a higher risk of hypercapnia, increased work of breathing, the potential for respiratory muscle fatigue, prolongation of the weaning process (if the rate is not decreased appropriately), and a greater risk of hemodynamic instability during withdrawal of ventilatory support.[16] Presently available data indicate that when SIMV and A/C are compared during full ventilatory support, SIMV provides for better hemodynamic function (higher mean arterial pressure, cardiac output, pulmonary artery occlusion pressure and oxygen delivery) without increased oxygen consumption, carbon dioxide production or resting energy expenditure.[17] Despite these statistically significant differences, however, there are really no clinically significant differences between the modes and all of them have been used successfully. Therefore, it would appear that it is primarily personal preference that determines the mode of mechanical ventilation that is best for the provision of full ventilatory support.[18] However, if partial ventilatory support is planned, and a volume preset mode is desired, then IMV/SIMV must be used.

Pressure preset (volume variable)

Modes of positive pressure ventilation that are not volume limited will deliver variable tidal volumes. The advent of microprocessor controlled ventilators has made volume variable modes more adaptable as intermittent positive pressure ventilation (IPPV) devices because they offer variable inspiratory flow capability, finite control of the preset airway pressure, and extensive monitor and alarm systems. Thus, 'new' modes of mechanical ventilation have become available recently that are both interesting and promising. The following presentation is intended as an overview of these volume variable modes with an emphasis on how each *may* improve patient care.

Pressure support (PS)

This technique was originally described in 1982 and was reported as a new ventilatory support modality in 1984 when it was applied independent of other positive pressure techniques.[19,20] Pressure support overcomes high circuit resistance and demand valve inertia by providing additional gas flow to achieve an adjustable pressure limit during spontaneous inspiration.

Figure 10.1 illustrates the function of a pressure

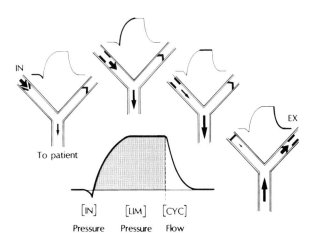

Fig. 10.1 Schematic illustration of pressure support mechanics. **IN** = initiation; **LIM** = limit; **CYC** = cycle; **EX** = exhalation. Reproduced from ref. 2 with permission.

support circuit. During spontaneous ventilation a subbaseline pressure is detected near the proximal airway and a positive pressure generator is activated. A very rapid flow enters the ventilator circuit and continues until a predetermined pressure is reached. Microprocessor analysis of flow and pressure characteristics determines the required variation of flow necessary to maintain the predetermined circuit pressure. Thus, as the patient begins to inspire the ventilator delivers flow sufficient to rapidly attain and maintain a predetermined inspiratory airway pressure. A feedback loop assures that a constant airway pressure is maintained until the inspiratory flow falls below a predetermined level. The ventilator continually monitors the airway pressure and adjusts flow to maintain the same pressure throughout the active inspiratory phase. Hence, an adjustable level of inspiratory pressure assist is provided with every spontaneous inspiratory effort. When gas flow reaches some predetermined minimum (set by the manufacturer), inspiratory flow stops and the exhalation valve opens.

Pressure support was initially used to ablate the increased work of breathing associated with the flow delay factors inherent in demand flow systems. Indeed, $3-8$ cm H_2O pressure support is comparable to a continuous flow system in reference to imposed WOB during spontaneous ventilation.[21] Thus, 5 cm H_2O pressure support, while not providing support sufficient to significantly decrease the WOB in most patients, does allow a demand flow system to function without imposing additional WOB due to the device. The routine use of 3–5 cm H_2O pressure support with SIMV should be considered no different than IMV with a properly functioning continuous flow system. However, this 3–5 cm H_2O pressure support with SIMV should not be confused with higher pressure support levels. Although many clinicians presently combine SIMV and PS, the practice is confusing in terms of the level of support being applied and lacks documented advantages. Utilizing the continuous positive airway pressure (CPAP) mode via a demand flow ventilator runs the risk of imposing detrimental work of breathing.[22] Provision of 3–5 cm H_2O PS appears to obviate this problem.

Pressure support appears to be a far better mode for partial ventilatory support than IMV or SIMV. The work of breathing is assisted with every breath (and throughout every breath), in contradistinction to IMV/SIMV where the patient must perform unassisted breaths interspersed with full positive pressure breaths. Preliminary data suggest that in patients capable of doing the vast majority of their own WOB, 30 cm H_2O pressure support provides full support, 20 cm H_2O pressure support provides partial support comparable to 4–6 breaths/min IMV/SIMV.[23]

Pressure control/inverse ratio ventilation (PC-IRV)

Interest in pressure control has always been as a mode for providing inverse ratio ventilation.[24, 25] When compared with 'conventional ventilation' in severe adult respiratory distress syndrome (ARDS), PC-IRV has been shown to improve oxygenation, decrease peak airway pressure, decrease required positive end expiratory pressure (PEEP), increase mean airway pressure and not adversely affect cardiovascular function.[26]

The number of ventilatory cycles per minute is preset and determines the time intervals at which a new inspiratory cycle will begin. The mechanism is similar to pressure support in that a rapid flow pressurizes the system after which a decelerating flow is provided to maintain the system pressure at the preset level. Most commonly, a portion of the ventilatory cycle is predetermined as inspiration (e.g. 80% inspiratory time). Thus, the positive pressure is cycled off when a predetermined time has elapsed from the start of inspiration. Thus, an 80% inspiratory time would provide an I:E ratio of 4:1.

This demand flow, volume variable technique for providing inverse ratio ventilation does not allow the patient to take spontaneous breaths and cannot provide partial ventilatory support. The patients must be sedated and neuromuscular blockade is often necessary in order to permit use of this ventilatory technique. In certain clinical situations, such as ARDS, it is sometimes difficult to maintain adequate carbon dioxide excretion,

especially with inverse ratio ventilation. In this circumstance, the practice of allowing the carbon dioxide level to rise while maintaining adequate oxygenation and pH control has been advocated. This technique is known as 'permissive hypercapnia'. Judgment concerning the utility and effectiveness of this technique must await appropriately designed and controlled clinical studies; however, there are some very preliminary indications that the technique may have some promise.

Airway pressure release ventilation (APRV)

APRV is a ventilatory support technique designed to augment alveolar ventilation in patients who require ventilatory assistance despite reduction of ventilatory work with CPAP.[27, 28] The APRV system (Figure 10.2)

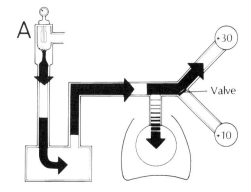

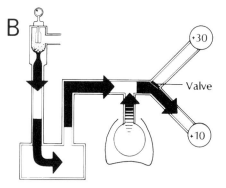

Fig. 10.2 Schematic representation of APRV. (**A**) The inflation pressure generated by a continuous flow system with a threshold resistor set at +30 cm H_2O. Flow into the lungs will be determined by the inflation pressure and the forces impeding flow (resistance and compliance). The inspiratory lung volume will be determined by the inflation pressure and the pulmonary compliance. (**B**) The release valve positioned to allow flow through the threshold resistor set at +10 cm H_2O. The resultant release pressure in the circuit allows exhalation. Reproduced from ref. 2 with permission.

includes an independent CPAP circuit in which baseline airway pressure is maintained above ambient pressure using a threshold resistor valve and either a high gas flow or a pressurized volume reservoir. A release valve is situated in the expiratory limb of the CPAP circuit to allow airway pressure to rapidly decrease. The release valve is driven by a timing device that allows adjustment of the extent, length, and frequency of pressure release. Closing of the release valve by a timing mechanism initiates the inspiratory phase. During this phase, the continuous gas flow exits through a threshold resistor with a preset pressure greater than that during expiration. Opening of the release valve by a timing mechanism cycles the mechanism from inspiration to expiration. This allows the continuous gas flow to exit through a threshold resistor with a lower preset pressure. Thus, airway pressure falls rapidly, gas exits the lungs, and carbon dioxide excretion occurs.

The lung volume at end inspiration will be primarily determined by the preset pressure and the pulmonary compliance. The end-exhalation lung volume will be determined by lung compliance, airway resistance, release time, and the gradient between the inspiratory and expiratory preset pressures. The patient can breathe spontaneously at all times. This means that APRV can provide both full and partial ventilatory support. Partial support is accomplished by lowering the frequency of airway pressure release until the patient is breathing with CPAP and with no APRV breaths.

Mandatory minute ventilation (MMV)

Mandatory minute ventilation is a technique that permits the patient to breathe spontaneously, measures the spontaneous minute ventilation, and maintains minute volume at a preset mandatory minimum level. The method, as initially developed, adjusted the ventilatory rate to maintain the desired level of ventilation.[29] Tidal volumes were preset at normal levels (10–15 cm^3/kg). Unfortunately, a pitfall of the system is that the preset minute ventilation can be maintained with very rapid and shallow breaths, thus leaving a patient who is in significant respiratory distress to breathe spontaneously until fatigue occurs. Presently available microprocessor technology has allowed the development of MMV systems that adjust pressure support levels in order to maintain the preset minute volume. Various ventilators implement MMV with either rate, pressure support or a combination thereof, depending upon the manufacturer.[30] The method used should be understood before the mode is activated. The MMV mode does not adjust PEEP, CPAP or FiO$_2$ levels; therefore, these factors must be set and changed manually as clinically indicated.

This mode is designed for use with spontaneously breathing patients who are judged appropriate for ventilator discontinuance. Its use with unstable patients or patients with abnormal patterns of ventilation is questionable. The automatic titration of ventilatory support that this mode offers may speed the 'weaning' process; however, clinical studies of this mode of ventilation are very limited and conclusions concerning efficacy are not possible.

Biphasic positive airway pressure (BiPAP)

CPAP applied by full face mask or nasal mask has been used for respiratory support in patients with various types of pulmonary pathology ranging from congestive heart failure to obstructive sleep apnea. Effectively, BiPAP is the combination of CPAP with pressure support augmentation of spontaneous inspiration. This method permits mechanical support of spontaneous ventilatory efforts without the need for intubation. This mode of ventilatory support has been demonstrated to be efficacious in the support of patients demonstrating hypoxemia and/or hypercapnia due to chronic obstructive pulmonary disease, congestive heart failure, adult respiratory distress syndrome, and *Pneumocystis carinii* pneumonia.[31–33] Although pressure injury to the nose has been reported,[32] the potential complications of gastric distention and aspiration do not appear to be significant problems.[33] Of course, this mode of ventilatory support would not be appropriate in patients with a compromised ability for airway protection. Additionally, patients must be observed carefully to ensure that the device does not become displaced and that spontaneous ventilation continues. At present, this device should not be considered for use in acute life-sustaining circumstances.

High-frequency ventilation (HFV)

Traditional positive pressure ventilators deliver greater than normal tidal volumes, whereas high-frequency ventilators provide tidal volumes less than the anatomic dead space at rates much greater than normal. Classification of HFV techniques by frequency reflects historical patterns of development more than functional differences. Frequencies are stated as either cycles/min or Hertz (Hz). One Hz equals 1 cycle per second, or 60 cycles/min. For purposes of simplicity and clarity, only the three major techniques with the greatest potential clinical applicability will be discussed. More complete discussions are available.[34, 35]

High-frequency positive pressure ventilation (HFPPV)

High-frequency positive pressure ventilation refers to the delivery of small tidal volumes through an insufflation catheter or endotracheal tube with circuitry having a minimal internal compressible volume. The characteristic rate is 60–100 breaths/min with inspiration taking 20–30% of the cycle.[34,36]

High-frequency jet ventilation (HFJV)

High-frequency jet ventilation refers to the delivery of a pulse of gas from a high-pressure source (5–50 psi) through a small-bore cannula with an interposed cycling mechanism allowing high frequencies. Solenoid valves are the most common cycling mechanisms,[37] although fluidics have been used.[38] Gas entrainment can occur around the jet and contribute significantly to inspiratory flow. The optimal catheter gauge and positioning within the endotracheal tube have not been established.[39] Inadequate humidification of delivered gas remains a major problem during HFJV, resulting in tracheal mucosal damage and thickened secretions blocking the airways. Attempts at humidification have included nebulization of a saline infusion by the jet stream, entrainment of humidified gases, and humidification of the jet gases.[35]

High-frequency oscillation (HFO)

High-frequency oscillation delivers gas to a reciprocating pump that actively transports the gas both into and out of the lungs. Thus, the desired inspired oxygen concentration can be delivered to an endotracheal tube in a sinusoidal waveform.[35] Since only high-frequency oscillators have *active expiration* as an intrinsic part of their design, they are much less prone to pulmonary hyperinflation because the ventilator actively pulls gas out of the system on each expiration.[40] Therefore, HFOs can be used at rates of 5–40 Hz. The commonly used frequencies of 10–15 Hz have evolved empirically.

Mechanisms of gas transport

The mechanisms of gas transport in high-frequency ventilation is an interesting but not well-defined entity. Early studies of gas transport mechanisms during HFV were accomplished with high-frequency oscillators which produce a sinusoidal waveform and an active expiratory phase. Generalizations to other waveforms (HFJV, HFPPV, etc.) in which expiration is passive may not be accurate. In any case, several mechanisms are believed to work in combination to produce carbon dioxide elimination during HFV.[41]

Molecular diffusion is the mechanism by which gases cross the alveolar–capillary membrane and is believed to be the dominant mechanism of gas movement distal to the terminal bronchioles. However, simple diffusion appears to be responsible for less than 10% of the total gas transport occurring with HFV.[42] The diffusion process is influenced by increased dispersion of gas molecules resulting from the high-velocity convective flows generated during HFV; this phenomenon is known as Taylor dispersion. The importance of this physical phenomenon in enhancing molecular diffusion during HFV is unknown.

Convection flow is another mechanism of gas flow that must be considered when considering high-frequency ventilation. When gas pressure at one end of a tube is greater than the pressure at the other end, convective forces cause gas to move longitudinally through the tube. Traditional physics of pulmonary function is based on convective factors such as resistance, viscosity, density, tube length and radius. Familiar clinical entities such as tidal volume and minute volume assume that gas movement is essentially convective, a valid assumption with spontaneous breathing and conventional PPV.

Although convection appears to remain the primary factor in HFV, the precise contributions of both convective and diffusive mechanisms have not been fully defined. It appears that both convection and diffusion interact and summate to produce the total gas transport picture in HFV.

Clinical applications of HFV

Although there are numerous reports of the successful use of HFV in various clinical situations, seldom do these reports describe HFV as having a distinct advantage over other methods. The clearest indication for use of HFV is in patients with massive air leaks and in whom conventional ventilation fails to provide adequate alveolar ventilation owing to loss of tidal volume through the fistulous tract.[37,43,44] Since the fistula represents a region of large effective compliance, much of the tidal volume is lost through the fistulous tract during conventional ventilation. At higher frequencies, the distribution of ventilation depends more on resistance while compliance becomes relatively unimportant.[35,45] It has been demonstrated that patients with a massive air leak from a fistulous tract can be ventilated and oxygenated with HFV when conventional techniques have failed.[37,43] Although the literature lacks controlled randomized prospective studies comparing conventional ventilation with HFV in the management of patients with airway rupture, cross-over studies done in the animal laboratory support the conclusions derived from clinical trials of HFV in life-threatening circumstances.[44]

Any advantage of HFV must be carefully weighed against the added hazards to the patient incurred by this technique. These dangers are inherent in the use of a very high pressure source to deliver pulses of gas in rapid succession into the airways and lungs. Massive barotrauma, in the form of injection injury, and over-distension injury can result. Injection injuries occur when a high-pressure jet of gas is directed against the airway mucosa, resulting in penetration into submucosal tissues and even perforation of the wall.

Tension pneumothorax occurs more readily with HFV than with conventional ventilation owing to the 'stacking' of breaths that so rapidly occurs if insufficient time or space for gas escape is allowed.

POSITIVE END EXPIRATORY PRESSURE (PEEP) AND CONTINUOUS POSITIVE AIRWAY PRESSURE (CPAP)

Positive end expiratory pressure (PEEP) exists whenever the airway pressure is greater than ambient pressure just prior to the next inspiration. PEEP is effectively independent of inspiratory mode or mechanics.

The application of PEEP has two primary effects on the pulmonary system. Firstly, PEEP increases functional residual capacity (FRC) by distending small patent alveoli and by recruiting previously collapsed alveoli. Low levels of PEEP (10 cm H_2O or less) are primarily responsible for alveolar distention, whereas levels of PEEP greater than 10 cm H_2O are generally required for alveolar recruitment. Secondly, PEEP facilitates the movement of water from the less compliant interstitial spaces (between the alveolar epithelium and capillary endothelium where gas exchange occurs) to the more compliant interstitial spaces (towards the peribronchial and hilar areas).[46] This interstitial water redistribution improves oxygen diffusion across the alveolar–capillary membrane and may play a major role in improving pulmonary mechanics and oxygenation in severe noncardiogenic pulmonary edema.[47] A number of other mechanisms have been proposed to explain the beneficial pulmonary effects of PEEP, but they seem to be limited to specific circumstances and are beyond the scope of this chapter.

Perfusion of a collapsed alveolus (zero V/Q) produces a 'true shunt' unit (Fig. 10.3). The hypoxemia that this shunting (Qs/Qt) creates is not responsive to oxygen therapy because the blood never comes in contact with alveolar gas. As discussed above, application of PEEP therapy may result in alveolar distension of poorly ventilated alveoli and the recruitment of collapsed alveoli; thus, the Qs/Qt is decreased and a more responsive hypoxemia results. It is reasonable to expect that expansion of collapsed alveoli and avoidance of alveolar hyperoxia to create an advantageous milieu for lung repair. The level of PEEP required to accomplish this is primarily determined by the underlying pathology. The overall clinical goal of PEEP therapy is to achieve adequate arterial oxygenation with nontoxic oxygen concentrations and without significant impairment of tissue perfusion. More specifically, it has been suggested[4,8] that 'enough' PEEP is the least amount that will result in a PaO_2 greater than 60 mm Hg

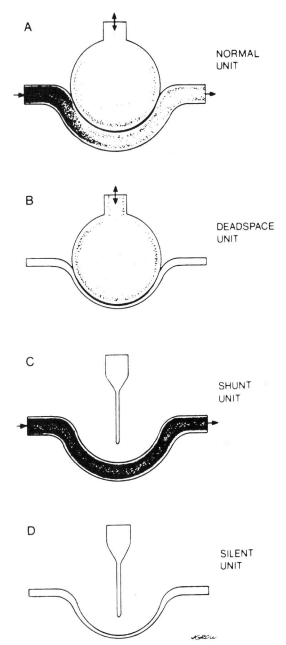

Fig. 10.3 The theoretic respiratory unit. (**A**) Normal ventilation, normal perfusion; (**B**) normal ventilation, no perfusion; (**C**) no ventilation, normal perfusion; (**D**) no ventilation, no perfusion. Reproduced from ref. 2 with permission.

(with adequate hemoglobin and adequate perfusion) with an FiO_2 less than 0.5.

The degree of PEEP therapy that provides the greatest benefit while producing the fewest detrimental effects is difficult to define and complex to monitor clinically. Impairment of cardiac output with PEEP therapy is a well-known phenomenon. Since oxygen delivery to the tissues is determined by the arterial oxygen content and the cardiac output, oxygen delivery may be compromised if reductions in cardiac output occur to a greater degree than improvement in arterial oxygen content. The reduction in cardiac output induced by PEEP is attributable to at least three factors:

1. decreased venous return to the right heart;
2. right ventricular dysfunction; and
3. alterations in left ventricular distensibility.

The primary mechanism responsible for reduction in cardiac output appears to be impedance to systemic venous return due to increased intrathoracic pressure. Right ventricular dysfunction occurs because PEEP increases right ventricular afterload due to increased pulmonary vascular resistance. Increases in right ventricular afterload can result in an increase in right ventricular end diastolic volume (RVEDV). This increase in RVEDV has been associated with a leftward shift in the intraventricular septum[2,6] and subsequent left ventricular dysfunction due to limitation of the distensibility of the left ventricle. Decreased distensibility of the ventricle during PEEP therapy also appears to be directly related to the transmission of increased pressures to the pericardium. This cardiac output reduction is considerably less with CPAP than with PPV and PEEP. Spontaneous ventilation with PEEP requires less fluid loading to maintain cardiac output and enhances the transpulmonary pressure gradient resulting from any level of PEEP.

Seven factors are commonly considered when monitoring PEEP therapy; these are discussed below. Some of the factors are considered for obvious reasons, while the rationale behind the need for the others is less obvious. These other, less clearcut factors are discussed in more detail.

1. Arterial oxygen tension (PaO_2).
2. Cardiac output (Qt).
3. Arterial–venous oxygen content difference (A-VDO_2).
   This calculation represents the volume of oxygen extracted from 100 ml of blood and is not necessarily reflective of total body oxygen extraction per minute (VO_2). Normal A-VDO_2 values are 4.5–6.0 ml/dl, however, acute stress has been demonstrated to commonly result in cardiac output increases in excess of increased oxygen demand, resulting in an A-VDO_2 of 3–4 ml/dl.[48]
4. Oxygen delivery (DO_2).
   This calculation is cardiac output multiplied by the arterial oxygen content multiplied by 10. It is expressed as ml/min and represents the total oxygen volume presented to the tissues per minute. Since this calculation encompasses the two most critical

factors affected by PEEP therapy, DO_2 should be evaluated after each change in PEEP level.
5. Intrapulmonary physiologic shunting (Qs/Qt).
   This calculation requires measurement of FiO_2 plus arterial and pulmonary artery blood samples. It is a mathematical calculation of the amount of the cardiac output that is not exchanging with functional alveoli.
6. Dead space ventilation (Vd).
   Dead space ventilation can be quantified by calculation of the dead space to tidal volume ratio (Vd/Vt) or monitored by noting changes in the difference between the arterial and the end-tidal PCO_2. PEEP applied to normal lungs will increase alveolar pressure and alveolar dead space ventilation; however, as PEEP is applied to diseased lungs and collapsed alveoli are recruited to functional status there is a redistribution of ventilation that improves the overall V/Q matching and results in a decrease in dead space ventilation.
7. Lung compliance (Cl).
   A reflection of total pulmonary compliance is available by calculating the effective static compliance (ESC). Lung compliance and ESC are severely diminished in ARDS. As alveoli are expanded and recruited in acute lung injury (ALI) with PEEP therapy, ESC will improve until overdistension of the alveoli occurs.

PEEP devices

The safety and efficacy of PEEP therapy is partly dependent upon understanding the basic technology being utilized. Inappropriate technical application may increase peak and mean expiratory airway pressures, increase WOB, alter cardiac output, and increase the incidence of barotrauma. PEEP devices used for adults are usually threshold resistors that theoretically do not alter pressure as flow increases. However, available PEEP devices tend to increase airway pressure when flow increases to very high levels (i.e. they have orificial or flow resistor characteristics).

Gravity-dependent devices

These threshold resistor devices demonstrate the lowest degree of flow resistor characteristics but require an upright and stable position, which severely limits portability and safety.

Water column

PEEP is established by maintaining a constant hydrostatic force over a diaphragm that separates the water column from the expiratory limb of the circuit. Thus, pressure exceeding the PEEP level is required to lift the diaphragm and allow gas to exit the valve. The PEEP level can be adjusted from 0–25 cm H_2O by the addition of water. A major problem is that PEEP levels fluctuate significantly at higher system flows due to vibrations of the water column created by gas movement under the diaphragm.[49]

Weighted ball valve

The threshold resistance is created by the weight of a precision-ground ball atop a calibrated orifice; the heavier the ball, the greater the expiratory pressure. Flow resistance is dependent upon the surface area of the calibrated orifice. Valves are available preset to 2.5, 5, 10 and 15 cm H_2O. They are unidirectional and will cause obstruction if aligned backward in the circuit. These devices are so gravity dependent that even a 10° tilt from vertical may cause changes in PEEP level.

Non-gravity-dependent devices

The most popular type of threshold resistors that operate independent of gravity and position are spring-loaded valves in which expiratory pressure is maintained by the compression of a spring below its no-load length. Flow resistance properties of these valves depend on the surface area available at the point of seating of the valve's diaphragm. Because of variation in design, the flow resistance properties of each valve must be evaluated separately.

Ventilator exhalation valves

Valves used with mechanical ventilators are balloon-type or diaphragm-type devices, both of which function in a similar manner. These valves establish PEEP by maintaining a force either in the balloon or on the diaphragm, which must be exceeded in order for exhalation to occur (Fig. 10.4).

There is a tremendous variation in the flow resistance properties of these devices. Many are designed with very small exhalation port surface areas. This is particularly true of many of the inexpensive disposable valves that are available for use on a number of ventilators. Nondisposable valves produced by manufacturers of ventilators normally perform better. However, in most, as flow rates are increased, PEEP is significantly elevated.

CPAP systems

CPAP systems may be divided into demand systems and continuous flow systems. The inability of demand systems to meet inspiratory demands is well documented and can impose a significant work of breathing.[50–52]

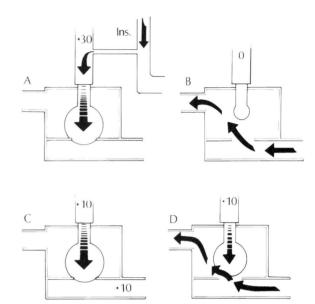

Fig. 10.4 Schematic representation of balloon-type exhalation valve under varying conditions of pressure. (**A**) The situation during positive pressure ventilation. The balloon is pressurized equal to the inspiratory line and therefore completely occludes the exhalation line. (**B**) Exhalation without PEEP. The balloon is collapsed, and there is free flow from the exhalation line to the outlet port without added resistance. (**C**) and (**D**) represent the circumstance where +10 cm H_2O pressure is applied to the balloon during exhalation. When exhalation line pressure is >+10 cm H_2O, the balloon will be displaced (**D**), and the gas will flow to the outlet port. When the exhalation line pressure is ⩽+10 cm H_2O, the balloon will occlude exhalation line and stop flow (**C**). As illustrated in (**D**), there is a potential restriction to flow resulting from the partially expanded balloon. This may be a clinically significant factor at relatively greater flow rates. Ins: Inspiration. Reproduced from ref. 2 with permission.

Continuous flow CPAP

Numerous variations on the design of 'continuous flow' CPAP systems exist but all stress that the circuit must be designed to minimize imposed work of breathing. One must be concerned with changes in pressure during inspiration, which are reflections of imposed inspiratory work on the patient, and changes in system pressure during expiration, which are reflective of imposed expiratory work. With all circuits, some fluctuations in system pressure is noted, the acceptable range being about ±2 cm H_2O. Fluctuations of greater magnitude during inspiration may be corrected by increasing system flow and/or increasing the size of the circuit reservoir. Changes in baseline pressure during exhalation are primarily affected by the flow-resistance properties of the PEEP device employed.

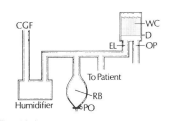

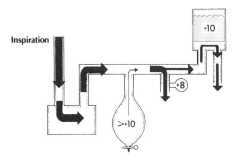

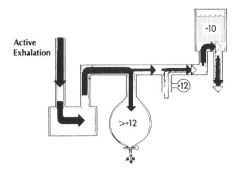

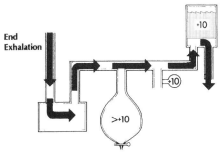

Fig. 10.5 Schematic representation of a CPAP device. **CGF** = continuous gas flow source; **RB** = elastic reservoir bag; **PO** = pop-off mechanism, which is an open nipple with an adjustable clamp; **WC** = water column determining the threshold pressure of $+10\,cm\,H_2O$; **D** = diaphragm of the PEEP device: **EL** = exhalation line of the patient circuit; **OP** = outlet port of the PEEP device. The continuous gas flow must be great enough to force some gas to continuously enter the reservoir bag except during peak inspiratory flow. Through adjustment of the pop-off mechanism, the pressure in the bag is maintained equal to or greater than the threshold pressure. Thus, gas will always flow through the outlet port of the PEEP device.

A typical continuous flow CPAP system is illustrated in Fig. 10.5. This system includes a medium volume, high compliance reservoir bag (5–10 liters) and maintains system flow in excess of patient peak inspiratory flow demands. Characteristically, system continuous flows are maintained at 60–90 l/min. The adequacy of continuous flow is evaluated by observing gas continuously exiting from the system, even during peak inspiratory flow periods. A system pressure manometer and, ideally, an oxygen analyzer, should be included in all CPAP circuits. Finally, a pressure pop-off is included in all systems to prevent excessive pressure (patient coughing with high flow resistance PEEP device or system obstruction) from building up in the system.

Physiologic PEEP

The term 'physiologic PEEP' has been applied to the application of $5–10\,cm\,H_2O$ of PEEP in intubated patients without identifiable pulmonary pathology. Several studies have shown beneficial effects of these low levels of PEEP with respect to maintenance of FRC and gas exchange in spontaneously ventilating intubated patients recovering from acute restrictive pulmonary pathology.[53,54] These data do not support the claim that all intubated patients require $5–10\,cm\,H_2O$ of PEEP. Although placement of an endotracheal tube is frequently associated with a reduction of FRC,[55] there are no data to suggest that physiologic PEEP may be beneficial in all patients who require intubation.

Ventilator discontinuance

Mechanical ventilation should be discontinued at the earliest time consistent with patient safety; however, careful assessment of the clinical situation is imperative because early attempts at ventilatory withdrawal without rationale usually result in unnecessary cardiopulmonary stress without shortening the ventilator

Note that the patient's airway pressure fluctuates not more than $\pm2\,cm\,H_2O$ of the threshold pressure. *Inspiration*: the majority of gas flow will enter the patient's airway without added impedance while the remainder flows through the outlet port of the PEEP device. Note that at the moment of the patient's peak inspiratory flow there may be a small amount of gas entering the patient circuit from the reservoir bag. *Active exhalation*: airway pressure is greater than threshold, causing more of the continuous gas flow to enter the reservoir bag. The increased expiratory flow may create increased pressure if the PEEP device has orificial resistor properties and thus increase the work of breathing. *End exhalation*: the continuous gas flow and reservoir bag maintain the circuit pressure at the threshold pressure.
Reproduced from ref. 2 with permission.

course. Ventilator discontinuance should be attempted only when:

1. the underlying indication for ventilatory support is reversed or significantly improved;
2. measurements of the cardiopulmonary reserves are judged adequate for spontaneous ventilation; and
3. general clinical examination and laboratory measurements suggest no factors that significantly increase ventilatory demand.

Assessment of cardiopulmonary reserves

1. A vital capacity (VC) greater than 15 ml/kg is encouraging because it reflects an adequate ventilatory muscle reserve. Do not rule out a trial of discontinuance for a VC between 10 and 15 ml/kg since VC often improves dramatically over several hours of spontaneous breathing. These guidelines apply to patients with previously normal pulmonary mechanics, chronically diseased patients (e.g. chronic obstructive pulmonary disease, quadriplegics) can breathe spontaneously with an extremely limited VC.
2. Immediate spontaneous tidal volumes (Vt) of greater than 2 ml/kg are encouraging. The adequacy of the Vt is often difficult to evaluate before the patient is breathing spontaneously for a period of time.
3. Spontaneous ventilatory rates of less than 25/min are encouraging; significant tachypnea demands re-evaluation.
4. Significant tachycardia on the ventilator is discouraging because the work of breathing will place an additional stress on the heart. Partial ventilatory support may prove a helpful step in evaluation.
5. Hypotension on the ventilator is discouraging; hypertension must be carefully evaluated.
6. Cardiac arrhythmias must be evaluated.
7. Hemoglobin content should be optimized.
8. Factors that increase ventilatory demand, e.g., acidemia, hypoxemia and high metabolic rates, should be corrected.

Evaluation of the respiratory status is best accomplished by blood gas evaluation before attempting removal from PPV:

1. arterial blood gas measurements must be acceptable on the ventilator;
2. no evidence of acute increased dead space ventilation should be present; and
3. intrapulmonary shunt measurement should be less than 30% and preferably less than 20%.

A conscious patient requires a thorough explanation of the procedure so that the activity around them is not alarming. Forewarning patients of the expected sequence of events results in less apprehension and reassures them that the clinician supervising the process is competent.

It has been clearly demonstrated that the method by which ventilatory support is withdrawn is not important in patients with adequate ventilatory reserves.[56] Experience indicates that this encompasses approximately 80% of patients who have had adequate reversal of the pathologic process that caused the need for mechanical ventilatory support. In these patients the ventilatory challenge is a reasonable approach to the withdrawal of ventilatory support.[57,58] In this circumstance, a competent practitioner (physician, respiratory therapist or nurse) removes the patient from the ventilator and provides a manual breath every 30 seconds with a manual resuscitation device delivering an FiO_2 of 0.5–0.8. This prevents hypoxemia, even if the patient makes no ventilatory efforts, while allowing the $PaCO_2$ to rise gradually.

The patient must be closely observed for clinical signs of detrimental WOB (tachypnea, tachycardia, diaphoresis, recruitment of accessory muscles of ventilation, etc.) and an ABG should be obtained after 5 minutes. If the patient shows evidence of cardiopulmonary instability, he is placed back on whatever level of ventilatory support is deemed appropriate until further improvement in the overall physiologic status is achieved. If the patient does well clinically and ABG analysis reveals appropriate ventilatory homeostasis, the patient is allowed to breathe spontaneously, observed for approximately another 5 to 10 minutes, and a similar clinical and ABG evaluation is carried out. If the patient remains stable, he is placed on CPAP, a T-piece or extubated as the clinical situation dictates. In this manner, one can safely withdraw ventilatory support from a stable patient in less than 15 minutes rather than over hours or days. However, the safety and efficacy of this method relies on a competent practitioner at the bedside making moment-to-moment evaluations of the patient's clinical work of breathing and cardiopulmonary stability.

The 20% of the patient population who require gradual withdrawal of ventilatory support usually include patients with severely compromised cardiac, pulmonary or neuromuscular function. Severe nutritional depletion is also a problem that may be encountered in severely ill patients. In these circumstances it may be necessary for the WOB to be assumed gradually in order to permit 'endurance training' to occur. Additionally, a sudden change from pure positive pressure ventilation to pure negative pressure ventilation may cause a rapid increase in venous return and cardiovascular compromise in certain patients.

Extrapulmonary gas exchange

In critically ill patients, acute respiratory failure is often secondary to acute lung injury (ALI), a pathologic response of lung parenchyma to severe systemic insults[59] that encompasses a spectrum of lung disease ranging from noncardiogenic edema (NCE) to the adult respiratory distress syndrome (ARDS).[60,61] The application of various types of airway pressure therapy has become the primary supportive modality for such patients because we have developed both the ability to safely establish and maintain artificial airways and the mechanical means by which to effectively apply positive pressure ventilation (PPV) and positive end expiratory pressure (PEEP).[60-65] There is good evidence and a general acceptance of the fact that the timely application of appropriate airway pressure therapy improves survival in patients with moderate to severe ALI.[64,66] However, patients with acute respiratory failure who require mechanical ventilatory support often require airway pressures high enough to be associated with pulmonary damage[60,67,68] and oxygen concentrations that are known to have toxic effects on lung parenchyma.[69-77] Therefore, any technique that would permit gas exchange (arterial oxygenation and carbon dioxide removal) at sites other than the lung could help avoid or diminish these detrimental effects of airway pressure and oxygen therapy and would be a welcome means by which to provide respiratory support for these patients.

EXTRACORPOREAL MEMBRANE OXYGENATION

Following the development of extracorporeal membrane oxygenators for open heart surgery, it was a logical step to the application of similar techniques to the treatment of severe acute respiratory failure. In the 1970s, extracorporeal membrane oxygenation (ECMO) was demonstrated to be capable of completely replacing the respiratory functions of the lung,[78-89] but its use failed to decrease mortality in adults with severe acute respiratory failure.[81] The technique was all but abandoned as a supportive modality for adults by 1980; however, investigation of ECMO for use in infant respiratory distress syndrome (IRDS) continued on the supposition that immature lungs, if protected from the damaging effects of toxic oxygen concentrations and high airway pressures, would gradually mature and assume near normal function. It appears that this approach has been successful in that the survival rate of neonates with IRDS who are treated with ECMO approaches 80%.[82] Additionally, improved survival rates have been noted when ECMO has been compared with conventional therapy in neonates suffering with severe respiratory compromise of other etiologies as well.[83]

EXTRACORPOREAL CARBON DIOXIDE REMOVAL

Extracorporeal carbon dioxide removal ($ECCO_2R$) was introduced in 1980 as a simplified veno-venous technique to provide significant carbon dioxide removal and minor augmentation of oxygenation in adults.[84] Unlike ECMO, which provides gas exchange for a volume of blood that approaches the total cardiac output, $ECCO_2R$ provides gas exchange for only a portion of the cardiac output (approximately 1 l/min). There is some evidence to suggest that this technique decreases mortality in severe acute respiratory failure in adults by allowing adequate carbon dioxide removal and arterial oxygenation to be achieved with significantly reduced airway pressures and oxygen concentrations.[85]

INTRAVASCULAR OXYGENATOR

The lack of efficacy of extracorporeal techniques for improvement of lung healing and the resource requirements (surgeons, technicians, support facilities, etc.) have relegated these techniques primarily to research endeavors at a few academic medical centers. In order to permit routine utilization, an extrapulmonary respiratory support device must be:

1. readily initiated at the bedside by an intensivist;
2. readily maintained by routine intensive care personnel (nurses, respiratory therapists, etc.); and
3. safe enough to be utilized as an alternative to exposure of the lungs to excessive pressures, volumes and oxygen concentrations.

No device with all of these characteristics is presently available. However, an *intracorporeal* respiratory support device that meets some of the above criteria, and has the potential to eventually meet them all, does presently exist.

The term intravascular oxygenator (IVOX) is somewhat of a misnomer because the device does not simply oxygenate, it removes carbon dioxide as well. The position of the device *in vivo* and the basic structure of the device are illustrated in Figs 10.6a, b. It is comprised of a bundle of hollow fibers which are inserted into the vena cava via the right internal jugular or femoral vein. The left-sided vessels cannot be used because of the angles that must be negotiated to allow placement in the vena cava. Pure oxygen is pulled through the hol-

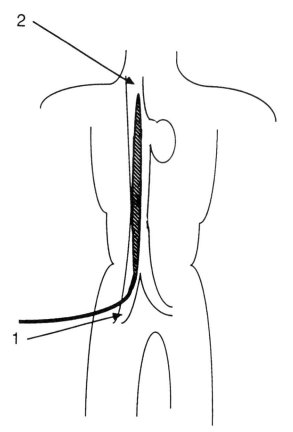

Fig. 10.6a The IVOX in place in the venous system. It may be placed by direct vessel cut-down from the right femoral vein (1) or the right internal jugular vein (2). Reproduced from ref. 86 with permission.

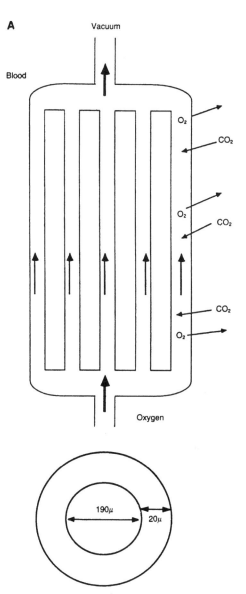

Fig. 10.6b A schematic representation of the IVOX device. The fibers are crimped to increase length and surface area and create disturbed blood flow in the vena cava. Oxygen is sucked through the fibers to effect gas exchange. (**B**) Fiber in cross-section. Reproduced from ref. 86 with permission.

low fibers under a vacuum and diffuses into the venous blood while carbon dioxide rapidly diffuses into the lumen of the fibers and is removed. The primary limitation of the device is its ability to exchange only about 25% of the total oxygen consumed and carbon dioxide produced by the body. Future refinements in the structure of the device may permit improved gas exchange capabilities and expand the usefulness of the method.

Conclusions

The complexity of intensive care has expanded with our technologic capability to support critically ill patients. As such, the complexity of the disease process that we now face requires an expanded armamentarium of support modalities. It is important to always remember and properly implement the basic techniques, but it is also important to be aware of new, more advanced methods and to understand under which circumstances they should be applied.

References

1. Schacter EN, Littner MR, Luddy P *et al*. Monitoring of oxygen delivery systems in clinical practice. *Crit Care Med* 1980; **8**: 405–9.
2. Shapiro BA, Kacmarek RM, Cane RD, Peruzzi WT, Hauptman D (eds). Oxygen therapy. In: *Clinical Application of Respiratory Care*, 4th edn. Chicago: Mosby Year Book, 1991: 123–34.

3. American College of Chest Physicians – Heart, Lung and Blood Institute. National Conference of Oxygen Therapy. *Chest* 1984; **85**: 234–47.

4. Scacci, R. Air entrainment masks: jet mixing is how they work; the Bernoulli and Venturi principles are how they don't. *Respir Care* 1979; **24**: 928–31.

5. Shim C *et al.* Cardiac arrhythmias resulting from tracheal suctioning. *Ann Intern Med* 1969; **71**: 1149–53.

6. Sloan HE. Vagus nerve in cardiac arrest. *Surg Gynecol Obstet* 1950; **91**: 257–64.

7. Ward JJ, Helmholz HF. Applied humidity and aerosol therapy. In: Burton GG, Hodgkin JE, Ward JJ (eds) *Respiratory Care: A Guide to Clinical Practice*, 3rd edn. Philadelphia: JB Lippincott, 1991: 355–96.

8. Radford R. Rational basis for percussion – augmented mucocilliary clearance. *Resp Care* 1982; **27**: 556.

9. Shapiro BA, Kacmarek RM, Cane RD, Peruzzi WT, Hauptman D. Applying and evaluating bronchial hygiene therapy. In: Shapiro BA, Kacmarek RM, Cane RD, Peruzzi WT, Hauptman D (eds). *Clinical Application of Respiratory Care*, 4th edn. Chicago: Mosby Year Book, 1991: 85–108.

10. Shapiro BA. When is an increase in work of breathing clinically significant? *Crit Care Med* 1990; **18**: 681.

11. Shapiro BA, Harrison RA, Cane RD, Templin R (eds). Respiratory acid–base balance. In: *Clinical Application of Blood Gases*, 4th edn. Chicago: Mosby Year Book, 1989: 38–56.

12. American Association for Respiratory Care. Consensus conference of the essentials of mechanical ventilators. *Resp Care* 1993; **37**: 999–1008.

13. Marinii JJ, Capps JS, Culver BH. The inspiratory work of breathing during assisted mechanical ventilation. *Chest* 1985; **87**: 612–18.

14. Marini JJ, Rodriquez RM, Lamb V. The inspiratory workload of patient-initiated mechanical ventilation. *Am Rev Respir Dis* 1986; **134**: 902–9.

15. Marcy TW, Marini JJ. Controlled mechanical ventilation and assist/control ventilation. In: Perel A, Stock MC (eds) *Handbook of Mechanical Ventilatory Support*. Philadelphia: Williams & Wilkins, 1992: 81–99.

16. Weisman IM, Rinaldo JE, Rogers RM, Sanders MH. State of the art: intermittent mandatory ventilation. *Am Rev Respir Dis* 1983; **127**: 641–7.

17. Groeger JS, Levinson MR, Carlon GC. Assist control versus synchronized intermittent mandatory ventilation during acute respiratory failure. *Crit Care Med* 1989; **17**: 607–12.

18. Peruzzi WT. Full and partial ventilatory support: the significance of ventilator mode. *Resp Care* 1990; **35**: 174–5.

19. Norlander O. New concepts of ventilation. *Acta Anaesthesiol Belg* 1982; **33**: 221.

20. Hansen J, Wendt M, Lawin P. Ein neus Weaning-Verfahren (inspiratory flow assistance-IFA). *Anesthetist* 1984; **33**: 428–32.

21. Kacmarek RM. The role of pressure support ventilation in reducing work of breathing. *Respir Care* 1988; **33**: 99–120.

22. Katz JA, Kraemer RW, Gjerde GE. Inspiratory work and airway pressure with continuous positive airway pressure delivery systems. *Chest* 1985; **88**: 519–26.

23. Van de Graaff WB, Gordey K, Dornseif SE *et al.* Pressure support. Changes in ventilatory pattern and components of the work of breathing. *Chest* 1991; **100**: 182–9.

24. Gurevitch MJ, Van Dyke J, Young ES *et al.* Improved oxygenation and lower peak airway pressure in severe adult respiratory distress syndrome. *Chest* 1986; **89**: 211–13.

25. Tharratt RS, Allen RP, Albertson TE. Pressure controlled inverse ratio ventilation in severe adult respiratory failure. *Chest* 1988; **94**: 755–62.

26. Abraham A, Yoshihara G. Cardiorespiratory effects of pressure controlled inverse ratio ventilation in severe respiratory failure. *Chest* 1989; **96**: 1356–9.

27. Stock MC, Downs JB. Airway pressure release ventilation: a new approach to ventilatory support during acute lung injury. *Respir Care* 1987; **32**: 517–24.

28. Stock MC, Downs JB, Frolicher DA. Airway pressure release ventilation. *Crit Care Med* 1987; **15**: 462–6.

29. Hewlett AM, Platt AS, Terry VG. Mandatory minute volume: a new concept in weaning from mechanical ventilation. *Anaesthesia* 1977; **32**: 163–9.

30. Thompson JD. Mandatory minute ventilation. In: Perel A, Stock MC (eds) *Handbook of Mechanical Ventilatory Support*. Baltimore: Williams & Wilkins, 1992: 137–43.

31. Meduri GU, Conoscenti CC, Menashe P, Nair S. Non-invasive face mask ventilation in patients with acute respiratory failure. *Chest*, 1989; **95**: 865–70.

32. Brochard L, Isabey D, Piquet J *et al.* Reversal of acute exacerbations of chronic obstructive lung disease by inspiratory assistance with a face mask. *New Engl J Med* 1990; **323**: 1523–30.

33. Pennock BE, Kaplan PD, Carlin BW, Sabangan JS, Magovern JA. Pressure support ventilation with a simplified ventilatory support system administered with a nasal mask in patients with respiratory failure. *Chest* 1991; **100**: 1371–6.

34. Froese AB, Bryan AC. State of the art: high frequency ventilation. *Am Rev Respir Dis* 1987; **135**: 1363–74.

35. McCulloch PR, Froese AB. High frequency ventilation. *Anesthesiol Clin North Am* 1987; **5**: 873–91.

36. Sjostrand U. High-frequency positive-pressure ventilation (HFPPV): a review. *Crit Care Med* 1980; **8**: 345–64.

37. Turnbull AD, Carlon GC, Howland WS *et al.* High frequency jet ventilation in major airway or pulmonary disruption. *Ann Thorac Surg* 1981; **32**: 468.

38. Klain M, Smith RB. High-frequency percutaneous transtracheal jet ventilation. *Crit Care Med* 1977; **5**: 280–7.

39. Gallagher TJ, Klain MK, Carlon GC. Present status of high frequency ventilation. *Crit Care Med* 1982; **10**: 613–7.

40. Carlon GC, Ray C Jr, Griffin J *et al.* Tidal volume and airway pressure on high frequency jet ventilation. *Crit Care Med* 1983; **11**: 83–6.

41. Chang HK. Mechanisms of gas transport during ventilation by high-frequency oscillation. *J Appl Physiol* 1984; **56**: 553–63.

42. Knopp TJ, Kaethner T, Meyer M *et al.* Gas mixing in the airways of dog lungs during high-frequency ventilation. *J Appl Physiol* 1983; **55**: 1141–6.

43. Carlon GC, Kahn RC, Howland WS *et al.* Clinical

experience with high frequency jet ventilation. *Crit Care Med* 1981; **9**: 1–6.

44. Mayers I, Long R, Breen PH *et al*. Artificial ventilation of a canine model of bronchopleural fistula. *Anesthesiology* 1986; **64**: 739–46.

45. Drazen JM, Kamm RD, Slutsky AS. High-frequency ventilation. *Physiol Rev* 1984; **64**: 505–43.

46. Cheney F *et al*. Effects of ultrasonically produced aerosol on airway resistance in man. *Anesthesiology* 1968; **29**: 1099–106.

47. Scacci R. Air entrainment masks: jet mixing is how they work; the Bernoulli and Venturi principles are how they don't. *Respir Care* 1979; **24**: 928–31.

48. Cherniack RM. Intermittent positive pressure breathing in management of chronic obstructive disease: Current state of the art. *Am Rev Respir Dis* 1974; **110**: 188–92.

49. Shim C *et al*. The effect of inhalation therapy on ventilatory function and expectoration. *Chest* 1978; **73**(6): 798–801.

50. Noehren T. Is positive pressure breathing overrated? *Chest* 1970; **57**: 507–9.

51. Martin RJ, Rogers RM, Gray BA. Mechanical aids to lung expansion: the physiologic basis for the use of mechanical aids to lung expansion. *Am Rev Resp Dis* 1980; **122**: 105–7.

52. Shapiro BA, Peterson J, Cane RD. Complications of mechanical aids to intermittent lung inflation. *Respir Care* 1982; **27**: 467–70.

53. Cournand A, Motley HL, Werko L. Physiologic studies of the effects of intermittent positive pressure breathing on cardiac output in man. *Am J Physiol* 1948; **152**: 162–74.

54. Price HL *et al*. Some respiratory and circulatory effects of mechanical respirators. *J Appl Physiol* 1954; **6**: 517–30.

55. Werko L. Influence of positive pressure breathing on the circulation in man. *Acta Med Scand* 1947; **193** (Suppl):1–125.

56. Tomlinson JR, Miller S, Lorch DG *et al*. A prospective comparison of IMV and T-piece weaning from mechanical ventilation. *Chest* 1989; **96**: 348–52.

57. Cane RD, Shapiro BA. Ventilator discontinuance. *Anesthesiol Clin North Am* 1987; **5**: 749–55.

58. Peruzzi WT. The ventilatory challenge in weaning. *Chest* 1990; **97**: 1024.

59. Weisman IM, Rinaldo JE, Rogers RM. Positive end-expiratory pressure in adult respiratory failure. *New Engl J Med* 1982; **307**: 1381–84.

60. Shapiro BA, Cane RD, Harrison RA. Positive end-expiratory pressure therapy in adults with special reference to acute lung injury: a review of the literature and suggested clinical correlations. *Crit Care Med* 1984; **12**: 127–41.

61. Suchyta MR, Clemmer TP, Orme JF *et al*. Increased survival of ARDS patients with severe hypoxemia: ECMO criteria. *Chest* 1991; **99**: 951–5.

62. Shapiro BA, Cane RD. Positive airway pressure therapy: PPV and PEEP. *Anesthesiol Clin North Am* 1987; **5**: 797–806.

63. Cane RD, Shapiro BA. Mechanical ventilatory support. *J Am Med Assoc* 1985; **254**: 87–92.

64. Kolobow T, Moretti MP, Fumagalli R *et al*. Severe impairment in lung function induced by high peak airway pressure during mechanical ventilation: an experimental study. *Am Rev Respir Dis* 1987; **135**: 312–15.

65. Weisman IM, Rinaldo JE, Rogers RM. Positive end-expiratory pressure in adult respiratory failure. *New Engl J Med* 1982; **307**: 1381.

66. Pierson DJ. Alveolar rupture during mechanical ventilation: role of PEEP, peak airway pressure, and distending volume. *Respir Care* 1988; **33**: 472–86.

67. Montgomery AB, Stager MA, Carrico CJ *et al*. Causes of mortality in patients with adult respiratory distress syndrome. *Am Rev Respir Dis* 1985; **132**: 485–9.

68. Deneke SM, Fanburg BL. Normobaric oxygen toxicity of the lung. *New Engl J Med* 1980; **303**: 76–86.

69. Shapiro BA, Cane RD. Metabolic malfunction of lung: noncardiogenic edema and adult respiratory distress syndrome. *Surg Ann* 1981; **13**: 271–98.

70. Shapiro BA, Cane RD, Harrison RA. Positive end-expiratory pressure in acute lung injury. *Chest* 1983; **83**: 558–63.

71. Nash G, Blennerhassett JB, Pontoppidan H. Pulmonary lesions associated with oxygen therapy and artificial ventilation. *New Engl J Med* 1967; **276**: 368–74.

72. Collins JF, Smith JD, Coalson JJ *et al*. Variability of lung collagen amounts after prolonged support of acute respiratory failure. *Chest* 1984; **85**: 641–6.

73. Witschi HR, Haschek WM, Klein-Szanto AJP *et al*. Potentiation of diffuse lung damage by oxygen: Determining variables. *Am Rev Respir Dis* 1981; **123**: 98–103.

74. Davis WB, Rennard SI, Bitterman PB *et al*. Pulmonary oxygen toxicity: Early reversible changes in human alveolar structure induced by hyperoxia. *New Engl J Med* 1983; **309**: 878–83.

75. Fox RB, Hoidal JR, Brown DM *et al*. Pulmonary inflammation due to oxygen toxicity: involvement of chemotactic factors and polymorphonuclear leukocytes. *Am Rev Respir Dis* 1981; **123**: 521–3.

76. Kistler GS, Caldwell PEG, Weibel ER. Development of fine structural damage to alveolar and capillary lining cells in oxygen-poisoned rat lungs. *J Cell Biol* 1978; **32**: 605–28.

77. Crapo JD, Barry BE, Foscue HA *et al*. Structural and biochemical changes in rat lungs occurring during exposures to lethal and adaptive doses of oxygen. *Am Rev Respir Dis* 1980; **122**: 123–43.

78. Davis WB, Rennard SI, Bitterman PB *et al*. Pulmonary oxygen toxicity: early reversible changes in human alveolar structures induced by hyperoxia. *New Engl J Med* 1983; **309**: 878–83.

79. Hill JD, O'Brien TG, Murray JJ *et al*. Prolonged extracorporeal oxygenation for acute post-traumatic respiratory failure (shock lung syndrome). *New Engl J Med* 1972; **286**: 629–34.

80. Hill JD, Ratliff JL, Fallat RJ *et al*. Prognostic factors in the treatment of acute respiratory insufficiency with long-term extracorporeal oxygenation. *J Thorac Cardiovasc Surg* 1974; **68**: 905–17.

81. Bartlett RH, Gazzinga AB, Fong SW *et al*. Prolonged extracorporeal cardiopulmonary support in man. *J Thorac Cardiovasc Surg* 1974; **68**: 918–32.

82. Zapol WM, Snider MT, Hill JD *et al*. Extracorporeal

membrane oxygenation in severe acute respiratory failure. *J Am Med Assoc* 1979; **242**: 2193–6.

83. Toomasian IM, Snedecor SM, Cornell RD. National experience with extracorporeal oxygenation (ECMO) for newborn respiratory failure: data from 715 cases. *Ann Arbor, Mich: ECMO Data Registry, Department of Surgery and Biostatistics.* University of Michigan, 1986.

84. Bartlett RH, Roloff DW, Cornell RG *et al.* Extracorporeal

circulation in neonatal respiratory failure: a prospective randomized study. *Pediatrics* 1985; **76**: 479–87.

85. Gattinoni L, Agnostoni A, Pesenti A *et al.* Treatment of acute respiratory failure with low frequency positive pressure ventilation and extracorporeal CO_2 removal. *Lancet* 1980; **2**: 292–4.

86. Durbin J Jr. Intravenous oxygenation and CO_2 removal device: IVOX. *Respir Care* 1992; **37**: 147–53.

CHAPTER 11

Cardiac Support for Acute Cardiac Failure

GINA PRICE LUNDBERG, JE CALVIN

Pathophysiology of cardiogenic shock 156
Predictors of cardiogenic shock 157
Prognosis after development of cardiogenic shock 157
Types of cardiac support 158
Nonpharmacological treatment 161
Ventricular assist devices/total artificial heart 163
Comprehensive hemodynamic management of cardiogenic shock and pump failure 171
Summary 173
References 173

Cardiogenic shock (CGS), defined by the presence of hypotension, altered mental status and oliguria in addition to obvious signs of cardiac failure such as left ventricular (LV) dilatation, an S_3 gallop, elevated jugular venous pressure (JVP), and peripheral or pulmonary edema, complicates the clinical course of approximately 5–10% of patients admitted with acute myocardial infarction[1] and 4% of patients after coronary bypass surgery.[2] The hospital mortality rate historically exceeds 80%.[1]

Over the last decade newer approaches have been introduced in an attempt to improve this dismal prognosis, and preliminary reports are indeed encouraging. The purpose of this chapter is to review the current means of acute cardiac support and critically evaluate their efficacy.

Pathophysiology of cardiogenic shock

CARDIAC ABNORMALITIES

The clinical syndrome of CGS can result from any single or any combination of the following physio-logical abnormalities complicating an acute myocardial infarction:

1. Depressed left ventricular contractility from myocardial infarction itself or cardiomyopathy.[3–7]
2. Reduced left ventricular compliance from myocardial infarction or ischemia.[8–10]
3. Mechanical complications of myocardial infarction such as severe mitral regurgitation (MR)[11–15] resulting in pump failure, interventricular septal defect (IVSD),[11,13,14,16,17] or free wall rupture resulting in cardiac tamponade.
4. Electrical disturbances such as severe bradycardia or tachyarrhythmias.
5. Depressed right ventricular (RV) contractility from RV infarction[18–20] leading to decreased preload of the left ventricle (because of reduced RV stroke output and reduced LV compliance produced by a direct mechanical ventricular interaction mediated by the pericardium and possibly the interventricular septum).[21,22]
6. Volume depletion (reduced preload) from excessive diuresis or drugs with venodilator capabilities.[23]
7. Depressed myocardial performance by a number of other reversible factors including hypoxemia, acidosis and negative inotropic medications.[24,25]

The most important of these abnormalities is the loss of systolic function from the loss of more than 40% of effective muscle mass. Most new therapies are aimed at either reducing muscle damage or supporting myocardial failure.

Predictors of cardiogenic shock

The Multicenter Investigation of Limitation of Infarct Size (MILIS)[26] study group followed 845 patients admitted for acute myocardial infarction prospectively for the development of CGS. They found that CGS developed in 7.1% of the patients hospitalized for acute myocardial infarction. Of note, half of these patients developed CGS at least 24 hours after their admission. The in-hospital mortality rate was 65% for patients with CGS as compared to 4% for patients without CGS. The study group found five independent predictors for in-hospital development of CGS. These were:

1. age greater than 65 years;
2. left ventricular ejection fraction on hospital admission less than 35%;
3. large infarct as estimated from serial enzyme determinations with a peak CK MB isoenzyme greater than 160 IU per liter;
4. history of diabetes mellitus; and
5. previous myocardial infarction.

The investigators found that the more risk factors a patient had, the greater the risk of mortality, with five risk factors giving a mortality of 55%. The most important determinate of in-hospital mortality in

patients with CGS was left ventricular dysfunction as reflected by a left ventricular ejection fraction less than 35% and the severity of left ventricular wall abnormalities.

Prognosis after development of cardiogenic shock

The first study which evaluated prognosis after myocardial infarction used three clinical signs to stratify patients: lung crackles, an S_3, and blood pressure.[27] Mortality ranged from 6% in uncomplicated myocardial infarction to 81% in patients with signs of clinical CGS using this classification.

With the introduction of flow-directed right heart catheterization in the early 1970s,[28, 29] ventricular function curves could be constructed on individual patients. By correlating significant physiological abnormalities such as pulmonary congestion and tissue hypoperfusion, optimal ranges of left ventricular filling pressure (so-called pulmonary capillary wedge pressure, PCWP), and cardiac index (CI) were determined. Analysis of such data allowed Forrester and colleagues[1] to develop a new classification based upon CI and filling pressures. This classification was not only useful for prognosis, but also for guiding therapy based on hemodynamic values observed in survivors. It seemed intuitive that if therapy could correct both physiological and hemodynamic abnormalities, prognosis could be improved. The original hemodynamic subgroups are shown in Table 11.1. It is important to note that this classification, although based on ventricular function, does not take into account the independent effects of

Table 11.1 Prognosis after myocardial infarction based upon clinical and hemodynamic parameters

	% Patients	Mortality (%)
Clinical class of acute MI (Killip and Kimball)[27]		
Class 1 No signs of congestive heart failure	40–50	6
Class 2 S_3, pulmonary congestion	30–40	17
Class 3 Acute pulmonary edema	10–15	81
Class 4 Cardiogenic shock	5–10	81
Clinical subsets of acute MI (Cedars-Sinai)[1]		
Subset 1 No pulmonary congestion or tissue hyperfusion	25	1
Subset 2 Pulmonary congestion only	25	11
Subset 3 Tissue hypoperfusion only	15	18
Subset 4 Tissue hypoperfusion and pulmonary congestion	35	60
Hemodynamic subsets (Cedars-Sinai)[1]		
Subset 1 PCWP ≤ 18; CI > 2.2	25	3
Subset 2 PCWP ≥ 18; CI > 2.2	25	9
Subset 3 PCWP ≤ 18; CI ≤ 2.2	15	23
Subset 4 PCWP ≥ 18; CI ≤ 2.2	35	51

PCWP: pulmonary capillary wedge pressure. CI: cardiac index.

mechanical defects, RV infarction, degree of coronary artery disease, severe hypertension, or comorbid conditions. Nonetheless, sound principles of therapy can be based upon it. This led to active research programs investigating the role of medical therapy in acute myocardial infarction and CGS.

Types of cardiac support

MEDICAL THERAPY

Historically, the major therapeutic emphasis has been placed on increasing blood pressure and cardiac output and relieving pulmonary edema through medical therapy, although mortality was never convincingly reduced. Nonetheless, medical therapy is of benefit in a small number of patients and allows stabilization in many patients awaiting diagnostic tests and more definitive therapies. Inotropic drugs such as catecholamines, phosphodiesterase inhibitors and vasodilator agents are commonly used to optimize hemodynamic endpoints.

Inotropic agents

Catecholamines

Catecholamines, by their interaction with adrenergic receptors,[30,31] stimulate cAMP production and are frequently used to treat patients with cardiogenic shock (see Table 11.2). The main goals of catecholamine therapy are to increase CI index and blood pressure. With selected agents, the PCWP can also be lowered.

Table 11.2   Catecholamine receptors stimulation

Drug	Receptor				
	α_1	α_2	β_1	β_2	DA_1
Epinephrine	+++	+++	+++	0	0
Norepinephrine	+++	+++	++	0	0
Isoproterenol	0	0	+++	+++	0
Dopamine	++	++[c]	+++[b]	+	+++[a]
Dobutamine	+	0	+++	+	0

α_1: postsynaptic receptor in vascular smooth muscle; α_2: presynaptic receptor; β_1: largely cardiac; β_2: largely smooth muscle of vasculature and bronchial tree; DA_1: dopaminergic postsynaptic receptors in renal, splanchnic, cerebral and coronary vessels; +: stimulation; 0: no effect.
[a] At doses <5 µg/kg/min.
[b] At doses between 5 and 15 µg/kg/min.
[c] At doses >5 µg/kg/min.

Dopamine

Dopamine is a complex drug given the fact that its effects are dose dependent.[32-34] It is capable of dopaminergic stimulation[35] with the resultant effects of increased renal and splanchnic blood flow at low doses of 1–5 µg/kg/min (Tables 11.2 and 11.3). There is mild beta-1 agonist[36] activity producing a small increase in stroke volume. At higher doses of between 5 and 15 µg/kg/min, beta-1 receptor stimulation predominates, resulting in increases in stroke volume, cardiac output (CO) and heart rate (HR). Because of its low beta-2 receptor agonist activity, little peripheral or pulmonary vasodilation occurs. As a result, neither systemic vascular resistance (SVR) nor the PCWP change significantly. Doses greater than 15 µg/kg/min cause alpha-1 receptor stimulation with the resultant effect of peripheral vasoconstriction. Although this aids in maintaining or increasing blood pressure, it has potential deleterious effects on cardiac output and renal blood flow.

Dobutamine

Dobutamine is a synthetic cardioactive sympathomimetic amine that stimulates beta-1 activity predominately over beta-2 and alpha adrenoceptors (Table 11.2).[32,33,37-39]

In patients with heart failure, dobutamine produces a reduction in SVR and a rise in cardiac output. It has been shown to decrease PCWP and increase stroke work (SW). It can cause increases in heart rate and its effect on blood pressure is variable.[34,39] In general, doses between 2.5 and 15 mg/kg/min are recommended (Table 11.3).

By increasing HR and SW, dobutamine also increases myocardial oxygen consumption (MVO_2). Dobutamine also increases coronary blood flow and myocardial oxygen delivery.[40] While dobutamine increases blood flow in patients with normal coronary arteries, in patients with coronary artery disease (CAD), these increases are inhomogeneous.[41] This suggests that dobutamine should be used with caution in patients with severe CAD. To further elaborate on dobutamine's potential to induce ischemia, another study of 18 patients with congestive heart failure (CHF) complicating CAD and seven patients with primary cardiomyopathy (1° CM) showed improved hemodynamics in both groups.[42] However, 22% of the patients with CAD showed abnormal lactate extraction with doses of dobutamine up 15 µg/kg/min. This potential for producing ischemia may be related to excessive increases in heart rate.[43,44]

Norepinephrine

Norepinephrine is the neurotransmitter of the sympathetic nervous system and is the biosynthetic

Table 11.3 Dose ranges for drugs used in cardiogenic shock

Drug	Usual doses	Intended hemodynamic action	Major side effects
Nitroglycerin	10–200 µg/min	↓ ↓ PCWP ↓ ischemia	Hypotension, headache
Nitroprusside	15–400 µg/min	↓ SAP, afterload, PCWP, ↑ CI	Hypotension, thiocyanate toxicity, ↓ PO$_2$ methemoglobinemia ischemia
Phentolamine	0.25–1 µg/min	↓ SAP, afterload, PCWP, ↑ CI	Hypotension
Norepinephrine	1–8 µg/kg/min	↑ SAP	↑ afterload; variable effect upon CO
Dopamine	2.5–15 µg/kg/min 5–15 µg/kg/min >15 µg/kg/min	↑ RBF ↑ CI, ↑ SAP ↑ CI, ↑ SAP	↑ HR, arrhythmia
Dobutamine	2.5–15 µg/kg/min	↑ CI, ↓ PCWP	↑ HR, arrhythmia (less common) ↑ ischemia
Amrinone	2.5–10 µg/kg/min	↑ CI, ↓ PCWP, ↓ MVO$_2$	↑ ischemia (rare)

CI: cardiac index; CO: cardiac output; HR: heart rate; MVO$_2$: myocardial oxygen consumption; PCWP: pulmonary capillary wedge pressure; RBF: renal blood flow; SAP: systolic arterial pressure.

precursor of epinephrine. It is both an alpha and beta agonist (Table 11.2). However, it has less beta-2 agonist activity than dobutamine; it therefore causes more peripheral vasoconstriction. It is generally used to treat a primary decrease in systemic blood pressure or an exacerbation of right ventricular ischemia and/or failure. In acute left heart failure, it is most commonly used with an alpha-2 blocker such as phentolamine to counteract the peripheral vasoconstricting effects which increase LV afterload.[45]

Isoproterenol

Isoproterenol[36] can be used when a chronotropic response is required in addition to an inotropic effect. Its powerful beta-1 effects increase heart rate significantly, making it useful in treating symptomatic bradycardias or complete heart block. However, it is well known to produce or aggravate ventricular arrhythmias and increase MVO$_2$. Therefore, it is used cautiously in patients with CAD.

Phosphodiesterase inhibitors

Amrinone

Amrinone is a bipyridine guanide that exerts its inotropic effect through inhibition of the enzyme phosphodiesterase III, thereby increasing cyclic adeno-

sine monophosphate (cAMP) and increasing cytosolic calcium. In addition to its inotropic properties, amrinone causes vasodilation, both arterial and venous, and thus reduces the SVR and workload (preload and afterload) of the heart.

Intravenous administration of the agent has been shown to increase cardiac output by 30–69% in patients with heart failure, and augment compliance (dP/dt) without causing significant changes in heart rate or blood pressure.[46–48] These effects are accompanied by a reduction in LV filling pressure (preload), mean pulmonary artery pressure (MPAP), right atrial pressure (RAP), and systemic (SVR) and pulmonary vascular resistance (PVR). Amrinone has been shown to reduce PCWP by an average of 27%, while a similar decrease has been reported for SVR. Stroke work is not changed.

Of particular significance is the effect of amrinone on MVO$_2$. Unlike the sympathomimetic amines, amrinone appears to produce a 20–30% decrease in MVO$_2$.[49,50] An explanation for this phenomenon may lie with amrinone's vasodilating capabilities. The effect of an inotropic agent on MVO$_2$ depends on its net effect on heart rate, contractile state, and mean systolic wall stress. Unless increased heart rate and contractile state are offset by decreased wall stress, MVO$_2$ will rise. A reduction in cardiac preload and afterload, achieved through amrinone's vasodilating properties, may produce the necessary fall in resting wall tension required to decrease MVO_2.

Findings from clinical studies appear to support this explanation. Intravenous amrinone was administered to nine patients with ischemic cardiomyopathy, and it decreased MVO_2 by 30%, despite a 69% increase in cardiac output.[50] Coronary sinus blood flow decreased by 17% and arterial-coronary sinus oxygen difference fell by 16%.

The beneficial effects upon hemodynamics appear to be sustained longer with amrinone than with dobutamine. In a comparison of both agents in patients with chronic congestive heart failure, the hemodynamic effects were found to be comparable. However, the initial increment in cardiac output produced by dobutamine decreased after 8 hours of therapy, whereas the increase produced by amrinone was sustained over 24 hours of infusion.[47] This apparent tachyphylaxis of dobutamine is probably due to beta receptor down-regulation.[51]

Combination therapy with amrinone and dobutamine has been found to decrease PCWP and increase cardiac output to a greater extent than when either of the drugs is used alone. A synergistic effect between dobutamine and amrinone has been demonstrated, resulting in greater increases in left ventricular dP/dt (from 1202 ± 376 to 1319 ± 419 mm Hg/s) and cardiac index (from 3.04 ± 0.67 to 3.56 ± 0.78 l/min/m^2) and greater reductions in left ventricular end-diastolic pressure (from 18.2 ± 10.3 to 15.3 ± 11.3 mm Hg) in 11 patients with chronic congestive heart failure.[52]

Common side effects of inotropic agents

Arrhythmias and hypotension can occur with either amrinone or dobutamine. Amrinone induces reversible thrombocytopenia in 2.4–4% of cases and arrhythmias in 3%. Gastrointestinal upset, chest pain and elevated liver enzymes have been reported on rare occasions.[53]

Dobutamine's side effect profile is similar to amrinone's. Increased premature ventricular beats have been reported in 5% of patients receiving dobutamine. Arrhythmias constitute the most common serious side effect of this agent.

Vasodilators

In the last two decades, vasodilators have taken on a more important role in the treatment of patients with acute heart failure. Patients with reduced pump performance have a critical dependence on low afterload; hence, drugs that reduce peripheral resistance increase stroke volume. Furthermore, pump performance is improved by the reduction in myocardial oxygen consumption through reduced systolic pressure or reduced wall stress.

In addition to the effect of vasodilators in reducing LV afterload, patients manifesting reduced left ventricular compliance due to acute myocardial ischemia may also benefit from sodium nitroprusside, nitroglycerin and phentolamine.[54–60] By virtue of their effects to shift the left ventricular end-diastolic pressure–volume relationship down and to the right,[54] left ventricular diastolic function improves (Fig. 11.1).

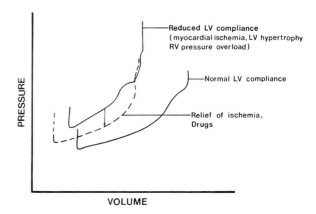

Fig. 11.1   Effects of reduced left ventricular (LV) compliance upon the LV diastolic pressure–volume relationship. Myocardial ischemia can acutely shift the relationship upwards. Venodilators can shift the relationship downwards, reducing the filling pressure with little disturbance in LV end-diastolic volume.

Without this effect on left ventricular end-diastolic pressure–volume relationships, much of the potential benefits of afterload reduction associated with the use of vasodilators might be opposed by these agents' effects of reducing venous tone and venous return, and thereby reducing left ventricular preload and stroke volume. However, as shown in Fig. 11.1, the concomitant shift downward of the left ventricular diastolic pressure–volume relationship observed with these vasodilators both maintains end-diastolic volume and reduces end-diastolic pressure. However, to gain the maximum benefit from administration of systemic vasodilators, the patient must first be adequately volume-resuscitated.[61,62] In chronic congestive failure, hydralazine mediates an increase in improved forward flow only in those patients with a larger than normal left ventricular preload prior to administration.

Types of vasodilators

Sodium nitroprusside

Sodium nitroprusside is an extremely important vasodilator that affects both the arterial and the venous circulation.[62] The balanced effect on the venous capacitance and arterial resistance vessels results in both afterload reduction and reduction in pulmonary congestion.[58,59,63] Heart rate, in general, increases and arterial blood pressure is reduced in normal patients; however, in heart failure this is not seen regularly. Nitroprusside is given in a dose between 15 and 400 mg/min (Table 11.3). The side effects include hypotension and the accumulation of thiocyanate. Prolonged administration of high doses, especially in the presence of renal failure, can result in cyanide toxicity. Thiocyanate levels should be determined under any of these conditions. Acute cyanide poisoning can be treated with amyl nitrite inhalations and intravenous administration of sodium thiosulfate.

Nitroglycerin

Intravenous nitroglycerin is a commonly used agent in treatment of pulmonary edema. Nitroglycerin has a profound effect on the venous circulation and therefore results in a reduction in venous return and pulmonary capillary wedge pressure.[25,54] Cardiac output is usually unchanged. The usual dose range is between 10 and 200 μg/min (Table 11.3) titrated to a hemodynamic response (usually decreasing PCWP to 14–18 mm Hg and decreasing systolic blood pressure by 10%.

Nitroglycerin may have advantages over diuretics in the treatment of acute pulmonary edema. Recent studies have demonstrated that furosemide, a potent loop diuretic, can result in a reduction in cardiac output and an elevation in systemic vascular resistance and pulmonary capillary wedge pressure within 15–20 minutes of administration.[64] Eventually the diuretic effect dominates. It is in this early phase that the use of a venodilator may result in a more immediate reduction in pulmonary venous pressure and congestion.

Nonpharmacological treatment

REPERFUSION TECHNIQUES

Beyond using supportive therapy aimed at improving cardiac output and optimizing LV preload, the last decade has witnessed major innovations in therapy aimed at restoring myocardial blood flow and improving ventricular function.

Thrombolytic therapy

Thrombolytic therapy is now associated with decreased mortality in patients with myocardial infarction.[65,66] The Society for Cardiac Angiography reported in 1985[67] a 42% in-hospital mortality rate for cardiogenic shock in patients who were successfully reperfused. This represents a significant improvement over earlier observations. Although the GISSI study clearly showed a benefit from intravenous streptokinase (IVSK) in acute

myocardial infarction, the one subgroup that did not show improved survival was the CGS group, the patients in Killip Class IV.[68] In patients with acute myocardial infarction complicated by CGS treated with thrombolytics, the mortality rate was 70% in both the IVSK-treated group as well as the control group. Large series with both intracoronary and intravenous administration of streptokinase have failed to show any significant benefit in patients with CGS.[69,70]

Intra-aortic balloon pumping

Intra-aortic balloon pumping (IABP) has been used in treating cardiogenic shock over the last two decades. Early experience demonstrated its usefulness as a bridge to early surgery aimed at establishing reperfusion or repairing mechanical defects. As a sole therapy, it was associated with a low salvage rate of approximately 15%.[71] More recently, DeWood et al.[72] demonstrated that intra-aortic balloon pumping alone had an in-hospital mortality of 52%, not significantly different from the in-hospital mortality of patients treated with IABP and coronary artery bypass grafting (CABG) combined (42%). However, long-term mortality was much higher in patients treated with IABP alone (71%) compared to patients who had both IABP and CABG (47%).

Despite its limitations as sole therapy, IABP is the only therapy that can achieve both systolic unloading of the left ventricle and improvement of coronary perfusion pressure (hence, it is a form of reperfusion therapy). These two observations result in a lowering MVO_2 (myocardial oxygen consumption) and an increased myocardial oxygen delivery. Therefore, IABP is indicated in any patient with CGS, especially when the patient is a candidate for other aggressive interventions. Cardiogenic shock and refractory pump failure are current American College of Cardiology (ACC)/American Heart Association (AHA) Class I indications[73] for IABP (usually indicated, always acceptable, Table 11.4). Two major contraindications to IABP are aortic regurgitation and suspected aortic dissection. Relative contraindications are peripheral vascular disease and a small body habitus.

Percutaneous transluminal coronary angioplasty

Since IABP as a sole therapy does not greatly improve survival in CGS, other studies[74–77] have emphasized the need for a more aggressive intervention including both IABP and restoring coronary perfusion by either percutaneous transluminal coronary angioplasty (PTCA) or coronary bypass grafting. Successful angioplasty is associated with survival benefits in several studies of patients with acute MI complicated by CGS. The Multi-Center Registry of Angioplasty Therapy of Cardiogenic

Shock[74] showed that successful emergency PTCA improves initial and long-term survival in patients with CGS complicating myocardial infarction. The 7-day survival rate after angioplasty for acute MI complicated by CGS was 70% in the patients in whom angioplasty was successful as compared to 20% in whom angioplasty was unsuccessful. The long-term survival in these same patients was 55% when angioplasty established reperfusion and 20% when reperfusion was not established with angioplasty (Fig. 11.2).

Ghitis also showed a decreased mortality from CGS complicating acute MI when angioplasty was successful.[78] Similar results have shown an in-hospital mortality rate of 19% when angioplasty was successful as compared to 60% when angioplasty was unsuccessful. Lee *et al.*[75] also evaluated early and long-term survival benefits in patients with CGS from myocardial infarctions when treated with PTCA and determined that successful angioplasty was associated with a 30-day survival of 77% compared to 18% in the group of patients where angioplasty had been unsuccessful. The results in patients who experienced unsuccessful intervention with PTCA were the same in patients treated with conventional therapy alone. In patients with multivessel disease, despite successful angioplasty, the mortality rate continues to be about 83%.

Although angioplasty failure and death were associated more frequently with proximal left anterior descending artery occlusions, other univariate predictors of hospital mortality were advanced age and elevated left ventricular end-diastolic pressure.

Hibbard *et al.*[79] identified other factors influencing mortality after PTCA which included:

1. the combination of age greater than 70 years and unsuccessful angioplasty (all died);
2. left main coronary artery disease (no survivors regardless of angioplasty outcome); and
3. a history of previous myocardial infarction (31% survived to hospital discharge and only 15% were alive at the 2-year follow-up).

Current ACC/AHA guidelines[73] designate PTCA for CGS of less than 18 hours duration as a Class IIa indication (acceptable, weight of evidence in favor of efficacy, Table 11.4).

Coronary artery bypass grafting

Several studies[72, 80–82] have evaluated the efficacy of emergency coronary artery bypass graft (CABG) surgery in patients with CGS, especially in conjunction with intra-aortic balloon pumping. The combined data from four surgical series suggest an average in-hospital

Table 11.4 ACC/AHA guidelines for the use of interventional devices or procedures for cardiac support early after myocardial infarction[102]

Device/intervention	I Usually indicated, always acceptable	IIa Acceptable evidence favours efficacy	IIb Uncertain, can be helpful	III Not indicated
IABP	CGS or RPF	VSD/MR PPF		Stable severe PVD
Primary PTCA	<6 h with contraindication to thrombolytics	CGS <18 h		
CABG	PTCA failure VSD MR Aneurysm Infarct with VT and RPF VT	CGS not suitable for PTCA[a]		
VAD	None		Bridge to transplant for RPF	

CABG: coronary artery bypass grafting; CGS: cardiogenic shock; IABP: intraaortic balloon pump; MR: severe mitral regurgitation; PPF: progressive pump failure; PTCA: percutaneous transluminal coronary angioplasty; PVD: peripheral vascular disease; RPF: refractory pump failure; VAD: ventricular assist device; VSD: ventricular septal defect; VT: ventricular tachycardia.
[a] Left main coronary artery disease; triple vessel disease; double vessel disease including proximal LAD with depressed LV function.

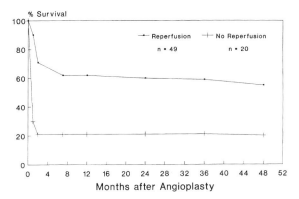

Fig. 11.2 Short-term and long-term survival after PTCA for cardiogenic shock. Group 1 had successful reperfusion of infarct-related artery and Group 2 had unsuccessful reperfusion.[75]

survival of 72.5% (range 58–88%). Studies by DeWood *et al.*[72] and Allen *et al.*[83] have shown that when inotropic support, IABP support and emergency CABG were used, in-hospital and long-term mortality were greatly decreased.

Early and late mortality seem to be related to four factors:

1. time to operation from onset of infarction;
2. time to operation from the development of CGS;
3. preoperative organ failure; and
4. history of previous myocardial infarction.[83]

Of these factors, Allen and colleagues also found that early revascularization (CABG < 18 hours) had the greatest benefits with the mortality rate decreasing to only 7% (Fig. 11.3). If surgery was delayed more than 18 hours after the onset of CGS, the mortality rate rose to 31%.

The major cause of early death post-CABG was multisystem organ failure. Preoperative organ failure progressed despite revascularization and reversal of hypotension; all the patients with preoperative organ

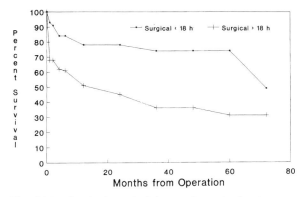

Fig. 11.3 Surgical survival for cardiogenic shock. Two groups are identified by shock duration.[83]

failure died within 12 months of revascularization. Previous myocardial infarction was related to an increased mortality rate in patients with CGS regardless of the time period to revascularization. For patients with early revascularization, the mortality rate was 27% with previous myocardial infarction (MI) compared to 22% with no previous MI. In the delayed revascularization group, mortality rose to 76% in patients with previous MI and increased to 57% in patients with no previous MI. Current ACC/AHA guidelines[73] indicate CABG for angioplasty failure, acute ventricular septal defects, papillary muscle rupture, aneurysm, infarcts with progressive heart failure or ventricular tachycardia, and infarction with incessant ventricular tachycardia as Class I indication. Cardiogenic shock less than 18 hours in duration and low probability of successful PTCA is a Class IIa indication for coronary bypass grafting (Table 11.4).

Table 11.5 summarizes the in-hospital mortality rates from published series on the efficacy of IABP, PTCA and CABG. Analysis is by intention to treat and survival rates are expressed as average ± the 95% confidence interval. These studies have no randomized controls and the medical therapy differs substantially among studies. Given those stipulations, CABG had the best results overall and is probably the procedure of choice for multivessel disease and left main coronary artery disease. PTCA results are better than IABP alone, but only successful PTCA approaches the results of emergency CABG for improved survival after myocardial infarction complicated by CGS.

Ventricular assist devices/total artificial heart

TYPES

A variety of ventricular assist devices (VAD) have been developed for the management of CGS complicating acute MI, open heart surgery and severe cardiomyopathy.

Pierce–Donachy VAD

The Pierce–Donachy prosthetic ventricle (Thoratec)[2,84,85] is an extracorporeal pneumatic pump (Fig. 11.4). During left heart assistance, blood is either removed from the left atrial appendage via a 51F cannula or the ventricular apex via a wire-reinforced segmented polyurethane large-caliber (13 mm internal diameter) end-hole cannula with outer coverings of nylon velour. Blood is returned to the ascending aorta via a 14 mm composite segmented polyurethane-woven Dacron prosthesis. When right ventricular assistance is

Table 11.5 In-hospital survival of cardiogenic shock by intervention

Study author	Total no.	Survived (n)	Survived (%)	Pooled average survival[a] (%)
Intra-aortic balloon pump				
Scheidt et al.[109]	87	15	17	
Hajemeijer et al.[40]	25	20	80	
DeWood et al.[72]	21	11	48	
				35 (33–37)
PTCA				
Lee et al.[75]	24	12	50	
Ellis et al.[111]	61	41	68	
Lee et al.[74]	69	40	55	
Stack et al.[112]	43	25	58	
Hibbard et al.[60]	45	25	56	
Ghitis et al.[78]	62	45	73	
				62 (59–65)
CABG ± intra-aortic balloon pump				
DeWood et al.[72]	19	11	58	
Guyton et al.[80]	17	15	88	
Allen et al.[83]	80	66	83	
Phillips et al.[113]	16	12	75	
Subramanian et al.[114]	20	11	55	
Kirklin et al.[115]	4	4	100	
				76 (74–77)

[a] 95% confidence interval given in parentheses.

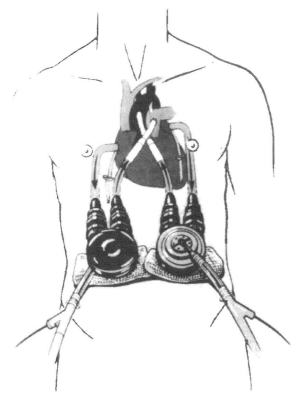

Fig. 11.4 Biventricular Pierce–Donachy VAD with atrial cannulation. Adapted from ref. 84.

needed, blood is removed from the right atrial appendage and returned to the pulmonary artery. A flexible segmented polyurethane blood sac which is seam-free and smooth internally is enclosed in a rigid polysulfone case. Two Bjork–Shiley tilting disc valves ensure unidirectional blood flow. Flow rates range from 2 to 6.5 1/min.

Hemopump VAD

The Hemopump VAD (Nimbus)[86-88] is a 9F intravascular device placed via the femoral or external iliac artery and inserted into the left ventricle under fluoroscopy (Fig. 11.5). It can also be placed directly in the aorta during open heart surgery. The inflow cannula removes blood from the left ventricle, and the blood is returned to the descending thoracic aorta by the transvalvular axial flow pump. The pump impeller spins at 15 000 to 27 000 (pump speed 1 to 7) revolutions per minutes, providing unidirectional, nonpulsatile flow. Maximum flow through the pump is 3.5–4.0 l/min. The pump assembly is attached to a high-speed motor and control console.

Symbion total artificial heart

The Symbion total artificial heart (TAH)[89,90] is an intrathoracic pneumatic device which incorporates a flexible diaphragm inside a semirigid housing (Fig. 11.6).[91] The inflatable diaphragm is made of four layers

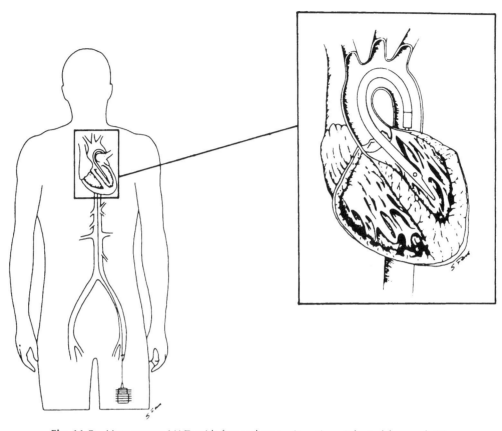

Fig. 11.5   Hemopump VAD with femoral artery insertion. Adapted from ref. 88.

of 0.18 mm Biomer. Air is pulsed through a single port in the base of each ventricle to inflate the diaphragm, thereby ejecting blood from the ventricle. Air exhaustion through concentric rings in the base of the ventricles allows diaphragmatic collapse and diastolic filling. Four Medtronic–Hall valves provide unidirectional blood flow. The valves join polycarbonate rings to form a ridged fitting that joins the atrial cuffs and great vessel grafts. The drive console (Utahdrive System) is a self-contained mobile system that provides continuous pulses of air to the diaphragms in TAH. It contains two independent controllers, a diastolic vacuum pump, two reserve high-pressure air tanks, backup battery systems, and a multiple tone alarm panel for mechanical and physiological emergency conditions. Cannulae from the pneumatic port in the base of each ventricle exit the patient's body at the left costal arch through velour-covered Silastic percutaneous leads. These cannulae join polyvinylchloride tubes that attach to the left and right air pressure fillings at the rear of each drive console. A smaller portable drive console (Heimes Portable Driver, Symbion) uses electrically driven reversing pistons in a valved cylinder to alternately pump the left and right ventricles. It has automatic electrical and mechanical backup mech-

anisms and a rechargeable nickel–cadmium battery pack that allows 3 hours of continuous use.

Novacor left ventricular assist device

The Novacor LVAD[92–94] is an implanted pump/drive unit consisting of a seamless polyurethane sac with Dacron inflow and outflow conduits connected to the left ventricular apex and the ascending aorta (Fig. 11.7). The conduits transverse the diaphragm and the pump/drive unit is positioned in the left upper quadrant of the anterior abdominal wall. A percutaneous vent tube connects the pump/drive unit to the external control console. The blood pump has symmetrically opposed pusher plates and pericardial tissue values with custom silicone flanges (Edwards) to maintain optimal flow throughout the pumping cycle. The Novacor LVAD has a stroke volume of 70 ml and can pump 10 l/min.

Percutaneous cardiopulmonary support

Percutaneous cardiopulmonary support (PCPS) has been used in cardiogenic shock as a bridge to revascularization by either CABG or PTCA.[95] Bypass cannulae (20F) are inserted into the femoral artery and vein

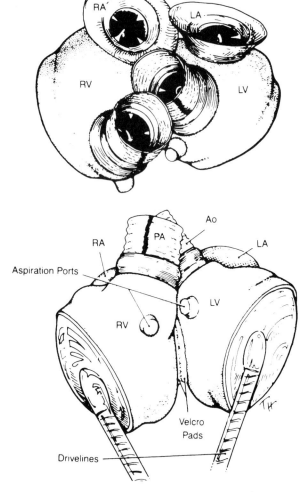

Fig. 11.6   Symbion total artificial heart. RA: right atrium; LA: left atrium; RV: right ventricle; LV: left ventricle; Ao: aorta. Adapted from ref. 91.

percutaneously via insertion of an 8F sheath followed by progressive dilatation with 12F and 14F dilators inserted over a guide wire. Then the cannulae are connected to the portable cardiopulmonary bypass support system (Bard), consisting of a nonocclusive blood pump, heat exchanger, oxygenator, connecting lines and supportive hardware.

Direct mechanical ventricular actuation

Direct mechanical ventricular actuation (DMVA) is a new experimental technique being used as a bridge to cardiac transplantation in patients with refractory

CGS.[96] The DMVA is a biventricular assist device that is an elliptically contoured cup that fits over the left and right ventricles. The cup consists of a semirigid outer shell made of Pyrex or Dacron-Reinforced Silastic and flexible inner diaphragm made of a Silastic membrane (Dow Corning Corp.). A continuous vacuum at the apex of the cup attaches the device to the ventricles by creating a constant diaphragm to epicardium seal (Fig. 11.8). The diaphragm is deflated and inflated pneumatically within the cup to allow blood to fill and eject from the ventricles, thereby enhancing diastole and systole. The DMVA is controlled by a pneumatic drive unit that has both pulsed pressure and sustained negative vacuum pressure systems. The device is applied via a small left anterior, sixth intercostal space thoracotomy. Since the device has no direct contact with blood, there is no need for anticoagulation. DMVA produces cardiac outputs of 4–11 l/min.[96]

INDICATIONS

At present, VADs have only a Class IIb indication (can be helpful, not well established by published evidence, Table 11.4) for acute pump failure or cardiogenic shock after myocardial infarction. They have mostly been used in the treatment of severe pump failure after cardiac surgery.

Because cardiac transplantation has become a widely accepted therapeutic intervention for end-stage chronic heart failure and refractory cardiogenic shock, and more than 20% of patients accepted for transplant die waiting for a suitable donor, temporary circulatory support as a bridge to cardiac transplantation is becoming a more frequent indication.[97] A ventricular assist device was first attempted by Cooley and colleague[98] in 1969 with an orthotopic artificial heart in a patient who could not be weaned from bypass. In 1978, Norman *et al.*[99] were among the first to use a VAD as a bridge to transplantation. In both of these reports, the patients died from infection within days of transplantation. In 1984, the first survival after transplantation following mechanical circulatory support with a VAD (Novacor) as a bridge to transplantation was reported by Portner and associates.[93]

Today, several VADs are used as a bridge to transplantation. The indications for VADs as a bridge to transplantation are:

1. acute cardiac decompensation while awaiting transplantation;
2. acute myocardial infarction with cardiogenic shock;
3. irreversible transplant rejection;
4. acute transplant graft failure; and
5. postcardiotomy pump failure.

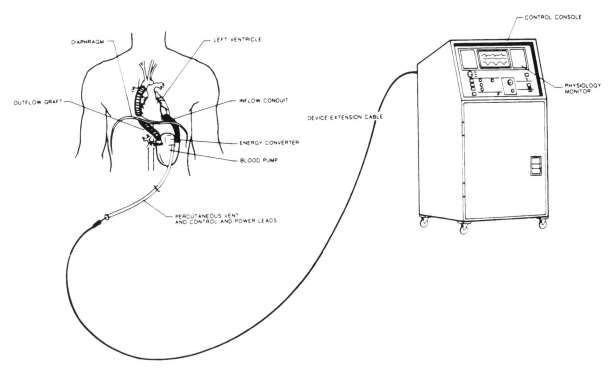

Fig. 11.7 Novacor LVAD showing both implanted pump/drive and external control console. Adapted from ref. 94.

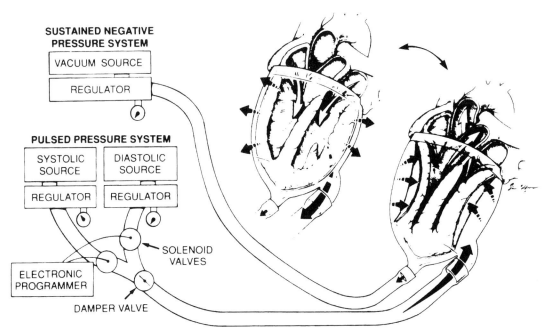

Fig. 11.8 Direct mechanical ventricular actuation device. Adapted from ref. 96.

OUTCOME

Thirty-day hospital mortality rates for all ventricular devices are summarized in Tables 11.6 and 11.7.

Pierce–Donachy VAD

Three separately reported studies with a total of 86 patients have shown a survival of 30–33% in patients with CGS when the Pierce–Donachy VAD was used.[2,84,85] In these patients, CGS was secondary to open heart surgery, myocardial infarction, end-stage cardiomyopathy (awaiting transplant), or postcardiac transplantation. These studies included patients with left or right ventricular assistance as well as bi-ventricular assistance.

In the largest series reported by Pennington, 48 patients with CGS were treated with the Pierce–Donachy VAD.[84] CGS was secondary to open heart surgery in 30 patients, acute MI in three patients, postorthotopic cardiac transplantation in four patients, and it was used as a bridge to transplantation in 11 patients. Of the 30 postcardiotomy patients, 14 received

a left VAD (LVAD), seven received only a right VAD (RVAD), and nine received biventricular VADs (BVADs). Sixteen patients (53%) had improvement in cardiac function, 15 (50%) were weaned from the VAD, and 11 (37%) were discharged from the hospital. Eight of the first 11 patients died in the operating room, but of the later 19 patients, 63% were weaned from the VAD and 47% survived to discharge. There were no intra-operative deaths. Of the 11 survivors, eight are still alive after a follow-up period of 6–55 months. The overall survival to discharge for the 48 patients treated with the Pierce–Donachy VAD was 33% and the survival to discharge for the 30 postcardiotomy patients was 36%.

When the Pierce–Donachy VAD has been used as a bridge to transplantation, survival has been better in patients with CGS who undergo successful transplantation. Pennington[84] used the Pierce–Donachy VAD as a bridge to transplantation in 11 patients with CGS. Four patients had an LVAD and seven patients required biventricular VADs. The duration of support ranged from 8 hours to 75 days (mean 15 days). Hemodynamic stability was achieved in all patients. Five patients

Table 11.6   Survival of cardiogenic shock using ventricular assist devices

Device	Study	Patient category	Total patients (*n*)	Survival at 30 days (*n*)	
Hemopump	Wampler *et al.*[88]	All patients with CGS:	41	13	(32%)
		Acute MI	17	7	(41%)
		Postcardiotomy	17	4	(24%)
		Other	7	2	(29%)
	Frazier *et al.*[86]	All patients with CGS:	7	5	(71%)
		Acute MI	1	0	
		Postcardiotomy	4	0	
		Transplant rejection	1	0	
		Acute donor CHF	1	0	
	Gacioch *et al.*[87]	All patients with CGS: (successful placement of device)	4	2	(5%)
Total			52	20	(38%)
Pierce–Donachy	Pennington *et al.*[84]	All patients with CGS:	48	16	(33%)
		Postcardiotomy	30	11	(36%)
		Bridge to transplantation	11	5	(45%)
		Acute MI	3	0	
		Post-transplant	4	0	
	Pennock *et al.*[2]	All patients with CGS:	30	9	(30%)
		Postcardiotomy	28	9	(32%)
		Acute MI	2	0	
Total			78	25	(32%)
Pierce–Donachy and Biomedicus	Zumbro *et al.*[85]	All patients with CGS:	33		
		Biomedicus device	25 }	10	(30%)
		Pierce–Donachy device	8 }		
PCPS as bridge to PTCA	Shaw *et al.*[95]	All patients with CGS:	10	8	(80%)
		(successful PTCA)	8	8	(100%)

Table 11.7 Overall survival with ventricular assist devices for cardiogenic shock

Study	Device	Total patients (n)	Survival at 30 days (n)	Average survival rate[a] (%)
Pennington et al.[84]	Pierce–Donachy	48	16[b] (33.3%)	
Pennock et al.[2]	Pierce–Donachy	30	9 (30%)	
Zumbro et al.[85]	Pierce–Donachy	8 ⎱	10 (30%)	
	Biomedicimus	25 ⎰		
Wampler et al.[88]	Hemopump	41	13 (31.7%)	
Frazier et al.[86]	Hemopump	7	5 (71%)	
Gacioch et al.[87]	Hemopump	4[c]	2 (50%)	
Portner et al.[94]	Novacor (LVAD and transplant	20	8 (40%)	
Joyce et al.[89]	Symbion TAH and transplant	100	47 (47%)	
Pooled results				39 (33–45)

LVAD: left ventricular assist device; TAH: total artificial heart.
[a] 95% confidence interval given in parentheses.
[b] Five of these 16 had transplant.
[c] Four of seven patients had successful placement of Hemopump.

received orthotopic cardiac transplant and four patients (80%) were alive following a mean of 17 months of follow-up.

Hemopump VAD

The largest study using the Hemopump LVAD was by Wampler et al. and consisted of 53 patients with refractory CGS.[88] The Hemopump was successfully inserted in 41 patients. Failure of insertion (22.6%) was due to severe peripheral vascular disease or inability to cross the aortic valve. CGS was secondary to acute MI in 42% of patients and postcardiotomy in another 42% of patients, with 26% of patients having CGS secondary to other causes. IABP had been used in 75% of patients prior to Hemopump insertion. Of the 41 patients with successful insertion of the Hemopump LVAD, 63% died on support or immediately after its removal. Thirty-six per cent of the patients were successfully weaned from support and 32% of the patients survived more than 30 days. The patients with CGS secondary to acute MI had a slightly better 30-day survival of 42% compared to patients with postcardiotomy CGS with a 30-day survival of 24%.

In two other small series of patients with CGS,[86,87] the 30-day survival was 50 and 71% when the Hemopump LVAD was used, and nearly half of these patients (five out of 11 total) had been discharged home. Overall, the survival of CGS with the Hemopump LVAD is approximately 38%.

In summary, both the Pierce–Donachy and the Hemopump VADs have survival rates of approximately 32%. This result is similar to the survival rates of CGS treated with IABP alone (35%). This is discouraging, but advances are being made technically and survival rates are improving with experience.

Symbion TAH

The Symbion TAH has been used as a bridge to transplantation since 1985 in at least 22 centers worldwide and has been implanted in over a 100 patients since 1985.[89] Of these, thirty were Symbion Jarvik-7–100 devices and 73 were Jarvik-7–70 devices for a total of 103 patients. Thirty-two patients (32%) died while being supported by the TAH. Of the 60 patients who received orthotopic human cardiac transplant, 47 (69%) survived at least 30 days postoperatively and 31 (16%) survived long term. The majority of deaths were due to multiple organ failure (MOF) with or without sepsis. Twenty-one patients (65%) who did not receive transplant and 18 patients (26%) who did receive transplant died of MOF.

Novacor LVAD

The Novacor LVAD has been used in 20 patients who had refractory CGS or were hemodynamically unstable as a bridge to cardiac transplantation.[94] All patients were stabilized hemodynamically and the device remained implanted a mean of 23 days. Orthotopic cardiac transplantation was performed in 10 patients with device implantation times ranging from 2 to 90 days. Eight patients survived to discharge, and after a mean follow-up of 16 months, there have been no late deaths.

Percutaneous cardiopulmonary support

Percutaneous cardiopulmonary support (PCPS) has been used as a bridge to PTCA in 10 patients with CGS with excellent results.[95] Eight patients had successful PTCA and all eight patients (80%) were alive at 10 months follow-up. The mean ejection fraction for patients with successful PTCA was 40%.

Direct mechanical ventricular actuation

DMVA has been used in two patients awaiting cardiac transplantation.[96] One patient received successful transplantation and is alive after more than a year of follow-up. DMVA has undergone limited clinical investigation in CGS as a bridge to transplantation.

COMPLICATIONS

Pierce–Donachy VAD

Complications are common in all patients receiving VADs (Table 11.8). Bleeding occurred in 22 of the 30 (73%) postcardiotomy patients receiving Pierce–Donachy VADs and required re-exploration in four patients.[84] One patient had disseminated intravascular coagulation (DIC). Thrombus was found in three VAD sacs during the time of removal, but none of these patients had embolic events. Cerebrovascular accidents (CVAs) occurred in three of the 48 patients receiving the Pierce–Donachy device (two of the 30 postcardiotomy patients). Of the total 48 patients, respiratory failure occurred in 12 (25%) patients. Renal failure occurred in 18 (38%) patients and required dialysis in 13 of these patients. Infection was a complication in 17 (35%) of the total 48 patients (8 of the 30 post-cardiotomy patients).[84]

Complications with the Pierce–Donachy device when used as a bridge to transplantation[84] are also common. Ten of the 11 patients had significant complications. Complications were severe enough to preclude transplantation in five patients. Bleeding occurred in 55%, necessitating mediastinal exploration. Infections occurred in four patients (36%), and renal failure occurred in three patients (27%). Significant right ventricular failure developed after implantation of the LVAD in two patients (18%). Both patients required an RVAD. Device malfunction occurred once.

Hemopump VAD

The most frequently seen complication with Hemopump VADs is dysrhythmia (Table 11.8) which is observed in 27.5% of patients, but none were associated with hemodynamic sequelae.[88] Cerebrovascular emboli with resultant hemiparesis occurred in two (5%)

Table 11.8 Reported complications from ventricular assist devices

Complication	Devices
Infection	TAH, PD, Novacor LVAD, HP
Thromboembolic events	TAH, PD, Novacor LVAD, HP
Renal failure	TAH, PD, Novacor LVAD
Multiple organ system failure	TAH, PD
Bleeding	TAH, PD, Novacor LVAD, HP, PCPS
Device failure	DMVA

DMVA: direct mechanical ventricular actuation; HP: Hemopump; LVAD: left ventricular assist device; PCPS: percutaneous cardiopulmonary support; PD: Pierce–Donachy device; TAH: Symbion total artificial heart.

patients and peripheral embolism occurred in one (2%) patient receiving Hemopump VADs. In all three circumstances, the patients had pre-existing mural thrombi. The total incidence of systemic thromboembolism during and after Hemopump implantation was 9.6%, despite heparin anticoagulation to a therapeutic range of 1.5–2.0 times control of either the activated clotting time or the partial thromboplastin time.

Symbion TAH

Infection was documented in 45% of patients.[89] Seventy-six per cent of those patients did not survive. Stroke or transient ischemic attack occurred in 9% of participants. No patient suffered from significant hemolysis (Table 11.8).

Novacor LVAD

The most common complication with the Novacor LVAD is bleeding which occurred in 40% of patients and necessitated reoperation in 20% of patients (five of 20).[94] Documented infection occurred in 30% of patients during the period of device implantation. Fatal cerebrovascular accidents occurred in 10% of patients, and transient ischemic attacks occurred in one other patient.

Percutaneous cardiopulmonary support

Percutaneous cardiopulmonary support caused bleeding complications, requiring blood transfusion in six of eight patients (75%), with one patient requiring surgical repair of the femoral artery.[95] Two patients (25%) had infection at the cannula site, requiring antibiotics and local treatment.

Direct mechanical ventricular actuation

DMVA caused no complications on one of the two patients reported.[96] In the other patient, the diaphragm developed a leak and a new device had to be implanted. This clinical failure of a small leak in the cup has been observed during prolonged experimentation *in vivo* and *in vitro*. There has been no report of sudden, complete cup failure. The cup can be replaced at the bedside using a standard thoracotomy tray.

Comprehensive hemodynamic management of cardiogenic shock and pump failure

The goals of treating cardiogenic shock include the following:

1. restoration of coronary blood flow;
2. achieving hemodynamic objectives of maintaining an adequate blood and cardiac output;

3. relieving hypoxemia; and
4. preventing other organ failures.

Figure 11.9 depicts a therapeutic algorithm for cardiogenic shock which emphasizes an evaluation of the candidacy for reperfusion therapy at the earliest stage even while hemodynamic objectives are being pursued. Based on the previous data, we recommend that all patients with cardiogenic shock less than 18 hours should have coronary angiography with a goal toward vascularization (Fig. 11.9). Patients with single vessel disease with a short duration of shock may be offered PTCA but should have surgery if the infarct-related artery cannot be opened. Patients with multivessel disease or left main disease should be offered surgery if this can be done in a timely fashion. Patients who cannot be operated on because of technical reasons should receive full medical support and should be considered for transplant if they can be initially stabilized with an IABP or a VAD (see below). Patients who have been in shock for more than 18 hours should have mechanical defects ruled out. In the absence of ongoing ischemia or a mechanical defect, transplantation bridged by either IABP or VAD should be considered.

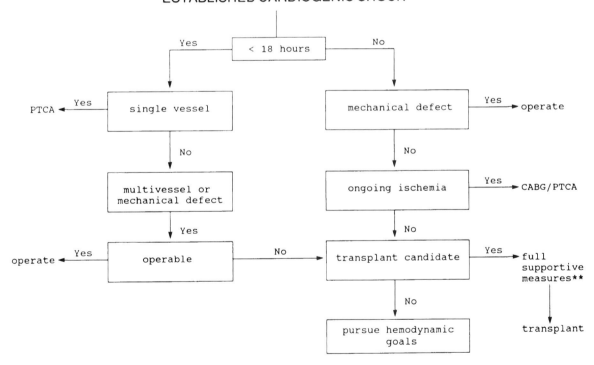

Fig. 11.9 Clinical algorithm for the management of cardiogenic shock based on shock duration, extent of disease and operability. PTCA: percutaneous transluminal coronary angioplasty; CABG: coronary artery bypass grafting.

As an aid to support the patient during diagnostic and therapeutic intervention, the pharmacological approach to CGS or acute pump failure and hemodynamic goals of pharmacological therapy will be reviewed.

The original description of hemodynamic subsets of myocardial infarction[1] consists of four groups:

1. patients with normal hemodynamics;
2. patients who have low CO with low PCWP (hypovolemia);
3. patients with high PCWP (pulmonary congestion) and normal CO; and
4. patients with both elevated PCWP and low CO (pump failure).

It did not specifically take into account patients with mechanical defects such as interventricular septal defect (IVSD) or papillary muscle rupture, patients with RV infarction, or patients with low cardiac output secondary to high LV afterload.

Table 11.9 provides a comprehensive therapeutic approach to the management of CGS based on a broader spectrum of hemodynamic profiles and should be implemented while patients are being evaluated for definitive therapy or when intraventional therapy has been ruled out. Uncompromised patients are designated as subset one requiring thrombolytic therapy if diagnosed early in their course (<6–24 hours). These patients require no further hemodynamic support. Subset 2 represents the patient who is hypovolemic and hypotensive. This is indicated by low PCWP in addition to a low CO. This derangement is often based on previous diuretic use, excessive nitrate use, or morphine administration. In this instance, a volume challenge is the most appropriate choice for therapy. Aliquots of crystalloid or colloid between 100 and 250 ml[100] to raise the PCWP to between 14 and 18 mm Hg are used (Fig. 11.10). The target range of PCWP must be individualized. Values between 14 and 18 are suggested as an initial target because in previous studies of myocardial infarction patients given either volume for low PCWP or afterload reduction for high PCWP,[101] cardiac output was optimized in range of filling pressures.

Subset 3 represents the patient who has an elevated PCWP either because of reduced compliance or poor contractility. In general, these patients are treated with diuretics or venodilators. Underlying myocardial ischemia manifesting itself as a primary diastolic abnormality may be responsible for the heart failure and should be sought out as a cause. If found, attempts to decrease MVO_2 with beta blockers or calcium blockers can be helpful.

Subset 4a represents a patient who is not hypotensive but has a depressed cardiac index and an elevated

Table 11.9 Therapeutic approach to patients with acute myocardial infarction based on hemodynamic subsets

Subset	Clinical situation	Arterial BP (mm Hg)	PCWP (mm Hg)	CI (l/min/m²)	Management
1	Normal	>100	<14	>2.2	Thrombolytics if <24 hours: Observe for arrhythmia Treat pain Noninvasive testing for long-term prognosis
2	Hypovolemia (clinically low output)	<100	<14	<2.2	Volume expansion algorithm
3	Pulmonary congestion (pulmonary edema)	>100	>18	>2.2	Diuretics/nitroglycerin
4a	Low output and pulmonary edema	>100	>18	<2.2	Arterial vasodilators
4b	Low output and pulmonary edema	<100	>18	<2.2	Inotropic agents and vasodilators Circulatory assist devices PTCA/CABG <18 hours
5	RV infarct	<100	<14 (CVP >10)	<2.2	Optimize PCWP; consider dobutamine early PTCA/CABG if <18 hours and poor response
6	Mitral regurgitation	Variable	>18 (V-wave)	Usually <2.2	As in 4: consider early surgery to replace valve
7	Ventricular septal defect	Variable	Usually high	Variable; O_2 step-up in RV	As in 4: consider early surgery to correct defects

BP: blood pressure.

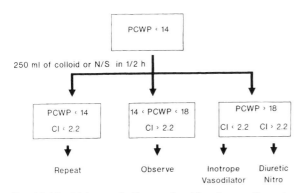

Fig. 11.10 Volume challenge algorithm for cardiogenic shock. PCWP: pulmonary capillary wedge pressure; CI: cardiac index.

PCWP. Vasodilators can be used initially in this situation, especially if the systolic blood pressure is greater than 100 mm Hg. Inotropic agents such as dobutamine or amrinone may be needed if the response to vasodilators is poor or the blood pressure is less than 90 mm Hg.

Subset 4b represents a patient that is hypotensive, has a low cardiac index, and an elevated PCWP. This patient has depressed inotropy resulting in true cardiogenic shock. The patient may also have a concomitant mechanical defect such as a papillary muscle rupture (Subset 6) or IVSD (Subset 7) which must be excluded. Both ACC/AHA and ACLS guidelines recommend dopamine as the initial drug of choice to restore the blood pressure and maintain coronary perfusion pressure.[73] Dopamine can be titrated to a systolic blood pressure greater than 70 mm Hg[102] as long as the heart rate is not excessive. Agents such as norepinephrine and phenylephrine should be used if the systolic blood pressure is less than 70 mm Hg or if there is significant tachycardia, since these agents have few chronotropic effects. In most cases, the patient will also require additional agents to decrease the PCWP and increase the cardiac output. If dopamine has resulted in an adequate BP response, vasodilators can be used. In instances where the blood pressure response has been poor, the use of inotropes such as dobutamine and amrinone is helpful. If severe hypotension persists, IABP should be placed. Consideration must be given to revascularization if the duration of shock is less than 18 hours.[71]

Subset 5 represents a patient with a predominant right ventricular infarction characterized by an elevated central venous pressure (CVP), low PCWP, and low CO. If the patient is not hypotensive and CVP is >12, a beta-1 agonist[103] or amrinone can be given. Volume challenge should be attempted if the CVP is less than 12 and the PCWP is less than 18.[18,46,103,104] Although ACC/AHA guidelines[73] recommend volume loading to achieve RAP or PCWP greater than 20 mm Hg, several

studies[18,103,105,106] show that this degree of volume loading is deleterious. If the patient is or becomes hypotensive, dopamine should be administered. Early in the course consideration should be given to either PTCA or CABG.

Complicating mechanical defects such as papillary muscle rupture (Subset 6) or IVSD (Subset 7) are best treated with surgical correction. Early surgical correction in conjunction with pharmacological therapy and IABP results in a survival of 50%.[12,13,15,16,107,108]

Summary

Acute pump failure and cardiogenic shock have been associated with a dismal prognosis for much of the last three decades. However, aggressive attempts to both support the failing myocardium and restore coronary perfusion, where appropriate, are yielding encouraging results. A review of both existing mortality data and suggested guidelines can provide the clinician with an effective diagnostic and therapeutic approach to such patients.

References

1. Forrester JS, Diamond G, Chatterjee K, Swan HJC. Medical therapy of acute myocardial infarction by application of hemodynamic subsets. *New Engl J Med* 1976; **295**: 1356-62–1404-13.
2. Pennock JL, Pierce WS, Wisman CB, Bull AP, Waldhausen JA. Survival and complications following ventricular assist pumping for cardiogenic shock. *Ann Surg* 1983; **198**: 469–76.
3. Alonso DR, Scheidt S, Post M *et al.* Pathophysiology of cardiogenic shock: quantification of myocardial necrosis, clinical, pathologic and electrocardiographic correlation. *Circulation* 1973; **48**: 588–96.
4. Bertrand M, Rousseau MF, LaBlanche JM *et al.* Cineangiographic assessment of left ventricular function in the acute phase of transmural myocardial infarction. *Am J Cardiol* 1979; **43**: 472–80.
5. Bigger JT, Fleiss JL, Kleiger R *et al.* The relationship among ventricular arrhythmias, left ventricular dysfunction, and mortality in the 2 years after myocardial infarction. *Circulation* 1984; **69**: 250–8.
6. Parmley WW, Tomoda H, Diamond G, Forrester JS, Crexells C. Dissociation between indices of pump performance and contractility in patients with coronary artery disease and acute myocardial infarction. *Chest* 1975; **67** (2): 141–6.
7. The Multicenter Postinfarction Research Group. Risk stratification and survival after myocardial infarction. *New Engl J Med* 1983; **309**: 331–6.
8. Glantz SA, Parmley WW. Factors which affect the

diastolic pressure–volume curve. *Circulation Res* 1978; **42** (2): 171–80.

9. Santamore WP, Carey R, Goodrich D, Bove AA. Measurement of left and right ventricular volume from implanted radiopaque markers. *Am J Physiol* 1981; **249**: H896–H900.

10. Serizawa T, Carabello BA, Grossman W. Effect of pacing-induced ischemia on left ventricular diastolic pressure–volume relations in dogs with coronary stenoses. *Circulation Res* 1980; **46** (3): 430–9.

11. Buckley MJ, Mundth ED, Daggett WM, DeSandis RW, Sanders LA, Austen WG. Surgical therapy for early complication of myocardial infarction. *Surgery* 1971; **70**: 814–20.

12. Clements SD, Story WE, Hurst JW *et al*. Ruptured papillary muscle, a complication of acute myocardial infarction: Clinical presentation, diagnosis and treatment. *Clin Cardiol* 1985; **8**: 93–103.

13. Gray RJ, Sethna D, Matloff JM. The role of cardiac surgery in acute myocardial infarction with mechanical complications. *Am Heart J* 1983; **106**: 723–8.

14. Meister SG, Helfant RH. Rapid bedside differentiation of ruptured interventricular septum from acute mitral insufficiency. *New Engl J Med* 1972; **287**: 1024–5.

15. Nishimura RA, Schaff HV, Shuh C *et al*. Papillary muscle rupture complicating acute myocardial infarction: analysis of 17 patients. *Am J Cardiol* 1983; **51**: 373–7.

16. Buckley MJ, Mundth ED, Daggett WM. Surgical management of ventricular septal defects and mitral regurgitation complicating acute myocardial infarction. *Ann Thoracic Surg* 1973; **16**: 598–609.

17. Mann JM, Roberts WC. Acquired ventricular septal defect during acute myocardial infarction: analysis of 38 unoperated necropsy patients and comparison with 50 unoperated necropsy patients without rupture. *Am J Cardiol* 1988; **62**: 8–19.

18. Calvin JE. Optimal right ventricular filling pressures and the role of pericardial constraint in right ventricular infarction in dogs. *Circulation* 1991; **84** (2): 852–61.

19. Cohn JN, Guiha NH, Broder MJ, Limas CJ. Right ventricular infarction: clinical and hemodynamic features. *Am J Cardiol* 1974; **33**: 209–14.

20. Lorrell B, Leinbach RC, Pohost GM *et al*. Right ventricular infarction: clinical diagnosis and differentiation from cardiac tamponade and pericardial constriction. *Am J Cardiol* 1979; **43**: 465–71.

21. Goldstein JA, Vlahakes GJ, Verrier ED *et al*. The role of right ventricular systolic dysfunction and elevated intra-pericardial pressure in the genesis of low output in experimental right ventricular infarction. *Circulation* 1982; **65**: 513–22.

22. Goto Y, Yamamoto J, Saito M *et al*. Effects of right ventricular ischemia on left ventricular geometry and the end-diastolic pressure–volume relationship in the dog. *Circulation* 1985; **72** (5): 1104–14.

23. Loeb HS, Pietas RJ, Tobin JR, Gunnar RM. Hypovolemia in shock due to acute myocardial infarction. *Circulation* 1969; **40**: 653–9.

24. Braunwald E, Sonnenblick EH, Ross JJR. Contraction of the normal heart. In: Braunwald E (ed.) *Heart Disease*. Philadelphia: WB Saunders, 1984: 409–46.

25. Smith TW, Braunwald E, Kelly RA. The management of heart failure. In: Braunwald E (ed.) *Heart Disease*. Philadelphia: WB Saunders, 1988: 485.

26. Hands ME, Rutherford JD, Muller JE *et al*. The in-hospital development of cardiogenic shock after myocardial infarction: incidence, predictors of occurrence, outcome and prognostic factors. *J Coll Cardiol* 1989; **14** (1): 40–6.

27. Killip T, Kimball JT. Treatment of myocardial infarction in a coronary care unit: a two year experience with 250 patients. *Am J Cardiol* 1967; **20**: 457–64.

28. Forrester JS, Ganz W, Diamond G *et al*. Thermodilution cardiac output determination with a single flow-directed catheter. *Am Heart J* 1972; **83**: 306–11.

29. Swan HJC, Ganz W, Forrester JS *et al*. Catheterization of the heart in man with the use of a flow directed balloon-tipped catheter. *New Engl J Med* 1976; **283**: 447–51.

30. Ahlquist RP. A study of adrenotropic receptors. *Am J Physiol* 1948; **153**: 586–600.

31. Letkowitz RJ, Stadel JM, Caron MG. Adenylate cyclase-coupled beta adrenergic receptors: structure and mechanisms of activation and desensitization. *Ann Rev Biochem* 1983; **52**: 159–86.

32. Goldberg LJ, Hsleh YY, Resnekov L. Newer catecholamines for treatment of heart failure and shock: an update dopamine and a first look at dobutamine. *Prog Cardiovascular Dis* 1977; **19**: 327–40.

33. Marcus FI, Opie LH, Sonnenblick EH. Digitalis, sympathomimetics and inotropic dilators. In: Opie LH (ed.) *Drugs for the Heart*. Philadelphia: WB Saunders, 1987: 91–110.

34. Wynands JE. Amrinone: Is it the inotrope of choice? *J Cardiothoracic Anaesth* 1989; **3**: 45–57.

35. Goldberg LI, Rafzer SI. Dopamine receptors. Applications in clinical cardiology. *Circulation* 1985; **72**: 245–8.

36. Watanabe AM. Recent advances in knowledge about beta-adrenergic receptors: application to clinical cardiology. *J Am Coll Cardiol* 1983; **1**: 82–9.

37. Baim DS. Effect of phosphodiesterase inhibition on myocardial oxygen consumption and coronary blood flow. *Am J Cardiol* 1989; **63**: 23A-26A.

38. Pozen RG, DiBianco R, Katz RJ, Bortz R, Myerburg RJ, Fletcher RD. Myocardial metabolic and hemodynamic effects of dobutamine in heart failure complicating coronary artery disease. *Circulation* 1981; **63** (6): 1279–85.

39. Sonnenblick EH, Frishman WH, LeJemtel TH. Dobutamine: a new synthetic cardioactive sympathetic amine. *New Engl J Med* 1979; **300** (1): 17–22.

40. Bendersky R, Chatterjee K, Parmley WW, Brundage BH, Ports PA. Dobutamine in chronic ischemic heart failure: alterations in left ventricular function and coronary hemodynamics. *Am J Cardiol* 1981; **48** (3): 554–8.

41. Goldstein RA. Clinical effects of intravenous amrinone in patients with congestive heart failure. *Am J Cardiol* 1985; **56** (3): B16–B18.

42. Gillespie TA, Ambos HD, Sobel BE, Roberts R. Effects of dobutamine in patients with acute myocardial infarction. *Am J Cardiol* 1977; **39**: 588–94.

43. Vatner SF, Baig H. Importance of heart rate in determining the effects of sympathomimetic amines on regional myocardial function and blood flow in conscious dogs with acute myocardial ischemia. *Circulation Res* 1979; **45**: 793–803.

44. Willerson JT, Hutton I, Watson JT, Platt MR, Templeton GH. Influence of dobutamine on regional myocardial blood flow and ventricular performance during acute and chronic myocardial ischemia in dogs. *Circulation* 1976; **53** (5): 828–33.

45. Abrams E, Forrestor JS, Chatterjee K *et al*. Variability in response to norepinephrine in acute myocardial infarction. *Am J Cardiol* 1973; **32**: 919–23.

46. Benotti JR, Grossman W, Braunwald E, Davalos DD, Alousi AA. Hemodynamic assessment of amrinone: a new inotropic agent. *New Engl J Med* 1978; **299** (25): 1373–7.

47. Klein NA, Siskind SJ, Frishman WH, Sonnenblick EH, LeJemtel TH. Hemodynamic comparison of intravenous amrinone and dobutamine in patients with chronic congestive heart failure. *Am J Cardiol* 1981; **48** (1): 170–5.

48. LeJemtel TH, Keung E, Sonnenblick EH *et al*. Amrinone: a new on-glycosidic, non-adrenergic cardiotonic agent effective in the treatment of intractable myocardial failure in man. *Circulation* 1979; **59** (6): 1098–1104.

49. Baim DS. Effects of amrinone on myocardial energetics in severe congestive heart failure. *Am J Cardiol* 1985; **56** (3): B16–B18.

50. Benotti JR, Grossman W, Braunwald E, Carabello BA. Effects of amrinone on myocardial energy metabolism and hemodynamics in patients with severe congestive heart failure due to coronary artery disease. *Circulation* 1980; **62**: 28–34.

51. Bristow MR, Ginsburg R, Umans B *et al*. Beta-1 and beta-2 adrenergic receptor sub-populations in non-failing and failing human ventricular myocardium: coupling sub-types to muscle contraction and selective beta-1 receptor down-regulation in heart failure. *Circulation Res* 1986; **56**: 297–309.

52. Gage J, Rutman J, Lucido D, LeJemtel TH. Additive effects of dobutamine and amrinone on myocardial contractility and ventricular performance in patients with severe heart failure. *Circulation* 1986; **74** (2): 367–73.

53. Treadway G. Clinical safety of intravenous amrinone – a review. *Am J Cardiol* 1985; **56** (3): B39–B40.

54. Alderman EL, Glantz SA. Acute hemodynamic interventions shift the diastolic pressure–volume curve in man. *Circulation* 1976; **54**: 662–71.

55. Berkowitz C, McKeever L, Croke RP *et al*. Comparative responses to dobutamine and nitroprusside in patients with chronic low output cardiac failure. *Circulation* 1977; **56**: 918–24.

56. Brodie BR, Grossman W, McLaurin MT. Effects of sodium nitroprusside on left ventricular diastolic pressure–volume relations. *J Clin Invest* 1977; **59**: 59–68.

57. Calvin JE, Driedger AA, Sibbald WJ. Phentolamine in low cardiac output states: an assessment with ECG-gated cardiac scintigraphy. *Crit Care Med* 1983; **11** (10): 769–74.

58. Chatterjee K, Swan HJC, Kanshik VS, Jobin G, Magnusson P, Forrester JS. Effects of vasodilator therapy for severe pump failure in acute myocardial infarction on short-term and late prognosis. *Circulation* 1976; **53**: 797–802.

59. Franciosa JB, Buiha NM, Limas CJ *et al*. Improved left ventricular function during nitroprusside infusion in acute myocardial infarction. *Lancet* 1972; **i**: 650–4.

60. Miller RR, Awan NA, Joye JA *et al*. Combined dopamine and nitroprusside therapy in congestive heart failure. *Circulation* 1977; **55**: 881–4.

61. Bakker J, Coffernils M, Leon M, Gris P, Vincent J-L. Blood lactate levels are superior to oxygen-derived variables in predicting outcome in human septic shock. *Chest* 1991; **99**: 956–62.

62. Pouleur H, Covell JW, Ross J. Effects of nitroprusside on venous return and central blood volume in the absence and presence of acute heart failure. *Circulation* 1980; **61**: 328–37.

63. Palmer RP, Lasseter KC. Sodium nitroprusside. *New Engl J Med* 1975; **292**: 294–7.

64. Francis GS, Siegel RM, Goldsmith SR *et al*. Acute vasoconstrictor response to intravenous furosemide in patients with chronic congestive heart failure. *Ann Intern Med* 1985; **103**: 1–5.

65. GISSI. Long-term effects of intravenous thrombolysis in acute myocardial infarction: Final report of the GISSI study. *Lancet* 1987; **ii** (2): 871–4.

66. International Study of Infarct Survival Collaborative Group (ISIS). Randomised trial of intravenous streptokinase, oral aspirin, both, or neither among 17187 cases of suspected acute myocardial infarction: ISIS-2. *Lancet* 1988; **ii** (1): 349–60.

67. Snell RJ, Parrillo JE. Cardiovascular dysfunction in septic shock. *Chest* 1991; **99**: 1000–9.

68. GISSI. Effectiveness of intravenous thrombolytic treatment in acute myocardial infarction. *Lancet* 1986; **i**: 397–401.

69. Kennedy JW, Gensini GG, Timmis GC, Maynard C. Acute myocardial infarction treated with intracoronary streptokinase: a report of the society for cardiac angiography. *Am J Cardiol* 1985; **55**: 871–7.

70. Rentrop P, Blanke H, Karsch KR *et al*. Selective intracoronary thrombolysis in acute myocardial infarction and unstable angina pectoris. *Circulation* 1981; **63**: 307–16.

71. McEnany MT, Kay HR, Buckley MJ *et al*. Clinical experience with intraaortic balloon pump support in 728 patients. *Circulation* 1978; **58** (Suppl. I): I-124–I-132.

72. DeWood MA, Notske RN, Hensley GR *et al*. Intraaortic balloon counterpulsation with and without reperfusion for myocardial infarction shock. *Circulation* 1980; **61** (6): 1105–12.

73. Gunnar RM, Bourdillon PD, Dixon DW *et al*. Guidelines for the early management of patients with acute myocardial infarction. *J Am Coll Cardiol* 1990; **16**: 249–92.

74. Lee L, Bates ER, Pitt B, Walton JA, Laufer N, O'Neill WW. Percutaneous transluminal coronary angioplasty improves survival in acute myocardial infarction complicated by cardiogenic shock. *Circulation* 1988; **78**: 1345–51.

75. Lee L, Erbel R, Brown TM, Laufer N, Meyer J, O'Neill WW. Multicenter registry of angioplasty therapy of cardiogenic shock: initial and long-term survival. *J Am Coll Cardiol* 1991; **17** (3): 599–603.
76. O'Neill W, Erbel R, Laufer N *et al.* Coronary angioplasty therapy of cardiogenic shock complicating acute myocardial infarction. *Circulation* 1985; **72**: III-309.
77. Shani J, Rivera M, Greengart A, Hollander G, Kaplan P, Lichstein E. Percutaneous transluminal coronary angioplasty in cardiogenic shock. *J Am Coll Cardiol* 1986; **7**, 149A.
78. Ghitis A, Flaker GC, Meinhardt S, Grouws M, Anderson SK, Webel RR. Early angioplasty in patients with acute myocardial infarction complicated by hypotension. *Am Heart J* 1991; **122**: 380–4.
79. Hibbard MD, Holmes DR, Bailey KR, Reeder GS, Bresnahan JF, Gersh BJ. Percutaneous transluminal coronary angioplasty in patients with cardiogenic shock. *J Am Coll Cardiol* 1992; **19**: 639–46.
80. Guyton RA, Arcidi JM Jr, Langford DA, Morris DC, Liberman HA, Hatcher CR Jr. Emergency coronary bypass for cardiogenic shock. *Circulation* 1987; **76** (Suppl. V): V22–V27.
81. Laks H, Rosenbranz E, Buckberg GD. Surgical treatment of cardiogenic shock after myocardial infarction. *Circulation* 1986; **74** (Suppl. III): III-11–III-15.
82. Noble RJ. Myocardial infarction with hypotension: problems in management. *Chest* 1991; **99**: 1012–15.
83. Allen BS, Rosenkranz E, Buckberg GD *et al.* Studies on prolonged acute regional ischemia. *J Thoracic Cardiovascular Surg* 1989; **98**: 691–703.
84. Pennington DG, Kanter KR, McBride LR *et al.* Seven years' experience with the Pierce–Donachy ventricular assist device. *J Thoracic Cardiovascular Surg* 1988; **96** (6): 901–11.
85. Zumbro CL, Kitchens WR, Shearer G, Harville G, Bailey L, Galloway RF. Mechanical assistance for cardiogenic shock following cardiac surgery, myocardial infarction, and cardiac transplantation. *Ann Thoracic Surg* 1987; **44**: 11–13.
86. Frazier OH, Wampler RK, Duncan JM *et al.* First human use of the hemopump, a catheter-mounted ventricular assist device. *Ann Thoracic Surg* 1990; **49**: 299–304.
87. Gacioch GDM, Ellis SG, Lee L *et al.* Cardiogenic shock complicating acute myocardial infarction: the use of coronary angioplasty and the integration of the new support devices into patient management. *J Am Coll Cardiol* 1992; **19**: 647–53.
88. Wampler RK, Frazier OH, Lansing AM *et al.* Treatment of cardiogenic shock with the Hemopump left ventricular assist device. *Ann Thoracic Surg* 1991; **52** (3): 506–13.
89. Joyce LD, Johnson KE, Toninato CJ *et al.* Results of the first 100 patients who received Symbion total artificial hearts as a bridge to cardiac transplantation. *Circulation* 1989; **89** (Suppl. III): III-192–III-201.
90. Mays JB, Williams MA, Banker LE *et al.* Clinical management of Total Artificial Heart drive systems. *J Am Med Assoc* 1988; **259**: 881–5.
91. DeVries WC. Surgical technique for implantation of the Jarvik-7–100 total artificial heart. *J Am Med Assoc* 1988; **259**: 875–80.
92. McCarthy PM, Portner PM, Tobler HG, Starnes VA, Ramasamy N, Oyer PE. Clinical experience with the Novacor ventricular assist system. Bridge to transplantation and the transition to permanent application. *J Thoracic Cardiovascular Surg* 1991; **102** (4): 586–87.
93. Portner PM, Oyer PE, McGregor CCA *et al.* First human use of an electrically powered implantable ventricular assist system. *Artificial Organs* 1985; **9** (A): 36.
94. Portner PM, Oyer PE, Pennington DG *et al.* Implantable electrical left ventricular assist system: bridge to transplantation and the future. *Ann Thoracic Surg* 1989; **47**: 142–50.
95. Shawl FA, Domanski MJ, Wish M, Punja S, Hernandez TJ, Park T. Emergency percutaneous cardiopulmonary support in cardiogenic shock: long term follow-up. *Circulation* 1989; **80** (Suppl. II): II-258.
96. Lowe JE, Anstadt MP, Van Trigt P *et al.* First successful bridge to cardiac transplantation using direct mechanical ventricular actuation. *Ann Thoracic Surg* 1991; **52**: 1237–45.
97. Copeland JG, Emery RW, Levinson MM *et al.* The role of mechanical support and transplantation in treatment of patients with end-stage cardiomyopathy. *Circulation* 1985; **7** (Suppl. 2): 7.
98. Cooley DA, Liotta D, Hallman GL *et al.* Orthotopic cardiac prosthesis for two-staged cardiac replacement. *Am J Cardiol* 1969; **24**: 723–30.
99. Norman JC, Cooley DA, Kahan BD *et al.* Total support of the circulation of a patient with postcardiotomy stone-heart syndrome by a partial artificial heart (ALVAD) for 5 days followed by heart and kidney transplantation. *Lancet* 1978; **i**: 1125.
100. Weil MH, Henning RJ. New concepts in the diagnosis and fluid treatment of circulatory shock (Thirteenth Annual Becton, Dickinson and Company Oscar Schwidetsky Memorial Lecture). *Anesth Analg* 1979; **58** (2): 124–32.
101. Crexells C, Chatterjee K, Forrester JS *et al.* Optimal level of filling pressure in the left side of the heart in acute myocardial infarction. *New Engl J Med* 1977; **289**: 1263–6.
102. Emergency Cardiac Care Committee and Subcommittees American Heart Association. Guidelines for cardiopulmonary resuscitation and emergency cardiac care, III: Adult Advanced Cardiac Life Support. *J Am Med Assoc* 1992; **268**: 2199–241.
103. Dell'Italia LJ, Starling MR, Blumgardt R *et al.* Comparative effects of volume loading, dobutamine and nitroprusside in patients with predominant right ventricular infarction. *Circulation* 1985; **6**: 1327–35.
104. Goldstein JAB, Vlahakes GJ, Verrier ED *et al.* Volume loading improves low cardiac output in experimental right ventricular infarction. *J Coll Cardiol* 1983; **2**: 270.
105. Berisha S, Kastrati A, Goda A, Popa Y. Optimal value of filling pressure in the right side of the heart in acute right ventricular infarction. *Br Heart J* 1990; **63**: 98–102.
106. Dhainaut JF, Ghannad E, Villemant D *et al.* Role of tricuspid regurgitation and left ventricular damage in the treatment of right ventricular infarction-induced low

cardiac output syndrome. *Am J Cardiol* 1990; **66**: 289–95.

107. Cohn LH. Surgical management of acute and chronic cardiac mechanical complications due to myocardial infarction. *Am Heart J* 1981; **102**, 1049–60.
108. Errington ML, Rocha e Silva M Jr. On the role of vasopressin and angiotensin in the development of irreversible shock. *J Physiol* 1974; **242**: 119–41.
109. Scheidt S, Wilner G, Mueller H *et al*. Intra-aortic balloon counterpulsation in cardiogenic shock. *New Engl J Med* 1973; **288**: 979–84.
110. Hagemeijer F, Laird JD, Haalebos MMP, Hugenholtz PG. Effectiveness of intraaortic balloon pumping without cardiac surgery for patients with severe heart failure secondary to a recent myocardial infarction. *Am J Cardiol* 1977; **40**: 952–6.
111. Ellis SG, O'Neill WW, Bates ER *et al*. Implications for patient triage from survival and left ventricular func-

tional recovery analyses in 500 patients treated with coronary angioplasty for acute myocardial infarction. *J Am Coll Cardiol* 1989; **13** (6): 1251–9.
112. Stack RS, Califf RM, Hinohara T *et al*. Survival and cardiac event rates in the first year after emergency coronary angioplasty for acute myocardial infarction. *J Am Coll Cardiol* 1988; **11**: 1141–9.
113. Phillips SJ, Kongtahworn C, Skinner JR *et al*. Emergency coronary artery perfusion: a choice therapy for evolving myocardial infarction. Results in 339 patients. *J Thoracic Cardiovascular Surg* 1983; **86**: 679–88.
114. Subramanian VA, Roberts AJ, Zema JM *et al*. Cardiogenic shock following acute myocardial infarction. *New York State J Med* 1980; **80**: 947–52.
115. Kirklin JW, Naftel CD, Blackstone EH *et al*. Summary of a consensus concerning death and ischemic events after coronary artery bypass grafting. *Circulation* 1989; **79**: I-81–I-91.

CHAPTER 12

Renal Support

HUGH S CAIRNS, GUY H NEILD

Introduction   178
Manifestations of renal impairment   182
Management of acute renal failure   184
Conclusion   190
Recommended reading   191
References   191

Introduction

Acute renal failure (ARF) is the commonest form of renal disease in the intensive care unit (ICU). This chapter will concentrate on the problems presented by the patient with ARF, although the principles of management also apply to chronic renal failure (CRF). ARF in the ICU has an overall mortality of 50% or greater and this has not changed in the past 20–30 years despite improvements in the monitoring and care of such patients.[1-5] The failure to improve mortality almost certainly reflects a change in the type of patient developing ARF;[1,4] in the 1960s the typical patient developed ARF from a single identifiable cause such as a postpartum hemorrhage or rhabdomyolysis whereas in the 1990s ARF is seen most commonly in patients with multiple organ failure, often in association with disseminated infection. Patients with ARF and single system disease now have a mortality of only 10–20%.[4,5] Although the mortality of ARF is high, death from the immediate consequences of renal failure is unusual; most patients die of cardiovascular, respiratory or infectious complications of their underlying disease.[6]

The major problems associated with renal disease in the ICU occur as a result of a reduction in the glomerular filtration rate. A broad classification of renal disease is:

1. pre-existent renal disease of any cause
2. hemodynamically mediated ARF – also termed prerenal ARF
3. acute intrinsic renal disease, e.g. acute glomerulonephritis
4. obstructive nephropathy which may be either intra or extra renal
5. renovascular disease affecting the large renal arteries.

The management of patients with renal disease depends initially on identifying the underlying cause.

PRE-EXISTENT RENAL DISEASE

Patients with significant pre-existent impairment of renal function (a glomerular filtration rate (GFR) below approximately 25–30 ml/min) are more likely to develop a number of conditions which may result in admission to ICU; these include peptic ulceration, atherosclerosis affecting coronary, cerebral and peripheral vascular beds and infective illnesses. Some individual chronic renal diseases may have life-threatening complications leading to ICU admission; e.g. cerebral hemorrhage in adult polycystic kidney disease,[7] hypertensive crises and infectious and other complications of renal transplantation and dialysis.

It is therefore common, as the mean age of ICU

admissions increases, to encounter patients with CRF in the ICU. Aside from the problems involved in the care of patients with impaired renal function discussed below, patients with CRF, when compared with those with normal renal function, are more likely to develop an acute deterioration in their renal function in response to any given insult. Acute on chronic renal failure is also more commonly irreversible than ARF alone and, if there is a subsequent recovery of function, the final GFR is often less than that prior to the exacerbation. Unfortunately it is often difficult, if not impossible, to prevent an acute deterioration in renal function in these patients.

HEMODYNAMICALLY MEDIATED ARF

Hemodynamically mediated ARF occurs when renal perfusion is reduced. The etiology is varied, ranging from cardiac disease to hypovolemia secondary to fluid losses in a variety of ways (Table 12.1). The pathophy-

Table 12.1 Causes of hemodynamically mediated ARF

Hypovolemia
Trauma
Hemorrhage
Surgery
Burns
Gastrointestinal losses

Reduced cardiac output
Cardiogenic shock
Congestive cardiac failure
Cardiac tamponade
Massive pulmonary embolus

Impaired renal autoregulation
Nonsteroidal anti-inflammatory agents
Angiotensin converting enzyme inhibitors
Hepato-renal syndrome

siology is complicated, with a number of different mechanisms leading to oliguria or anuria; oliguria is defined as a urine volume of less than 400 ml/day (<20 ml/h) and anuria less than 100 ml/day.

A reduction in renal blood flow and renal perfusion pressure reduces intraglomerular capillary pressure, the driving force of glomerular ultrafiltration. The kidneys are however capable of autoregulation and maintain a relatively constant GFR over a wide range of renal perfusion pressures; the physiology of the autoregulation and the interaction of the various vasoactive systems on afferent and efferent glomerular arteriolar tone are fairly well understood.[8] The control and autoregulation of peritubular blood flow are much less well understood. A number of conditions (e.g. treatment with nonsteroidal anti-inflammatory drugs, Table 12.1)

can interfere with autoregulation and result in the development of ARF with mild reductions in renal perfusion.

Moderate reductions in renal perfusion result in oliguria as the kidneys conserve salt and water in the absence of histological damage; this is therefore termed prerenal oliguria and is the initial stage in the development of hemodynamically mediated ARF. Rapid correction of the hypovolemia or cardiac output may produce an increase in urine volumes and avert established ARF.

As renal blood flow falls further, ischemic damage to the tubular cells in the medullary thick ascending limb of the loop of Henle (mTAL) occurs;[9,10] These cells are metabolically active yet exist in a chronically hypoxic environment. Other tubular cells, particularly in the proximal tubule, are also subject to ischemic damage. Tubular epithelial cells die and are shed into the tubular lumen – hence the name acute tubular necrosis (ATN), which is a histological description of the final stage of a number of different pathological processes which produce ARF, not all of which are hemodynamically mediated. The further fall in renal blood flow also reduces intraglomerular capillary pressure to a critical level, leading to a fall in GFR. Tubular obstruction also induces a tubuloglomerular feedback which increases afferent glomerular arteriolar tone, leading to a further fall in glomerular capillary pressure and GFR. Indirect evidence in man suggests that GFR ceases when the transcapillary pressure gradient falls below 27–29 mm Hg;[11] this correlates with a capillary hydraulic pressure of approximately 50 mm Hg and a mean blood pressure (BP) of about 60 mm Hg.

The oliguria of hemodynamically mediated ARF occurs partially as a result of a reduction in GFR and also probably as a consequence of tubular obstruction by cellular debris and back leak of filtrate into the interstitium.

The hepatorenal syndrome (HRS) is a specific form of hemodynamically mediated ARF which occurs in patients with severe liver disease. Pathologically there is a profound reduction in cortical blood flow which is secondary to increased local renovascular resistance unrelated to changes in cardiac output. HRS is manifested by oliguria with very low urinary sodium (often less than 5 mmol/l), indicating preservation of tubular function. Histological changes are minimal and correction of the liver disease by hepatic transplantation or nephrectomy and renal transplantation into a patient without hepatic disease results in a rapid recovery of renal function. Most patients with jaundice and ARF however do not have HRS but renal failure secondary to hypovolemia and hypotension. Jaundice may sensitize the tubules to ischemic damage and may also impair cardiac function.[12]

Sepsis is an additional, potent stimulus to the development of hemodynamically mediated ARF.[4,5]

The pathophysiology is poorly understood but ARF develops against a background of systemic hypotension resulting from a reduction in systemic and renal vascular resistance.[13] Renal blood flow may fall or increase, although there is a redistribution of blood away from the cortex. The changes in intrarenal hemodynamics are the result of a complex interaction between the various vasoactive systems including cyclo-oxygenase products, leukotrienes, endothelium-derived relaxing factor,[14,15] renal nerves[13] and cytokines. Many patients who develop ARF in the ICU setting are septic.

ACUTE INTRINSIC RENAL DISEASE

Intrinsic renal disease producing ARF may result from either glomerular disease or conditions affecting the renal interstitium, most commonly the tubules. Glomerular disease which produces ARF is given the name rapidly progressive glomerulonephritis (RPGN). Causes are shown in Table 12.2 and include the microscopic vasculitides Wegener's granulomatosis and microscopic polyarteritis, autoimmune disease such as systemic lupus erythematosis and antiglomerular basement membrane (GBM) disease and postinfectious causes such as hemolytic uremic syndrome and post-streptococcal glomerulonephritis.

The recognition and diagnosis of acute GN depends, as always, on the history and examination; a careful search for nonrenal manifestations of systemic disease such as a vasculitic rash or joint involvement is vital. Urine testing for blood and protein and microscopy for red cell morphology and red cell casts may point towards a glomerular lesion. If an acute GN is suspected or the cause of ARF is unclear, autoantibodies should be measured; the presence of anti-GBM, antinuclear or antineutrophil cytoplasmic antibodies (ANCA) may indicate the diagnosis; ANCA may occasionally occur in nonglomerular disease.[16] Immunoglobulin electrophoresis and complement levels are also helpful.

If an acute GN is suspected either clinically or as the result of investigations, a renal biopsy should be performed. A biopsy is necessary for several reasons:

1. The diagnosis may be unclear without histology.
2. Even if the diagnosis is clear, the biopsy may indicate the prognosis for recovery of renal function.
3. As a correlate of 2, treatment decisions are often influenced by the severity of changes seen on biopsy; for example marked glomerular or interstitial destruction in a patient with acute glomerulonephritis will indicate a poor prognosis for renal recovery and should therefore temper enthusiasm for aggressive immunosuppressive regimes.

Acute interstitial renal disease occurs most commonly in response to drugs or toxins. Table 12.3 lists those agents which cause ARF and which fall into two main groups. Some are damaging in all patients by a direct toxic effect on tubules; the commonest are the aminoglycoside antibiotics and radiocontrast agents. The toxicity of these agents is dose related and occurs most commonly in the elderly, in patients who are sodium and volume depleted, in the presence of other tubular toxins and in those with pre-existent renal disease, particularly myeloma and diabetes mellitus.[17]

The second group is those drugs which produce an acute interstitial nephritis as a result of an idiosyncratic immunological response. The drug acts as a hapten, inducing either an antibody mediated or more commonly a T cell mediated immunological reaction against some component of the interstitium. The commonest drugs are antibiotics and nonsteroidal anti-inflammatory agents (NSAIs) (Table 12.3). As NSAIs are now available without prescription, it is

Table 12.2 Acute glomerular disease producing acute renal failure

Secondary glomerulonephritis

Microscopic vasculitis – ANCA related
    Wegener's granulomatosis – 90% cANCA positive
    Microscopic polyarteritis – c or pANCA positive

Anti-glomerular basement membrane (GBM) disease (with pulmonary hemorrhage – Goodpasture's syndrome)

Systemic disease
    Systemic lupus erythematosis
    Henoch–Schönlein purpura
    Cryoglobulinaemia
    Scleroderma

Infectious
    Post-streptococcal glomerulonephritis
    Infective endocarditis

Hemolytic uremic syndrome
    Epidemic – diarrhea related
    Sporadic

Neoplastic disease – commonly membranous glomerulonephropathy

Drug reactions
    Penicillamine
    Hydralazine
    Rifampicin

Primary glomerulonephritis – only rarely produces ARF

IgA nephropathy

Mesangiocapillary glomerulonephritis

Membranous glomerulonephropathy

cANCA = cytoplasmic antineutrophil cytoplasmic autoantibody;
pANCA = perinuclear antineutrophil cytoplasmic autoantibody.

important to ask patients specifically about such drugs as a cursory drug history may not elicit an accurate response.

The diagnosis of acute interstitial nephritis may be difficult. Eosinophiluria occurs in approximately 50% of cases[18] and occasional patients have heavy proteinuria, particularly in NSAI associated cases.[19] A renal biopsy may be necessary to make the diagnosis and steroid therapy may hasten recovery of renal function.[20] Discontinuation of the offending drug is important although identifying the culprit may be difficult.

Nondrug causes of tubular damage and ARF include multiple myeloma and the various syndromes associated with cell lysis. The commonest renal complication of myeloma is cast nephropathy; this is characterized by tubular casts which are composed of monoclonal immunoglobulin light chains and tubular proteins. The casts elicit a peritubular cellular reaction and renal

Table 12.3   Agents producing interstitial disease

Direct nephrotoxins
Antibiotics
  Aminoglycosides
  Sulphonamides
  Cephalosporins
  Amphotericin B

Radiocontrast

Chemotherapeutic drugs
  Cisplatinum
  Methotrexate
  Mitomycin

Poisons
  Paraquat
  Mushrooms
  Snake bites

Heavy metals, e.g. lead, bismuth, mercury

Organic solvents, e.g. carbon tetrachloride

Tubular toxicity and obstruction

Immunoglobulin light chains – 'cast nephropathy'

Rhabdomyolysis – myoglobin

Tumor lysis syndromes
  Urate, phosphate

Immunologically mediated – acute interstitial nephritis

Antibiotics
  Penicillins
  Cephalosporins

Nonsteroid anti-inflammatory agents

Diuretics
  Frusemide
  Thiazides

Anticonvulsants

impairment occurs as a consequence of tubular obstruction by the casts and tubular toxicity by the light chains.[21, 22] The diagnosis of cast nephropathy depends on finding a serum paraprotein and urinary monoclonal light chains (Bence Jones proteinuria) combined with the histological features on renal biopsy. Appropriate therapy with alkaline diuresis, plasma exchange and chemotherapy may improve renal function (see below).[23, 24]

The recognition of ARF secondary to cell lysis is usually straightforward. Rhabdomyolysis and tumor cell lysis are often apparent from the history and the characteristic biochemistry with elevated urate and phosphate, low calcium and often striking hyperkalemia. Urinanalysis may reveal myoglobinuria in rhabdomyolysis, although this may be short lived, and urine microscopy may show urate or calcium phosphate crystals in tumor lysis. A renal biopsy is not particularly helpful in these patients and may be contraindicated, e.g. by thrombocytopenia. Rather analogous to myeloma cast nephropathy, renal impairment occurs as a consequence of tubular obstruction by urate, calcium phosphate and/or myoglobin casts and direct tubular toxicity.[25] Prevention or reversal of renal impairment may be possible in these patients with a vigorous alkaline and saline diuresis (see below).[26]

The heavy metals, including lead and mercury, are also toxic to tubular cells and may produce ARF, although more commonly they result in chronic renal disease.

OBSTRUCTIVE NEPHROPATHY

Obstruction to the urinary tract may be symptomatic with unilateral or bilateral loin pain and acute anuria. Frequently however it is silent with the history providing few clues. Normal urine volumes do *not* preclude a diagnosis of obstructive ARF and the insidious development of obstruction will often be associated with polyuria. A renal ultrasound will demonstrate upper tract dilatation in almost all patients with significant obstruction.[27] Ultrasound will also often demonstrate the cause of the obstruction; ureteric calculi however are difficult to detect with ultrasound and a plain abdominal X-ray is important to demonstrate radio-opaque stones. All patients with ARF should have a renal ultrasound although the urgency with which it is performed will depend on clinical circumstances.

Bladder outflow obstruction is diagnosed and treated relatively easily with either a urethral or suprapubic catheter; gradual drainage of the chronically distended bladder is not necessary.[28] Obstruction to the upper urinary tract may require nephrostomy drainage followed by specialized approaches depending on the underlying pathology. Treatment decisions in patients with obstruction secondary to malignant disease may be particularly difficult.

RENOVASCULAR DISEASE

Atherosclerotic renal artery stenosis (ARAS) is increasingly recognized as a cause of both acute and chronic renal failure. Angiotensin converting enzyme inhibitors (ACEI) may produce an acute deterioration in renal function in patients with bilateral renovascular disease; the mechanism is not completely clear although inhibition of angiotensin II mediated increase in glomerular efferent arteriolar tone is probably the major factor.[29]

ARAS is common, being found in 20–40% of patients with significant coronary, cerebral or peripheral vascular disease,[30] and is responsible for approximately 10% of cases of end-stage renal failure in Europe. Clues to ARAS being the cause of renal failure may be present in the history; it is commoner in the elderly, smokers and those with concomitant vascular disease. Anuria in a patient with asymmetry of renal size should suggest ARAS, as should recent treatment with ACEIs.

The diagnosis of ARAS can be difficult. Doppler ultrasound is not particularly helpful and is very labor-intensive, whereas nuclear medicine scans with or without captopril as a stress are less useful in patients with ARF although they can confirm renal infarction. Intra-arterial digital subtraction angiography is probably the investigation of choice for suspected ARAS; it will provide information about both renal arteries and also other major vessels including the aorta which may influence treatment decisions re angioplasty versus reconstructive surgery. Magnetic resonance angiography can provide accurate and detailed information about renal arteries,[31] although this remains the province of specialized units for the moment.

CONCLUSION

The cause of ARF should usually be determined within 24 hours with the history and examination combined with renal ultrasound and urine examination. Even if the precise diagnosis is unclear, the etiological group should be apparent. The importance of urine examination with microscopy and testing for blood and protein cannot be overstressed.

Manifestations of renal impairment

Renal failure, whether acute or chronic, produces its clinical manifestations as a result of the disturbance of three separate, albeit interrelated, functions:

1. reduction in the GFR
2. impairment of tubular function
3. disturbance of renal synthetic functions.

REDUCTION IN GFR

The normal GFR in an adult is approximately 80–120 ml/min/1.73 m^2, which is equivalent to 150 litres per day. GFR falls with age such that a 70-year-old can be expected to have a GFR approximately 50% of normal. It is, of course, the filtration of such large quantities of fluid that provides adequate clearance of the traditional markers of renal function, urea and creatinine. The plasma concentrations of urea and creatinine remain within the 'normal' range until the GFR falls to below 50% of normal (i.e. 50 ml/min).

Creatinine is a product of skeletal muscle and its production is relatively constant from day to day for a given muscle mass; its release is not affected by normal muscle use although death of skeletal muscle may increase plasma creatinine acutely. The plasma creatinine will be substantially higher in a muscular 80 kg man than in a 50 kg woman for a given GFR; for example two patients with plasma creatinine values of 130 and 250 μmol/l may have similar GFRs. Creatinine is freely filtered at the glomerulus and, in normal kidneys, tubular absorption and secretion is relatively unimportant; creatinine clearance as calculated from accurate urine collections or estimated from a patient's height, weight, sex and plasma creatinine is therefore a fair approximation of GFR. As GFR falls, tubular secretion of creatinine becomes increasingly important and creatinine clearance therefore overestimates GFR; this is significant only when GFR is less than 20 ml/min.

Urea is an hepatic product of protein catabolism and, in healthy patients who are in nitrogen balance, production directly reflects protein intake. A large protein meal, either intentional or inadvertent after an upper GI bleed, will increase plasma urea, often to supranormal levels. Conversely a low-protein diet or hepatic dysfunction will result in a low urea for a given level of renal function. Unlike creatinine, there is significant tubular handling of urea; antidiuretic hormone (ADH) increases the permeability of the collecting tubules to urea, reducing urea clearance. Patients who are desalinated or dehydrated will therefore frequently have a plasma urea which is elevated in disproportion to the plasma creatinine.

Neither urea nor creatinine, although easily measured markers of GFR, is particularly toxic and they are not the sole cause of the symptoms and signs of the 'uremic' state. Other products of protein metabolism which have been poorly defined and which have molecular weights between 5000 and 10 000 Daltons, are probably the main toxins; these have been termed the middle molecules of renal failure.[32]

The ability of the kidneys to maintain sodium and water homeostasis is perturbed as the GFR falls. Nevertheless this is only a major clinical problem at very low GFRs. Since a GFR of 15 ml/min is equivalent to greater than 20 l per day containing more than 3000 mmol of sodium, the kidneys, at this level of GFR, are able to maintain sodium and water balance relatively easily. However, at extremes of sodium and water intake, this may not be possible, in particular when tubular function is impaired (see below). As the GFR falls below 10 ml/min, sodium and water homeostasis becomes more precarious. Patients with nonoliguric ARF usually have a GFR in this range; sodium and water balance can then only be maintained with careful monitoring of clinical state and electrolyte balance, particularly in acutely ill patients who may have unusual, nonrenal losses. Oliguria with established ARF represents a GFR which approaches zero when control of sodium and water balance is nonexistent.

Calcium, phosphate and potassium homeostasis follow a similar pattern to sodium and water with respect to GFR, although for different reasons. The excretion of phosphate and potassium in the urine and the retention of calcium largely depend on tubular function, as does renal acid–base balance.

DISTURBANCE OF TUBULAR FUNCTION

The renal tubules are serially organized; i.e. each part of the nephron depends for its function on the operation of sections upstream. The proximal tubules reabsorb 60–80% of filtered sodium and water, most of the filtered bicarbonate and phosphate and virtually all of the glucose, amino acids and small molecular weight proteins. Although more distal nephron segments are able to compensate for reduced sodium and water reabsorption by the proximal tubules (this is why proximal tubular diuretics are only weakly diuretic), they cannot reabsorb glucose, amino acids, phosphate or bicarbonate. The loop of Henle primarily reabsorbs sodium and chloride, creating the interstitial hypertonicity that produces the countercurrent mechanism. The distal tubules reabsorb more sodium in exchange for potassium and hydrogen ions and the collecting tubules determine final urine concentration under the influence of ADH.

Depending on the cause of the renal failure, tubular function may be well preserved; this commonly occurs in glomerulonephritis. Alternatively GFR and tubular function may decline roughly in parallel as occurs with hemodynamically mediated ARF, or tubular function may be impaired prior to a significant reduction in GFR as seen with various tubular toxins.

Disturbance of tubular function in patients in the ICU setting is important in as much as it affects sodium and water balance. Although proximal tubular damage with resultant glycosuria, phosphaturia and leak of small molecular weight proteins and amino acids occurs in conditions such as myeloma and heavy metal poisoning, this usually has little clinical relevance. Distal tubular damage which affects the ability to retain sodium is much commoner, being seen in obstructive nephropathy and with tubular toxins. Damaged tubules which are unable to conserve sodium may produce significant desalination, reducing renal perfusion and GFR. Many patients with ARF therefore become desalinated as a secondary effect of their renal impairment.

RENAL SYNTHETIC FUNCTIONS

The kidneys also have a central role in erythropoiesis, vitamin D metabolism and blood pressure control. Both acute and chronic renal failure can lead to disturbance of these systems.

Erythropoietin (EPO) is a glycoprotein produced by specialized peritubular cells in the renal interstitium. EPO stimulates erythroid stem cells to divide, thereby increasing erythropoiesis and preventing anemia. Patients with chronic and end-stage renal failure are frequently anemic and the improvement following recombinant human EPO administration indicates that a major component of this anemia is deficient EPO generation.[33, 34] Serum EPO levels fall rapidly in ARF compared with those in patients with similar illnesses but normal renal function.[35] Although patients with ARF are frequently anemic, this is usually multifactorial and not, at least in the first week, a consequence of deficient EPO production. The use of recombinant EPO is therefore probably not justified early in the course of ARF but may have a role in prolonged cases.

Inactive vitamin D, either of dietary origin or from cutaneous synthesis, is hydroxylated in the liver and then the kidney to the active hormone 1,25-dihydroxycholecalciferol. Activity of renal 1α-hydroxylase is reduced in renal failure when the GFR falls below approximately 60 ml/min; this may lead to mild hypocalcemia and a compensatory increase in parathormone concentrations. In ARF this probably has little clinical relevance initially but may become clinically relevant in prolonged cases. Dietary supplementation with active vitamin D is relatively straightforward.

The kidneys play a central role in the control of systemic blood pressure. Hypertension is a common complication of CRF and may also, if long-standing, produce renal impairment. Hypertension complicating ARF is unusual; conditions affecting the renal microvasculature such as hemolytic uremic syndrome and scleroderma may however present with severe hypertension and ARF and the malignant phase of long-standing hypertension usually produces a rapid reduction in GFR. The presence of hypertension in a case of ARF should initiate a search for intrinsic renal disease.

Management of acute renal failure

The management of the patient with ARF can be considered in two parts:

1. strategies to reverse renal impairment or to speed recovery of useful renal function.
2. support of the patient until renal function recovers.
   (a) conservative measures to minimize the metabolic consequences of ARF
   (b) renal replacement with some form of dialysis.

REVERSAL OF ARF

Attempts to reverse ARF depend initially on identifying the cause. Most patients in the ICU with ARF have a hemodynamically mediated renal lesion, with ischemic damage secondary to reduced renal perfusion. The cause of this (Table 12.1) is usually clear and initial treatment should be directed at the underlying cause, if possible; e.g. antibiotics and fluids for sepsis, appropriate intravenous fluids for hypovolemia of any cause, support for the failing heart and surgery for underlying surgical problems. It is clear that nephrotoxic ARF can be reduced or prevented with adequate salination.[26, 36] The same may be true for hemodynamically mediated ARF and may depend on the positive correlation between renal energy requirements and sodium reabsorption;[37] increasing tubular sodium delivery may reduce energy requirements and consequent ischemic damage.

Traditionally urine biochemistry has been used to distinguish prerenal oliguria from established ATN; concentrated urine with a low sodium is taken to indicate poorly perfused, but nevertheless functioning, kidneys and a dilute urine with higher sodium is taken to indicate established renal damage (Table 12.4). The distinction was felt to be relevant with the former requiring intravenous fluid and the latter fluid restriction to prevent fluid overload. This is however an inappropriate response for a number of reasons. Renal hypoperfusion with oliguria is just one, albeit easily measured, manifestation of a systemic disturbance; hypoperfusion of other organs such as the gut, liver and myocardium is usually also present and may have more life-threatening short-term consequences. Therefore an

Table 12.4 Urine biochemistry

	Prerenal oliguria	Established ARF
Na$^+$	<10 mmol/l	>20 mmol/l
Urine/plasma urea ratio	>10	<10
Urine/plasma osmolality ratio	>1.3	<1.1

Urine concentration is also affected by diuretics which often prevent interpretation of urinary electrolytes.

inability to reverse renal impairment acutely does not override other indications for fluid replacement. Furthermore ARF secondary to ATN is not an all or none phenomenon and the rate of recovery of renal function depends, in part, on the speed with which renal perfusion improves.

Therefore patients who are oliguric require intravenous fluid replacement to optimize their tissue, including renal, perfusion; depending on their clinical state this may be no fluids as in cardiogenic shock or many litres of fluid as in rhabdomyolysis or septicemia. In oliguric or anuric patients, intravenous fluids may of course produce fluid overload; with careful monitoring, particularly in an ICU setting, this is not usually a problem. If the patient becomes overloaded and remains oliguric, this will merely hasten the need for some form of dialysis. Of course careful monitoring of fluid state with right- and left-sided central venous pressures will reduce the risk of fluid mismanagement. The development of pulmonary edema in a patient with ARF is usually due to fluid overload; adult respiratory distress syndrome (ARDS) should only be considered after fluid overload has been excluded.

Specific replacement fluids may be indicated in certain clinical situations. The intraluminal cast formation which occurs in myeloma cast nephropathy, urate and phosphate deposition in tumor lysis and myoglobin deposition in rhabdomyolysis is partially dependent on luminal pH; the solubility of these substances is markedly reduced below a pH of 6. Treatment should therefore be aimed at increasing urinary pH above 6–6.5. This is most easily obtained with bicarbonate solutions; a regime composed of one-third 0.9% saline, one-third isotonic sodium bicarbonate (1.26 or 1.4%) and one-third 5% glucose has been suggested for rhabdomyolysis.[38] Urine flow may need to be maintained with diuretics, preferably mannitol (see below). Light chains and the other toxins also have a direct toxic effect on proximal tubular cells[21] and increased delivery of and therefore reduced reabsorption of sodium and bicarbonate may further reduce nephrotoxicity. The appropriate use of intravenous fluids including bicarbonate can prevent renal impairment in all cases of rhabdomyolysis provided therapy is commenced early.[25, 26] This is unfortunately not always possible.

There are various therapies which have been attempted to protect kidneys from ischemic or toxic damage and which have a variable success.

Diuretics

Diuretics are frequently used in oliguric patients in an attempt to increase urine volumes and reverse renal damage. Two main groups are used, loop diuretics and the osmotic diuretic mannitol. Before discussing these agents, it is worth stressing that inappropriately increasing sodium and water excretion in a hypovolemic patient with a diuretic will merely exacerbate their condition and further reduce renal perfusion. Patients therefore must be adequately filled prior to the administration of a diuretic.

The loop diuretics frusemide and bumetanide are potent agents which reduce sodium reabsorption in the loop of Henle, thereby increasing urinary sodium and free water loss. As a consequence of increased sodium delivery to the distal tubule they increase Na^+/H^+ and Na^+/K^+ exchange, reducing urinary pH and increasing potassium losses. They are strongly protein bound, particularly to albumin, and for their tubular effect depend on active secretion into the lumen by proximal tubular cells; this process is partially blocked by bile acids, explaining the reduced effect of loop diuretics in patients with significant liver disease. Loop diuretics also relax vascular smooth muscle, producing a vasodilatory effect in the kidneys and other vascular beds.

The ability of loop diuretics to ameliorate hemodynamically mediated ARF is unclear. Studies in man have been equivocal[39] and are difficult to design and perform because of the heterogeneous nature of patients ARF. Animal studies have also produced conflicting results, with some demonstrating a beneficial effect and others failing to do so. A reasonable conclusion is probably that these agents will increase urine production, may convert oliguric ARF to nonoliguric ARF but do not have a potent renoprotective effect.

Frusemide in high doses is ototoxic, although the effect is reversible, and intravenous doses of 250 mg or more need to be given slowly – a maximum rate of 4 mg/min is suggested. For this reason it is often simpler to use bumetanide which is less ototoxic.

Mannitol, a complex sugar, acts as an osmotic diuretic, reducing tubular reabsorption of water throughout the nephron. Therefore, unlike loop diuretics, mannitol increases proximal tubular urine flow and does not alter urinary pH. Mannitol is widely used to prevent ARF in cardiac surgery and renal transplantation although its efficacy in these situations is unclear. The data are rather similar to those with loop diuretics although there is probably a greater benefit.[40] Mannitol is also useful as part of an alkaline diuresis in the treatment of rhabdomyolysis,[38] myeloma cast nephropathy[23] and tumor lysis syndromes as it does not reduce urinary pH.

The major problem with mannitol use is its retention in renal impairment. This may lead to an osmotic increase in the circulating volume and fluid overload in susceptible patients. Therefore the clinical condition and response to mannitol must be assessed frequently and treatment discontinued if necessary.

Renal vasodilators

Dopamine, which produces a positive inotropic effect at standard doses, is a vasodilator in various splanchnic vascular beds including the kidney at doses of 1.5–3.0 ng/kg/min. Studies in normal individuals indicate that dopamine increases GFR and renal plasma flow to a variable extent.[41] Low-dose dopamine is therefore commonly used in oliguria and ARF although evidence for its efficacy is lacking. One justification for its use is that dopamine may also protect other splanchnic beds such as the gut. Other dopaminergic agonists such as dobutamine and dopexamine may have similar effects; dopexamine in particular may reduce mortality in acutely ill patients.[42]

The stable prostacyclin analog iloprost is a potent vasodilator both in the kidney and elsewhere. In normal subjects prostacyclin increases renal plasma flow without increasing GFR.[43] There have been case reports of a dramatic effect of prostacyclin in individual cases of ARF, usually associated with microvascular disease such as hemolytic uremic syndrome and malaria. In hemodynamically mediated ARF prostacyclin probably has no role.

Other vasodilators such as the nitrovasodilators nitroprusside and nitroglycerin have not been shown to be of value in reversing ARF.[42]

Other strategies

Sepsis is a frequent cause of ARF. Attempts to reduce the mortality of Gram-negative septicemia have used antibodies against bacterial endotoxin.[44] There is controversy as to their efficacy[45] and their value in reducing the incidence and severity of ARF in these patients is unclear. Further attempts to influence sepsis with antiendotoxin and anticytokine approaches are being explored and may be shown to affect ARF.

It is beyond the scope of this chapter to discuss in detail the immunosuppressive protocols for the management of rapidly progressive glomerulonephritis (RPGN); most use a combination of steroids either as oral prednisolone or intravenous methylprednisolone and either cyclophosphamide or azathioprine. Plasma exchange is also commonly used in RPGN although its use in severe lupus nephritis has recently been shown to be of no value[46] and doubts have been raised in other conditions. Plasma exchange is nevertheless of value for lung hemorrhage associated with anti-glomerular basement membrane disease. It is also useful in hemolytic uremic syndrome[47,48] and probably in myeloma cast nephropathy.[23,24]

Conclusion

Overall the major approach of attempts to prevent hemodynamically mediated ARF depends on correcting, as rapidly as possible, the hemodynamic disturbance with appropriate intravenous fluid replacement combined with cardiac support. The reversal of nonhemodynamically mediated ARF depends on identifying the cause and removing or treating it.

CONSERVATIVE MANAGEMENT OF ARF

The major consequences of renal failure occur secondary to:

1. the accumulation of products of protein metabolism
2. electrolyte disturbances, particularly with acidosis and hyperkalemia
3. fluid overload due to reduced urinary volume.

Prior to the development of dialysis for ARF, the management of ARF was based on altering protein, electrolyte and fluid intake with the hope of an early recovery of renal function.[49] Renal replacement, in particular with hemofiltration, has rendered some aspects of the conservative measures unnecessary.

Fluid balance

Most patients with acute renal failure are anuric and even patients with nonoliguric ARF usually become oliguric when dialysis or hemofiltration is started. Daily fluid requirements therefore are (a) urine output plus (b) insensible losses (for an adult these are approximately 12 ml/kg/day, which is about 600–800 ml/day) minus (c) endogenous water production of some 300 ml/day. This usually works out at some 500 ml/day and cannot be calculated with greater accuracy. Monitoring of fluid balance should include, if possible, daily weights; most patients with ARF can be expected to lose 1 kg every 3–4 days.

Fluid restriction to 500 ml/day may be impossible in patients with ARF, especially on the ICU with the need for multiple intravenous drugs and often parenteral nutrition.

Electrolytes

Hyperkalemia is common in ARF, particularly when related to rhabdomyolysis or tumor lysis syndromes.

The danger of hyperkalemia is related to rate of rise in potassium and is best judged electrocardiographically by tall peaked T waves and widening of the QRS complexes. Initial therapy frequently involves intravenous glucose and insulin, calcium gluconate and potassium binding agents such as calcium resonium. Calcium resonium may cause severe constipation and should be given with a laxative which will also increase potassium losses. These measures only reduce potassium temporarily and definitive treatment of hyperkalemia depends on either improving renal function or dialysis.

In established ARF, hyperkalemia is rarely a problem. Nevertheless the kidneys are the major excretion pathway for potassium and therefore potassium intake needs to be minimized in most patients. Hypokalemia may occur during the recovery phase of ARF, especially in patients who have been very catabolic; enteral or parenteral supplements may therefore be necessary.

Sodium requirements will vary markedly in different patients; basal requirements are on average between 30–50 mmol/day. Plasma sodium is not an indicator of sodium balance but reflects alterations in free water intake and excretion. Total body sodium is best judged by evidence of fluid status; overloaded patients will require sodium removal and dry patients the reverse.

Daily H^+ production is approximately 1 mmol/kg, although this may increase in catabolic states or in lactic acid or ketoacid states. Reducing protein intake (see below) may reduce H^+ generation. Acidosis may be corrected with intravenous sodium bicarbonate alone although most patients with established ARF cannot tolerate the associated sodium and water load. Bicarbonate increases CO_2 production which may be problematic in patients with respiratory difficulties.

Dietary management

Reduction of protein intake to minimize the accumulation of products of protein metabolism is recognized as unsuitable in patients with ARF where dialysis is available. Patients in the ICU, and particularly those with ARF, have increased protein requirements due to:

1. increased activity of proteases and other proteolytic enzymes;[50]
2. hormonal alterations with elevated catecholamines and glucagon which, combined with insulin resistance, increase catabolism; and
3. renal replacement therapy leading to increased losses of amino acids, glucose and small peptides.

Patients with ARF who remain in neutral or positive nitrogen balance have a lower mortality than those in negative balance,[51] although there may be a variety of reasons for this which do not relate directly to nutrition.

Patients with ARF therefore should receive similar nutrition to any other patient on the ICU. The restrictions of fluids and electrolytes in an oliguric or anuric patient of course still apply unless renal replacement therapy can compensate for these.

RENAL REPLACEMENT THERAPY

The replacement of renal function in the ICU involves either dialysis, which may be peritoneal or hemodialysis, or the more recently introduced and widely used hemofiltration. The principles by which dialysis and hemofiltration alter plasma biochemistry are very different.

Dialysis

Dialysis utilizes two different physical processes: diffusion and convection. Diffusion is numerically more important and involves the movement of solutes down a concentration gradient across a semipermeable membrane. This depends on having a solution, called the dialysate, on one side of the semipermeable membrane and blood on the other side. Hemodialysis uses an artificial extracorporeal membrane through which the blood is pumped whereas peritoneal dialysis uses the peritoneum with dialysate being placed in the peritoneum. The dialysate is designed to produce large concentration gradients of those compounds which should be removed in large quantities, e.g. creatinine and urea, lower gradients where only moderate quantities should be removed, e.g. potassium, and a reverse gradient where a net positive balance is desired, e.g. calcium. Table 12.5 lists the composition of a typical hemodialysis solution. It is diffusion during dialysis which produces the clearance of urea, creatinine and the middle molecules and corrects any electrolyte disturbance.

Table 12.5 Composition of dialysate solutions

	Hemodialysate	Peritoneal dialysate	Hemofiltrate
Na^+	135	132	140
K^+	2.0	Variable	Variable
Ca^{2+}	1.5	1.75	1.6
Mg^{2+}	0.375	0.75	0.75
Cl^-	105	102	100
Lactate	–	35	45
Acetate	2.0[a]	–	–
HCO_3^-	35	–	–
Glucose	2.0	1.36/3.86%	–

All concentrations in mmol/l.
[a] Acetate concentration 40 mmol/l for acetate-based hemodialysis.

The other physical process that occurs during dialysis is convection. This is the movement of water (and any solutes) across a semipermeable membrane down a pressure gradient. This of course is what happens in the glomerulus with the glomerular basement membrane (GBM) being the semipermeable membrane. During hemodialysis a hydraulic pressure gradient can be created across the extracorporeal membrane and this leads to net fluid removal from the patient. Altering the transmembrane pressure, by changing pressure in either the blood or dialysate compartment, permits control of fluid removal. Modern volumetric hemodialysis machines are capable of measuring the rate of fluid removal during hemodialysis and altering transmembrane pressure to achieve a prescribed rate of fluid removal.

It is impossible to create a hydraulic pressure gradient during peritoneal dialysis and therefore an osmotic pressure gradient is created by altering dialysate composition. Typically glucose, as a cheap and relatively nontoxic osmotically active molecule, is used; dialysate with higher glucose concentrations (typical range 1.36–3.86%) produces greater fluid shifts into the peritoneum and therefore greater fluid removal from the patient (Table 12.5). Glucose of course is absorbed by diffusion across the peritoneal membrane and repeated use of dialysate with high glucose concentrations may result in hyperglycemia. Other osmotically active molecules such as maltose and amino acids have been used in peritoneal dialysis fluid in place of glucose but have not achieved wide use mainly because of expense.

The correction of acidosis by dialysis depends on using a bicarbonate source. In peritoneal dialysis this is typically lactate, whereas in hemodialysis it may be either acetate or bicarbonate. Lactate and acetate are metabolized in the liver to produce bicarbonate, thereby correcting the acidosis. Significant hepatic disease however may result in hyperacetatemia or hyperlactatemia with only partial correction of the acidosis.[52]

Hemodialysis

During hemodialysis (HD) blood is pumped through the extracorporeal artificial kidney, normally at a rate of 200–250 ml/min, whilst dialysate is pumped at a rate of 500 ml/min. This has a number of consequences which limit the use of HD to specialized units and the benefits in many patients with ARF. Hemodialysis produces very high clearance of urea, creatinine, phosphate, potassium, etc.; this of course is why patients with end-stage renal failure can dialyse for only 10–12 hours per week and maintain adequate biochemistry. Typical rates of urea or creatinine clearance during HD are 300–400 ml/min. Such rapid removal of osmotically active molecules may result in significant fluid shifts during dialysis and in acutely ill patients may produce hypotension. It can be impossible to dialyze patients who are already hypotensive although this has improved with changes in dialysate composition and improved membrane technology (see below).

A dialysate pump speed of 500 ml/min means that during a typical 4-hour dialysis session a patient will be exposed to 120 liters of dialysate. Therefore the water used must be very pure and dialysate composition must be monitored closely. This requires expensive and complicated equipment which is only available in specialized dialysis units.

The high clearances achieved during HD mean that even catabolic patients with ARF require no more than 2–3 hours per day of HD to maintain adequate biochemistry. Although substantial volumes of fluid can be removed during a 3-hour dialysis by alterations in the transmembrane pressure (see above), such a daily dialysis regime will result in a 20-hour period each day when there is no control over the fluid state of an anuric patient with ARF. For many patients fluid balance becomes impossible.

Vascular access

The removal of 200–250 ml blood per minute for HD requires access either to a central vein or the arterial circulation. Most long-term HD is via radial or brachial arteriovenous fistulae which are created surgically. Increased venous flow results in arterialization of superficial veins and after a period of weeks can be cannulated for each dialysis session. Such an approach is not feasible in ARF and other options need to be considered.

Central venous cannulation with double lumen catheters are the commonest first line option for acute HD in the UK. Catheters can be placed in the femoral vein where the risk of traumatic complications is lowest or in the subclavian or internal jugular veins. Flows for HD are usually satisfactory although local and systemic infections may be a problem; it is unclear whether elective line changes reduce infective complications although they increase traumatic complications.[53]

Cannulation of both the femoral artery and vein is used in some units although this is mainly employed for arteriovenous hemofiltration (see below). More commonly for HD, arteriovenous (AV) shunts are inserted in either the wrist, the elbow or the ankle. These involve the surgical insertion of Teflon cannulae into the relevant artery and vein with an extracorporeal connection; when not in use the arterial blood flows through the short extracorporeal connection. For dialysis the connection is broken. AV shunts require specialist surgical insertion but, once in place, are often very satisfactory with low complication rates including infections although documented evidence to support this clinical observation is lacking.

Dialysis membranes

Until the 1980s all hemodialysis membranes were cuprophane based – termed cellulosic. These provide adequate hydraulic clearances and are permeable to molecules up to molecular weight of approximately 5000 Da. There are a number of problems with these membranes which limit their use, particularly in ICU patients. They are, to a certain extent, bioincompatible; when blood comes in contact with the membrane there is complement activation, initiation of an acute phase response and white cell clumping. The major acute consequence is obstruction in the pulmonary micro-vasculature which results in hypoxia which may persist for several hours. Patients may also become hypoxic because of removal of CO_2 and bicarbonate into the dialysate with a resulting reduction in respiratory drive. Chronic consequences of cellulosic membrane use include increased hepatic B_2 microglobulin production which may result in dialysis related amyloid. The low hydraulic permeability of cellulosic membranes limits the rate of fluid removal with these membranes.

Recently semisynthetic cellulosic membranes have become available which are more biocompatible, although the relatively low hydraulic permeability and impermeability to higher molecular weight molecules are unchanged.

Synthetic, biocompatible membranes which are composed of either polyacrylonitrite (PAN) or polysulphone are now available. These have a high hydraulic permeability, remove molecules up to size 10 000–15 000 Da and are biocompatible with little complement or white cell activation. Their hydraulic permeability necessitates their use with volumetric HD machines (which measure rate of fluid removal) and also permitted the development of hemofiltration as an alternative to HD in ARF (see below). These membranes are more expensive than cellulosic membranes, costing approximately £30 ($40) per artificial kidney compared with £7 ($10).

Patients with ARF who have either cardiovascular or respiratory problems should probably have a PAN or polysulphone membrane for their first few dialyses in an attempt to minimize cardiorespiratory disturbance.

Dialysate

Bicarbonate is the ideal buffer to correct the acidosis of renal failure during dialysis. Dialysate however contains calcium, which is unstable in solution with bicarbonate. Acetate was therefore used for many years as an alternative, undergoing metabolism in the liver.[54] Acetate however is metabolized slowly in some patients and the resultant hyperacetatemia is felt to contribute to dialysis-related hypotension and post-dialysis hangover.[52] Bicarbonate-based dialysis is now possible with machines that mix bicarbonate and calcium containing solutions just prior to use and thereby avoid the precipitation of calcium carbonate. Bicarbonate dialysis reduces the incidence of significant hypotension although it is not yet available in all units.

Peritoneal dialysis

The composition of peritoneal dialysis (PD) dialysate is similar to hemodialysate (Table 12.5) with the exception of glucose which, in PD, is used in different concentrations to alter rates of fluid removal. PD will correct the metabolic disturbance and can provide volume control. The various techniques of PD have spawned a number of acronyms. Continuous ambulatory PD (CAPD) is the commonest form of PD for patients with ESRF; dialysate is infused into the peritoneum via a soft cuffed catheter and left *in situ* for 4–8 hours before being drained out and replaced with fresh dialysate – volumes of 1.5–2 litres are routinely used. In patients who cannot perform three to four evenly spaced exchanges daily, intermittent PD (IPD) may be done, for example at night. Machine control of drainage and dwell times is possible and this is termed continuous cycling PD (CCPD). PD via a soft catheter is not suitable for patients with ARF as the catheters are inserted surgically and, if used immediately, often result in leaks.

A semirigid catheter however can be inserted under local anesthetic, usually in the midline below the umbilicus, and is suitable for patients with ARF. PD may then be machine controlled as CCPD or controlled by the nursing staff; the latter of course is fairly labor-intensive. Exchange with 8–12 l/day will usually provide adequate biochemical control in anuric ARF and can rapidly correct hyperkalemia or fluid overload. If PD is continued for some time potassium may need to be added to the dialysate to prevent hypokalemia.

PD is associated with a number of problems which limit its use in patients with ARF. Technical or mechanical difficulties with semirigid catheters are common. Extravasation of dialysate, either through or into the anterior abdominal wall, is relatively common. Poor drainage of dialysate related to catheter position or obstruction by the omentum may occur and bowel trauma from catheter insertion is seen. The latter is more likely in patients who have had previous abdominal surgery and this may prevent PD altogether. Acute abdominal disease may be an absolute contraindication to PD. If PD is continued for any period, bacterial peritonitis becomes increasingly likely. This may necessitate removal of the PD catheter and can be a serious complication in the compromised ICU patient.

The significant morbidity and problems that occur with PD in patients with ARF have reduced its popularity as a form of treatment. Nevertheless unavailability of other forms of renal replacement may necessitate its use; if this is the case PD should be limited to a few days before transfer to another form of dialysis.

Hemofiltration

The introduction of hemofiltration (HF) has radically altered the management of patients with ARF in the ICU. Prior to HF, the development of ARF involved consultations with nephrologists, decisions about transfers to a unit with access to HD and often major difficulties in fluid balance in what was often an acutely ill patient. HF has changed all that.

As previously stated, HD and PD involve the removal of solutes and water by diffusion and convection, with diffusion providing the lion's share of solute clearance and convection being used for fluid removal. HF involves the removal of an ultrafiltrate of plasma by convection across the semipermeable membrane of the hemofilter; there is no diffusion. The fluid is replaced with a physiological solution that replaces the electrolytes (Table 12.5) and water but not the substances which the kidneys normally remove, e.g. urea, creatinine, phosphate and, to a lesser extent, potassium. The rate of clearance (or GFR equivalent) is therefore merely the rate at which ultrafiltrate is produced, e.g. 900 ml/h is equivalent to a creatinine (or urea) clearance of 15 ml/min (i.e. 900 ml/h $\times$ 1 h/60 min = 15 ml/min). The rate at which replacement fluid is administered will determine the fluid balance of the patient and provides close control of fluid state.

The development of HF was made possible by the highly permeable biocompatible membranes, PAN and polysulphone, which produce high ultrafiltration rates.[55] Initial forms of HF used the patient's arterial blood pressure to drive the system (arteriovenous HF) whereas many units now use pumped venovenous HF via double lumen central venous catheters. Most patients with ARF are managed with HF removing 500–1500 ml/h.

There are several benefits of HF which make it particularly suitable for patients with ARF. Continuous HF permits close control of fluid balance in anuric or oliguric patients, simplifying drug regimes and enteral or parenteral nutrition. The use of biocompatible membranes minimizes respiratory difficulties. Since the clearance of osmotically active molecules is relatively low, fluid shifts and the resultant hypotension that may occur during HD are much less common with HF. It is possible to perform HF in persistently hypotensive patients requiring inotropic support whereas HD may be impossible.

There are however a number of minor problems associated with HF. Central venous or arterial access may result in traumatic or infectious complications. Continuous anticoagulation for the extracorporeal circuit may produce bleeding difficulties, although these are rarely severe. Continuous filtration will, of course, remove other low-molecular-weight molecules of which the most important seem to be amino acids. It has been estimated that, during parenteral nutrition and HF, 10% of administered amino acids are removed by the filter.

If patients are very catabolic, the clearances produced by routine HF may not provide adequate biochemical control. In specialized units with access to HD, continuous HF can be combined with short periods of HD. This has been termed continuous ultrafiltration with periods of intermittent dialysis (CUPID). A recently described alternative is to run hemofiltration fluid at a rate of 1 l/h through the dialysate compartment of the hemofilter.[56] This provides a small amount of dialysis (i.e. diffusive clearance) without using large quantities of dialysate (standard HD uses 500 ml/min). At a rate of 900 ml/min, clearances can increase from 15 ml/min to 25–30 ml/min, which provides much better biochemical control. This process has been termed hemodiafiltration (HDF).

Anticoagulation during dialysis

Extracorporeal circuits require the use of anticoagulants to prevent clotting in the circuit; clotted lines result in blood loss (volume 100–200 ml), reduced dialysis time and the expense of replacing the kidney and the lines. Heparin is used most commonly – a loading dose is given prior to dialysis and then a continuous infusion throughout dialysis or filtration. The major short-term complications are bleeding and thrombocytopenia. The use of low-molecular-weight heparin may reduce thrombocytopenia but does not seem to reduce the risk of bleeding. Patients at high risk of bleeding require low doses of heparin and dialysis can even be performed without heparin – blood flow needs to be kept as high as possible and lines should be flushed frequently with normal saline.

Prostacyclin which prevents platelet aggregation can be used instead of heparin. With prostacyclin the risk of bleeding during HD seems to be reduced[57] and it can also be used during HF.[58]

Adequacy of dialysis

Studies of patients with ESRF treated with dialysis indicate that there is a correlation between dialysis adequacy and morbidity and mortality; poorly dialyzed patients do worse. A series of complicated mathematical models have been developed to monitor chronic hemdialysis but a crude, but useful, conclusion is that, in a well-nourished patient, predialysis urea should be less than 27 mmol/l and mean urea less than 18 mmol/l. It is unclear whether the data apply to patients with ARF in the ICU but they do provide a guide.

DRUGS IN RENAL FAILURE

Renal failure may affect the handling of drugs in a number of ways. The commonest is by impairing excretion as a result of reduced GFR and disturbed tubular function although drug absorption, distribution, metabolism and pharmacodynamics may also be affec-

Table 12.6 Drug excretion affected by renal failure

Antibiotics
  Penicillins[a]
  Aminoglycosides
  Cephalosporins

Antiarrhythmics
  Digoxin
  Most other agents unaffected

Antihypertensives
  ACE inhibitors
  β-Blockers
  Minoxidil – may produce pericardial effusions

Miscellaneous
  Cimetidine – avoid in renal failure
  Ranitidine – reduce dose
  Allopurinol
  Antacids – some have a high sodium content
  Opiates

[a] Penicillin G is exclusively removed by glomerular filtration. In established renal failure, 2.4 g (4 M units) is the maximum daily dose.

ted. Table 12.6 lists some common drugs, the doses of which may need to be adjusted in renal failure. An additional complication is that clearance by hemo- or peritoneal dialysis or hemofiltration varies between different drugs and cannot be predicted intuitively.

There are several basic rules for drug prescribing in renal failure:

1. Don't assume that a normal plasma creatinine or urea indicates a normal GFR.
2. Whenever prescribing, decide whether each drug is excreted by the kidney and adjust the dose accordingly. If you don't know, look it up, e.g. in Bennett.[59]
3. Consider the nephrotoxic potential of all drugs in patients with renal disease. For example use of an NSAI may be catastrophic in a patient with borderline renal function.

Conclusion

Treatment of patients with ARF in the future will depend on further attempts to prevent the development of ARF, for example by blocking the mediators of sepsis, and improved treatment of the acutely ill patient, perhaps with assessment of regional blood flow and oxygen consumption. Reduction in the mortality requires better treatment of the underlying diseases, ARF being just a manifestation of a systemic upset in most cases.

Renal failure is nevertheless a very serious complication for patients in the ICU; many patients develop ARF as part of a terminal illness. The decision not to treat a patient with renal failure because of a predicted high mortality can only be taken with all the facts concerning the individual patient available; although some forms of ARF have a particularly high mortality (e.g. post acute aortic aneurysm repair), it has proved very difficult, if not impossible, to lay down guidelines permitting selection of patients for dialysis.

Recommended reading

Acute Renal Failure. Brenner BM, Lazarus JM (ed). New York: Churchill Livingstone, 1988.
Acute Renal Failure in the Intensive Therapy Unit. Bihari D, Neild G (eds). London: Springer-Verlag, 1990.

References

1. Stott R, Cameron JS, Ogg C, Bewick M. Why the persistently high mortality in acute renal failure. *Lancet* 1972; ii: 75–8.
2. Werb R, Linton AL. Aetiology, diagnosis, treatment and prognosis of acute renal failure in an intensive care unit. *Resuscitation* 1979; 7 (2): 95–100.
3. Beaman M, Turney JH, Rodger RS, McGonigle RS, Adu D, Michael J. Changing pattern of acute renal failure. *Quart J Med* 1987; 237: 15–23.
4. Turney JH, Marshall DH, Brownjohn AM, Ellis CM, Parsons FM. The evolution of acute renal failure, 1956–1988. *Quart J Med* 1990; 74: 83–104.
5. Groeneveld ABJ, Tran DD, van der Meulen J, Nauta JJP, Thijs LG. Acute renal failure in the medical intensive care unit: predisposing, complicating and outcome factors. *Nephron* 1991; 59: 602–10.
6. Woodrow G, Turney JH. Cause of death in acute renal failure. *Nephrol Dial Trans* 1992; 7: 230–4.
7. Chapman AB, Rubinstein D, Hughes R *et al*. Intracranial aneurysms in autosomal dominant polycystic kidney disease. *New Engl J Med* 1992; 327: 916–20.
8. Schnermann J, Briggs JP, Weber PC. Tubuloglomerular feedback, prostaglandins, and angiotensin in the autoregulation of glomerular filtration rate. *Kidney Int* 1984; 25: 53–64.
9. Epstein FH, Balaban RS, Ross BD. Redox state of cytochrome a,a3 in isolated perfused rat kidney. *Am J Physiol* 1981; 243: F257–F262.
10. Brezis M, Rosen S, Silva P, Epstein FH. Selective vulnerability of the thick ascending limb to anoxia in the isolated perfused rat kidney. *J Clin Invest* 1984; 73: 182–90.
11. Moran M, Kapsner C. Acute renal failure associated with elevated plasma oncotic pressure. *New Engl J Med* 1987; 317: 150–3.
12. Better OS. Renal and cardiovascular function in liver disease. *Kidney Int* 1986; 29: 598–607.
13. Henrich WL, Hamasaki Y, Said SI, Campbell WB, Cronin RE. Dissociation of systemic and renal effects of endotoxemia: prostaglandin inhibition uncovers an important role of renal nerves. *J Clin Invest* 1982; 69: 691–9.
14. Badr KF, Kelley VE, Rennke HG, Brenner BM. Roles for thromboxane A₂ and leukotrienes in endotoxin-induced acute renal failure. *Kidney Int* 1986; 30: 474–80.
15. Lugon JR, Boim MA, Ramos OL, Ajzen H, Schor N. Renal function and glomerular hemodynamics in male endotoxemic rats. *Kidney Int* 1989; 36: 570–5.
16. Falk RJ. ANCA-associated renal disease. *Kidney Int* 1990; 38: 998–1010.
17. Moore RD, Smith CR, Lipsky JJ, Mellits ED, Lietman PS. Risk factors for nephrotoxicity in patients treated with aminoglycosides. *Ann Intern Med* 1984; 100: 352–7.
18. Ten RM, Torres VE, Milliner DS, Schwab TR, Holley KE, Gleich GJ. Acute interstitial nephritis: immunologic and clinical aspects. *Mayo Clin Proc* 1988; 63: 921–30.
19. Clive DM, Stoff JS. Renal syndromes associated with non-steroidal antiinflammatory drugs. *New Engl J Med* 1984; 310: 563–72.
20. Neilson EG. Pathogenesis and therapy of interstitial nephritis. *Kidney Int* 1989; 35: 1257–70.
21. Cooper EH, Forbes MA, Crockson RA, MacLennan ICM. Proximal tubular function in myelomatosis: observations in the fourth Medical Research Council trial. *J Clin Pathol* 1984; 37: 852–8.
22. Coward RA, Mallick NP, Delamore IW. Tubular function in multiple myeloma. *Clin Nephrol* 1985; 24: 180–5.
23. Zucchelli P, Pasquali S, Cagnoli L, Ferrari G. Controlled plasma exchange trial in acute renal failure due to multiple myeloma. *Kidney Int* 1988; 33: 1175–80.
24. Johnson WJ, Kyle RA, Pineda AA, O'Brien PC, Holley KE. Treatment of renal failure associated with multiple myeloma. *Arch Int Med* 1990; 150: 863–9.
25. Odeh M. The role of reperfusion-induced injury in the pathogenesis of the crush syndrome. *New Engl J Med* 1991; 324: 1417–22.
26. Ron D, Taitelman U, Michaelson M, Bar-Joseph G, Bursztein S, Better OS. Prevention of acute renal failure in traumatic rhabdomyolysis. *Arch Int Med* 1984; 144: 277–80.
27. Webb JAW, Reznek RH, White FE, Cattell WR, Kelsey Fry I, Baker LRI. Can ultrasound and computed tomography replace high-dose urography in patients with impaired renal function. *Quart J Med* 1984; 53: 411–25.
28. Foster MC, Upsdell SM, O'Reilly PH. Urological myths. *Br Med J* 1990; 301: 1421–3.
29. Hricik DE, Browning PJ, Kopelman R, Goorno WE,

Madias NE, Dzau VJ. Captopril-induced functional renal insufficiency in patients with bilateral renal-artery stenoses or renal-artery stenosis in a solitary kidney. *New Engl J Med* 1983; **308**: 373–6.

30. Harding MB, Smith LR, Himmelstein SI. *et al.* Renal artery stenosis: prevalence and associated risk factors in patients undergoing routine cardiac catheterization. *J Am Soc Nephrol* 1992; **2**: 1608–16.

31. Debatin JF, Spritzer CE, Grist TM *et al.* Imaging of the renal arteries; value of MR angiography. *Am J Radiol* 1991; **157**: 981–90.

32. Ringoir S, Schoots A, Vanholder R. Uremic toxins. *Kidney Int* 1988; **33**: S4–S9.

33. Winearls CG, Oliver DO, Pippard MJ, Reid C, Downing MR, Cotes PM. Effect of human eryhtropoeitin derived from recombinant DNA on the anaemia of patients maintained by chronic haemodialysis. *Lancet* 1986; **2**: 1175–8.

34. Eschbach JW, Egrie JC, Downing MR, Browne JK, Adamson JW. Correction of the anaemia of end-stage renal disease with recombinant human erythropoeitin. *New Engl J Med* 1987; **316**: 73–8.

35. Lipkin GW, Kendall R, Haggart P, Turney JH, Brownjohn AM. Erythropoeitin in acute renal failure. *Lancet* 1989; **i**: 1029.

36. Brezis M, Epstein FH. A closer look at radiocontrast-induced nephropathy. *New Engl J Med* 1989; **320**: 179–81.

37. Cohen JJ. Relationship between energy requirements for Na^+ reabsorption and other renal requirements. *Kidney Int* 1986; **29**: 32–40.

38. Better OS, Stein JH. Early management of shock and prophylaxis of acute renal failure in traumatic rhabdomyolysis. *New Engl J Med* 1990; **322**: 825–9.

39. Brown CB, Ogg CS, Cameron JS. High dose frusemide in acute renal failure. A controlled trial. *Clin Nephrol* 1981; **15**: 90–6.

40. Dawson JL. Post-operative renal function in obstructive jaundice: effect of a mannitol diuresis. *Br Med J* 1965; **1**: 82–6.

41. ter Wee PM, Rosman JB, van der Geest S, Sluiter WJ, Donker AJM. Renal hemodynamics during separate and combined infusion of amino acids and dopamine. *Kidney Int* 1986; **29**: 870–4.

42. Leier CV. Regional blood flow responses to vasodilators and inotropes in congestive cardiac failure. *Am J Cardiol* 1988; **62**: 86E–93E.

43. Bolger PM, Eisner GM, Ramwell PW, Slotkoff LM, Corey EJ. Renal actions of prostacyclin. *Nature* 1978; **271**: 467–9.

44. Ziegler EJ, Fisher CJ Jr, Sprung CL *et al.* Treatment of gram-negative bacteremia and septic shock with HA-1A human monoclonal antibody against endotoxin – a randomized, double-blind, placebo-controlled trial. *New Engl J Med* 1991; **324**: 429–36.

45. Warren HS, Danner RL, Munford RS. Anti-endotoxin monoclonal antibodies. *New Engl J Med* 1992; **326**: 1153–6.

46. Lewis EJ, Hunsicker LG, Lan S-P, Rohde RD, Lachin JM. A controlled trial of plasmapheresis therapy in severe lupus nephritis. *New Engl J Med* 1992; **326**: 1373–9.

47. Bell WR, Braine HG, Ness PM, Kickler TS. Improved survival in thrombotic thrombocytopenic purpura-hemolytic uremic syndrome – clinical experience in 108 patients. *New Engl J Med* 1991; **325**: 398–403.

48. Rock GA, Shumak KH, Buskard NA *et al.* Comparison of plasma exchange with plasma infusion in the treatment of thrombotic thrombocytopenic purpura. *New Engl J Med* 1991; **325**: 393–7.

49. Berlyne GM, Bazzard FJ, Booth EM, Janabi K, Shaw AB. The dietary treatment of ARF. *Quart J Med* 1967; **36**: 59–83.

50. Horl WH, Heidland A. Enhanced proteolytic activity – cause of protein catabolism in acute renal failure. *Am J Clin Nutr* 1980; **33**: 1423–7.

51. Mault JR, Bartlett RH, Dechert RE, Clark SF, Swartz RD. Starvation: a major contribution to mortality in acute renal failure. *Trans Am Soc Artif Intern Organs* 1983; **29**: 390–4.

52. Mansell MA, Wing AJ. Acetate or bicarbonate for haemodialysis. *Br Med J* 1983; **287**: 308–9.

53. Cobb DK, High KP, Sawyer RG *et al.* A controlled trial of scheduled replacement of central venous and pulmonary-artery catheters. *New Engl J Med* 1992; **327**: 1062–8.

54. Mion CM, Hegstrom RM, Boen ST, Scribner BH. Substitution of sodium acetate for sodium bicarbonate in the bath fluid for hemodialysis. *Trans Am Soc Artif Intern Organs* 1964; **10**: 110–13.

55. Kramer P, Seegers R, De Vivie D, Matthaei D, Trautmann M, Scheler F. Therapeutic potential of hemofiltration. *Clin Nephrol* 1979; **11**: 145–9.

56. van Geelen JA, Vincent HH, Schalekamp MADH. Continuous arteriovenous haemofiltration and haemodiafiltration in acute renal failure. *Nephrol Dial Trans* 1988; **3**: 181–6.

57. Swartz RD, Flamenbaum W, Dubrow A, Hall JC, Crow JW, Cato A. Epoprostol (PGI_2, prostacyclin) during high risk hemodialysis: preventing further bleeding complications. *J Clin Pharmacol* 1988; **28**: 818–25.

58. Davenport A, Davison AM, Will EJ. Anticoagulation with prostacyclin in patients treated by continuous haemofiltration. *Nephrol Dial Trans* 1988; **3**: 547.

59. Bennett WM. Guide to drug dosage in renal failure. *Clin Pharmacokinetics* 1988; **15**: 326–54.

CHAPTER 13

Medical Staffing and Training

United Kingdom
A R WEBB————————————————
Required skills of intensive care medical staff   193
Training intensive care medical staff   195
References   197

United States of America
DAVID R GERBER, CAROLYN E BEKES————
Medical staffing in ICUs   202
Training   204
Conclusion   206
References   206

Australia
GEOFFREY J DOBB————————————————
Staffing   197
Training   199
The future   201
References   201

Canada
**BRIAN P EGIER, CINDY M HAMIELEC,
JOHN R HEWSON**————————————————
The resource model   207
The people   208
Training   210
Bibliography   211

United Kingdom

A R WEBB

Intensive care has been defined as a service for patients with potentially recoverable conditions who can benefit from more detailed observation and treatment than is generally available in standard wards and departments.[1] Intensive care has evolved from the early success in simple mechanical ventilation of the lungs of polio victims to the present day where patients admitted to intensive care will usually have failure or dysfunction of one or more organ systems requiring mechanical support and monitoring. It is an expensive specialty which must, for financial viability, become rationalized, involving centralization to concentrate the medical, nursing and other specialist (including laboratory) support required. The current status of UK intensive care is that specialty recognition has not yet been achieved although many of the larger units are run by senior medical staff whose role can only be adequately described as that of an intensive care specialist. The majority of UK intensive care specialists are also practicing anesthetists[2] but a strong emphasis on the multidisciplinary demands of critically ill patients has seen increasing numbers of physicians and occasionally surgeons adopting the role of intensive care specialists. Experience in the USA has demonstrated a reduction in patient mortality when intensive care is managed by a trained specialist.[3,4] It has been recommended by the UK Intensive Care Society that a 10-bedded intensive care unit should have 15 consultant sessions allocated (1 session = 3.5 hours) with additional allocation for management and audit activities. These sessions should be divided between several intensive care specialists. In addition the intensive care specialist should be supported by junior doctors in training. Unfortunately the achievement of these recommendations and the training of junior doctors in intensive care methods still requires considerable expansion of specialist posts.

Required skills of intensive care medical staff

MANAGEMENT

The technical requirements of intensive care medicine have advanced greatly in the past 10 years. This, coupled with an increasing demand for intensive care, has inevitably led to an increase in costs. In a climate of increasing financial constraints there is a need to rationalize the consumption of scarce resources which, in effect, means improved efficiency. Much of the activity of the UK intensive care unit is predictable;

most postoperative admissions are booked such that beds and staff can be made available appropriately. Whilst the availability of nursing staff is the variable which provides the greatest scope for adjustment in the quest for efficient rostering, it is also possible to adjust the working patterns of junior medical staff to ensure availability when most booked admissions arrive. Senior intensive care medical staff, together with their senior nursing colleagues, command the primary responsibility for the financial management of the intensive care unit. It is through their actions that treatment of the critically ill is initiated and perpetuated; they are ultimately responsible for the activity of the unit and patient outcome. The needs of the population served and the clinical skills necessary to maintain the life of the critically ill must be balanced with an ability to manage staff, to cope with predicted peaks and troughs of activity, to liaise with admitting medical staff, to ensure patients are admitted early and discharged on time, and to liaise with hospital management to ensure that costing information is up to date. The intensive care specialist requires training in the principles of management and medical audit in order to maintain efficiency. Adequate time must be allocated to this role, which should not devolve to those with the right management training but no clinical responsibility.

DECISION MAKING

In the intensive care unit most decisions are ultimately made by a team of personnel. Unlike most other medical specialties in the UK, patients in the intensive care unit are under the shared care of the admitting team and the intensive care specialist. In addition the complex nature of the disease process suffered by the critically ill may warrant clinical input from other specialists. Intensive care is also unique among the medical specialties in that the boundaries between medicine and nursing are notoriously gray and the relationships with paramedical staff assume special importance. The intensive care ward round features active discussion with all members of staff involved with the patient. Clinical decisions in the intensive care unit can be thought of under three categories:

1. decisions relating to common or routine problems for which a unit policy exists;
2. decisions relating to uncommon problems requiring discussion with all currently involved; and
3. decisions of an urgent nature taken by intensive care staff without delay.

Although category (1) decisions will often be taken by the intensive care unit staff, the policies will have been discussed and agreed previously by a team of interested

parties. Such policies may be written but many form such a stable part of daily intensive care life that they are accepted by default. Problems with policy decisions arise when there is disagreement from another involved specialist. Although there may have been previous agreement the interpretation of the current problems may differ. Such conflict often leads to frustration and, if frequent, harms the morale of all members of the intensive care staff. Hence the intensive care specialist requires arbitration skills and the ability to compromise whilst defending the position of his staff. Category (3) decisions must, by their nature, be taken without much discussion. Thus the intensive care specialist must also take the occasional dogmatic lead.

PRACTICAL SKILLS

With the explosion in technology available for monitoring the critically ill and for the support of failing organ systems the intensive care specialist must acquire expertise in the use of these techniques and the procurement and maintenance of sophisticated machinery. Whilst many techniques are common to other medical specialties and training can therefore be gained by rotation through these specialties, their concentration in the intensive care unit demands consolidation of such experience with particular reference to the management of the critically ill. The most basic practical skill demanded of all intensive care medical staff is the maintenance of the airway and ventilation. There is no doubt that this skill is best learnt as a junior anesthetist with hands-on experience of manual ventilatory support, intubation and basic mechanical ventilation in the operating theater. In addition time spent as a junior anesthetist provides a valuable opportunity to master other practical techniques such as central venous and arterial cannulation and insights can be gained into the role of monitoring in the unconscious patient. Further expertise in the management of complex ventilators and weaning problems commonly found in the intensive care unit, mechanical ventilation of diseased lungs, the management of tracheostomy and the monitoring requirements of patients with multiple organ failure can only be gained in the intensive care unit after the basics have been provided in anesthesia. Techniques used for cardiovascular monitoring share a great deal with those used in the cardiac catheter laboratory. Here the rotating trainee can learn the practical aspects of manipulation of catheters through the cardiac chambers and the interpretation of pressure and flow data usually relating to structural cardiac defects. These basics again require development through experience in the intensive care unit before skills acquired can be applied to the dynamic circulatory changes occurring as a result of critical illness and therapeutic manipulations in intensive care. Similar statements can be made for the role of training in respiratory and renal medicine; whilst valuable experience in pulmonary diagnosis can be gained via the chest radiograph or bronchoscopy, or dialysis in renal failure, it is in the intensive care unit that trainees will gain expertise in the interpretation of portable anteroposterior chest radiographs, bronchoscopy of ventilator and oxygen-dependent patients, and renal support for the patients with an unstable circulation.

TECHNICAL KNOWLEDGE

The intensive care specialist has an important role in the choice of equipment used in the intensive care unit. These choices must encompass the capital and revenue costs of the machinery, ease of use and maintenance and the effectiveness of the equipment in achieving the task for which it is proposed. Such choices can only be made through experience of what is available coupled with the experience of critical illness for which the equipment is to be used. Costs of equipment can be reduced by bulk purchasing and in-house maintenance; thus the intensive care specialist must be involved in the choice of equipment for other hospital departments. Knowledge of how the equipment works is important for a proper understanding of how it will interact with the patient, how to interpret data from monitoring equipment and what to do when the equipment does not appear to work. In today's microchip world a healthy understanding of the concepts of computer technology is required. As this knowledge is fundamental to the practice of anesthesia the important of time spent in this specialty is highlighted; time spent with medical physics and technical staff provides useful additional experience.

PHARMACEUTICAL KNOWLEDGE

Drug therapy in the critically ill often involves complex therapeutic regimens to support failing organ systems, to sedate patients for tolerance of mechanical support systems, to provide analgesia after surgical interventions and for specific treatment of the underlying diagnosis. Such regimens are clearly open to the problems of drug interactions and, in addition, pharmacokinetics are often severely altered by the effects of major organ system dysfunction, particularly involving the liver and kidneys. As with practical training above, much of the basics of this therapeutic knowledge can be gained by rotation through anesthesia and the major medical specialties with which aspects of these therapeutic interventions are shared. However, in view of the limited knowledge of pharmacokinetics in the critically ill and the wide individual variations in drug handling in the face of organ dysfunction, it is only

through considerable experience in the intensive care unit that such knowledge can be consolidated. Although many aspects of specific treatment for the underlying diagnosis are largely controlled by other specialists, it falls to the intensive care medical staff to coordinate and ensure the safety of a therapeutic approach. Through a process of repeated questioning of the value of individual components of a therapeutic strategy with a clear expectation of what acute effects should be achieved and a healthy suspicion of the role of drugs in contributing to aspects of a patient's illness, pharmaceutical education is something which is ongoing and never complete in the intensive care specialist.

TEACHING AND TRAINING

It should be clear from the above that the modern intensive care specialist must acquire a number of skills that cannot be gained outside the intensive care unit. It is therefore necessary to be able to provide this education to junior doctors in training for intensive care. In addition, nursing and paramedical colleagues require a program of education which consolidates basic skills and updates knowledge as new practices and treatments emerge. Furthermore, colleagues from other disciplines who have contact with intensive care would benefit from a better understanding of the specialist requirements of critically ill patients. Such teaching would reduce conflict in decision making as well as facilitating earlier transfer of patients to intensive care, whilst there is still a chance of recovery!

Training intensive care medical staff

The intensive care unit can be one of the most stressful environments for any staff to work in. Junior doctors often rotate into intensive care posts with little preparation for what is expected of them. It becomes clear to these doctors that patients are totally dependent on intensive care staff and procedures for survival, that time available for the care and treatment of these patients is limited, yet much of this time can be taken up by difficulties with communication with patients and the many other members of staff involved in their care; unexpected and emergency events are frequent requiring rapid decisions and actions. The following are key points towards avoidance of junior staff stress:

1. Supervision of junior doctors by experienced staff including the intensive care specialist and senior nursing staff.

2. Whilst it is not practical to have the intensive care specialist on site for 24 hours per day, there should be continuous availability for discussion and a clear expectation for early contact to be made.
3. Clear guidelines available for management of common and routine intensive care problems.
4. Hands-on training for management of resuscitation, practical procedures, effective use of monitoring techniques available and therapeutic strategies for management of organ dysfunction. This is most effectively achieved via small group workshops.
5. Management of the working period to allow regular breaks and adequate sleep. In common with other acute medical specialties there have been moves to reduce junior doctors' hours of work, recognizing that periods of unbroken sleep are necessary to ensure safe practice. In order to achieve this some intensive care units have already designed working shift systems (Table 13.1).

Table 13.1   Four-person partial shift system rotating on a 4-week cycle

Week	Mon	Tues	Wed	Thur	Fri	Sat	Sun	Total hours
1	D1	S + N		D2	D1	D1	D1	72
2	N		D2	D1	N	N	N	82
3		S + D2	D1	N				36
4	D2	D1	N		D2			40

D1 Day shift with main responsibility for patient care	0800–2000	12 h
D2 Day shift for practical help during busy period	1200–1800	6 h
N Night shift	1900–1100	16 h
S Teaching session	1000–1200	2 h
Average hours per week	57.5 h	
Long periods of duty	72 h and 63 h	
Average teaching seminars per week	1 h	

Overlap between shifts allows handover.

Ideally junior staff should not be asked to combine intensive care with responsibility for other activities. Often anesthetic and medical junior staff are expected to cover the intensive care unit in addition to their anesthetic and emergency medical responsibilities. As a consequence continuity of care is lost, involvement in intensive care often becomes peripheral, and adequate training cannot be facilitated. In essence stress may be coped with by avoidance thus shifting stress to others.

In view of the multidisciplinary nature of the requirements, training recommendations are provided jointly by the Royal College of Anaesthetists, the Royal College of Physicians, the Royal College of Surgeons and the Intensive Care Society. There is no separate College of Intensive Care Specialists. The Joint Advisory Committee on Training in Intensive Therapy (JACIT) was formed to develop higher professional training programs in intensive care.[5] These programs are of 2 years duration and are open to trainees of all specialties who hold a higher postgraduate qualification and are undertaking a higher professional training program in their own specialty. More recently another such committee, the Intercollegiate Committee for Intensive Therapy, under the above bodies, has been formed to discuss and design shorter training programs at a more basic, junior level. Such programs would be undertaken at the senior house officer or registrar grades. Many agree that exposure to intensive care should begin at the undergraduate level, allowing newly qualified doctors to recognize critically ill patients and thus invoke the urgent attention that they require. In addition such exposure provides valuable insight into the applied physiology involved in management of these patients building on the understanding of physiology acquired in the preclinical years. The difficulty with providing bedside teaching of intensive care to undergraduates relates to the imbalance of intensive care specialists and beds in a teaching hospital and the large numbers of undergraduates needing to receive this teaching in a short period of time. Undergraduates may spend up to 2 weeks attached to the intensive care unit. During this time they have to cope with the differences between the organ system and problem-oriented approach adopted by most intensive care units and the traditional diagnosis-oriented approach of general medical training; they cannot hope to be exposed to the wide spectrum of critical illness dealt with in intensive care. During general professional training those who aspire to a career in intensive care medicine will benefit from rotation through anesthesia and the major general medical specialties as outlined above. In addition, all general professional trainees would benefit from rotation through intensive care to improve recognition of critical illness and resuscitation skills. Again the relatively small size of intensive care provides severe practical limitations to such a goal; an attachment of 3 months is the minimum necessary for a trainee to become familiar with the environment and practices of intensive care whereas an attachment of 6 months is necessary to gain useful experience in the practices. It has been argued that a period of anesthetic training is mandatory prior to intensive care attachment but this may be impractical.

Training of junior doctors in intensive care must be formalized and made available throughout the training grades. Training will not become adequate until specialists are appointed in sufficient numbers to provide the training. This in turn requires the formulation of a unified program with or without examination as is being developed by the intercollegiate committees. This aspect of UK intensive care is in a state of flux but the current process of change should do much to improve the present situation.

References

1. *The Intensive Care Service in the UK*. London: The Intensive Care Society, 1990: 2.
2. *Intensive Care Services: Provision for the Future*. London: Association of Anaesthetists of Great Britain and Ireland, 1988: 4.
3. Knaus WA, Draper EA, Wagner DP, Zimmerman JE. An evaluation of outcome from intensive care in major medical centers. *Ann Intern Med* 1986; **104**: 410–18.
4. Brown JJ, Sullivan G. Effect on ICU mortality of a full-time critical care specialist. *Chest* 1989; **96**: 127–9.
5. Hanson GC. The future of medical manpower in the intensive therapy unit. *Care Crit Ill* 1989; **5**: 115–16.

Australia

GEOFFREY J DOBB

In Australia and New Zealand the value of highly developed intensive care units (ICU) with consultants responsible for the intensive care phase of patients' management has been recognized since at least the early 1960s.[1,2] From the outset it was appreciated that a larger general ICU made better use of resources than a multiplicity of mono-specialty units. These early units were also clearly distinguished from 'recovery rooms', 'admission rooms' or 'special care' areas. That is, they were designed for patients who were critically ill and in need of constant medical and nursing supervision. Most needed support of their ventilation or circulation.

The workload imposed by larger, general ICUs justified a separate senior and junior medical staff dedicated to the care of their patients. The trend toward centralization of intensive care facilities has been accentuated by Australia's geography with the population concentrated in the cities and sparsely populated country areas. As a result, the major intensive care facilities of the less densely populated states of Northern Territory, South Australia and Western Australia are confined to the cities. Highly developed aero-medical systems bring critically ill patients, sometimes over distances of thousands of kilometers, to those facilities. In the more populous states there are major ICUs in the larger towns as well as the state capital cities. Smaller towns may have limited intensive care facilities, but even here the tendency is to transfer patients needing a long stay, more complex care or tertiary services to the major centers.

The range of needs has resulted in a variety of units being covered by the designation 'intensive care.' In practice these include short-term facilities with the

capability of resuscitating the more critically ill patients before their transfer, units that might more properly be called 'high dependency units' which provide intensive nursing care and observation but lack immediate medical cover, and ICUs with a full range of facilities. A classification of 'intensive care units' accepted by the Australian and New Zealand College of Anaesthetists is shown in Table 13.2 and an alternative from the Health Department of New South Wales in Table 13.3. While there is no generally accepted definition of an ICU in Australia, one that has been widely discussed is:

> A recognised intensive care unit is a separate hospital area, equipped and staffed so as to be capable of mechanical ventilation for a period of several days, and invasive cardiovascular monitoring. It must be supported by at least one specialist or consultant in intensive care, immediately available during normal working hours, and a registered medical practitioner must be present in the hospital and available immediately to the unit on a 24 hour-a-day basis. Registered nursing staffing should provide a minimum of 16 hours per patient and more where appropriate and according to the dependency of the patient. There must be defined admission and discharge policies.

Such units are found in medical school general teaching hospitals, major country centers and some of the larger private hospitals. Intensive care training in Australia and New Zealand is designed to prepare doctors for work in units like this, and it is this training and the staffing of these units that is described.

Table 13.2 Classification of intensive care units (modified from Faculty of Anaesthetists RACS 'Minimum Standards for Intensive Care Units', 1991)

Level I
Capable of providing immediate resuscitative management for the critically ill, short-term cardiorespiratory support, and having a major role in the monitoring and prevention of complications in 'at risk' medical and surgical patients.

Level II
Capable of providing a high standard of general intensive care which supports the hospital's other delineated roles. Capable of providing ventilatory support and with ECG, pulse oximetry, monitoring and support equipment to sustain the unit's delineated role, e.g. invasive hemodynamic monitoring and dialysis support.

Level III
Provides the widest level of care, monitoring and therapy as required by its referral role as well as that required by the delineated role of the hospital. Such a referral intensive care unit should be capable of managing all aspects of intensive care medicine.

Table 13.3   Health Department of New South Wales classification of intensive care facilities

Level I
No service.

Level II
Recovery area for postoperative patients or high dependency area for general ward patients. Registered nursing equivalent to 4 h/patient/day desirable. Quality assurance activities.

Level III
As Level II, plus 24-hour access to a medical officer on site or available within 10 minutes. Registered nursing equivalent to 6 h/patient/day. Separate area preferable. Formal quality assurance program. Liaison psychiatry available.

Level IV
As Level III, plus separate area of 4–6 beds minimum. Admission and discharge policies and patient care review. Nominated specialist director and designated day time medical officer, plus medical registrar on site or available within 10 minutes. Specialist on-call 24 hours. Registered nursing equivalent to 8 h/patient/day desirable or according to patient dependency. Capable of short- to medium-term ventilation. Simple invasive monitoring.

Level V
As Level IV, plus designated medical officers on site 24 hours and specialist director on site during day. Capable of medium-term ventilation and external life supports. Can provide limited isolation facilities. Registered nursing equivalent to 16 h/patient/day desirable or according to patient dependency. Formal audit and review or procedures. Link with Level V rehabilitation services.

Level VI
As Level V, plus medical and/or ICU registrar on site 24 hours. Supported by ICU consultants and full-time specialists. Capable of all forms of intensive care monitoring and therapy of critically ill patients. Registered nursing equivalent to 24 h/patient/day desirable or according to dependency of patients. May provide specialty training posts for ICU registrars.

Staffing

CONSULTANT

From the outset[1,2] it was recognized that having senior specialists or consultants who devoted substantially the whole of their working time to intensive care was an important part of the delivery and process of intensive care. Experienced medical staff are then always available for critically ill patients and to support the junior medical staff. Today it would be very unusual for a consultant appointed to a major ICU not to have completed training with a Fellowship through the

Australian and New Zealand College of Anesthetists endorsed in Intensive Care (FANZCA) or through the Intensive Care Specialist Advisory Committee of the Royal Australasian College of Physicians (FRACP). It has been estimated that close to a third of the membership of the Australian and New Zealand Intensive Care Society of approximately 450 has one of these diplomas of Fellowship (P. Byth, personal communication).

The details of consultant staffing vary between units but virtually all use a team approach to patient care in order to provide the 24 hours a day, 7 days a week, care needed by critically ill patients and still allow time for teaching, research, family and recreational needs. This also makes it possible for consultants to provide services outside the ICU (e.g. occasional anesthetic lists, a ward-based parenteral nutrition service, a consultative service outside the ICU or participation in long-distance patient retrieval and transport) without compromising the service available to patients in the ICU. There are almost as many approaches to the rostering of intensive care consultants as there are ICUs but the concept of shared care is a common one. This requires agreement between all the consultants involved on the preferred management of common clinical problems. Significant benefits include a very intimate form of peer review and close psychological and professional support when dealing with the many stressful, emotionally demanding or politically sensitive problems that frequently arise from episodes of critical illness.

The College of Anaesthetists minimum standards for a Level III unit (Table 13.2) require it to have a medical director with specialist intensive care qualifications and sufficient supporting specialists so consultant support is always available for medical staff in the unit. A postgraduate qualification in intensive care is recommended for senior medical staff appointed to both Level II and III units. The guidelines for hospitals on the duties of an intensive care specialist refer to both clinical duties and the administrative and educational duties. It is recommended that a unit's director and deputy director should need to provide no more than ten half days of clinical duties in the ICU between them each week in order to provide time for other duties. For other intensive care specialists it is recommended that the clinical duties should not exceed seven half days a week. Financial and other constraints prevent these recommendations being achieved in many units. By one calculation[3] a director and 6.7 full-time equivalent consultants are needed to staff a unit of ten or so beds. In practice, a ratio of one full-time equivalent consultant to every three to five ICU beds is commonly found.

OTHER MEDICAL STAFF

The other medical staffing of Australian ICUs may include fellows, senior registrars, registrars and residents. Patterns of staffing vary widely between units depending on the way they have evolved, whether they are part of departments of 'Anaesthesia and Intensive Care' or independent departments, and the Industrial Awards governing the terms and conditions of employment. These awards are different in each state, but generally limit the number of hours that may be worked continuously and provide penalty payments (i.e. standard rate plus a loading) for hours worked over 38–42 per week on average. Continuous cover for an ICU at reasonable cost is provided by rotating shift systems. During normal working hours a ratio of one registrar or resident to every five or six ICU beds is common with slightly higher ratios of beds to doctors at other times.

Fellows

The status of Fellows varies between states. In New South Wales the term is often used for intensive care physicians who have completed their training. Their role may be that of a junior consultant or similar to that of a senior registrar. The term 'Fellow' is also applied to overseas research and training Fellows who come to ICUs in Australia for a defined period with defined objectives in research and/or training from other countries. Some Australian units have long-standing links with particular units elsewhere. Most of these links are with units from the Western Pacific region where medical services, including the provision of intensive care, are developing at a rate matching their economic growth.

Senior registrars

Senior registrar status is generally reserved for those who have completed the requirements for specialist registration of the Medical Board in each state. In practice, this may not be in intensive care with some posts being occupied by physicians who have still to complete the requirements for the FANZCA endorsed in intensive care or the requirements of the Specialist Advisory Committee on Intensive Care of the RACP. They will however, have completed the requirements for the FANZCA in anesthesia or the Specialist Advisory Committee in general internal medicine or thoracic medicine, for example. In addition to their clinical duties, a senior registrar would be expected to provide some supervision of more junior medical staff and participate in teaching and research.

Registrars

These represent a very varied group in experience and training, but usually they have passed the primary examination of whichever postgraduate training program they are in (unless training in internal medicine) and have four or more years' experience since gradua-

tion. The more senior of the internal medicine trainees will have passed the Part I examination for the diploma of FRACP.

While some registrars are primarily training in intensive care, the majority fill this post on rotation for 3–6 months from a training scheme in anesthesia, internal medicine, surgery, accident and emergency medicine or another specialty. This provides some experience of the more common acute medical emergencies causing critical illness, practice in the priorities of resuscitation, some limited experience of invasive hemodynamic monitoring, central venous cannulation and other practical procedures, and an opportunity to participate in the care of unconscious or highly dependent patients. Perhaps more importantly, it provides an opportunity for registrars from a variety of backgrounds to gain an appreciation of the scope, capabilities and limitations of intensive care that can guide appropriate referral of patients for intensive care in the future.

Residents

Doctors within 2 or 3 years of qualification are closely supervised during periods working in the ICU. Hospitals usually construct their resident posts so that they rotate through four or five different specialties during a 1-year appointment. This is to provide a breadth of exposure appropriate to general medical training before acceptance into a specialty training programme. Some residents may be undertaking the Family Medicine Training Programme. Inevitably, much of the more routine work is done by the resident with their contribution to clinical decision making increasing with experience and consultants' assessment of capabilities. A post in intensive care also provides residents with an opportunity to have supervised teaching and to practice various practical procedures such as insertion of chest drains and central venous catheters.

Training

In the early 1970s it was recognized that intensive care was a multidisciplinary specialty.[4] However, all but one major ICU in Australia and New Zealand was staffed by Fellows of either the Faculty of Anaesthetists of the Royal Australasian College of Surgeons or the Royal Australasian College of Physicians.[5] These two groups, with support from the Australian and New Zealand Intensive Care Society, met to consider the possibility of a conjoint training program for trainees in intensive care.[6] However, because of very significant discrepancies in the training requirements and examination systems between the Faculty and the College, rather than any lack of good will from those involved in intensive care from the two groups, it was not possible to reach agreement on a single diploma. There are therefore two routes to recognition of completion of training in intensive care: through what is now the College of Anaesthetists and through the College of Physicians. The opportunity for a unified training system may have been lost but both appear to be producing a high caliber of training intensive care physicians. Having two schemes available also offers trainees a choice, introduces an element of healthy competition and provides a degree of flexibility that might be hard to match with a single scheme.

COLLEGE OF ANAESTHETISTS TRAINING SCHEME

The primary examination in basic sciences is common to anesthesia and intensive care. This covers pharmacology, physiology and relevant physics and clinical measurement. A minimum of 5 years recognized clinical experience (4 years if training started before January 1985) after at least 2 years of general medical and surgical experience as a resident is then needed together with success in the final examination which is specific to intensive care, before the diploma of Fellowship endorsed in intensive care can be awarded. The clinical experience must include a minimum of 2 years of intensive care, 18 months of anesthesia and an elective year. Posts recognized for training are inspected by the College and must meet their guidelines to be approved. These guidelines cover the clinical workload, investigative facilities available, level of supervision and the physical facilities and equipment available in the unit. Training units must have a program of education, review and research, and training appointments must be entirely in intensive care with provision for trainees to take part in out of hours rosters. The number of posts approved for training in each unit is specified and it is only when occupying one of these posts that recognition is given to the training received. The objectives of training are clearly defined in a document available to each trainee. The final examination is traditional in format (Table 13.4).

Two surveys have been conducted of successful candidates in this examination.[7,8] In both there has been some indication that additional experience in internal medicine would have been useful. A mandatory 6-month medical rotation is now a minimum requirement during training. Some respondents to the second survey thought it would be desirable to have additional short formal courses available which covered the objectives of the final examination. At the present time such a course is held only once a year in Adelaide, South Australia. Other comments related to the potential lack of training in research methods in what is a

clinically oriented training program and the difficulties in training in an adult oriented program when their professional goal was pediatric intensive care. However, most of the doctors surveyed perceived the final examination as being of a high standard with the work towards a successful attempt being useful in their preparation for intensive care practice. Indeed, all found the intensive care component of their training for the final Fellowship examination as being suitable for their present occupational role.[8]

One of the interesting aspects of those obtaining the final Fellowship endorsed in intensive care is the frequency with which other vocational training diplomas are held (Table 13.5). Only eight of the 59 respondents to the survey had obtained the Fellowship

Table 13.4 Format of the final examination for the diploma of Fellowship of the Australian and New Zealand College of Anaesthetists endorsed in intensive care

Two written papers:
  Short answers
  Essay type

Clinical examination

Two oral examinations

Assessment of investigations

Table 13.5 Postgraduate diplomas of Membership or Fellowship of a College or Faculty held by 59 respondents to a survey of successful candidates for the Final Fellowship of the Australian and New Zealand College of Anaesthetists (or FFARACS) endorsed in intensive care (modified from ref. 8)

Diploma	Number with diploma	Number obtaining this diploma first
FFARACS – Intensive care	59	8
FFARACS – Anaesthesia	40	31
FFARCS	12	6
FFARCSI	4	3
FRACP	3	3
MRCP	5	4
Other	4	?

FFARACS:	Fellow of the Faculty of Anaesthetists of the Royal Australasian College of Surgeons (now Australian and New Zealand College of Anaesthetists).
FFARCS:	Fellow of the Faculty of Anaesthetists of the Royal College of Surgeons (now Royal College of Anaesthetists).
FFARCSCI:	Fellow of the Faculty of Anaesthetists of the Royal College of Surgeons, Ireland.
FRACP:	Fellow of the Royal Australasian College of Physicians.
MRCP:	Member of the Royal College of Physicians.

in intensive care first. The common components between the training schemes in anesthesia and intensive care make it possible for doctors to obtain both diplomas by extending the period of training and successfully completing both final examinations.

COLLEGE OF PHYSICIANS TRAINING SCHEME

The College of Physicians require a minimum 4-year period of basic training after qualification before the Part I examination of their Fellowship can be taken. At least two of the years after completion of an internship must be in internal medicine or its subspecialties, which include intensive care. As appropriate for an examination at this point in training, the Part I is very broadly based. The components include multiple choice questions, clinical examination with long and short cases, and oral examination sections.

After successfully completing the Part I examination a trainee can undertake at least three years of 'advanced training' before the Fellowship is awarded. This is overseen by the Specialist Advisory Committee in each subspecialty of medicine, and general internal medicine. Intensive care has had its own Specialist Advisory Committee (SAC) since 1977. Trainees who register with the SAC in intensive care must do two of their three years in intensive care medicine. The third, elective, year may be spent in anesthesia, research, another subspecialty of medicine, intensive care, a combination of these or other activities accepted by the SAC. During the advanced training period it is necessary to complete a project, the nature of which is flexible and loosely defined. It must, however, be acceptable to the supervisor of training. Each advanced trainee has a supervisor of training who advises the SAC on whether the overall 3 years of training are completed successfully. Subject to this, the diploma of Fellowship is awarded at the end of advanced training without further examination.

In contrast with the College of Anaesthetists' scheme there is no recognition of specific training posts and no 'exit' examination on completion of training.

OUTCOMES OF TRAINING

It is the policy of the Australian and New Zealand Intensive Care Society that those who have successfully completed training under either the College of Anaesthetists or College of Physicians programs are regarded as absolutely equivalent in every respect. Many Australian ICUs have consultants who have trained through both of these programs, have trainees in both programs and have those with a Fellowship diploma from the College of Anaesthetists involved in the training of advanced trainees through the College of Physicians and vice versa.

The survey of Fellows of the College of Anaesthetists endorsed in intensive care[8] reported that over 80% of respondents spend 50% or more of their working time in clinical intensive care. There were 36% working as Directors of ICUs, 15% as Deputy Directors and 34% as staff specialists. Only 7% had no intensive care appointment. The survey found that Fellows endorsed in intensive care generally maintained long-term involvement in clinical intensive care practice.

The future

Intensive care units in larger Australian hospitals have already achieved a high degree of autonomy. Dedicated, well-qualified and experienced consultant staff with specific training in intensive care are normal in such units. There has been a tendency in Australia towards fragmentation of the medical colleges, with individual colleges to cover the specialties and subspecialties (e.g. dermatologists, ophthalmologists, venereologists, emergency medicine, etc.). The concept of an Australian and New Zealand College of Intensive Care Medicine has been widely canvassed but is not an immediate prospect. There is however, considerable support for a Faculty of Intensive Care Medicine within the Australian and New Zealand College of Anaesthetists for Fellows with diplomas endorsed in intensive care.*

Both the College of Anaesthetists and the College of Physicians are currently addressing the issues involved in recertification. Aspects of this remain controversial, but there is general recognition that 'training' is not something that ends with the award of a College's Fellowship. Instead, and especially in a rapidly developing specialty such as intensive care, training in its broadest sense, continuing medical education and peer review should continue throughout a medical career.

* The Faculty of Intensive Care, Australian and New Zealand College of Anaesthetists, has now been establiished.

References

1. Galbally B. The planning and organization of an intensive care unit. *Med J Aust* 1966; **1**: 622–4.
2. Spence M. An organization for intensive care. *Med J Aust* 1967; **1**: 795–801.
3. Smallwood RW, Sando MJW, Holland RB. Medical staff needed in a hospital to service anaesthesia and intensive care. *Anaesth Intensive Care* 1981; **9**: 3–14.

4. Editorial. Intensive care medicine: new specialty, new journal. *Med J Aust* 1975; **2**: 583–4.
5. Baker AB. Intensive care – the Australasian approach. *Intensive Care Med* 1983; **9**: 41–2.
6. Worthley LIG. Training in intensive care. An Australian view. *Crit Care Med* 1981; **9**: 69–70.
7. Byth PL, Harrison GA. A survey of successful FFARACS candidates in Australasia. *Crit Care Med* 1986; **14**: 583–6.
8. Harrison GA, Byth PL. A survey of Fellows of the Faculty of Anaesthetists of the Royal Australasian College of Surgeons endorsed in intensive care by examination in the first 10 years of final examinations in intensive care. *Anaesth Intensive Care* 1992; **20**: 203–10.

United States of America

DAVID R GERBER, CAROLYN E BEKES

The use of special care units dates back over 100 years to the mid-1800s. For most of the first 100 years these facilities were used principally in the care of sick postoperative patients and were attended primarily by surgeons and later also by anesthesiologists.

In 1958, specialized respiratory care units were established at hospitals in the USA, Canada, and the UK. In the 1950s the first shock unit was also established at the University of Southern California, USA, and in 1962 the forerunner of the modern coronary care unit opened in Kansas City, USA.

In the 30 years since then, critical care units have become ubiquitous in hospitals throughout the USA and much of the world. These units vary in size and scope, from small multidisciplinary units to large, highly specialized ones. Along with the expansion of numbers and types of units has come the development of critical care medicine as a distinct clinical discipline. This specialty has evolved from its origins in the care of the postoperative patient to include the treatment of a wide variety of patients and conditions by a diverse group of clinicians.

Medical staffing in ICUs

EARLY RECOMMENDATIONS

In 1971 Safar and Grenvik developed a comprehensive plan for organizing and staffing intensive care units (ICUs).[1] They provided recommendations for the organization, administration, and staffing of ICUs which contained several key points. A full-time medical director, chosen on the basis of interest and qualifications, rather than specialty, was suggested. It was

further recommended that (at least in major referral hospitals) this be a full-time geographic position. Twenty-four-hour in-house coverage of the ICU was deemed necessary to provide an appropriate level of patient care. They also proposed that all ICU clinicians be trained in a principal medical discipline (medicine, surgery, pediatrics or anesthesia) and have particular competence in the management of acute situations such as airway emergencies, resuscitation, shock and arrhythmias. It was further recommended that the provision of medical care to critically ill patients be delivered using a team approach. In large or tertiary hospitals they suggested that the team, led by the medical director, consist of attendings from internal medicine, surgery and anesthesia, as well as members of the house staff from these disciplines.

These authors also addressed the issue of training physicians for the practice of critical care medicine (CCM). They advocated the development of fellowship programs in CCM, as well as the establishment of departments of critical care medicine in medical schools.

RECOMMENDATIONS OF THE SOCIETY OF CRITICAL CARE MEDICINE

In 1988 the Society of Critical Care Medicine (SCCM) published a set of guidelines for services and personnel in ICUs.[2] Recommendations regarding the position of medical director included (for major facilities) critical care or equivalent board certification, 24-hour availability or acceptable coverage, and a variety of academic and administrative qualifications. Additional criteria were established regarding the level of coverage and qualifications of physicians covering the ICU. In 1992 the Society published guidelines formally defining an 'intensivist'.[3] Educational, clinical, and administrative parameters were established. Among these were formal training and/or certification in CCM, devotion of greater than 50% of professional time to the practice of CCM, and competence at a variety of critical care procedures. A spectrum of competencies in clinical and management areas were also key criteria in the definition of an intensivist as presented in the guidelines.

JUSTIFICATION FOR DEDICATED CRITICAL CARE STAFF

In 1982 Li *et al.*[4] compared the outcomes of ICU patients managed by clinicians located on-site in the ICU on a full-time basis with the outcome of patients managed by private practice physicians. They found no significant difference in overall mortality between the two groups; however, when patients were stratified according to their predicted likelihood of death, those treated by an ICU clinician had significantly lower ICU and hospital mortality rates, compared to the group treated by the private doctors.

In 1988 a study by Hainer and Lawler[5] compared critical care as provided by family practitioners (FP) with that provided by internists for a variety of parameters. Outcomes were statistically identical in both groups for all the criteria evaluated, most notably mortality, length of stay, and rate of ICU readmission. It was, however, noted by the authors and by subsequent reviewers[6] that both groups were managed largely by 'house staff' from the same institution and it was therefore not surprising that the outcomes were similar.

In 1988 Reynolds *et al.*[7] evaluated the effect of CCM physician staffing on patients with septic shock, comparing such patients treated by non-CCM-trained internists with a subsequent group of patients managed by a CCM-trained ICU staff. Patients were evaluated for the frequency of a variety of invasive interventions as well as for mortality. There was no significant difference in APACHE II (Acute Physiology and Chronic Health Evaluation) scores between the two groups. The CCM-treated group had a significantly higher frequency of invasive vascular procedures (pulmonary artery and arterial catheters) performed. This group also had a significantly lower death rate (57% vs 74%, $p < 0.01$).

In 1989 Brown and Sullivan[8] compared two groups of patients with similar APACHE scores, one treated by their attending physicians, the second by a full-time, fellowship-trained critical care specialist. They noted a 52% decrease in ICU mortality ($p < 0.01$) and a 31% decrease in overall hospital mortality ($p < 0.01$) in the group treated by the critical care specialist.

Studies such as these support the argument for the use of trained critical care specialists and dedicated clinical directors for ICUs. However, although agreement regarding the desirability of ICU coverage by critical care clinicians continues to grow, it is still not universally accepted.

ORGANIZATION AND STAFFING

Research on staffing and organization

The first extensive statistical review of ICU personnel, facilities and services in the USA was published by Greenbaum in 1984 under the sponsorship of the SCCM.[9] At that time 73% of ICUs were directed by internists, with less than 15% being run by surgeons. Family practitioners were noted to direct 6.5% of units, and anesthesiologists 2.3%. However, there was a significant variation depending upon the size of the hospital and the number of ICUs within the hospital.

Under the auspices of the Society of Critical Care Medicine's Task Force for the Distribution of ICU Resources in the United States, a comprehensive report on critical care units in the US was published by Groeger *et al.* in 1992.[10] This exhaustive review studied American ICUs with regard to medical and nonmedical personnel, size, distribution, facilities, and other parameters. Responses were obtained from 2876 ICUs, representing a total of 1706 hospitals out of 4233 contacted (40%).

Administration and organization

The information obtained from the SCCM's 1992 survey indicates that just over one-third of ICUs are administratively located within a department of medicine. Twenty-two per cent were identified as independent of any specialty, 12% in a department of pediatrics, and 10% within a department of surgery. The remainder are divided among a variety of departments but only 3% of ICUs identified themselves as part of a separate critical care department.

In only 12% of responding units was authorization by the medical director or attending intensivist required to admit a patient. This was most often the case in pediatric and neonatal units (31 and 30%, respectively) and least common in combined medical/surgical/CCUs (3%).

Physician staffing and direction

The 1992 survey revealed that 63.3% of ICUs were now directed by physicians from internal medicine disciplines, including 95.4% of medical ICUs and 72.4% of medical–surgical units. Surgeons were noted to direct 18.1% of units overall. They are responsible for 20.6% of medical–surgical units, 59.5% of neurological units, and 75.8% of surgical ICUs. Pediatricians are responsible for the direction of 16.9% of units overall, 93.7% of which are pediatric or neonatal ICUs. Anesthesiologists were noted in this report to be responsible for 4.7% of ICUs. The remaining units are directed by emergency medicine physicians, family practitioners, neurologists, multiple specialists, or other specialists not specifically identified.

The extent to which both medical directors and staff physicians in an ICU are certified in CCM correlates with hospital size (Tables 13.6 and 13.7). The average number of certified physicians per unit was also found to be quite variable depending on the type of unit, ranging from a low of 1.4 in neurological units to a high of 3.6 in neonatal ICUs. The average number of certified physicians per unit was 2.4 (Table 13.8).

Coverage of ICUs by house staff (residents and fellows) has increased in the interval between the two

Table 13.6 Percentage of CCM-certified ICU medical directors by hospital size

No. of hospital beds	% Certified directors
<100	19.9
101–300	37.9
301–500	51.6
>500	55.9
Overall	44.1

Adapted from ref. 18 with permission.

Table 13.7 Number of CCM-certified ICU physicians by hospital size

No. of hospital beds	No. of certified physicians
<100	1.2
101–300	2.2
301–500	2.5
>500	2.8

Adapted from ref. 18 with permission.

Table 13.8 Average number of CCM-certified ICU physicians by type of unit

Type of unit	CCM-certified physicians
Neurological	1.4
Surgical	2.4
Medical/surgical	2.5
CCU	2.5
Medical	2.8
Neonatal	3.6
Average	2.4

Adapted from ref. 18 with permission.

reports. In 1984, although 76.6% of large hospitals (more than 401 beds) were identified as having house staff participation in the management of ICU patients, 62.7% of these hospitals reported that these house officers also had responsibilities outside the unit. The 1992 survey revealed that in large hospitals (defined here as greater than 500 beds), 95% had dedicated ICU residents. In 1992, only 5% of smaller hospitals were found to have house staff dedicated to the ICU. Data were not provided regarding the availability of non-dedicated resident coverage in the smaller hospitals. The 1992 report also identified a median of one fellow assigned to each ICU in large hospitals.

Nonphysician staffing

Dubayo et al.[11] published a report on the use of physician assistants (PAs) in the ICU in 1991. Their performance was compared to that of medical house officers. Although there was a slight increase in length of ICU stay (p <0.05) and a slight decrease in the number of ICU admissions per month (p <0.05) with the PAs, there was no difference in mortality or complications. The authors of this paper concluded that when properly trained, PAs may have an appropriate role in the ICU.

Training

HISTORICAL ASPECTS

The training of specialists in CCM has continued to evolve over the last two decades. Even today clinicians may come to this field through a variety of specialties and pathways.

In 1980 the American Board of Medical Specialties (ABMS) attempted to develop a unified CCM certification process with the participation of the specialties of internal medicine, surgery, pediatrics, anesthesia, obstetrics and gynecology, and neurology. In 1983 this cooperative effort was abandoned due to the inability of these groups to arrive at a mutually acceptable curriculum and certification process. Since that time, however, several specialty boards have developed independent certification processes in CCM.

A survey in 1986 by Kruse and Carlson[12] of members of the Internal Medicine Section of the SCCM revealed that 85% of the respondents had some form of formal postresidency training. Thirty-nine per cent were trained in pulmonary medicine, 35% in critical care, and 9% in both.

THE CERTIFICATION PROCESS

The most current data available indicate that in the USA there are 6023 physicians certified in CCM by the individual boards of Internal Medicine, Surgery, Anesthesiology, Pediatrics, and Obstetrics and Gynecology. A breakdown of the number of intensivists by primary specialty is shown in Table 13.9. Although authorized to do so by the ABMS, the American Board of

Table 13.9 Number of certified specialists in CCM by primary specialty

Specialty	No. of certified physicians
Internal medicine	4150
Surgery	882
Anesthesia	554
Pediatrics	446
Obstetrics/gynecology	1

Source: Society of Critical Care Medicine and Specialty Boards.

Neurosurgery has never granted certification in CCM. A small number of intensivists have also been certified by the American Osteopathic Association; however, complete data are not available from that organization at this time.

Certification by the American Board of Internal Medicine (ABIM) has been offered through a number of pathways (designated A–F). These represented a variety of combinations of training and clinical experience (Table 13.10).

Table 13.10 Requirements for ABIM certification in CCM

Criteria	Pathway					
	A	B	C	D	E	F
CCM training (years)	1	3[a]		2		
Subspecialty training (years)	2		2[b]			
Subspecialty certification	Yes	Yes			Yes	
Internal medicine certification						Yes
Years of CCM practice					2	4

[a]CCM and other subspecialty training totalling 3 years.
[b]General Internal Medicine including 6 months of CCM.

The first ABIM certification examination in CCM was conducted in 1987. Only 9% of those taking the examination at that time had any fellowship training in CCM; of 2712 examinees, 1725 were successful. Of those applying through the CCM training pathways, 80% passed the examination. Sixty-four per cent of applicants with prior subspecialty certification and 2 years of critical care experience passed, as opposed to only 46% of those with 4 years' clinical experience and internal medicine certification.[13] Subsequent examinations in 1989 and 1991 resulted in the certification of 1115 of 1814 (61%) and 1310 of 2104 (62%) applicants, respectively.[14] From 1993 onwards, all applicants for the examination will have to have satisfied the requirements for formal training in CCM to be eligible for the boards.

In 1992, 181 applicants registered for the certification examination in pediatric critical care. Fifty-two registrants entered by the training route, 19 by a combination of training and practice, 34 by practice experience alone, and eight by certification in another specialty plus 2 years of pediatric CCM training. One hundred and fifty-one registrants took the exam and 100 passed (66%) (personal communication, American Board of Pediatrics). The American Board of Surgery reports that 208 examinees passed the surgical boards in CCM for the most recent examination. Of these, 62 were fellowship trained (personal communication, American Board of Surgery). The American Board of Anesthesiology does not have information regarding the fellowship training of its diplomates (personal communication, American Board of Anesthesiology).

Certification for physicians trained in obstetrics and gynecology as their primary specialty is contingent upon at least 1 year of additional training in a surgical or anesthesiology critical care program.

FELLOWSHIP TRAINING

The SCCM Guidelines Committee presented an extensive series of guidelines for the content of CCM fellowships in 1992[15] which updated the previously published guidelines (1986 and 1973). A detailed outline of the recommended topics was broken down into four major categories:

* Credentials
* Cognitive skills
* Procedural skills
* Patient care experience.

A fifth category of additional requirements for pediatric CCM trainees was also included.

The Credentials designation includes items such as Advanced Cardiac and Advanced Trauma Life Support certification. Under the heading of Cognitive skills is a broad array of pathophysiologic, clinical, technical and administrative topics. The Procedural skills and Patient care categories are self-explanatory.

The Guidelines Committee also published a set of guidelines for the qualifications of a director of a CCM training program.[16] These include academic, clinical and administrative qualities recommended in a fellowship director.

At the present time, fellowship training in critical care is offered in programs accredited by the American Boards of Anesthesiology, Internal Medicine, Pediatrics and Surgery. Although there are many similarities in the requirements mandated by each board, they have all established their own criteria for eligibility for training and certification, as well as specific program content and educational requirements.[17] An overview of these programs is presented in Table 13.11. Currently there are a total of 204 training programs accredited by the Accreditation Committee on Graduate Medical Education: 43 in anesthesiology, 111 in internal medicine, 17 in surgery, and 33 in pediatrics (personal communication, SCCM). The guidelines for these programs, as stated in the Directory of Graduate Medical Education Programs, contain details regarding required facilities, faculty, patient populations, and academic and procedural skills for these programs. Although these guidelines list acceptable additional areas of clinical experience for trainees (e.g. rotations through other types of ICUs in addition to the core program), none specifically detail the required critical care rotations (either by number or unit) necessary for training in that specialty. Within the general framework

Table 13.11 Comparison of specialty board requirements for training in CCM

	Specialty			
	Anes	Med	Peds	Surg
Duration of training	12 months	2 years[a]	2 years	1 year
Completion of residency	Yes	Yes	Yes	Yes[b]
Trainee : patient ratio	1 : 5	1 : 5	1 : 4	1 : 5
Research experience	No[c]	Yes	Yes	Yes
Required rotations stated	No	No	No	No

Anes: anesthesia; Med: medical; Peds: pediatrics; Surg: surgical.
From ref. 17.

[a]One year of CCM if certified in another subspecialty by ABIM.
[b]May be performed after completion of regular 5-year residency or after 3 years if the remainder of residency requirements are ultimately satisfied.
[c]Opportunities for research must be available.

established by each specialty board, individual programs are free to determine the specific structure and content of their training programs.

Conclusion

Despite the increasing numbers of critical care physicians in the USA and their growing numbers as directors and primary attendings in intensive care units, a number of significant issues remain unresolved.

Although the number of formally trained and certified clinicians in CCM is increasing rapidly, their numbers as directors of ICUs remain small, with only 44.1% of units in the USA being directed by such physicians (only 19.9% in hospitals with less than 100 beds).

Details regarding the training of critical care clinicians would also seem to be unresolved. Clinicians can enter the discipline from a variety of specialties and via myriad pathways. As a result there is the potential for great disparities in the type and quality of training provided to different individuals, as well as the emphasis which may be placed on various aspects of critical care medicine. Nevertheless, the formalization of training in CCM is clearly a major step toward improving the quality of critical care education and presumably its practice as well.

Since the practice of CCM remains fragmented, divided between practitioners from various different specialties, as well as among critical care specialists and nonspecialists, disagreements regarding authority and autonomy are inevitable. Hopefully, with the growing acceptance of CCM physicians these 'turf battles' will disappear as the primary responsibility for the management of critically ill patients is ultimately given over to specially trained clinicians.

In the USA in particular all these issues are influenced by physician reimbursement. Acting sometimes as a consultant, sometimes as the primary attending, sometimes as a specialist, and sometimes as a generalist orchestrating the care of the patient, the intensivist is caught up in the complicated web of payments which exists in the USA, being required to charge for a variety of different levels and types of service under different circumstances. The establishment of CCM as a recognized and independent specialty may help to organize better the process of payment.

Despite these ongoing problems and 'growing pains', the specialty of critical care medicine has grown significantly, and has established a place for itself in the medical community in a relatively short period of time. Its role in the delivery of health care to critically ill patients in the USA is almost certain to increase in coming years.

References

1. Safar P, Grenvik A. Critical care medicine: staffing intensive care units. *Chest* 1971; **59**: 535–47.
2. Task Force on Guidelines, Society of Critical Care Medicine. Recommendations for services and personnel for delivery of care in a critical care setting. *Crit Care Med* 1988; **16**: 809–11.
3. Guidelines Committee, Society of Critical Care Medicine. Guidelines for the definition of an intensivist and the practice of critical care medicine. *Crit Care Med* 1992; **20**: 540–2.
4. Li TCM, Phillips MC, Shaw L, Cook EF, Natanson C, Goldman L. On-site physician staffing in a community hospital intensive care unit. *J Am Med Assoc* 1984; **252**: 2023–7.
5. Hainer BL, Lawler FK. Comparison of critical care provided by family physicians and general internists. *J Am Med Assoc* 1988; **260**: 354–8.
6. Carlson RW, Haupt MT, Kruse JA. Comparison of critical care by family physicians and general internists (letter). *J Am Med Assoc* 1989; **261**: 243.
7. Reynolds HN, Haupt MT, Thill-Baharozian MC, Carlson RW. Impact of critical care physician staffing on patients with septic shock in a university hospital medical intensive care unit. *J Am Med Assoc* 1988; **260**: 3446–50.
8. Brown JJ, Sullivan G. Effect on ICU mortality of a full time critical care specialist. *Chest* 1989; **96**: 127–9.
9. Greenbaum DM. Availability of critical care personnel, facilities, and services in the United States. *Crit Care Med* 1984; **12**: 1073–7.
10. Task Force for the Distribution of ICU Resources in the United States, Society of Critical Care Medicine. Descriptive analysis of critical care units in the United States. *Crit Care Med* 1992; **20**: 846–63.
11. Dubayo BA, Samson MK, Carlson RW. The role of physician-assistants in critical care units. *Chest* 1991; **99**: 89–91.
12. Kruse JA, Carlson RW. Training and practice patterns of

society of critical care medicine internists. *Crit Care Med* 1987; **15**: 1065–6.

13. Norcini JJ, Shea JA, Langdon LO, Hudson LD. First American board of internal medicine critical care examination: process and results. *Crit Care Med* 1989; **17**: 695–8.

14. American Board of Internal Medicine. Performance on the 1990 pulmonary disease and 1989 and 1991 critical care medicine (CCM) examinations. *ABIM Newsline* 1992; Spring/Summer: 4.

15. Guidelines Committee, Society of Critical Care Medicine. Guidelines for program content for fellowship training in critical care medicine. *Crit Care Med* 1992; **20**: 875–82.

16. Guidelines Committee, Society of Critical Care Medicine. Guidelines for the qualifications of a director of a fellowship training program in critical care medicine. *Crit Care Med* 1992; **20**: 883.

17. American Medical Association. Essentials of accredited residencies. In: *Directory of Graduate Medical Education*. Chicago: American Medical Association, 1992: 28–9, 51–3, 104–5, 140–1.

18. Groeger JS *et al.* Descriptive analysis of critical care units in the United States. *Crit Care Med* 1992; **20**: 846–63.

Canada

BRIAN P EGIER, CINDY M HAMIELEC, JOHN R HEWSON

Intensive care medicine began in Canada, as in many other countries, out of the necessity to satisfy two needs. The beginning of major surgical interventions involving the heart and great vessels coincided with the poliomyelitis epidemics in the 1950s. To satisfy such needs, these early intensive care units (ICUs) began as outgrowths of the postoperative recovery rooms. While internists (in particular respirologists) and surgeons were involved, anesthetists had a prominent role in the creation of these units, a relationship which grew naturally from their intraoperative skills and responsibilities.

Initially, continuous staffing of these early units was provided largely by nurses, resulting in care by crisis intervention rather than crisis prevention. By the mid-1960s, the ICUs in university teaching hospitals had not only become distinctly recognized formal entities but were by then starting to be staffed around the clock by residents 'floating' in from other services (anesthesia, medicine, surgery) for finite shifts. Although these residents did not know the patients in detail because of the transient nature of their coverage, at least there was a physician in the ICU.

Growth in technology, increases in the complexity of surgical intervention and anaesthetic management as well as changing expectations of the public in terms of what the 'miracles' of modern medicine could and should provide led to the growth and dissemination of ICUs by the 1970s.

Parallel with this growth came the recognition that effective crisis prevention required organized physician input. Experienced physicians fully trained in a traditional 'primary' specialty (anesthesia, medicine, surgery) with a special interest in critical care medicine (CCM) made themselves continuously available to the tertiary (university) ICU on a rotational basis (e.g. one week in four) for clinical and educational activities within the unit including regular, structured bedside rounds on all patients. One of these physicians assumed the role of ICU director, thereby taking responsibility for a greater proportion of the administrative, research and didactic educational functions within the unit.

In conjunction with this emerging role of the intensivist came the dedication (again, in teaching centers) of residents to the ICU for defined rotations, rather than the previous floating shift model. This made possible the provision of around the clock physician presence by individuals who were familiar with the details of the patients, thereby moving significantly away from crisis intervention and towards crisis prevention. Such a role for the residents was dictated by their educational requirements for gaining experience in intensive care as well as by the necessity of providing this essential in-house service.

Thus evolved from the 1950s through the 1980s a system initiated by need in turn satisfied by informal and finally increasingly formal function. With escalating costs and in an increasingly top-down government-run health care system, a task force created by the federal government issued a blueprint for intensive care services in the mid-1980s. In many ways this report simply formalized the direction into which the system had already been evolving. While not being a directive for implementation *per se*, it has been and will likely continue to be the model for continuing development.

We will therefore summarize major aspects of this report in order to give a bird's eye view of how Canada's critical care system is currently structured. We will then go on to describe how we are presently staffed and the trends for the future. Finally, we will describe our future in terms of Canada's training programs for future intensivists.

The resource model

DEFINITIONS

Current practice in Canada enables a general categorization into three types of specialized units, as defined by Health and Welfare Canada in 1986.

Level I

A Level I unit has monitored beds designed to care for patients who require intensive nursing care and medical interventions of a noninvasive nature. If invasive techniques and respiratory support are used, it is usually for stabilization prior to transfer to a Level II or Level III unit and/or of short duration. A facility with a Level II or Level III unit may also have a monitoring unit designed to accommodate less critically ill patients who have not yet reached the status where they can be transferred to a regular nursing unit.

Level II

Level II units have capabilities for invasive monitoring and respiratory support. A physician-director coordinates support and consultative services which are less comprehensive than those at Level III.

Level III

This unit has a comprehensive and multisystem intensive care capability; supplies a broad range of consultative services, and 24-hour medical coverage by qualified physicians available in the hospital. The unit has a medical director with additional training in critical care medicine. Teaching and research is an integral part of this unit.

Hospital size and levels of care

A Level I (monitoring) unit is usually established in a hospital with less than 300 active treatment beds. A hospital with 300 beds or more requires a Level II or Level III intensive care unit. In special circumstances such as geographic isolation or specialized case mix, a Level III unit may be required in smaller facilities.

The percentage of the total hospital bed complement that should constitute intensive care beds depends on the type of hospital and cases that are being treated. Presently in Canadian hospitals, the number of intensive care beds (including coronary care) is appropriately based on the utilization of 3–5% of the total active treatment beds. The applicable percentage in any particular situation is determined by the size of the hospital's geographic catchment area and whether the hospital provides special services and programs such as trauma care, neurosurgery, or open heart surgery; as well as the availability of medical expertise and specialist consultation.

The average occupancy rate in an Intensive Care Unit should be at least 75% with most ICUs averaging 80–85%. (Current occupancy rates are frequently approximately 90% or higher.) The average length of stay will depend, to a significant degree, on the kind of patient being treated in a particular unit.

In most institutions, there exists an interdisciplinary ICU committee with representation from medical staff (including the unit medical director), nursing, hospital administration, and allied health care professionals. This facilitates interdisciplinary input into: the organization of the unit; setting policies governing admissions, discharges, procedures and standards of patient care; utilization, including interunit transfer policies and regular case reviews; medical education; budgeting; assessment of new products, techniques and equipment; development of treatment protocols, policies and protocols for organ and tissue donations; emergency evacuation and disaster planning.

GRADED REFERRAL SYSTEM

This system of differential resources depending on the size, function and expertise available is coupled with an increasingly formal graded referral grid to move patients to the level of care required. Thus community hospitals with Level I or II units can and do refer appropriate patients onwards to more specialized facilities. This occurs even from one tertiary hospital to another. While there is clearly a long way to go to accomplishing such regionalization of resources, Canada is moving towards not only graded referral from primary through secondary and tertiary levels of care but also from tertiary to tertiary centers. In an attempt to maximize efficiency of resources (and thereby minimize costs), there is increasing demand by governments for and movement towards specialization within tertiary centres. Not all tertiary care hospitals will offer all services on site but will have 'easy' access to, for instance, dialysis, cardiovascular surgery or MRI scanning. While clearly reducing costs and perhaps creating greater expertise through sheer volume of experience, the ease of access is not always as safe and smooth as might be optimal. For example there is the occasional need to transfer critically ill patients simply because no one tertiary care hospital in a city has all the services that the patient requires.

The transportation facilities necessary to make such a grid work include both land and air, all run by the provincial health ministries. While available, there is increasing pressure on the system in terms of timely access and appropriate support (e.g. availability of suitably trained individuals to transport the patient).

The people

STAFFING: THE TWO TIERS

In Level I units, patients are often managed primarily by their family physician or general internist with consultative input from available subspecialists as required.

There is no in-house ICU physician and emergency coverage may be provided by a physician on call in the emergency room (where available) or via call-back of the primary physician.

While the level of illness in a Level II unit may be less than that in a Level III unit, crisis prevention may be of even greater importance since there is less physician availability for crisis management. Level II ICUs are currently staffed either by dedicated rotating physicians trained in anesthesia, medicine, surgery or pediatrics (in an open or semiclosed administrative structure) or in an open scenario by the patient's primary physician, be it internist or surgeon, perhaps with limited anesthesia input regarding ventilatory therapy. Increasingly there is a movement, partly driven by medical–legal risk management concerns, for a critical care trained individual to be the director of such a unit. Off hours emergency intervention is provided by the on-call emergency physician and/or anesthetist. Such a system requires intense and effective communication between the various players as the patients may find themselves being cared for by multiple physicians each with a specific area of interest and expertise. With the possible exception of the ICU director, physicians in Level II units are unlikely to have either specific critical care training or see themselves as intensivists. Indeed, they define themselves as surgeons, internists or anesthetists.

The patients in Level III ICUs, through filtering and selection, tend to require 24 hour a day physician availability for both crisis prevention and intervention. In order to provide such coverage by physicians who know the patients, a two-tiered system of staffing evolved first informally and is now increasingly formally recognized as being vital to the provision of optimal care.

Tier I

'Tier I' is composed of attending intensivists, all fully qualified in anesthesia, medicine, surgery or pediatrics (a few being certified in more than one) who rotate through the ICU for a defined but dedicated time period (frequently one week in four). With the passage of time and the recent advent of formal training in CCM in Canada increasingly larger numbers of these physicians have specific training and qualifications in critical care medicine.

While formal critical care trained specialists are relatively recent on the Canadian scene (the first group having finished training in 1990), a significant number of practicing intensivists in the tertiary care centers have completed additional, albeit not officially recognized, training in critical care medicine of one to two years' duration post certification in their 'primary' specialty.

These intensivists function in varied environments in terms of administrative and political structure. Canada's tertiary ICUs run the gamut from virtually open units where the intensivist functions largely without formal recognition and only at the tolerance of the patient's primary surgeon or internist, to closed structures where the intensivist formally assumes primary responsibility for the patient's care while in the unit. Recognition of the intensivists' additional skills, knowledge and experience is variable and is made worse by the part-time nature of how they function. With few exceptions, such individuals practice critical care only part-time, with the majority of their clinical practice and perhaps their teaching and/or research focused on their 'primary' specialty. While this has the acknowledged benefit of providing 'a way out' for the physicians wanting to leave the practice of critical care medicine and return full-time to their base specialty, it also limits the dedication and commitment to critical care medicine in terms of both clinical and academic development. This is further reinforced by the lack of any vertical department of critical care medicine in a Canadian university. Thus the intensivist enters and progresses through an academic faculty by way of commitment to (and recognition by) one of the 'traditional' departments, be it anesthesia, medicine, surgery or pediatrics. Needless to say, critical care medicine can only advance in this setting through the hard work of a few individuals and the enlightened good nature (when it exists) of the traditional university structure.

Remuneration of intensivists varies across the country as such structures are province-based. Everything from flat salaries to per-diem rates per patient or bed to pure fee for service is seen. These result in wide variations in the adequacy of remuneration and working conditions (e.g. hours) across the country. Indeed, in some provinces it is almost impossible to earn a reasonable income doing full-time CCM (which obviously promotes the part-time model with its inherent limitations in terms of specialty development). On the other hand, remuneration in another province is such that everyone wants to be part of it, resulting in occasional political battles and turf wars between individuals with and without additional critical care qualifications.

The make-up of such tertiary-care intensivists has changed over the years. Whereas anesthesia-based individuals were a major force both in numbers as well as prominence in the earlier years, the mix is shifting towards a greater proportion of internal medicine-based, usually respiratory physicians. Surgeons as well are entering critical care in larger numbers. While a phase-out of physicians who are shifting back to their primary specialties over time explains part of this demographic trend, the mix of people entering critical care training and practice is clearly altering the balance, with fewer anesthetists, more surgeons, and many more internists.

Tier II

The intensivist provides expertise as well as continuity of patient care. However, he or she cannot be physically at the bedside for days at a time. Therefore, to provide the hands-on availability of continuous care, a second tier of physicians is needed. This 'Tier II' was traditionally filled by residents from anesthesia, medicine, surgery, pediatrics and occasionally emergency medicine who rotated through ICU for a dedicated period of 1–3 months, as part of their mandated training. The past several years, however, has seen two forces at work to change the make-up of Tier II. First, the absolute numbers of residents has been dwindling as a result of cutbacks in availability of training positions by the provincial Ministries of Health. Second, the distribution of trainees has changed as educational requirements are increasingly focusing away from tertiary care and are taking precedence over service needs. The result has been an increasingly critical shortfall in the availability of adequate numbers of residents to maintain a two-tiered system. The solution to this problem has focused on defining, creating and supporting 'resident equivalents' or critical care clinical assistants (CCCAs).

Such clinical assistants have become vital to the functioning of many tertiary level ICUs. These individuals vary from general practitioners who are trained on site or fully qualified specialists (not CCM trained) working part-time to supplement their incomes during research years or early in their practices. Indeed, such a hospital-based position, usually paid on an hourly or straight salaried basis, may well be defining a new alternative to private independent practice. These physicians have none of the costs or problems associated with setting up and maintaining an independent practice, are involved in providing an exciting level of tertiary care, and are paid competitively.

The CCCA functions under the guidance and supervision of the attending intensivist, akin to the way in which a surgical assistant interfaces with the surgeon in the operating room. The formalized recognition and support of these resident equivalents is one vital aspect of the ability of tertiary care ICUs to continue to function in Canada, a process which is still evolving.

Specific mention must be made of the Tier I staffing of pediatric ICUs. These physicians emanate from either a pediatric or anesthesia background and like the current situation on the adult side increasing numbers of these individuals have completed additional training in pediatric critical care.

Training

There are two levels of trainee in Canadian teaching ICUs. The rotating residents come from such programs as anesthesia, medicine, surgery, pediatrics, and emergency medicine. They have dedicated rotations of generally from 1–3 months' duration in usually either a medical, surgical or combined ICU, depending on the structure in that training center. During their rotation, they function under the attending physicians (usually the intensivist but there are still a few tertiary ICUs where care is supervised directly by the primary surgeon) providing hands-on care and gaining skills through experience. The educational objectives are primarily the responsibility of the parent residency program.

In the 1980s, the newly formed Canadian Critical Care Society invested a great amount of effort in defining the domain of knowledge and skills making up the newly emerging specialty of CCM. Ultimately the specialty was recognized by The Royal College of Physicians and Surgeons of Canada, the body responsible for specialist training and certification in Canada. This led to the development of training programs in critical care medicine which have two characteristics setting them apart from those of most other countries.

The first of these characteristics is educational. Faced with the burgeoning requests for recognition of increasing numbers of specialties and subspecialties, The Royal College in the late 1980s established a new program entitled 'Accreditation Without Certification.' In distinction from the traditional process of not only accrediting programs but also ultimately independently examining the trainees for certification, the College under this new process vigorously examines the structure, educational process, including in particular the evaluation process and the resources of the university-based program. However, the ultimate decision regarding success or failure in completing the training programme is left to the program itself (i.e. there is no external examination for certification). Critical care is but one of several specialties whose training is governed by this structure.

The second and crucial characteristic of CCM training in Canada is that it reflects the philosophical tenet that critical care medicine is a truly multidisciplinary specialty. Although there is a separation into adult and pediatric training programs, within each of these pathways the training is truly multidisciplinary. There are no divisions into medicine, surgery or anesthesia programs. All programs will train qualified individuals from any of the specified base specialties. In turn, the qualifications and recognition of the successful graduate is a generic multidisciplinary one. The challenge of having physicians from such varied backgrounds in the same program in fact gives our programs great strengths and fosters the kind of multidisciplinary understanding and cooperation that is vital to the care of our patients. Two years of training in critical care and successful completion of the trainee's certification in his/her base specialty is the requirement for recognition as an intensivist in Canada.

We have tried to provide the reader with an overview of critical care medicine in Canada. It is a system which arose out of need, and has evolved through an informal to a now increasingly formal structure. Many challenges remain both in the provision of clinical care and the academic development of critical care medicine in Canada.

Bibliography

Dubaybo BA, Samson MK, Carlson RW. The role of physician-assistants in critical care units. *Chest* 1991; **99**: 89–91.

Guidelines Committee, Society of Critical Care Medicine. Guidelines of the care of patients with hemodynamic instability associated with sepsis. *Crit Care Med* 1988; **16**: 809–11.

Hewson JR. Toward national standards for physician staffing of critical care units. Newsletter – The Canadian Critical Care Society, 1988.

Jeffrey SG, Strosberg MA, Halpern NA *et al*. Descriptive analysis of critical care units in the United States. *Crit Care Med* 1992; **20**: 1057–9.

Knaus WA, Draper EA, Wagner DP *et al*. An evaluation of outcome from intensive care in major medical centres. *Ann Intern Med 1986;* **104**: 410–18.

Pollack MM, Katz RW, Ruttiman VE *et al*. Improving the outcome and efficiency of intensive care: the impact of an intensivist. *Crit Care Med 1988;* **16**: 11–17.

Report of the Subcommittee on Institutional Program Guidelines. *Guidelines for Establishing Standards for Special Services in Hospitals*. Intensive Care Services, Health Services Directorate, Health Services and Promotion Branch. Published by authority of the Minister of National Health and Welfare, 1979. Revised, 1986.

Task Force on Guidelines, Society of Critical Care Medicine. Guidelines for standards of care for patients with acute respiratory failure on mechanical ventilatory support. *Crit Care Med* 1991; **19**: 275–8.

Task Force on Guidelines, Society of Critical Care Medicine. Guidelines for categorization of services for the critically ill patient. *Crit Care Med* 1991; **19**: 279–85.

Task Force on Guidelines, Society of Critical Care Medicine. Recommendations for services and personnel for delivery of care in a critical care setting. *Crit Care Med* 1992; **20**: 1057–8.

Wilson RF. Surgical intensive care units. In: Parrillo JE, Ayres SM (eds) *Major Issues in Critical Care*. Baltimore: Williams & Wilkins, 1984:17–33.

CHAPTER 14

Nursing Staffing and Training

United Kingdom
MANDY SHEPPARD————————————
Staffing   212
Training   215
References   217

Europe
AM TIMMERMANN————————————
Intensive care nursing in the EC   223
ICU staffing in Belgium   224
Conclusions   225
Bibliography   225

Australia
MICHELLE KELLY, FRANCES MONYPENNY————
Preregistration education   218
Postregistration education   219
Continuing education   219
Competency standards   219
Registering bodies   221
Career paths and remuneration   221
Staffing   221
Conclusion   222
References   222

United Kingdom

MANDY SHEPPARD

The specialty of critical care has undergone rapid development over the last three decades. Despite this progress there is a significant variation in intensive care units (ICUs) across the UK in terms of size, staffing, structure and available services.[1] This lack of uniformity has obvious implications for the nursing structure within critical care areas and underlines the importance for nurse staffing and training to be tailored to the demands of individual units.

Staffing

While it is indisputable that the number and skills of staff are predominant when discussing a critical care nursing establishment, there are in addition a number of key elements that must be addressed to ensure a stable foundation. Without this the nursing contingent will not work as a team, development or progression will be difficult, and any prospect of change can precipitate unease.

There are many styles of management and it would be wrong to be prescriptive; however, it would be correct to state that the chosen style has tremendous influence on the behavior and functioning of the nursing team. The ability to provide strong leadership, to motivate and to sincerely value staff are all important qualities of the nurse manager.

The nursing team is a comparatively large one; this serves to highlight and focus on accepted management strategies. One such example is communication. It is understandable that misinterpretation or a lack of information can lead to unrest. Therefore it is necessary to institute both formal and informal communication channels for the dissemination of information and to allow the nursing group to air views or discuss concerns.

Another example is regular performance review which enables feedback concerning performance to be given and an opportunity for individuals to set objectives and goals. This not only enhances job satisfaction for the nurses but also helps the manager realize the potential of the staff and have some control over the accepted standard of performance.

A nursing philosophy that states the views, beliefs and goals of the nursing team is essential. It should be a working document, evident in daily practice and not merely a paperwork exercise. The development of a philosophy is a fundamental step in bringing the team together and fostering a sense of cohesiveness and purpose.

A 'framework' around which nursing care can be planned, delivered and evaluated should be formulated. This framework, sometimes referred to as a 'model,' must be able to meet the needs of the particular unit and its patients. It should reflect the philosophy and facilitate a consistent approach to the management of care.

A good standard of clinical care necessitates the utilization of research-based findings. The nursing team should be encouraged to question the rationale for practice and furthermore to justify it in terms of research, not by the time-honored method of custom and tradition. This necessitates the staff being well informed and abreast of current issues. The identification of educational needs, accessibility to journals, books, study days and a commitment to on-going training are all important.[2] Perhaps of greater importance is the initial desire of staff to maintain their knowledge and ability. This can vary between individuals but can also be significantly influenced by example and by the general environment and ethos of the unit.

As initially stated, the nursing complement must meet the needs and demands of the particular unit. While broad guidelines can be useful they can also be detrimental if interpreted too rigidly and not adapted for specific areas. It is important to be in possession of accurate and meaningful information when embarking upon such an exercise. It will, as recommended by the Kings Fund report entitled 'Intensive Care in the United Kingdom 1989', emphasize the need for data collection, accurate record keeping and audit mechanisms to be in place.[3] Health Service reforms in latter years have focused on cost-effective care and have encouraged managers to scrutinize and justify their use of resources. As the nursing component of any unit budget is usually the largest in monetary terms, nurse managers in particular are being asked to question their practice, to exercise imagination and to be adaptable in the work environment. This encouragement to develop a flexible approach now may pay dividends in the future as it is predicted that the traditional face of the workforce will change. It is proposed that more part-time workers will be employed and that there will be increased mobility in and out of the work market.[4]

There are a number of factors to be considered in the pursuit of an ideal nursing establishment.

BED OCCUPANCY

The number of nurses required should in part be dictated by the bed occupancy of the unit, and not the actual number of beds. For example, it would be quite unnecessary to fully (100%) staff a ten-bedded unit if on average only five of the beds were occupied at any one time. It would be more sensible to employ, on a permanent basis, a 'core staffing', i.e. 50% in this case, sufficient to meet the needs of the average bed occupancy. Many units that subscribe to this method keep one or two nursing positions vacant; this maneuver provides the finance to employ part-time staff during above average or peak bed occupancy periods.

It is not uncommon for critical care nurses in some units to voice dissatisfaction when frequently redeployed to busy wards or departments if the ICU is quiet. If this is a regular occurrence, firstly the need for an ICU in that area must be questioned and secondly the possibility of an artificially high nursing establishment in relation to bed occupancy must be considered.

ACTIVITY PATTERNS

It would be ideal to be able to exercise control over the bed occupancy but, due to the nature of the speciality, this is almost impossible. The monitoring of activity patterns, while not providing discrete predictions of staffing needs will at least detect possible trends and allow staff to be rostered in a manner that mirrors the changes in workload.

Variations in activity can be seen on small and extended time scales. In surgical units, the variation can be noted through the day. This usually reflects the discharge of patients who underwent surgery the previous day and patients being admitted from the operating theatres. A knowledge of the timing and structuring of the theater lists is invaluable in this respect. ICUs situated in areas that experience fluctuations in population can have activity variations perhaps on a monthly or seasonal basis. For example, if near a seaside resort the summer months are likely to be busier. If near a popular conference venue, increased activity may be seen when meetings are held. This emphasizes the need to monitor over a significant time period to detect all variations.

PATIENT DEPENDENCY

The Intensive Care Society has recommended the need for a 1:1 nurse to patient ratio over a 24-hour period[5] and furthermore there will be some patients who for certain parts of the day will require more than one nurse. This refers to intensive care patients; those requiring high dependency care do not require such levels of nursing input. It is therefore necessary to measure the dependency of the patients admitted and to relate this information to the bed occupancy rate and any variations in activity. For example, the ten-bedded unit experiencing an average occupancy of 50% (five beds) during the week may decrease to 10% (one bed) at weekends. This immediately suggests that the manpower should be concentrated during the week and reduced on Saturdays and Sundays. Additionally if, of the 50% occupancy during the week, only 80% require intensive care (four beds) and the remaining 20% require high dependency care (one bed), the 1:1 ratio should only apply to four beds and a 1:2 or even 1:3 ratio to the remaining one bed. The efficient use of nursing resource can be lost in this sort of unit. If there is only one highly dependent patient, requiring 0.5 or 0.3 of a nurse, the remaining half or two-thirds of that nurse can be redundant. It is far more efficient to concentrate patients of a similar dependency in one area. However, many units in the UK provide both intensive and high dependency care, highlighting the need for flexible manpower strategies to avoid underutilization of staff.[1]

A major shortcoming of dependency scoring is that it sometimes takes no account of the varying capabilities of the differing levels of staff. One nurse with 2 years of critical care experience may be more competent in caring for a particular patient than a nurse of 6 months experience who may not be able to manage. This introduces the dimensions of skillmix and quality into the equation. Skillmix is often misinterpreted as grademix, which merely reflects the numbers at each grade employed; true analysis of skillmix requires close examination of the skills within those grades.[6]

The major determinant of skillmix required will be the type and dependency of patients admitted. Units that frequently admit critically ill patients, perhaps with multiple organ failure requiring invasive monitoring and advanced therapeutic techniques, will require a relatively high proportion of intensive care trained nurses. Within this overall requirement for appropriately trained staff, more specific skills can be identified. For example, if hemofiltration is regularly performed, there need to be nurses who are capable of managing extracorporeal methods of renal replacement.

A further important factor is the provision of training. Many ICUs supply clinical experience for nurses undertaking postregistration intensive care training. In these centers, staff must be clinically competent, the staff levels must reflect the associated supervisory roles, and a proportion of the nurses have to be trained to teach and assess the learners.

It is advisable to analyze all the activities in a unit, from clerical work through to the delivery of all aspects of care. This should include all groups of staff, in particular the medical and technical; the function of the nursing structure cannot be viewed in isolation. The information gained from such an analysis can be used to determine the proportionate skill levels needed and therefore the personnel required. Job descriptions that accurately reflect roles should be produced and when fitted together (rather like the pieces of a jigsaw puzzle) should provide an overall picture of the unit activities. Duplication of duties must be minimized and omissions guarded against.

Although a clear distinction between roles is often difficult to identify in critical care areas, it is essential that in broad terms the 'right person is doing the right job.' A failure to do so results in staff feeling threatened if not appropriately skilled to undertake certain tasks and, conversely, others may feel frustration and demoti-

vation if they are performing tasks that are not fitting to their level of expertise; the possible benefit of a support worker should be considered in the latter case. It is recognized that in some areas the trained staff spend considerable amounts of time performing tasks that could be done by support workers.[7] This applies to all groups of staff in an ICU and not only to nurses.

The Intensive Care Society has recommended that each ICU has a nurse manager who also acts in a clinical capacity, providing resource and support.[5] Commonly, the manager is supported by a group of shift managers (sisters/charge nurses) who are primarily concerned with the shift-to-shift and day-to-day organization of the unit. These two levels are further supported by a body of staff nurses, the majority of whom possess a postregistration critical care qualification. Some of the nurses within this group will be relatively senior, possessing much clinical expertise and wishing to develop management skills. Most units also employ a small number of nurses who possess their basic registration and wish to gain critical care experience. Many units provide the clinical placements for nurses who are enrolled in critical care courses but to maintain their true training status these should not be included in the establishment numbers.

Job descriptions and an understanding of skillmix will make selection and recruitment of new staff more specific and the appointment of inappropriate staff less likely. Good management of a unit will improve the retention of staff. A degree of regular staff turnover is helpful, but it can be unsettling if it is too great.

In summary, to decide the ideal nursing complement for a particular unit the following must be established:

1. *The average bed occupancy* – essentially employ a core number of staff to deal with this workload.
2. *The peaks and troughs of activity – the pattern.* Roster the core staff accordingly, any part-time hours to cover peak activity times.
3. *The dependency of the patients admitted; when, how many and in what proportion* – to determine the skills required by the nursing team, in what proportion and when to be supplied.
4. *A complete view of the activities undertaken in the unit* - to decide how the multidisciplinary team members will work together and to allocate activities appropriately.

In addition to the number of nurses required to provide care, the management of a unit on a shift basis must also be accounted for. This can be influenced by the physical layout of the unit; for example in small, open-planned areas the shift manager may care directly for a low dependency patient whilst acting as the shift manager. Larger units, perhaps with some beds in side rooms, require the manager to be free from the demands of direct patient care. Similarly spare staff or 'runners' may be required in the latter type of unit to assist with care, fetch supplies and relieve staff for breaks. This can often be achieved without extra nurses in open-planned units.

Lastly, when calculating the number of nurses required, in addition to recognizing the actual contracted hours, annual leave entitlement must also be accounted for in the equation. For example, if a nurse is contracted to work 150 hours per month, of those hours he or she is allowed approximately 22 hours of holiday. If it were decided that 20 nurses were required for the unit, their total leave amounts to some 438 hours. This number of hours represents nearly three additional nurses and therefore 23 nurses should be employed to provide cover.

It is traditional to allow also for sickness, in the same manner as for annual leave. This is best achieved by retrospectively calculating average sickness rates for the individual area as there can be immense variation between units. It is important to remember that sickness should be monitored closely and any predisposing factors addressed.

The pattern of shifts worked on a unit should mirror the activity to enable the provision of staff at the correct times. A degree of flexibility is essential and the staffing resource has to be used fully. One answer to this is to minimize the length of time that shifts overlap, when doubling of staff numbers occurs.

All aspects of the nursing structure must be regularly evaluated and reanalyzed. Bed occupancy rates, activity patterns and patient dependencies can change; this must be reflected and catered for.

Sadly, financial restrictions are often the catalyst for nurse managers to examine their establishment. This type of scenario should not necessarily equate with a decrease in staff numbers or a perceived reduction in patient care. Moreover, the inappropriate use of nursing staff in a climate of limited resource is inexcusable and if bed occupancy and activity patterns are assessed, skillmix appropriately matched to dependencies and the shift patterns used to maximum effect, patient care can often be maintained and even enhanced. In addition, nurses may become more influential in the health care setting if able to demonstrate their capacity to react to financial pressures.[8]

We still know very little about the relationship between nursing numbers, skillmix and patient outcome[6] and in future, every effort must be made to correlate these variables.

Training

The formal training of nurses in critical care is well accepted. In 1972, the Joint Board of Clinical Nursing Studies (JBCNS) was established and provided specific postregistration intensive care training. In 1979 the English National Board (ENB) replaced the JBCNS and instituted the ENB 100 General Intensive Care Nursing course of 6 months duration. In 1990 the ENB recommended that this course, along with others, should be decreased to 24 weeks.[9] This reduction, which shortened clinical exposure considerably, caused much concern. It became apparent that nurses needed critical care experience before embarking on the 24-week course and furthermore needed to consolidate their courses for a longer period of time. At both ends of this spectrum, there were implications for the clinical areas. Perhaps most importantly, nurses finishing the shortened ENB 100 course could not, in general, be regarded as being as competent as those in previous times.

Until recently, the majority of ICUs that provided clinical placements for the ENB 100 course members had minimal involvement in the content or structuring of the courses. This is now changing with the Colleges of Nursing becoming the 'providers' of education and the ICUs the 'purchasers'. This new purchasing power has meant increased flexibility and freedom for the clinical areas in choosing the most appropriate education for critical care nurses of the future. In many senses, the changes have allowed units to almost demand certain requirements from the educational establishments. This has led to improved assessment of clinical needs and a closer working relationship between the managers of both clinical care and education.

Many colleges of nursing are becoming affiliated with higher education establishments and a number of nursing courses can be attributed points to reflect the academic achievement. This is known as the Credit Accumulation and Transfer System (CATS) and is recognized throughout higher education. This serves to increase the credibility and profile of nurse education. In addition, the ENB has introduced the ENB Higher Award. This system is also awarded CATS points and begins at Certificate level (120 points), moves onto Diploma levels (240 points) and finally reaches Degree level (360 points). Nurses can accumulate these points by both attending courses and by a system of accreditation for previous experiential learning (APEL). Therefore, the traditional ENB 100 course in some institutions may be a component of a diploma or degree program. This improved level of education has given rise to the possibility of advanced practitioners within the clinical areas.[10] While this may have indisputable benefits for patient care, it does cause some nurses concern in light of the current financial climate. Many fear a potential future scenario of one advanced practitioner in relation to a number of support workers caring for a set group of patients. The practitioner would act in a supervisory role, interpreting patient data and directing therapy. This method of organizing care is alien and threatening to British nurses who have traditionally enjoyed a more holistic approach to practice.

The revision of basic nurse training in the form of Project 2000 does have implications for critical care. A small number of nursing students in the past have been allocated to spend a period of their training in ICUs, however these have been in the minority. This lack of exposure to the specialty during training is known to have a detrimental effect on recruitment[11] and the advent of Project 2000 which does not incorporate critical care only serves to exacerbate the situation. This perhaps emphasizes the need for units to develop their own recruitment strategies and not to rely on the throughput of students. Certainly, those units accommodating post-registration students seem to enjoy more successful recruitment programs.[12]

Informally, there is tremendous variation in the training provided by individual units and, as for staffing, the training must meet not only the needs of the nurses but also the requirements of the unit. If certain techniques, are not routinely addressed in critical care courses, yet are regularly undertaken, then the unit must provide appropriate in-house training.

At the very least, when commencing employment in a unit, the nurse must receive help in becoming oriented to the new workplace,[2] in terms of geography and practice. Some units operate a mentor or 'buddy' system that allows the new nurse to associate with one particular member of staff.

At an early stage the nurse must be allowed to express his or her needs and objectives. This can be achieved through a performance review system. Commonly, the nurse is directly interviewed by a senior member of staff, often a sister or charge nurse. The nurse manager should have a secondary input to prevent personal bias exerting any effect, to ensure consistency of judgment and to have a global view of the abilities and needs of the staff. This allows the training requirement to be assessed and will alter according to the level of nurse. At a junior level, objectives usually center around the acquisition of clinical skills and knowledge, whereas at a more senior level, the opportunity to practice management or teaching skills is expressed. In some cases training will be individually directed where special needs are identified. The nurse manager can in addition recognize common needs and supply these in the form of general teaching sessions, the provision of literature and the attendance at relevant study days.

It should be remembered that the simplest method of learning is to copy others. This is particularly pertinent to the more junior nurse who has little experience on which to base informed judgments. In essence the practice of each nurse as an individual will always be copied by others and thus each nurse needs to act as a suitable role model. The achievement of this relies in part on a cascade effect from the top of the nursing group. Appropriate selection of recruits, management style and performance appraisal should help to maintain certain standards of practice and ensure that all staff act as role models.

As previously stated, training must be directed towards the needs of individuals and the unit as a whole. There are many factors that may attract a nurse into the critical care environment. The satisfaction to be gained from nursing patients on a one to one basis is important to many, as is the unique opportunity to combine nursing skills, knowledge and technology in the care of the critically ill patient.[13] The skills required range from those that are fundamental to physical and emotional human needs through to advanced technical abilities. The requirement for advanced skills has resulted in nurses extending their traditional roles. It is possible that to ensure continuity of patient care, the varying degrees of role extension seen in ICUs has been a reflection of the differing medical and technical availability. Indeed, one study of over 250 units in the UK confirms this variation and the difficulty in defining the boundaries of nursing roles.[14]

Extended role has always caused much controversy and many nurses hold the view that their roles are expanded as opposed to extended and are integral to critical care nursing.[15] In practical terms this has necessitated nurses gaining certificates in competency for each extended role. Examples include the administration of intravenous drugs, venepuncture or defibrillation. Furthermore, these certificates are not recognized nationally, requiring nurses to be reassessed as competent each time the nurse changes hospitals.

In June 1992, the United Kingdom Central Council for Nursing, Midwifery and Health Visiting (UKCC) produced the document 'The Scope of Professional Practice'.[16] This has recognized the ridiculous situation in relation to certification of extended role that has been in operation. In addition the document advises that practice should reflect patient needs and not be restrictive, as extended role has been in the past. While this is a welcome development, the impact on clinical areas in terms of training needs must be appreciated. Although the responsibility for practice rests firmly with the nurse as an individual, the nurse manager must also accept responsibility for deciding patient needs and the consequent role of the nurse, and also must provide the associated training. It is unreasonable to expect nurses to undertake roles, regardless of their willingness, unless they are adequately prepared.

The importance of on-going training can often be overlooked, especially during busy times and when resources seem stretched. With careful rostering and inventive planning, time can, and indeed must, be put aside for education. Many colleges of nursing have recognized the increasing constraints and offer continuing education courses in the evenings and on a part-time basis. This will have to become more widespread in future to ensure that critical care nurses continue to develop and remain updated.

The staffing of critical care areas is inextricably linked to the preparatory and subsequent on-going training of the nurses. Both nurse education and the clinical environment are currently undergoing great change; it is difficult to predict the future. Critical care nursing must always be in a position to meet the requirements of the patients, be responsive to any changes in need and be specific to the immediate environment. Regardless of the uncertainty, the nursing population within critical care has the opportunity now to step back, assess in which direction it would prefer to develop and, most importantly, justify that decision.

References

1. The Association of Anaesthetists of Great Britain and Ireland. *Intensive Care Services – Provision for the Future.* London: The Association of Anaesthetists of Great Britain and Ireland, 1988.
2. Stones JN. A survey of continuing educational needs of nurses working in an intensive care unit. *Intensive Care Nursing* 1986; **1**: 130–7.
3. Kings Fund Centre. *The Intensive Care Services in the UK.* London: Kings Fund, 1989.
4. Davies C. *The Collapse of the Conventional Career: The Future of Work and its Relevance for Postregistration Education in Nursing, Midwifery and Health Visiting.* London: ENB, 1990.
5. Intensive Care Society. *The Intensive Care Service in the UK.* London: Intensive Care Society, 1990.
6. Gibbs I, McCaughan D, Griffiths M. Skillmix in nursing: a selective review of the literature. *J Adv Nursing* 1991; **16**(2): 242–9.
7. Ball J, Hurst K, Booth M, Franklin R. But who will make the beds? A research based strategy for determining nursing skillmix for the 1990's. The Nuffield Institute and Mersey Regional Health Authority, 1989.
8. Ashworth P. Economics, effectiveness, evidence, ethics and education – five essentials for intensive care. *Intensive Care Nursing* 1989; **5**(2): 49–51.
9. Post-basic Clinical Nursing Studies Courses. *Revised Outline Criteria for Certificate Courses in General Nursing.* London: ENB, 1990.
10. Ball C. Education and staffing in ICU: past, present and future. *Br J Nursing* 1992; **1**(8): 399–401.
11. Hall S. Nursing as a career. *Nursing Standard* 1989; **3**(40): 35.
12. Atkinson BL. Training nurses for intensive care. *Intensive Care Nursing* 1990; **6**(4): 172–8.
13. Sheppard AJ. Career development in intensive care 1. *Br J Nursing* 1992; **1**(9): 467–9.
14. Last T, Self N. Kassab J, Rajan A. Extended role of the nurse in ICU. *Br J Nursing* 1992; **1**(13): 672–5.
15. Atkinson B. The current state of critical care. *Intensive Care Nursing* 1991; **7**(2): 73–9.
16. United Kingdom Central Council for Nursing, Midwifery and Health Visiting. *The Scope of Professional Practice.* London: UKCC, 1992.

Australia

MICHELLE KELLY, FRANCES MONYPENNY

Australian nurses work in a variety of settings, from the extremes of remote areas to highly technological specialist units. There are two levels of nurses, registered nurses (Level 1) and enrolled nurses (Level 2). All registered nurses (Level 1) are educated in universities to bachelor degree level while enrolled nurses gain their qualification at technical and further education (TAFE) colleges.

In 1989, of the 230 600 registered nurses only 145 800 were actually working in nursing. A similar ratio is seen in the enrolled nurse figures with only 30 100 of the 56 000 enrolled working in nursing.[1] Statistics for the critical care nurse population are difficult to obtain because of the lack of uniform definitions of specialist nursing across Australia.

Nursing has been molded by the nation's history, its people, its geography and its climate. It has derived its roots from the British Florence Nightingale nursing system but is now rapidly developing its own body of knowledge, character and achievements that are uniquely Australian.

Australia is a vast country with a land area of over 7.5 million square kilometers. Its 17.5 million population is primarily concentrated around the eastern, southern and south western coastal areas. It is divided into two territories and six states (Fig. 14.1). Federation in 1901 established a federal government with the existing states maintaining a degree of autonomy. Responsibility for nursing education lay within state government jurisdiction under the respective health departments.

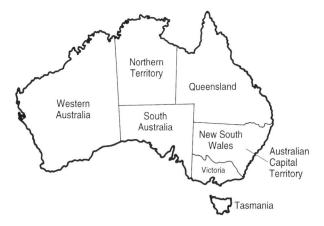

Fig. 14.1   States and territories of Australia.

Over the last decade there has been a shift of responsibility for nursing education funding from the health to the education departments at state level. From 1994, the federal government will take over the funding aligning nursing with all other tertiary courses.

This chapter will concentrate on education and staffing issues of registered nurses only, as enrolled nurses are not generally employed in critical care areas in Australia, or if they are, do not undertake patient care except under strict supervision.

In order to understand the current issues in relation to education of critical care nurses and staffing of critical care areas, it is necessary to review some of the influences which affect nursing in general. Some of these issues will be highlighted in this chapter.

Preregistration education

In 1973, nurses decided to formulate a policy from within the profession which would guide future government planning of nursing education. A working party was formed in which four leading nursing organizations were represented (The Royal Australian Nursing Federation, National Florence Nightingale Committee of Australia, Royal College of Nursing (Australia) and The New South Wales College of Nursing). A series of workshops with nurses were held over the subsequent years. The information gathered in these workshops was used to formulate the policy statement, 'Goals in Nursing Education' – released in 1976. The policy highlighted the need for a change in nursing education from the hospital-based 'apprentice' style education to tertiary studies with a minimum undergraduate two qualification ((UG2/diploma) for registration.[2]

The struggle for tertiary education for nurses dates back many decades. As early as 1967 a combined nursing and degree course was introduced in New South Wales (NSW) at the University of New England, run in association with two hospitals. During the four years, students undertook half their studies in the hospital and the other half at the university. However, the two programs were not integrated, resulting in the students studying two courses concurrently – an arts degree and a general nursing course. Despite changes in the programs over the following years, there were many problems and student retention rate was low so the course was discontinued in 1975. It was not until 1989 that further preregistration bachelor degree programs were available in Australia for those wishing to become nurses.[3]

Renewed hope in this struggle for tertiary education emerged when colleges of advanced education were established in the early 1970s. These colleges were to provide vocational courses with close links to industry. As other health professionals were educated within this system it gave nurses renewed hope that they would be educated in the same way.[3]

Success finally came in 1975 when the first full-time preregistration nursing course at diploma level was commenced at the College of Nursing (Australia) in Melbourne, itself, at that time a College of Advanced Education. That year the federal government funded six, 3-year full-time diploma nursing courses, two in NSW, two in Victoria and one each in South Australia and Western Australia. By 1978 there were 461 students enrolled in these six courses, a very small number compared with the 23 495 undertaking general nursing courses offered at the 226 hospital-based schools of nursing around the country.[3] The popularity of these diploma courses continued to grow and by 1983, the students enrolled in these programs accounted for 5% of the total student nurse population throughout Australia.[4]

The NSW state government was the first to make a firm commitment to the future of nursing education. In 1983 it announced the complete transfer of NSW nursing programs to the tertiary sector to occur as of January 1985.[3] It was not until 1984 that the federal government agreed, in principle, that all preregistration nursing programs throughout Australia would be transferred to the tertiary sector over a 9-year period, to be completed by 1993.[4] Two years after its initial announcement, the NSW state government, confronted with an acute nursing shortage, attempted to reverse its decision on the transfer, sparking a rapid and astonishing response from the profession. Thousands of nurses at all levels marched to state parliament to express their objection and were successful in preventing the move of nursing education back to the hospitals.

The Queensland state government was, in 1988, the last to implement the transfer. The last intake of nurses to hospital-based courses was in 1990. Following the transfer, not all hospital-based schools of nursing closed. Those that remain now offer postregistration and continuing education courses for nurses.

In 1988 the 1976 education policy statement was reviewed by both the reconvened working party of the groups that formulated the original 1976 education policy statement and the profession. The new policy – 'Nursing Education Targets 1989–2000' – stressed that the nursing profession should be 'accountable for the promotion, development, implementation, and evaluation of nurse education programs which ensure the maintenance of standards of nursing practice that are acceptable to the profession and satisfy the health care needs of society' and that the basic nursing qualification be a bachelor degree.[5] The bachelor degree programs were to replace existing diploma programs as of 1991 and the transition is to be completed by 1996.[5] The policy statement also included recommendations for the implementation of higher degree postregistration programs (postgraduate diploma, master and doctor of nursing).

The profession's goals in this regard were assisted by federal government rationalization of the tertiary education sector as a result of the Dawkins White Paper which recommended the amalgamation of universities and colleges of advanced education as the first step to a more streamlined and cost-effective national education system.[6] The policy statement's recommendations were implemented and since 1992 the undergraduate qualification to become a registered nurse is a bachelor program.

Postregistration education

At present, postregistration education may either be undertaken in hospital-based programs or in the tertiary sector. With a bachelor degree being the initial nursing qualification, it would follow that further education should be at a higher degree level. The courses currently available at tertiary level are conversion courses (from diploma to degree), postgraduate diploma, masters and doctor of nursing. However, specialist courses within this framework are developing but are limited and may never be able to cater fully for all the specialist nursing education needs. Therefore, hospital-based postregistration certificate courses, which have for many years been the only way to gain specialist qualifications, may continue to play an important role. The value of these programs is recognized not only in Australia but also in the United States of America (USA), Canada and the United Kingdom (UK), where they continue to be developed. In Australia, the whole issue of postregistration education is currently being reviewed at a national level through the National Nursing Consultative Committee. The future of postregistration education is therefore in a state of flux.

Specialization in Australia has evolved, as it has in the USA, with the proliferation of specialized health care. Australian nurses are grappling with issues of nomenclature and credentialling in relation to specialist practice. As in other specialties, critical care nurses need to develop advanced standards of practice which will, in the first instance, identify what it is they do and therefore help define critical care nursing as a discrete specialty. The standards can then be used to assess the competency of critical care nurses, determine the education requirement of the specialty, and help align remuneration with the level of expertise, as well as becoming the benchmark for the credentialling of critical care nurses as specialists (see 'Competency standards').

Critical care nursing as a specialty in Australia has evolved with the growth and expansion of intensive care units since the 1960s. The critical care nursing courses developed in acute care hospitals to aid recruitment of staff. Historically these courses have ranged from 26 to 52 weeks duration. Participants are employed by and gain experience in the intensive care unit throughout the course. Currently, nurses seeking critical care qualifications have several options available to them. They can undertake a course which is hospital-based (certificate) or a combined hospital and university course (certificate/graduate diploma) or a solely tertiary course (graduate diploma/masters). The recognition of the value of clinical experience in specialist nursing training has meant that some graduate diploma programs require concurrent full-time employment within the specialty of the university affiliated hospitals.

Because of this diversification of education, the need for advanced standards of practice is heightened as they will stipulate the requirements for entry to specialty practice. Education programs can be developed with these requirements in mind.

Continuing education

Non-award continuing education programs offered by hospitals and professional bodies play an important role in the development of nurses at all levels, including critical care nurses. The growing continuing education activities are due to advances in technology, changing skills mix and multiskilling of employees which has resulted from the rationalization of health care services in this country. Continuing education programs within employer settings have also gained importance in order to meet the requirements of the government's 'Training Guarantee Act 1990' which decrees that a percentage of the employer's payroll is expended on training.[7]

Competency standards

The Australian government, as part of its plan for microeconomic reform, especially labor market reform through award restructuring, is attempting to make vocational education and training more responsive to the needs of industry. In 1989, the National Training Board (NTB) was established. The NTB released a policy describing the Australian Standards Framework (ASF). This is 'a set of eight competency levels which provide reference points for the development and recognition of competency standards.'[8] Another body, the National Office of Overseas Skills Recognition (NOOSR), has extended its role of assessing overseas professionals to that of supporting the professions during the development of competency standards for entry level to that profession.[9] The NOOSR's interest in helping professional groups develop national standards is to facilitate their work in the recognition of the skills of overseas people attempting to enter the Australian workforce.

Nursing was well on its way to developing its own competencies prior to government initiatives. The development of these competencies was instigated in part by the national move to tertiary education (i.e. to ensure uniform entry standards) and to facilitate overseas entry of nurses to meet the shortfall in the nursing workforce created by the move of nursing education out of hospitals.

Prior to 1986, each state's Nursing Registration Board (NRB) had its own set of competency standards. These standards guided curriculum development and accreditation of nursing programs and were the benchmark for registration (see 'Registering bodies'). With the desire of the Australian nurse registering authorities to establish recognition of registration/enrolment across states/territories, the Australia Nursing Assessment Council (ANAC) highlighted at the 1986 Australian Nurse Registering Authorities Conference (ANRAC), the need for a single set of competencies which would be acceptable by all state registering authorities as the basis for registration/enrolment.[10]

At ANRAC 1990 validated lists of competencies were approved as the minimum requirements for entry to practice as a registered or enrolled nurse (including those nurses returning to practice or overseas nurses requiring registration or enrolment in Australia).[11] These lists are now known as the ANRAC competencies and guidelines for their use and assessment were distributed in 1992.[11] Competency in this context is defined as:

> ... the ability of a person to fulfil the nursing role effectively and/or expertly ... These competencies are defined as personal attributes which, when taken as a whole, result in effective and/or superior performance.[12]

Competencies are not just skills and, as Cameron (1989) suggests, 'A set of competencies should represent the behavioural repertoire of a competent practitioner.'[10]

With nursing education now based at tertiary institutions, ANRAC competencies provide the framework for the planning and curriculum development of nursing courses as the graduates will be required to demonstrate these competencies to gain registration/enrolment. The

ANRAC competencies have also paved the way for reciprocal recognition across Australia and on the first of March 1993, two states and the two territories instituted mutual recognition agreements.

The foresight of nursing in developing nationally accepted (ANRAC) competencies has placed it in good stead for fulfilling the entry level standards for nurses within the Australian Standards Framework (ASF). In Fig. 14.2, Andrews (1993) suggests how nursing may fit

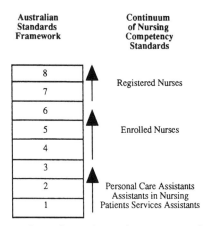

Fig. 14.2 The relationship of nursing work to the Australian Standards Framework. Reproduced with permission of *Australian Critical Care.*

into the ASF with registered nurses coming in at Level 7–8.[13] Andrews states though that 'much remains to be done in regard to their (competencies) implementation, the development of advanced competencies within the eight level NTB framework and the alignment of the various State awards and career structures to the National Framework'.[14]

The responsibility of developing advanced competencies rests with the specialty nursing groups such as the Confederation of Australian Critical Care Nurses (CACCN) which is at present embarking on this project. However, there is no consensus on the definition of a nursing specialty, therefore not all areas of nursing are represented by specialty groups who would be responsible for developing these competency standards (see 'Postregistration education').

While critical care nurses require advanced competencies above registered nurse entry level, the Australian nursing profession in general has concerns regarding the changing skills mix of the health care workforce with much nursing work being undertaken by other categories of health care workers at lower levels on the ASF. Nurses must work towards preserving nursing work at all levels of practice and this work can only be enhanced/supported by clear and concrete competency standards.

Registering bodies

Each state/territory has its own Nurses Registration Board (NRB). On qualifying, nurses register with their state registration board which enables them to practice within that state. In the past, if they wished to work in another state they were required to seek additional registration within that state. As part of the profession's desire for 'self-governance' and establishment of mutual recognition across states/territories, 1992 saw the establishment of the Australian Nursing Council (ANC).

The council is made up of representatives from each nursing registration board, the ANF, Royal College of Nursing (Australia) and federal and state government bodies. Some of the key functions of the ANC are to 'co-ordinate all matters relating to regulation of nursing in Australia, including the education, registration and/or enrolment, practice and professional conduct of nurses' and to 'establish and maintain a national register of nurses in Australia.'[15]

It has taken the nursing profession many years to accomplish this goal – the establishment of a national regulatory body. With the foresight of nurse leaders in establishing the ANC, nurses have pre-empted the heads of government decision on the need for national professional bodies who would facilitate recognition of skills across states/territories. As stated earlier, nurses have already implemented reciprocal recognition of registration in some states/territories.

Career paths and remuneration

Australian nurses work under an award system. Conditions of work and salary are negotiated by nursing unions with the state industrial commissions. It was not until 1988 that nursing was regarded as a profession rather than a trade. This helped bring nursing salaries into line with other health professionals, e.g. physiotherapists.[16]

Prior to 1989 there were three separate nursing union bodies in Australia – the Australian Nurses Federation (ANF), the New South Wales Nurses Association (NSWNA) and the Queensland Nurses Union (QNU). They have now joined together and each is a state branch of the ANF.

Part of the government's plan for economic reform is also via award restructuring and career development opportunities. Nursing is well ahead of this agenda with the ANF working towards defining a 'national' award which would align nursing award structure, wages and conditions across states and territories. This move would not only improve the position of nurses but would also facilitate the movement of nurses across the country by reducing local and/or state variations in work conditions and pay.

Staffing

Determination of nursing staffing needs in critical care areas in Australia is currently based on historical data, predictable workload, tradition and the severity of patient illness. This generally allows for one registered nurse for each one or two patients. Enrolled nurses are usually not employed in the critical care areas.

The patient dependency tools in use in hospitals do not adequately assess the nursing needs for the critically ill population. With the growing need to restrain the health care expenditure, there is increasing pressure to provide more health services for less dollars and therefore a push for services to be more accountable for their expenditure. Nursing is not immune to this pressure and methods based on historical data and tradition will be difficult to sustain. Some intensive care units are using computerized patient dependency tools developed overseas but due to their expense, it is unlikely they will be widely used in Australia. Locally designed tools are needed and are being developed.

In 1988, the Commonwealth Department of Health, Housing and Community Services embarked on a 5-year program to develop a method that would facilitate the measurement of hospital performance. The Casemix Development Program was set up to study and develop casemix information systems.[17] 'The term casemix is used to describe the mix and type of patients treated by a hospital. In other words it is a hospital's workload or throughput'.[18] To obtain this casemix information for the acute hospital setting, the Diagnosis Related Group (DRG) system developed by Professor R Fetter at Yale University (USA) in the late 1960s is being adapted for Australian needs. 'The DRG system is designed to classify each acute hospital inpatient into one group within the classification system at the end of their hospital episode.'[17] This information will show the volume and mix of patients treated in a hospital and in the clinical units within that hospital (i.e. casemix). It can also be used to examine trends in treatment practices and resource utilization.

At government level, the DRG-based casemix information will be used in strategic planning and service development and in determining funding for hospitals. The hospitals will use this information for resource allocation, to review utilization, predict resource need and for quality assurance.[18]

One of the major weaknesses of DRGs is that it does not account for factors associated with the intensity of nursing care. Therefore, current methods fail to determine staffing needs accurately and also fail to identify the cost of nursing, particularly in critical care areas. This is at present being addressed by the National Nursing Service Weight Study, which is validating data collected from two states on nursing time (nursing weights). The study will determine the nursing weights/ intensity per DRG (including those DRGs under which the critically ill individuals are classified).[17] When the information of nursing service weights is available the nurse manager will be able to predict nursing requirements relative to the patient casemix in their unit.

Conclusion

Every aspect of nursing in Australia is undergoing rapid change. These changes are influenced by many factors such as government health and education policies, greater public awareness and expectations of health care issues, as well as the growth and refinement of nursing as a profession. Because of the state of flux resulting from these ever-changing influences, the issues highlighted in this chapter may well change direction. One thing that is unlikely to change, though, is that nursing is moving forward and is gaining greater recognition as a profession and therefore education is of utmost importance.

With greater recognition, nursing takes on a more influential role in health care planning and must be accountable for its consumption of the health care dollar. One of the major challenges for nursing is the ability to provide effective and competent patient nursing care based on accurate identification of the patient's needs while remaining within budgetary constraints and maintaining a high standard of care. Critical care nurses have a greater challenge in this sense, as the critically ill individual requires high-intensity care which equates with expensive care.

References

1. Castles I. *Career Paths of Qualified Nurses, Australia 1989*. Australian Bureau of Statistics, Canberra: Commonwealth Government Publishing Service, 1990.
2. Royal Australian Nursing Federation, College of Nursing Australia, National Florence Nightingale Committee of Australia, New South Wales College of Nursing (1976). Goals in nursing education. In: Nursing Targets Working Group, *Proceedings of the Nursing Educational Targets Project*. Canberra: Royal College of Nursing, 1990: Appendix 1.1.
3. Russell RL. *From Nightingale to Now, Nurse Education in Australia*. Sydney: WB Saunders, 1990: 181–96.
4. Wood P. *Nursing: Progress Through Partnership 1921–1991*. Canberra: Australian Government Publishing Service, 1990: 191–231.
5. Royal Australian Nursing Federation, College of Nursing Australia, National Florence Nightingale Committee of Australia, New South Wales College of Nursing (1976). Goals in nursing education. In: Nursing Targets Working Group, *Proceedings of the Nursing Educational Targets Project*. Canberra: Royal College of Nursing, 1990: Appendix 3.1.
6. Dawkins JS. *Higher Education: A Policy Statement*. Canberra: Australian Government Publishing Service, 1988.
7. Mascord P. The career structure and lifelong education. In: Gray G, Pratt R (eds) *Issues in Australian Nursing 3*. Melbourne: Churchill Livingstone, 1992: 281–95.
8. Department of Employment, Education and Training. *Competency Standards*, Higher Education Series. Canberra: Australian Government Publishing Service, August 1992, Information Paper No. 1.
9. Heywood L, Gonczi A, Hanger P. *A Guide to Development of Competency Standards for Professions*. National Office of Overseas Skills Recognition, Canberra: Australian Government Publishing Service, April 1992: Research Paper No. 7: 14.
10. Cameron S. Competencies for registration of nurses in Australia. In: Gray G, Pratt R (eds) *Issues in Australian Nursing 2*. Melbourne: Churchill Livingstone, 1989: 209–23.
11. Percival E. The ANRAC competencies. *The Lamp* 1992; **49**(4): 14–16.
12. ANRAC Nursing Competencies Assessment Project. *The Report to the Australasian Nurse Registering Authorities Conference*, Vol. 1, The Project Report. Queensland: University Press, 1990: 22.
13. Andrews J. Specialisation and competency standards, issues and developments. *Austral Crit Care* 1993; **6**(1): 13–15.
14. Andrews J. Specialisation and developing standards within the National Standards Framework. *Austral Crit Care* 1992; **5**(3: 6–9.
15. Beaumont M. Australian Nursing Council. *Austral Nurses J* 1992; **22**(5): 9.
16. McCoppin B. The use and abuse of industrial power – the profession's dilemma. In: Gray G, Pratt R (eds) *Issues in Australian Nursing 2*. Melbourne: Churchill Livingstone, 1989: 263–82.
17. Ferguson L. Casemix update. *Austral Crit Care* 1992; **5**(4): 11–13.
18. Picone D, Britt M, Kidd J. DRGs and casemix based hospital management, an introduction. *The Lamp* 1991; **48**(5): 19–22.

Europe

AM TIMMERMANN

At present there is no official information regarding staffing and training in intensive care units (ICUs) in

European countries. This chapter provides information gleaned from two sources:

1. Information gathered from the countries of the European Community (EC)
2. The results of an inquiry carried out at our institution, the University Hospital of Liège, concerning the hospital's ICU personnel.

Intensive care nursing in the EC

The EC is a supranational power, acting through community-agreed policies that will ultimately become law in the various member countries. With respect to nursing, the EC has worked toward producing directives concerning the recognition of the various nursing diplomas and so to facilitate free movement of nursing personnel among the member states.

To work as a nurse in an EC member country, a minimum level of basic training is necessary to obtain the title 'nurse responsible for general care'. This training consists of 2 years of basic studies and a third year of specialized work, or 4600 hours of both theoretical and practical courses. The title 'nurse responsible for general care' implies a level of function that is unanimously accepted by the EC countries, but it has no legal standing.

During the postwar years, nursing education has developed along comparable lines to the medical model. Thus, several specialized areas have been created. All 'further' nursing education, beyond the basic training, depends entirely on each country's own regulations and educational programs. The EC has not yet intervened to codify this period of continuing postregistration education, which has two important consequences:

1. Specialization is not regulated for all EC countries.
2. Specialized nurses may not have their status recognized in all countries of the EC.

To date, specific training in intensive care has not been standardized by the EC and does not have official community recognition. Each member nation can require and/or organize such training but many anomalies exist. For instance, the special training need not even be recognized within the country itself (e.g. Belgium). The implication of this is that such specialized training will not be recognized by any increase in salary, and will not be a legal requirement of anyone wishing to work in an ICU.

Intensive care training now exists in Belgium, Germany, Greece, Ireland, Italy, the Netherlands, Portugal and the United Kingdom (UK). In Luxembourg, France and Denmark, it is a specialization for the anesthetist

nurse. So, although ICU training is not officially recognized, it does nonetheless exist in the majority of EC countries. The implementation of training is a response to the needs of nursing staff working in the ICU, where the ever-increasing technology, combined with an expanding knowledge base, demands a formal training program and justifies the creation and development of the specialty of intensive care nursing.

Guidelines for nurse staffing levels for ICUs are scarce at national level and proposals vary significantly from country to country. Within a given country there is wide variation from hospital to hospital. Standards for the number of personnel are often below the real needs for a particular unit and official information concerning these standards amongst the EC member states are almost nonexistent; in Belgium no official standard has been published although several sets of recommendations are in the project stage. The semiofficial guideline is to provide three nurses for two intensive care beds (1.5/bed), which seems somewhat inadequate. Financial considerations currently allow two nurses for each type of intensive care bed (intensive care beds make up 2% of acute care beds).

A poll conducted by the Belgian Minister of Public Health in 1980, studying all hospitals, gave information about staffing levels in university hospitals. The number of on-site nurses was then used as a basis for financing these hospitals. These staffing levels are presented in Table 14.1. On average there were 2.45 nurses/bed, but

Table 14.1 Staffing levels in university hospitals

Type of ICU	Nurses/bed
CCU	1.3–1.5
ICU	2.5–3.7
Adult medical ICU	1.9–2.8
Adult surgical ICU	1.8–3.1
Cardiac surgical ICU	3.0–3.4
Pediatric ICU (especially surgical ICU)	3.5–3.7
Sterile unit ICU	2
Neonatal ICU	2.5–2.7

it can be seen that different types of unit had different staffing levels. The poll confirms that staffing levels must be adapted to each different type of unit, as determined by the department head. The intensity and proximity of care and surveillance required is a function of the patient's degree of autonomy, which itself is a function of the medical condition and age of the patient.

Each country has its own terms and conditions of service concerning the number of hours of work each week, holiday allowances, sick leave, etc. For this reason it is prudent to start any analysis of staffing requirements with the personnel needed for a 24-hour period. In doing this the related tasks such as administration which are added to patient care must not be forgotten.

Once the staff required for 24 hours coverage is defined, then the total number of personnel per unit can be easily calculated, taking into account the local regulations of employment and levels of absenteeism. The total personnel necessary for the unit would thus be the sum of:

- the personnel necessary for 24 hours coverage given the statutory defined number of hours of work per week;
- the personnel necessary to cover holidays;
- the personnel necessary to cover unexpected events (illness, absenteeism);
- the necessary support and administrative personnel for the unit.

It is for this reason that it is preferable to speak in terms of the number of nurses necessary per patient and per shift, rather than in terms of a global standard.

ICU staffing in Belgium

Given the lack of official information concerning staffing standards in intensive care, the following relates to the current situation in Belgium.

In order to take into account the opinions regarding staffing and training of people who are working in intensive care units, we made poll of the ICU personnel at our institution, the University Hospital of Liège. This has a capacity of 635 beds, which include 34 intensive care beds, with a staff of 83.75 full-time equivalents – an average of 2.46 nurses per bed. The distribution of nurses is as follows:

- CCU   (coronary care unit):   8 beds 2.1 nurses/bed
- MICU (medical ICU):   8 beds 2.5 nurses/bed
- SICU (surgical ICU):   18 beds 2.6 nurses/bed

Ninety-five questionnaires were distributed to personnel who were working or who had worked in intensive care; the response was 85%. The professional experience of such nurses is very important: 83% already have significant experience of working in this type of unit (mean time 8 years).

In order to assess the staff's perception of staffing requirements each nurse was asked to define the staff necessary for each shift of the day, for weekdays, weekends and holidays. We compared the results with the actual conditions of work defined by the hospital directorate. The numbers provided by the staff were quite close to the actual situation, except for certain shifts which were felt to be a little understaffed. The staff estimates of their requirements and the present staffing situation for the different shifts are given in Tables 14.2 to 14.4. The working hours are based on the legal conditions of work of 38 hours/week, 5 days/week.

Table 14.2 Staffing on A shift (06:45–14:51, with 30 minutes lunch break)

Unit	Weekdays		Weekend	
	Estimated (E)	Present (P)	E	P
CCU	4	4	3.5*	3
MICU	4.35*	4	4.05	4
SICU	4.3*	4	4	4

Table 14.3 Staffing on B shift (14:24–22:00)

Unit	Weekdays		Weekend	
	Estimated (E)	Present (P)	E	P
CCU	3	3	2.6	2.3
MICU	3.35*	3	3.2	3
SICU	3.95*	4	3.53*	3

Table 14.4 Staffing on the night shift (21:30–07:15)

Unit	Weekdays		Weekend	
	Estimated (E)	Present (P)	E	P
CCU	2.35*	2	2.35*	2
MICU	2.9	3	2.9	3
SICU	3	3	3	3

From the tables it can be seen that an increase in staff was felt to be needed on A shift on weekdays for the medical and surgical ICUs and at the weekend for the coronary care unit (CCU). An increase in staffing on B shift was wanted on weekdays in the medical ICU and at weekends for the surgical ICU, while on the night shift staff increases were felt to be needed in the CCU.

The heavy workload on the medical ICU is largely a result of the increasing number of hematology patients admitted in an advanced state of illness and requiring protective isolation. In the surgical ICU the increasing number of organ transplantations further increases the workload. The personnel requirements of the CCU are relatively high with respect to the national average because increasing numbers of noncoronary medical ICU patients are cared for in our CCU.

The results of the poll concerning training are quite interesting and clearly show the relationship between training and staffing in intensive care. The basic training of nurses was considered insufficient by 51% of respondents. Practical experience in the ICU was deemed to be too short, and the time devoted to basic techniques was thought to be too long relative to that devoted to major techniques. The elements necessary for rational decision making in the ICU were not required. Certain desires were expressed with respect to the basic aspects of training:

1. Increasing the length of time given to practical work in the ICU in the last year of training;
2. improving the supervision of students in the ICU with 'monitors' trained in intensive care;
3. increasing the training concerning relational and communication aspects of intensive care (patient's family) and difficult situations (death, therapy for hopeless situations, etc.).

Ninety-three per cent of respondents were involved in the supervision of newly graduated nurses. For 91.5%, the valid way to train a new nurse is to take him or her under the direct supervision of one or more fully qualified nurses. The period of supervised work should last for at least 1 month, with the new trainee as an additional team member during this period. Correctly accomplished, this period increases the utility and quality of new personnel and favors their integration into the team.

Extra training in intensive care was judged necessary by 46% of the respondents. Because the basic level of training has decreased, while the level of technology in the ICU has increased, specific, supplementary knowledge is required. Forty-two per cent of respondents felt that specific training was not necessary, because in their view coursework is often too theoretical, and because they believe that the best training takes place on-site. Twelve per cent had mixed opinions. The best period for supplementary training was thought to be during the first year of work. Only 6% of personnel saw this supplementary education as requiring an extra year of study; this is in contradiction to what is now organized by the nursing schools.

The positive aspects of supplementary training are:

1. a better understanding of certain pathologies and their treatment, enabling a better surveillance of the patient and greater staff confidence;
2. learning new techniques and use of new materials;
3. revision of certain aspects of work that were previously misunderstood or forgotten.

Thus this training increases the motivation of the personnel and decreases stress levels.

The negative aspects evoked were:

1. there was no legal or financial compensation for working in ICUs;
2. the time allocated to coursework was additional to normal working hours and family requirements. This lack of 'protected' time led to long hours and inevitable fatigue.

Conclusions

Staffing and training are interrelated and cannot be considered separately. Staffing requirements should be filled 24 hours per day throughout the year and new personnel should not be counted as full staff for the first few months of their work, so allowing for proper and thorough training.

Any supplementary training, however it is organized, must be based on practical aspects with a theoretical basis that will stimulate thought and understanding of the particular aspect under consideration; the human aspects must not be neglected.

Let us hope that the creation of the Europe of tomorrow will help us to develop these different elements, to increase the quality of care offered to our patients, and to improve the working conditions of our ICU personnel.

Bibliography

Anrys H, Dubois P, Gemelli A *et al. Les Hôpitaux dans le marché commun.* Brussels: Maison Larcier.
Bonnet F. *Technologies Hospitalière.* University of Liège
De Wever A. *Les Hôpitaux en Europe.* Cliniques Universitaires Saint Luc, Hôpital Erasme.
Formation Supérieure en Soins Infirmiers. Société de Réanimation de Langue Française, 1992.
Leroy X. *L'enseignement des soins infirmiers et l'exercice de la profession.* Brussels: AIMS.
Stinglhamber-van der Borght B. *Infirmière: genèse et réalité d'une profession.* Brussels: Edition De Boeck-Wesmael, 1991.

CHAPTER 15

Respiratory and Physical Therapy

Physical Therapy, USA
NANCY D CIESLA————————————
History 226
Governing bodies 227
Education and training 227
Treatment and training specific to critical care 227
Scope of practice 228
Staffing 229
Future 230
References 230

Canada
MARGARET E FIELDING, H RONALD WEXLER——
Education 235
Scope of practice 236
References 236

Australia
JILL C NOSWORTHY, LINDA DENEHY,
ROSEMARY P MOORE————————————
History 239
Governing bodies 239
Physiotherapy education and training 240
Staffing 242
Research and the future 243
References 243

Respiratory Care, USA
ANTHONY L BILENKI————————————
History 231
Governing bodies 231
Sponsoring organizations 232
Education and training 232
Scope of practice 232
Staffing 233
Future of respiratory therapy 234
References 234

Education and Training of Respiratory Therapists in Canada
PAUL ROBINSON, H RONALD WEXLER————
Current standards (scope) of practice 237
Current educational process 237
Continuing education 238
Future of respiratory therapy 238
References 238

Physiotherapy EC/UK
BERNADETTE HENDERSON, DIANA DAVIS———
Governing and professional bodies in the UK 244
Education 245
Clinical practice 247
Future of critical care physiotherapy in the UK 249
Physiotherapy in the EC 250
Acknowledgements 254
References 254

Physical therapy, USA

NANCY D CIESLA

History

The first reported use of physical therapy in the United States (US) was at the Children's Hospital in Boston, Massachusetts in 1898.[1] Treatments were delivered by reconstruction aides. Nineteen years later, in 1917, the US government established the Division of Special Hospitals and Physical Reconstruction.[2]

After evaluating the European model for rehabilitation, the Surgeon General asked colleges and universities in the US to establish physical therapy schools. Initial training was to provide rehabilitation to victims of World War I. 'Physiotherapy' was defined as the use of physical measures – hydrotherapy, electrotherapy, mechanotherapy, active and passive exercises and massage.[3] Breathing exercises were used in the United Kingdom to treat patients with chest injuries as early as 1915, and in 1918 postural drainage was described in the American literature.[4,5] Two years later the first neurosurgical recovery room was opened at Johns Hopkins Hospital in Baltimore, Maryland. The first multidisciplinary critical care service opened in 1958 at Baltimore City Hospital under the direction of Dr Peter Safar.[6]

Miss Winifred Linton at the Brompton Hospital in London is credited with the development of physiotherapeutic techniques for the treatment of chest disease, in 1934. However, it was not until the polio epidemic in the 1950s that physical therapists in the USA became primarily involved with children and adults with respiratory failure. Physical therapists provided assessment and designed treatment programs to improve both respiratory and extremity muscle strength. The treatment techniques used at the Brompton Hospital and during the polio epidemic are the basis for our current practice of chest physical therapy.[7] Although the indications and contraindications for active and passive exercises of the extremities used in the intensive care unit are different, the actual techniques differ little from those described in the early 1900s.

Governing bodies

The first professional organization for physical therapists, the American Women's Physical Therapeutic Association, was formed in 1921 by 274 charter members. By the late 1930s, the 1000-member association included men and changed its name to the American Physiotherapy Association. By 1947, the name was changed to the American Physical Therapy Association (APTA) which now represents over 67 168 physical therapists, physical therapy assistants, and physical therapy students. It is estimated that slightly more than half of all licensed therapists belong to the APTA. The goal of the Association is to foster improvements in physical therapy education, practice, and research.

Education and training

Formal education programs in physical therapy have existed since 1928. The medical profession began to recognize the importance of physical therapy in 1925, when the Council on Physical Therapy was established. In conjunction with the American Medical Association (AMA), the American Physiotherapy Association developed educational requirements.[2] Between 1936 and 1956 the AMA assumed responsibility for accreditation and recognition of programs. The first educational standards required graduation from a school of physical education or nursing and an additional 9

months of coursework. Accreditation responsibility was shared between the Physical Therapy Association and the AMA from 1956 until 1977. In 1977, the Commission on Accreditation in Education of the APTA was recognized as an independent accrediting agency by the US Department of Education and the Council of Postsecondary Accreditation. Since 1983, the commission has been the sole accrediting agency for entry-level education programs for the physical therapist and physical therapist assistant in the USA.[8] The physical therapist has 4–6 years of college education and training; the physical therapist assistant receives an associate's degree after 2 years of training at the community college level. All physical therapists are licensed at the state level after passing a national examination. Physical therapy assistants work under the direction of a licensed physical therapist and provide treatment after patient evaluation by a therapist. Licensure is required in some states.

Today there are 141 entry-level physical therapy and 165 physical therapy assistant accredited programs in the USA. The profession is moving from an entry-level baccalaureate to master's degree. Seventy-three programs currently offer an entry-level master's in physical therapy. All physical therapy programs require clinical experience in a variety of practice settings following didactic instruction.[8]

The profession has moved into clinical specialization in cardiopulmonary, neurological, orthopedic, and pediatric physical therapy. To sit for the specialty examination, the applicant must submit evidence of 3 years of full-time practice within the past 10 years. For cardiopulmonary specialization, 2 years of cardiopulmonary experience is required. Evidence of teaching, participation in scientific research, and administrative experience are also required.[9] Although increasing numbers of physical therapists are entering the intensive care unit (ICU) as part of the medical team providing care to critically ill and injured children and adults, there is no critical care specialty. The skills required to work in this setting include expertise in cardiopulmonary care and general musculoskeletal treatment. Patients treated by physical therapists in the ICU include those with neurological or orthopedic injury or disease.

Treatment and training specific to critical care

The polio epidemic and opening of special units to serve patients following cardiac surgery, neurosurgery, and for treatment of shock brought physical therapy into the critical care arena. Although chest physical therapy treatments were provided, patients in the intensive care unit were often considered too sick for rehabilitative services. In 1972, at the request of Dr Crawford McAslan, a British anesthesiologist, this author began working in the Shock Trauma ICU, in Baltimore, Maryland. Dr McAslan's insight led to early rehabilitation for the critically injured adult.

It is now well established that physical therapy can be initiated within days of admission to the ICU. The goals of treatment are to prevent pulmonary infection, reduce secondary complications related to immobility, prevent permanent physical deformity and decrease overall rehabilitation time. Beginning rehabilitation shortly after brain or spinal cord injury decreases total hospitalization time.[10,11] The Society of Critical Care Medicine in the USA now includes physical therapists as an essential part of the health care team for all critical care units.[12]

In the early 1970s, formal physical therapy training did not include the rationale for and types of equipment and hemodynamic monitoring unique to the ICU. The physical therapy educational curriculum has since responded to the increasing number of physical therapists working in the ICU, and to the changes in technology that have occurred with the development of critical care medicine. The Department of Education of the APTA identifies cardiopulmonary physical therapy as an integral part of the curriculum. An understanding of the cardiac and pulmonary systems as well as musculoskeletal and neurological pathophysiology is emphasized. Students are trained to recognize the influence of pathology, pathophysiology, and hemodynamic alterations associated with immobility and exercise. To prepare for clinical practice, students are trained in basic electrocardiography, auscultation of the lungs, monitoring of blood pressure and peripheral pulses. Students are introduced to the types of ventilators and specialty beds found in the ICU and the rationale for their use. Instruction in the placement and purpose of intravascular lines to measure arterial and venous pressures, the use of pulse oximetry, assessment of arterial blood gases, and airway suctioning are recommended for entry-level curricula.[13]

There are regional differences as to the type and extent of physical therapy services in the ICU. In the USA physical therapists tend to be more involved in respiratory care on the East coast and in cardiac and rehabilitative procedures on the West coast. There are more physical therapy services in the ICU at major medical centers than community hospitals. National statistics are not available on the number of therapists working in intensive care. However, the R Adams Cowley Shock Trauma Center in Baltimore has provided comprehensive physical therapy to the ICU trauma patient since 1974. The Shock Trauma physical therapy department sponsors an annual course for training of therapists working with the adult ICU patient. Over the past 12 years the attendance has

included representation from the majority of states and the number of course participants quadrupled.

Scope of practice

The following section is an overview of physical therapy services commonly provided in the ICU (Table 15.1). The plan of care is developed and modified in concert with the medical staff's daily assessment of patient stability and prognosis. Specific variations in the treatment approach according to age, illness, or disease are beyond the scope of this chapter.

Table 15.1 Physical therapy treatment in the ICU

Intervention	Rationale
Chest physical therapy	Clear atelectasis, prevent pulmonary infection, increase respiratory muscle strength
Range of motion: passive, active, resistive	Prevent joint contracture, prevent muscle atrophy, maintain functional muscle strength
Bed positioning	Prevent postural deformities Maintain normal joint range of motion Decrease the influence of abnormal muscle tone
Transfers from supine to sitting/standing.	Minimize effects of immobility on all body systems, e.g. increase vital capacity, prevent bone demineralization, prevent orthostatic intolerance
Ambulation: while ventilating patient via manual resuscitator bag, supplemental oxygen and intravascular lines accompanying patient	Assist in weaning from mechanical ventilation, minimize effects of immobility on all body systems
Serial casting/splinting	Prevent joint contracture, maximize functional positioning

From ref. 16, with permission.

CHEST PHYSICAL THERAPY

Chest physical therapy is best incorporated into the total rehabilitation plan of the patient. Based on a clear-cut indication for treatment such as an atelectasis, infiltrate,

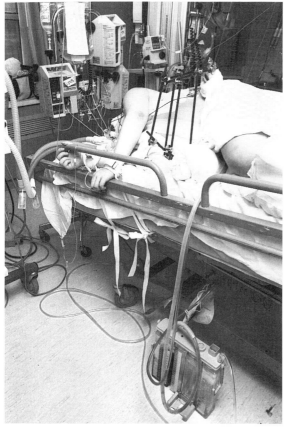

Fig. 15.1 Even the most critically injured patients can usually be positioned for segmental postural drainage.

clinical evidence of secretion retention, or decrease in arterial oxygenation thought to be a result of secretion retention; postural drainage, percussion and vibration are performed. Even the most critically injured patients can usually be positioned for segmental postural drainage (Fig. 15.1). Patients are taught breathing exercises and cough stimulation techniques. Initial assessment includes determination of the patient's level of mobility. After a clinical assessment and evaluation of the patient's response to treatment; patient mobilization, breathing exercises and cough instruction may replace segmental postural drainage with manual techniques. Nurses and respiratory therapists are also part of the team of health care professionals assisting with airway clearance – postural drainage, percussion, vibration and suctioning.

REHABILITATION

Patients at high risk for contracture and motor deficit are assessed very early in the ICU. The rehabilitative phase of ICU physical therapy includes a comprehensive

assessment of range of motion, muscle strength, movement patterns and functional mobility. The goal of therapy in the ICU is to maintain functional mobility, not increase muscle strength. Treatment interventions include range of motion exercises, bed positioning, transfers from supine to sitting and standing, and ambulation training. Active, passive and resistive range of motion exercises are utilized, depending upon the patient's clinical status. Multiple catheters and lines may inhibit spontaneous movement, for example the presence of a chest tube may increase shoulder pain and restrict shoulder motion. Subclavian catheters may cross the shoulder joint and limit shoulder range of motion. Tightness of the shoulder capsule can be minimized through gentle active range of motion exercises or passive stretching with joint mobilization techniques.

Occasionally, a noncompliant patient or patient exhibiting severe abnormal muscle tone cannot be assessed accurately for joint versus muscle contracture. Assessing joint motion following a scheduled operative procedure, while the patient is under general anesthesia, will allow the therapist to discriminate between joint

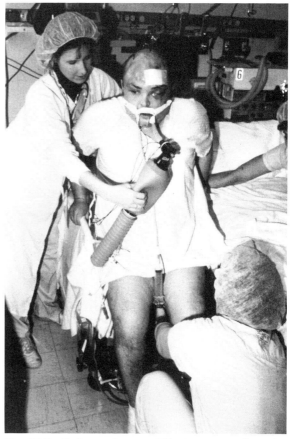

Fig. 15.2 Patients who are difficult to wean from the ventilator benefit from progressive mobilization while one therapist provides ventilation with a manual resuscitator bag.

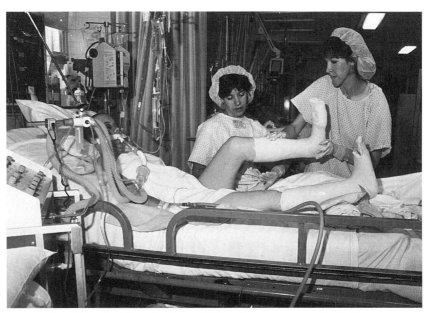

Fig. 15.3   Serial casting is used following acute severe brain injury.

and muscle pathology and thus select appropriate treatment interventions.

Therapeutic positioning, such as placing a brain-injured patient with increased extensor muscle tone in the sidelying position, is used to maintain normal range of motion. To minimize the systemic effects of immobility on all body systems, even the most critical patient can often be assisted with changing body position from supine to sitting or standing and taught to transfer from bed to chair. At the physician's discretion, patients requiring supplemental oxygen may ambulate despite the presence of intravascular lines, electrocardiogram leads, abdominal drains and chest tubes. Patients who are difficult to wean from the ventilator benefit from progressive mobilization while one therapist provides ventilation with a manual resuscitator bag (Fig. 15.2). Psychological as well as physical benefit is derived from this approach.

Serial casting is used following acute severe brain injury to prevent equinus deformity and to enhance rehabilitation (Fig. 15.3). Early casting does not appear to increase intracranial pressure or the incidence of deep venous thrombosis.[15] Physical therapists in the ICU also educate the staff, the patient, and the family to maximize the patient's performance in activities in daily living.

Staffing

Physical therapy staffing in the critical care unit varies depending upon staff availability, physician preference and hospital resources. Critical care medicine standards require a minimum of Monday through Friday services on the daytime shift. This is usually adequate for rehabilitative care. Hospitals providing chest physical therapy services usually offer additional coverage, ranging from daytime and evening coverage 365 days per year to daytime coverage 5 days per week and limited weekend services.

Future

The future holds an ever-expanding role for the physical therapist in critical care. Technological advances in respiratory and hemodynamic monitoring will allow ongoing assessment of treatment interventions and clinical research to better evaluate the efficacy of specific procedures. However, the fact that physical therapy is an art as well as a science should not be overlooked as our technology advances. In rehabilitative ICU care, the therapist's interpersonal skills may be more important that the use of one very specialized treatment technique over another. Patients' motivation and desire to return to a previous level of functioning are key factors in determining their functional outcome.

References

1. Kigin C. Evolution of pulmonary physical therapy in the United States. *Physiother Practice* 1986; **2**: 22–30.

2. The beginning of modern physiotherapy. *Phys Ther* 1976; **56**: 15–21.

3. Granger FB. The development of physiotherapy. *Phys Ther Rev* 1923; **3**: 14–19.

4. MacMahon C. Breathing and physical exercises for use in cases of wounds in the pleura and lung and diaphragm. *Lancet* 1915; **ii**: 769–70.

5. Bushnell GE. The treatment of tuberculosis. *Am Rev Tuberc* 1918; **2**: 259–74.

6. Weil MH, Von Planta M, Rackow EC. Critical care medicine: introduction and historical perspective. In: Shoemaker WC, Ayres S, Grenvik A, Halbrook PR, Thompson WL (eds) *Textbook of Critical Care*. Philadelphia: WB Saunders, 1989: 1–3.

7. Gaskell DV, Webber BA. *The Brompton Hospital Guide to Chest Physiotherapy*. Boston: Blackwell Scientific Publications, 1980: vii.

8. Evaluative criteria for accreditation of education programs for the preparation of physical therapists. Alexandria, Virginia: Commission on Accreditation in Physical Therapy Education, American Physical Therapy Association, 1992.

9. Cardiopulmonary Specialty Council. Alexandria, Virginia: American Physical Therapy Association, 1989.

10. Mackay LE, Bernstein BA, Chapman P, Morgan A, Milazzo LS. Early intervention in severe head injury: long-term benefits of a formalized program. *Arch Phys Med Rehabil* 1992; **73**: 635–41.

11. Oakes DD, Wilmot SB, Hall KM, Sherck. Benefits of early admission to a comprehensive trauma center for patients with spinal cord injury. *Arch Phys Med Rehabil* 1990; **71**: 637–43.

12. Guidelines for categorization of services for the critically ill patient. *Crit Care Med* 1991; **19**: 279–85.

13. American Physical Therapy Association. Department of Education Task Force on content of post baccalaureate degree entry-level curricula, April 1992.

14. Ciesla N. Postural drainage, positioning, breathing exercises. In: Mackenzie CF (ed.) *Chest Physiotherapy in the Intensive Care Unit*. Baltimore: Williams & Wilkins, 1989: 93–107.

15. Murdock K, Gerold K, Keller C, Ciesla N. Serial casting of the lower extremity is not associated with increased risk of DVT. Proceedings of National Trauma Symposium, Baltimore, Maryland, March 1992.

16. Imle PC. Changes with immobility and methods of mobilization. In: Mackenzie CF (ed.) *Chest Physiotherapy in the Intensive Care Unit*. Balitimore: Williams & Wilkins, 1989: 93–107.

Respiratory care, USA

ANTHONY L BILENKI

History

Respiratory care is defined as an allied health profession that provides treatment to persons with abnormalities and deficiencies of the cardiopulmonary system.[1,2] The profession was established in the late 1940s and early 1950s. Prior to this, hospitals were staffed by oxygen technicians trained on the job who supplied oxygen, mixed gases and respiratory equipment to patients with cardiopulmonary disease. As equipment and technology improved, the oxygen technician became the ideal person to deliver inhalation therapy. By 1959 education and training were still hospital based, but the oxygen technician was now eligible to sit for an examination given by the American Registry of Inhalation Therapists (ARIT). A candidate successfully completing the testing became known as a Registered Inhalation Therapist (RIT).[2]

Scientific and technological advances allowed more and more hospitals to open critical care units and critical care medicine became a specialty in itself. This resulted in increased responsibilities for the inhalation therapist from the late 1960s to 1980s. Improvement in cardiopulmonary and mechanical ventilation techniques and the introduction of central venous pressure and pulmonary artery pressure monitoring required the addition of a trained clinician to manage the patient in the critical care setting. A respiratory therapist with formal training was the best candidate to face the challenges of patient care in the critical care setting. In 1962 the American Medical Association (AMA) approved criteria for inhalation therapy programs under their Council of Medical Education.[2]

The respiratory care practitioner's responsibilities continued to expand as techniques such as independent lung ventilation (ILV), pressure-controlled inverse ratio ventilation (PCIRV) and extracorporeal membrane oxygenation (ECMO) all became therapies that the respiratory therapist was able to provide. This expansion of the practitioner's scope of clinical practice came about due to the clinicians' increasing knowledge of pathophysiology, patient assessment, and use of equipment such as microprocessor ventilators, oscillation ventilators and extracorporeal support devices.[2]

Governing bodies

In 1947, in Chicago, Illinois, a group of oxygen technicians and pulmonary physicians incorporated the Inhalation Therapy Association (ITA). The association began to coordinate the activities of the practitioners and allowed them to be more responsive to the needs of their patients. The ITA created a forum for the exchange of ideas and interaction between the disciplines. Specific criteria for credentialing were also established[2–4] (see Table 15.2).

The American Association for Respiratory Care (AARC) has grown in responsibility over the years, and

Table 15.2 Chronology of the AARC and NBRC[1,5,6]

1947	Inhalation Therapy Association (ITA) incorporated
1948	ITA named
1954	Name changed to the American Association for Inhalation Therapy (AAIT)
1959	American Registry of Inhalation Therapists (ARIT) formed
1973	Name changed to the American Association for Respiratory Therapy (AART)
1974	National Board for Respiratory Therapy (NBRT) formed
1976	ARIT designation changed to RRT
1983	The NBRT name changed to The National Board for Respiratory Care (NBRC)
1986	AART Name changed to the American Association for Respiratory Care (AARC)[2]

has established standards for the practice of respiratory care in the USA.[1,4] The National Board for Respiratory Care (NBRC) is the agency that administers the credentialing examination for both registered therapists and certified technicians.[5,6]

Sponsoring organizations

Respiratory care organizations such as the ITA, AARC and ARIT began with support of physicians with backgrounds in pulmonary medicine.[2,3] Table 15.3 lists the bodies that comprise the Board of Medical Advisors (BOMA) for the AARC.[3] The NBRC, which administers the national credentials, is sponsored by a variety of medical organizations[5,6] (see Table 15.4).

Table 15.3 AARC sponsoring organizations[1]

American College of Chest Physicians (ACCP)
American Society of Anesthesiologists (ASA)
American Thoracic Society (ATS)
Society for Critical Care Medicine (SCCM)
American Academy of Pediatrics (AAP)
American Academy of Allergy and Immunology (ACAI)[5]

Table 15.4 NBRC sponsoring organizations[5,6]

American Association for Respiratory Care (AARC)
American College of Chest Physicians (ACCP)
American Society of Anesthesiologists (ASA)
American Thoracic Society (ATS)
National Society for Cardiovascular Technology/Pulmonary Technology (NSCT/NSPT)[5]

Education and training

There are two types of respiratory care practitioners in the USA, registered respiratory therapists (RRT) and certified respiratory therapy technicians (CRTT). As of 1992 there were approximately 44 000 RRTs and 66 000 CRTTs.[5,6]

An individual may enter the profession by pursuing the following educational pathways:

1. *RRT*: After high school, a college/university based program is followed that results in a 2-year associate or a 4-year bachelor degree. Course work in anatomy and physiology, microbiology, chemistry, biology, mathematics and physics must be included in the respiratory care curriculum.[5,6]
2. *Other pathways*: Individuals who have other associate or bachelor degrees with the previously mentioned course work can be eligible for credentialing by completing 4 and 2 years, respectively, of full-time clinical experience, and successful completion of the CRTT test as an entry level credential.[5–7]
3. *CRTT*: A 1-year program is followed after high school. This program must be approved by the AMA committee on allied health education and accreditation. This individual must also successfully complete the CRTT examination. The CRTT credential is the minimum that an individual should possess in order to practice respiratory care.[2,6,7]

Scope of practice

The scope of practice for the respiratory therapist depends in part on institutional/physician preference. Respiratory therapy practice includes obtaining and analyzing blood samples for pH and blood gas analysis, oxygen administration, mechanical ventilation, care of the artificial airway, bronchopulmonary hygiene, administration of inhaled medications and cardiopulmonary resuscitation.

The respiratory therapist may be responsible for obtaining blood samples by percutaneous or capillary punctures, from peripheral arterial and venous lines, and from pulmonary artery catheters. These blood samples are used to determine acid–base and blood gas levels.[1]

The respiratory therapist may also be responsible for obtaining hemodynamic data from patients with Swan–Ganz catheters in the critical care setting. The use of noninvasive monitors such as pulse oximeters, end-tidal carbon dioxide monitors, and transcutaneous oxygen and carbon dioxide monitors is increasing, enabling the practitioner to observe trends in oxygenation and ventilatory status.

Oxygen administration is a primary focus of the respiratory therapist. The devices used range from simple low-flow systems such as the nasal cannula, a simple face mask and partial and non-rebreathing face masks, to high-flow oxygen systems that provide exact concentrations of oxygen to the patient. High-flow systems are configured to meet the patient's inspiratory flow demand and their demand for oxygen at a predetermined oxygen concentration. These systems usually include a Venturi device and systems where gases are blended and analyzed to deliver the desired concentration.

Continuous positive airway pressure (CPAP) is used in situations where a patient may need additional support to improve oxygenation and may be indicated instead of mechanical ventilation. Nasal CPAP can also be used in patients with chronic lung disease and/or muscle fatigue, avoiding intubation and mechanical ventilation.

Respiratory therapists may also be responsible for the delivery of mixed gases like helium and oxygen. Helium, a gas that is less dense than air, is used to carry oxygen molecules past an obstruction. This type of therapy may be used to treat patients with croup or epiglottitis.

Innovations in mechanical ventilation have widened the role of the respiratory therapist significantly. The therapist is responsible for operating, monitoring, and maintaining the patient–mechanical ventilator interface, including adjustment of the ventilator to maintain physiologic parameters as directed by a physician. Ventilators have evolved over the years from machines that were once simple devices that delivered preset amounts of pressure at predetermined times with little consideration for patient response or effort, to microprocessor-controlled devices that sense patient effort and even provide ventilatory support only when necessary.[7,8]

Respiratory therapists also participate in the care of the artificial airway. In rural/community hospitals they may perform endotracheal intubation in the critical care and emergency room setting. In the university hospital setting, endotracheal intubation is the responsibility of anesthesiology and/or critical care staff; here the respiratory therapist may assume responsibility for manipulation, and maintenance of the position of the endotracheal tube, and routine changing of tracheostomy tubes for patients with established tracheostomies.[9–11]

In the USA the respiratory therapist, physical therapist and nurse perform bronchopulmonary hygiene. The health care professional involved in airway clearance varies with available personnel and institutional practice. Different techniques are used to facilitate the removal of secretions such as postural drainage, percussion, vibration, breathing exercises, incentive spirometry, positive expiratory pressure (PEP) therapy and tracheal aspiration. The respiratory therapist evaluates each patient and, in consultation with the physician, formulates a plan of care.[12,13]

Respiratory therapists assume an active role in the administration of inhaled pulmonary medications. These drugs may be delivered by small volume nebulizer, positive pressure breathing device, continuous nebulization system, metered dose inhaler or ultrasonic nebulizer. Medications such as bronchodilators, mucolytics, steroids, antibiotics, antiviral agents and bland aerosols may be administered in this manner; the respiratory therapist determines with a physician the most effective method.

Respiratory therapists perform cardiopulmonary resuscitation and participate in trauma management in many hospitals. The therapist may perform any one of many duties such as endotracheal intubation, airway management, closed chest massage, oxygen administration, bag–valve–mask ventilation, drug administration via tracheal instillation, patient transport, mechanical ventilation, or hemodynamic monitoring. The therapist is thus an important member of the health care team.[9,10]

Respiratory therapists perform other duties in addition to direct patient care duties. They may act in a consultant role to determine the most beneficial type of respiratory care for patients. They may serve as a faculty member in critical care medicine with teaching and research responsibilities. The respiratory therapist may also administer and maintain extracorporeal gas exchange in the critical care setting. The duties performed vary from hospital to hospital and state to state.

Staffing

Staffing requirements differ from hospital to hospital. Generally, a hospital will have at least one respiratory therapist for each critical care unit. This may be based on the severity of illness of the patients so that a university hospital will have more respiratory therapists available in critical care areas. Smaller community hospitals on the other hand may only have one therapist assigned to staff an entire hospital on a night shift. All hospitals provide coverage for respiratory care 24 hours a day, 365 days a year.

As hospitals look for ways to optimize their use of manpower, the respiratory therapist may be identified as an individual capable of assuming additional responsibility for other cardiopulmonary technologies. Future health care will see increased technology requiring a

unified entry level for all respiratory practitioners which
may promote increased consistency in job responsibilities of respiratory clinicians throughout the USA. As
a result, the care delivered by respiratory therapists
will be maintained at a safe and acceptable level of
quality.

This may necessitate more delegation of routine
procedures to subordinates with supervision by an RRT.
At present many hospitals allow both CRTTs and RRTs
to perform the same duties in the critical care setting.
The CRTT should be viewed as an entry-level clinician
and will perform basic forms of therapy while the RRT
will be left to perform the more complex duties that
may include extracorporeal membrane oxygenation
(ECMO), intravascular oxygenation (IVOX), all types
of mechanical ventilation, and maintenance of indwelling arterial blood gas monitors.

Future of respiratory therapy

Future changes in science and medicine will result in
more sophisticated advances in technology. These
advances will require appropriate practitioners to plan,
implement and evaluate the changes and will place
more demands on the respiratory therapist.

References

1. The American Association for Respiratory Care. *Statement of Principles/Position Statements*. Dallas, Texas:
   The American Association for Respiratory Care, 1978.
2. Eubanks DH, Bone RC. Professional growth and interaction. In: *Comprehensive Respiratory Care: A Learning
   System*, 2nd edn. St Louis: CV Mosby, 1990: 3–7.
3. Masferrer R. History of the inhalation therapy – respiratory care profession. In: Burton GC, Hodgkin JE (eds)
   Respiratory Care: A Guide to Clinical Practice, 2nd edn.
   Philadelphia: JB Lippincott Company, 1984: 5–10.
4. Eubanks DH, Bone RC. Professional growth and interactions. In: *Comprehensive Respiratory Care: A
   Learning System*, 2nd ed. St Louis: CV Mosby, 1990:
   7–8.
5. The National Board for Respiratory Care. *NBRC Directory*. Lenaxa, Kansas: The National Board for Respiratory
   Care, 1992: vii.
6. The National Board for Respiratory Care. *Standards of
   Excellence*. Lenaxa, Kansas: The National Board for
   Respiratory Care, 1989.
7. Kigin C. Evolution of pulmonary physical therapy in the
   United States. *Physiother Practice* 1986; **2**: 22–30.
8. Masferrer R. History of the inhalation therapy – Respiratory therapy profession. In: Burton GC, Hodgkin JE (eds)
   Respiratory Care: A Guide to Clinical Practice, 2nd edn.
   Philadelphia: JB Lippincott, 1984: 11.
9. Kacmarek RM. AARC Program Committee Lecture.
   Respiratory Care Practitioner – Carpe Diem. *Respir Care*
   1992; **37**: 264–9.
10. Kacmarek RM. The role of the respiratory therapist in
    emergency care. *Respir Care* 1992; **37**: 523–30.
11. Barnes TA, Durbin CG [editorial]. ACLS skills for the
    respiratory therapist: time for a mandate. *Respir Care*
    1992; **37**: 516–19.
12. Mahlmeister MJ, Fink JB, Hoffman GL, Fifer LF.
    Positive-expiratory-pressure mask therapy: theoretical
    considerations and a review of the literature. *Respir Care*
    1991; **36**: 1218–30.
13. Lewis RM [editorial]. Chest physical therapy: time for a
    redefinition and a renaming. *Respir Care* 1992; **37**:
    419–21.

Canada

MARGARET E FIELDING, H RONALD WEXLER

Physiotherapy has been recognized as an integral part of
health care in Canada since World War I. The profession emerged in response to the identified need for
rehabilitation for the returning men and women of
Canada's air force, army and navy.

Physiotherapists provide treatment to patients with
dysfunction of all body systems – musculoskeletal,
neurological, cardiovascular and dermal. They are also
involved in the management of all stages of disease and
dysfunction from the acute or intensive care level to the
chronic and the rehabilitative stages. Physiotherapists
provide care throughout the life cycle from prenatal and
neonatal through to geriatric.

The practice of physiotherapy is regulated in Canada
in all ten provinces. The profession is self-regulating
and is governed by the respective provincial regulatory
bodies. In addition the Canadian Physiotherapy Association–L'Association canadienne de physiotherapie,
with its provincial branches, has developed rules of
conduct and a code of ethics for the profession.

In order to practice in Canada physiotherapists must
obtain a 4-year baccalaureate degree in physical therapy
from a Canadian Physiotherapy Association accredited
university program and meet provincial statutory regulations. Currently there are 13 universities in Canada
that offer courses leading to a physical therapy or
physiotherapy degree. In some instances the title of the
degree is rehabilitation.

In 1992 there were 4800 physiotherapists registered
to practice in Ontario, with in excess of 10 000 in
Canada. By nature of their education experience and
clinical skill, physiotherapists have much to offer the
patient who is critically ill.

Education

Although critical care is not specifically designated as an area for study at the undergraduate level, many of the courses in cardiology, respirology, pathology, human physiology and anatomy contain material that prepares the physiotherapists to treat this population.

The Canadian Physiotherapy Association Core Curriculum[1] indicates the expectations of what the student will be able to accomplish upon graduation. Those areas of particular import to critical care relate to the impact on the musculoskeletal, cardiovascular, respiratory, nervous and dermal systems of:

- physiological responses and functional outcomes when pathology develops;
- the etiology, pathology, clinical signs and symptoms and prognosis of systemic disease and common disorders including those due to congenital, developmental, degenerative, inflammatory and traumatic causes;
- the effects and complications of surgery, general anesthetic and prolonged bed rest;
- the degrees of burns and difference between superficial and deep burns as they relate to soft tissue structure and the body's response to skin loss.

Newly graduated physiotherapists are able to obtain an accurate history and a complete description of all pertinent problems. They select, apply and interpret evaluation procedures and identify problems and dysfunctions that are susceptible to physiotherapeutic intervention. Physiotherapists plan, select, apply and modify as necessary the physiotherapy management program for the patients.

At the same time they are able to discuss the indications and merits of the various interventions with their colleagues, as well as the patient and family members, to ensure that they consent to and will comply with these interventions. Physiotherapists are aware of the legal and ethical considerations that affect the delivery of their care.

Prior to graduation physiotherapy students are required to complete between 1000 and 1200 hours of clinical practice. During this time they learn to establish interpersonal relationships based on respect for the dignity of each individual, to respect the patient's right to confidentiality and to modify theories and principles when dealing with the various age groups and acuity of the disease, disorder or dysfunction.

During the early years of clinical practice many physiotherapists will work in various settings to gain a variety of experience before deciding on an area of concentration. In the area of critical care, physiotherapists would normally be those specializing in cardiopulmonary or cardiorespiratory physiotherapy and who also develop an interest or subspecialty in critical care. In small institutions physiotherapy for patients in critical care may be part of a general specialization in medical and surgical management of patients.

Since medical knowledge is continuously expanding, one of the major challenges for the graduate physiotherapist is to stay abreast of current knowledge. There are various routes open to those seeking to enhance their level of knowledge.

LITERATURE REVIEW

The Canadian Physiotherapy Association publishes a scientific journal, as do many other national associations, such as the American Physical Therapy Association, the Chartered Society of Physiotherapy (of Great Britain) and the Australian, New Zealand and South African associations. In addition there are many interest groups that publish newsletters and publications from other professional groups that can be accessed.

CONTINUING EDUCATION

Most of the universities in Canada now offer a masters level program in physiotherapy or rehabilitation. Many of these programs encourage clinical enquiry and have a research component as a requirement. Although at present there are no doctorate level courses specifically in physiotherapy, a significant number of physiotherapists have pursued doctor of philosophy programs in related fields such as anatomy, physiology or epidemiology.

Short continuing education courses are a way of life for the practicing physiotherapist. These courses and seminars may be offered by the national professional association, one of its many special interest divisions, or provincial or local branches. In addition many health care or educational institutions and consulting companies offer these short programs. Many physiotherapists also find programs offered by other professional groups assist them in increasing their knowledge base. Many of these short courses are offered over a weekend which allows the physiotherapists to participate without interrupting their availability to provide patient care.

NETWORKING AND CONSULTATION

Networking and consultation with colleagues from both within and outside the profession at conferences, seminars, teaching and patient care rounds, and supervising the clinical practice of student physiotherapists provides the new graduate and the more experienced physiotherapists with opportunities to be aware of new developments both within the physiotherapy scene and health care in general.

TEXTBOOKS

Textbooks on such subjects as *Chest Physiotherapy in the Intensive Care Unit* by CF Mackenzie,[2] *The Essentials of Respiratory Physiology* by West[3] or Kryger's *Introduction to Respiratory Medicine*[4] and *Chest, Heart and Vascular Disorders for Physiotherapists* by Cash,[5] to name but a few, become ready references for physiotherapists in critical care.

Scope of practice

As currently practiced in Canada, chest physiotherapy includes the assessment of chest movement, breathing patterns, respiratory rate and rhythm, breath sounds and adventitial sounds, as well as chest X-ray and blood gas information. The selection and performance of physiotherapeutic techniques is made to improve and correct malfunctions detected in the assessment, according to the patient's tolerance.

These techniques will usually include breathing exercises with shaking, vibrations, squeezing, clapping and positioning. It may also include teaching the patient to use an incentive spirometer and mechanical vibration to the chest wall.

If the patient is unable to cooperate with breathing exercises some facilitation techniques may be applied. These will attempt to alter breathing patterns. If there are increased or retained secretions, positioning or postural drainage could be used with manual or mechanical vibrations, shaking, springing, or clapping to expedite removal of these secretions. If the patient is unable to eliminate the secretions himself they may be removed by nasotracheal or endotracheal suction. Moving the patient in bed, transferring out of bed or ambulating may also be used to improve respiratory status. Ventilatory and general muscle training may be used to assist in weaning the patient from a ventilator. The type and frequency of treatment selected and performed is directly related to the assessment and on how the patient responds to and tolerates the treatment.

In addition to the general mobilization of the patient in bed and transferring out of bed, the patient will be encouraged to perform foot and ankle exercises, active range of motion and muscle strengthening exercises. As soon as able the patient will be assisted to standing and walking activities. If necessary the patient may be ambulated with or without walking aids and, if necessary, using a portable ventilator.

An active rehabilitation program will be initiated when appropriate. This will frequently involve transporting the patient to the physiotherapy gym. Noted effects include a lightening of the patient's affect, facilitation of the weaning process from the ventilator and the eventual rehabilitation of the patient. It has been shown that exercise directed toward development of strength and endurance of the arms and upper body musculature, in association with adequate nutrition, leads to earlier weaning from mechanical ventilator support.

All assessment findings, treatments, and the patient's response and appropriate modifications are documented on the patient record.

References

1. Canadian Physiotherapy Association. *Recommended Core Curriculum for Physiotherapy Education Programs.* Canadian Physiotherapy Association, 1985.
2. Mackenzie CF, Imle PC, Ciesla N. *Chest Physiotherapy in the Intensive Care Unit,* 2nd edn. Baltimore: Williams & Wilkins, 1989.
3. West JB. *Respiratory Physiology – The Essentials,* 4th edn. Baltimore: Williams & Wilkins, 1985.
4. Kryger MH. *Introduction to Respiratory Medicine,* 2nd edn. New York: Churchill Livingston Inc, 1990.
5. Cash JE. *Chest, Heart and Vascular Disorders for Physiotherapists.* London: Faber & Faber, 1975.

Education and training of respiratory therapists in Canada

PAUL ROBINSON,
H RONALD WEXLER

Respiratory therapy is an allied health profession that has seen exceptional growth in the past 30 years. Physicians and allied health workers alike are often unfamiliar with the scope of practice and role of the Registered Respiratory Therapist (RRT).

The Respiratory Therapy Act, passed by the Province of Ontario, defines the practice of respiratory therapy as 'the providing of oxygen therapy, cardio-respiratory equipment monitoring and the assessment and treatment of cardio-respiratory and associated disorders to maintain or restore ventilation.'[1] A RRT requires skills in patient care and the ability to operate and interface highly technical medical equipment with these patients.

The combination of these skills makes the RRT an essential person in today's technically oriented health care system.

RRTs practice their profession primarily in the following areas: critical care (for adults, children and neonates), anesthesia, cardiopulmonary diagnostics, routine therapeutics and home care.[2] Presently, respiratory therapy is one of 24 newly recognized medical disciplines recognized under the new Ontario Regulated Health Professionals Act.[3]

Current standards (scope) of practice

At the time of writing, the Canadian Society of Respiratory Therapists (CSRT) Education Committee is in the process of creating the Scope of Practice Document for Respiratory Therapy on a national level. Several provinces have already completed Scope of Practice Documents for their own provincial bodies.[4] The challenge for any Respiratory Therapy Scope of Practice document, particularly on a national level, is to reflect the varying ranges of practice of the profession. As hospitals and technology have grown, respiratory therapists, with their specialized mix of clinical and technical training, have molded themselves to the needs of individual hospitals. Consequently the scope of practice for therapists varies markedly from region to region and hospital to hospital.

Standards of practice recently completed in Ontario have categorized the scope of practice into 'basic skills' and 'added skills'.[5] Basic skills are those which are taught in an accredited respiratory therapy program. Added skills require further theoretical instruction and clinical experience. Tables 15.6 and 15.7 represent a condensed outline of the standards for the practice of respiratory therapy in the province of Ontario. While standards for other regions across Canada may vary, the skills listed in Tables 15.6 and 15.7 represent the basic practice of respiratory therapy.

Current educational process

Respiratory therapy in Canada is offered at the community college level. Programs are accredited by the Canadian Medical Association through the Committee on Conjoint Accreditation. Conjoint accreditation is a process designed to ensure national standards for educational programs in designated health science professions.[6] Table 15.5 lists the collaborating organizations that comprise the membership of the Committee on Conjoint Accreditation specifically for respiratory

Table 15.5 Collaborating organizations comprising the Committee on Conjoint Accreditation for respiratory therapy[7]

Canadian Society of Respiratory Therapists
Canadian Thoracic Society
Canadian Anaesthetists' Society
Canadian Paediatric Society
Canadian Critical Care Society
Canadian Medical Association
Association of Canadian Community Colleges
Canadian Hospital Association

Table 15.6 Respiratory therapy scope of practice: basic skills[5]

Airway management
Endotracheal intubation
Endotracheal extubation
Endotracheal, nasophyryngeal and tracheostomy care
Suctioning
Maintaining and ventilating an airway manually
Blood gases
Bronchoscopy assistance, ventilation, instillation
Electrocardiography
Exercise testing
Monitoring devices – calibration, setup and surveillance
Pulmonary function testing
Specimen handling
Arterial puncture
Pulmonary artery lines
Medical gas therapy
Medical vacuum
Ambulatory care
Drainage devices
Drug administration – inhalation, topical
Patient assessment
Rehabilitation
Resuscitation
Transport of the critically ill adult, pediatric and neonate
Physical therapy – percussion, postural drainage, vibration
Ventilatory management – inhalation, management, assessment and weaning

Table 15.7 Respiratory therapy scope of practice: added skills[5]

Allergy testing and desensitization
Infusion pumps
Nutritional assessment
Hyperbaric therapy
Drug administration – intravenous
Electrical stimulation

Table 15.8 CSRT National Curriculum categories[9]

General anatomy and physiology
Respiratory system
Cardiovascular system
Respiratory pathophysiology
Disease of other systems
Pharmacology
Infection control
Applied science
Patient assessment
Professionalism
Therapeutic modalities
Auxiliary equipment
Adjunctive procedures
Cardiopulmonary function testing
Blood gas analysis
Ventilators
Ventilation
Anesthesia

therapy. Currently, there are 17 CMA accredited educational programs in Canada for respiratory therapy.[8]

While entry requirements for respiratory therapy programs vary according to individual institutions, a background in physics, chemistry and mathematics is required. Although some programs have a minimum preacceptance educational level of secondary school grade 12, due to limited enrolment and high numbers of applicants many successful applicants have some postsecondary education.

Programs in respiratory therapy must offer a minimum of 45 weeks of didactic teaching and a minimum of 40 weeks of clinical experience.[6] Course content for the programs is guided by the Canadian Society of Respiratory Therapists' (CSRT) National Curriculum. The curriculum is divided into 18 categories as listed in Table 15.8.[9] Graduates of accredited respiratory therapy programs may then challenge the National Registry Examination set by the Canadian Board for Respiratory Care (CBRC).

The CBRC was incorporated in 1991 to set, administer, and grade a bilingual national registry examination. Prior to 1990 the registry examination was under the jurisdiction of the CSRT. Today the examination process is completely independent of the CSRT, although the CBRC adheres to the CSRT National Curriculum.[8] Successful candidates of the CBRC registry examination become registered with CSRT and are allowed to practice as registered respiratory therapists (RRTs).

Continuing education

Until recently, continuing education for RRTs has been the responsibility of the individual therapists. The

CSRT has developed a program to credit the RRT for postdiploma educational experience through the use of CERT (Continuing Education for Respiratory Therapists). CERT is a program where the RRT can obtain and accumulate points for attending educational conferences, forums or workshops. Guidelines for postdiploma curricula in the areas of neonatology, cardiopulmonary diagnostics and anesthesia have been approved by the Medical Advisory Board of the CSRT.[10] This will allow institutions to begin postdiploma programs, giving the RRT the opportunity to formally specialize in a clinical area.

The CSRT, with the CMA, publishes one scientific journal, *Registered Respiratory Therapist*, which prints technical and medical papers of current value as well as establishing a medium to keep members informed of Society news. Several provincial Societies also publish their own journals.

Future of respiratory therapy

In light of current economic conditions and the restructuring of health care, the future of respiratory therapy is quite unpredictable. The rapid growth of the profession can be attributed to the special training and skills of the respiratory therapists, making them ideal practitioners in hi-tech medical areas.

Because technology appears to have no limits, there is optimism that respiratory therapy will continue to grow in the future. As the role of the RRT expands, community colleges are feeling pressure to comply with their educational mandates while complying with the educational needs of the RRT. As these educational needs continually grow, the current training process may have difficulties meeting the requirements for educating a competent RRT.[11] One program in Canada is now offering a postdiploma bachelor of health science in respiratory therapy (BHSc) as a 3-year program.[12] It remains to be seen what role a baccalaureate-level education for respiratory therapy may play.

References

1. Bill 64, Respiratory Therapy Act. Ontario Provincial Government, 1991.
2. Hughes J. Respiratory technology, 1950–1980: three decades of evolution and the effect on managerial planning. *Respir Technol* 1982.
3. MacDonald M, Quintieri G. The Regulated Health Professions Act, 1991. *Respir Ther* 1992.

4. Sevile C. Role definition, professional standards and scope of practice. *Reg Respir Therapist* 1992: letter.
5. Standards for the practice of Respiratory Therapy in the Province of Ontario, August 1992.
6. Discussion Paper on the Future of the Conjoint Accreditation Process. May 1992.
7. Basis of Accreditation for Educational Programs in Allied Medical Disciplines, June 1991.
8. Canadian Board for Respiratory Care: *Examination Information Manual*, 4th edn. CBRC, 1993.
9. Canadian Society of Respiratory Therapists. *National Curriculum*. CSRT, 1991.
10. Holmuth C. News from head office. *Reg Respir Therapist* 1992; **28**(4).
11. Von Der Heydt PA, Grossman GD. Education of respiratory care personnel. In: Burton GG, Hodgkin JE (eds) *Respiratory Care: A Guide to Clinical Practice*, 3rd edn. Philadelphia: JB Lippincott Co., 1991: 31.
12. Bachelor of Health Science (Respiratory Therapy). Draft Document. University College of the Cariboo, 1992.

Australia

JILL C NOSWORTHY, LINDA DENEHY,
ROSEMARY P MOORE

History

The practice of cardiothoracic physiotherapy within Australia has evolved from the treatment approaches used in England for the management of diseases such as bronchiectasis and pneumonia. Such treatment regimens have been well described in the literature.[1] The development in the 1950s of technology which enabled clinically based arterial blood gases analysis led to earlier identification of respiratory failure. Subsequently within the Australian public hospital system, specialist areas were created where patients in respiratory failure were managed. The introduction of technology such as positive pressure ventilation led to the development of intensive care units. All professionals involved in treating these patients used an empirical approach to develop effective treatment strategies. In addition to the physiotherapy techniques associated with postural drainage, manual hyperinflation with a hand-held bagging circuit was used to assist with improving ventilation and secretion clearance.[2] Physiotherapy management of the critical care patient is now increasingly being examined for its efficacy and is continually being modified to accommodate the advances in technology and the understanding of diseases. The published studies of Ellis *et al.* (1988)[3] and Stiller *et al.* (1990)[4] are a representative sample of Australian evaluative research in this area.

Governing bodies

REGISTRATION BOARD

All physiotherapists practicing in Australia are required by law to seek registration on an annual basis with the Physiotherapists Registration Board of the state or territory in which they intend to practice. Each board is responsible for administering the parliamentary act relating to physiotherapy registration in that state. The composition of the boards varies between states but includes a mixture of academic and clinical physiotherapists, medical practitioners and public consumers. To be eligible for registration, Australian-trained physiotherapists must hold a physiotherapy degree or diploma from a recognized institution. All foreign-trained physiotherapists must have a prescribed qualification granted in the UK or Hong Kong or have undertaken an examination process and gained a final certificate from the Australian Examining Council for Overseas Physiotherapists.

PROFESSIONAL ASSOCIATION

The Australasian Massage Association was formed in 1906 and became the Australian Physiotherapy Association (APA) in 1939 and has always had a strong commitment to professional development. The APA was a foundation member of the World Confederation for Physical Therapy and has been an active member country since 1952. In 1992, the APA had more than 7500 members throughout Australia which represented the majority of registered physiotherapists. All members of the APA are bound by the ethics of the Association irrespective of their individual area of practice.[5] Until the 1970s, Australian physiotherapy treatments were only provided on medical practitioner referral. After extensive debate within the physiotherapy profession, the APA changed its code of ethics in the mid-1970s to allow physiotherapists to provide treatment and advice without a medical referral. Although close interprofessional consultation has continued, the increased responsibility for decision making which directly affected patient care stimulated the educational institutions to expand the undergraduate curricula. A much greater emphasis on assessment, diagnostic practices and problem solving skills was built into all aspects of each curriculum.

With increasing knowledge, skills requirements and technology, special interest groups have been formed within the APA. These groups are now mostly responsible for the development of short courses for professional continuing education. Courses in critical care physiotherapy are usually convened by the Cardiothoracic Special Interest Group (CTSIG) in each state.

The continuing development of specialist areas in physiotherapy was recognized and a procedure established in 1982 which allowed APA members to undertake a four-stage process of clinical specialization. Successful completion of this procedure leads to the award of specialist fellow of the Australian College of Physiotherapists (FACP). Included in the specialization areas is cardiothoracic physiotherapy, which covers management of the critically ill, acute and chronic patient in the cardiothoracic area.

In the 1970s, three of the state APA branches initiated quality assurance committees with the aim of improving physiotherapy standards of practice. By 1986, a national APA quality assurance committee was formed. Its charter is to educate physiotherapists in all aspects of quality assurance in clinical practice. All state branches formed quality assurance subcommittees which then became responsible for conducting short courses and workshops in the processes of quality assurance.

HEALTH CARE FACILITY ACCREDITATION

Another organization which influences physiotherapy standards is the Australian Council on Healthcare Standards (ACHS). The Council was jointly established in 1974 by the Australian Medical and Australian Hospitals Associations to improve the quality of hospital patient care. It is a completely independent, nonprofit-making body which surveys hospitals and provides a 3- to 5-year certificate of accreditation if all criteria of the Council's published standards are met.[6] All aspects of the physiotherapy service are surveyed in relation to documentation, quality assurance, clinical practice standards and departmental organization. The development of hospital-wide clinical indicators which are used to evaluate the management and outcomes of patient care commenced in 1989.[7] From 1993, all hospitals surveyed by the ACHS will have their outcomes compared to the established thresholds for these clinical indicators. This development has led the APA national quality assurance committee to consider the gradual development of physiotherapy specific clinical indicators in all areas of clinical practice.

Some physiotherapists in private practice are surveyed by the ACHS accreditation process. In 1990, the APA commenced a private practice accreditation scheme which enabled all private practitioners to be assessed in relation to practice standards set by the APA.

Physiotherapy education and training

Physiotherapy education in Australia began in Melbourne, Victoria in 1896 when Eliza McCauley became the first student to undertake practice in massage at The Melbourne Hospital and anatomy studies at the University of Melbourne. By 1904 she had commenced training others and in 1906 the University of Melbourne enrolled its first students in massage. The University of Sydney followed in 1907 and University of Adelaide in 1908.[8]

The physiotherapy training courses remained the responsibility of the APA and registration boards until after World War II. Thereafter, it was recognized that the only possible path to educational development, including postgraduate education and research, was through the administration of courses by educational bodies. In 1958 the first degree course in physiotherapy was offered at the University of Queensland.[9]

As the centenary of physiotherapy education in Australia approaches, there are currently six institutions offering 4-year undergraduate programs leading to a physiotherapy qualification and these are summarized in Table 15.9. Discussions are in progress for the commencement of a seventh physiotherapy course at the University of Newcastle in New South Wales.

Historically, the Australian practice of physiotherapy in the critical care setting is based on the British model where physiotherapists are involved in the management of the patient's respiratory system, whether or not the patient is intubated. The cardiothoracic physiotherapist requires training in the theory and practice of ventilation and ventilatory support, tracheostomy management, suction techniques, all inhalational therapies including continuous positive airways pressure (CPAP) applied intermittently, and intermittent positive pressure breathing (IPPB), together with manual physiotherapy techniques. These manual techniques include specific patient positioning, manual hyperinflation, breathing exercises, postural drainage, vibrations and percussion, limb exercises, early positioning of neurological patients and early ambulation. The choice of technique is dependent upon the physiotherapist's assessment.

UNDERGRADUATE COURSES

In comparison with physiotherapy education programs offered in other countries, the annual intake of physiotherapy students to the six centers is large.[10] Physiotherapy courses attract large numbers of the most academically able students from the top 2% of those eligible to enter tertiary education. Over 95% graduate within the minimum period of study.[11]

Table 15.9 A summary of physiotherapy courses offered in Australia

State (city)	University	Title of degree conferred	Postgraduate courses
Victoria (Melbourne)	University of Melbourne	Physiotherapy	Diploma in Physiotherapy
(Melbourne)	La Trobe University	Applied Science (Physiotherapy)	Diploma in Cardiac Rehabilitation
New South Wales (Sydney)	University of Sydney	Applied Science (Physiotherapy)	
(Newcastle)	University of Newcastle	Proposed course	
South Australia (Adelaide)	University of South Australia	Applied Science (Physiotherapy)	Graduate Certificate in Physiotherapy
Queensland (Brisbane)	University of Queensland	Physiotherapy	Intensive Care Practicum
Western Australia (Perth)	Curtin University of Technology	Applied Science (Physiotherapy)	Diploma in Pulmonary Rehabilitation

Each 4-year undergraduate course in the Australian universities offers a thorough and broad medical science education in the initial years of study. This includes study in: medical biology, physics, behavioral science, physiology, anatomy, neuroscience, pathology and research methods. In addition, physiotherapy specific subjects including kinesiology and applied anatomy, measurement, electrotherapy and the principles and practice of physiotherapy treatment are studied in the first 2–3 years. All courses involve a large component of clinical education. The point at which this is introduced into the course and the manner in which it is developed varies from one institution to another. The fourth year of most courses is substantially clinic-based at the large teaching hospitals. Also, in this year, all institutions offer professional practice units covering issues in biomedical ethics, quality assurance and standards of practice.

Physiotherapy courses at the universities are subject to regular review of their structure, content and contact hours. This process begins when the course is initially set up, and is performed by the academic board of the university and its subcommittees. Review of courses is also undertaken by the physiotherapy registration board in each state.

CARDIOTHORACIC PHYSIOTHERAPY EDUCATION

The cardiothoracic physiotherapist in Australia is involved in the management of critical care patients in public and larger private hospitals. Cardiothoracic physiotherapy is taught in all training institutions as a major subject area along with neurological and orthopedic streams. In most courses, basic cardiothoracic teaching commences during or toward the end of second year, progressing on through the third and fourth years.

Respiratory and cardiac pathology related to medical and surgical conditions is taught in conjunction with the pathophysiological basis of physiotherapeutic management of these conditions. Cardiothoracic physiotherapy manual skills are taught on campus and put into practice in the clinical setting, supervised by clinicians or university staff. In the third year of most of the undergraduate programs, students become involved with physiotherapy management of general medical, respiratory medical and general surgical patients in the associated teaching hospitals.

The objectives of clinical teaching are to:

- develop an understanding of the terminology used in the patient record;
- develop skills in the assessment of cardiothoracic patients;
- develop skills in problem solving;
- develop the ability to perform basic cardiothoracic treatment techniques;
- appreciate the importance of basing treatment selection upon a sound knowledge of physiology and pathophysiology of the disease being managed, accurate initial assessment and reassessment procedures.

The progression to management of critical care patients begins in the final year of most courses. Management of patients in cardiothoracic surgery, transplantation, neurosurgical, coronary care and intensive care units requires the students to draw on previously acquired knowledge and to possess a commitment to learning in the clinical environment.

Physiotherapy students are taught a problem solving approach to patient management. This is achieved through teaching patient assessment and reassessment, the use of diagnostic tools such as arterial blood gas analysis, chest X-ray and cardiovascular monitoring.

The interpretation of patient problems is based on a sound knowledge of pathophysiology which has built upon the theory covered in physiology and pathology in earlier years of the course. Theory covered in the cardiothoracic subject areas includes respiratory failure, adult respiratory distress syndrome, cardiothoracic surgical procedures, major organ transplantation, diagnostic procedures, inhaled drug delivery systems, oxygen therapy and humidification, arterial blood gas analysis, physiotherapy management of neonatal, pediatric, head injured, spinal cord damaged and general intensive care patients.

At the completion of the 4-year undergraduate course, students are expected to be able to organize a full workload which may involve managing medical or surgical patients, and to safely and effectively execute cardiothoracic physiotherapy techniques at a basic level. In larger hospitals, new graduates work in association with more senior physiotherapists, however this situation, although ideal, is not always possible in smaller hospitals or in country centres.

POSTGRADUATE EDUCATION

The physiotherapy graduate diploma courses which are offered in some Australian states were developed in response to a professional need to enhance existing clinical knowledge and skills in specialist areas of physiotherapy practice. A graduate diploma in cardiothoracic physiotherapy is currently offered at the University of Melbourne as a 2-year part-time course. This course focuses on attainment of further knowledge and skills specific to cardiothoracic physiotherapy, particularly in the acute and critical care settings. The theoretical component of the course includes advanced physiology of the cardiovascular and respiratory systems, thoracic and applied anatomy and research methodology. Seminars and lectures in advanced cardiothoracic pathology and clinical issues are taken in the second year of the course in conjunction with a 120-hour clinical studies unit. Overseas and interstate clinical placements are encouraged. The University of South Australia offers a graduate certificate in cardiothoracic physiotherapy. This is a 6-month advanced theory course covering topics related to the acute and critical care areas. At La Trobe University, 2-year part-time postgraduate courses in cardiothoracic physiotherapy were conducted in 1983, 1984 and 1988. In 1993, a graduate diploma course in cardiac rehabilitation is proposed to be offered for the first time from La Trobe University. In Western Australia at Curtin University of Technology, a 2-year part-time graduate diploma in pulmonary rehabilitation is offered. An intensive care practicum of 4 weeks clinical work and lectures is offered at the University of Queensland for

Masters qualifying students with an interest in the cardiothoracic area.

FURTHER DEGREES

The University of Queensland has offered a doctorate of philosophy (PhD) program for some time. However, it was not until 1980 that such programs began at other universities. Today, research degrees both at masters and PhD level are offered at all Australian universities with physiotherapy schools.

The first PhD with a thesis in the area of cardiothoracic physiotherapy was awarded by the University of Sydney to Elizabeth Ellis.[3]

CONTINUING PROFESSIONAL EDUCATION

All state and territory branches of the APA conduct continuing professional development through short courses, seminars and lecture sessions. These courses are normally conducted in the larger population centers. However, as Australia is a large country with a small population, regular access to continuing education for all physiotherapists also requires approaches such as tele- and video-conferencing and interactive computer programs. Continuing education is undertaken voluntarily at present.

In the last 5 years, courses to upgrade or enhance skills in critical care physiotherapy management have been conducted in all Australian states. These courses are usually of 2–4 days duration over weekends and involve a mixture of theoretical and clinical practice. All courses are subjected to peer review processes by the APA before they are conducted, to ensure a uniformity of standards.

In 1988, the national CTSIG of the APA held the inaugural 2-day biennial cardiothoracic physiotherapy conference. The conference was intended to provide a regular forum within Australia for the presentation and examination of current clinical practice and research in the field of cardiothoracic physiotherapy. Two further conferences have been conducted at which this initial philosophy was upheld.

Staffing

Traditionally, physiotherapy staffing levels in critical care units were determined according to the preferences of the unit's medical team, but more recently they have been affected by changes in resource allocation. The only available studies in Australia of workforce staffing levels were conducted in 1981 and 1984 by a sub-committee of the APA (Victorian branch). In these studies, 102 different centers participated and a combined total of 5395 direct contact patient treatments from all areas of physiotherapy were recorded and analyzed. As a result of these surveys, a defined percentage of direct patient contact time was derived. In the critical care area this percentage amounted to 65% of the working day. A six-step formula was devised and based on that, a daily staffing level of 1.2 full time equivalents is required for a six-bed intensive care or high dependency unit.[12]

Recently a questionnaire survey comparing the application of chest physiotherapy in intensive care units in acute general hospitals within Australia, the UK and Hong Kong was published.[13] From the 32 Australian hospitals randomly surveyed, the authors concluded that the staffing ratio was one full-time therapist to six intensive care beds, which would suggest that staffing levels in Australia are, on average, slightly below that recommended by the APA survey formula.

However as Ntoumenopoulos and Greenwood (1991)[14] found, there is considerable variability in the provision of such physiotherapy services between the different Australian states. The results of this survey stated that in Western Australia, all hospitals provided a 24-hour, 7 days per week service, whilst 78% of Queensland and 67% of New South Wales and Tasmanian hospitals provided this level of service. No public hospitals in Victoria or South Australia provide a 24-hour service. An extended hours service, that is, up to 9 p.m., was provided in 9% of hospitals in Victoria and 50% of hospitals in South Australia. All centers provided a daily physiotherapy critical care service with more staffing available during Monday to Friday and a limited service on the weekends. Since this work was published, the increasing pressure to minimize the hospitalization period of patients has seen the introduction of more evening and weekend services in some of the Victoria hospitals. With changes in the industrial laws in 1992, the potential impact on service provision is not yet clear.

Research and the future

The need for objective measurement and analysis of current practices is of utmost importance in the 1990s. Justification of the physiotherapists' position in the health care team, and their value in clinical and financial terms has become increasingly necessary. Cardiothoracic, and indeed all, physiotherapists must be able to provide a sound rationale for the use of specific treatment techniques and regimens.

In Australia this is gradually being achieved through

the development of quality assurance projects, post-graduate education and clinical research. The establishment of the Physiotherapy Research Foundation (PRF) in 1990 to support research of a high caliber in all areas of physiotherapy demonstrates the APA commitment to furthering the development of efficient and effective patient care.

It is fitting to end a section on physiotherapy training with examples of the varied interests of clinical and research cardiothoracic physiotherapists in Australia. These include hemodynamic stability of ventilated intensive care patients; manual hyperinflation; intermittent CPAP; pulmonary and post transplant rehabilitation; aspects of management of cystic fibrosis; the role of manual vibrations and positioning for intensive care patient management; bronchial hyper-responsiveness; sleep disorders; and clinical decision making in cardiac rehabilitation. This list is by no means exhaustive and will no doubt grow and change, in response to the needs of the Australian community and physiotherapy profession, as the next century approaches.

References

1. Gaskell DV, Webber BA. *The Brompton Hospital Guide to Chest Physiotherapy.* Oxford: Blackwell Scientific Publications, 1973.
2. Clement AJ, Hubsch SK. Chest physiotherapy by the 'bag-squeezing' method: a guide to technique. *Physiotherapy* 1968; **54**: 355–9.
3. Ellis ER, Grunstein RR, Chan S, Bye PT, Sullivan CE. Non invasive ventilatory support during sleep improves respiratory failure in kyphoscoliosis. *Chest* 1988; **94**: 811–15.
4. Stiller K, Geake T, Taylor J, Grant R, Hall B. Acute lobar atelectasis. A comparison of two chest physiotherapy regimens. *Chest* 1990; **98**: 1336–40.
5. Australian Physiotherapy Association. Ethical principles. *Australian Journal of Physiotherapy* 1990, **36**:117–21.
6. The Australian Council on Healthcare Standards. *The ACHS Accreditation Guide: Standards for Australian Healthcare Facilities.* Zetland, NSW: The Council, 1991: 1–10.
7. The Australian Council on Healthcare Standards. *Clinical Indicators – A Users' Manual: Hospital-wide Medical Indicators.* Zetland, NSW: The Council, 1991.
8. McMeeken J. *Physiotherapy – Movement for Life.* University of Melbourne Dean's Lecture Series, 1992.
9. Cosh P. The challenge of physiotherapy education in Australia. *Austral J Physiother* 1971; **17**: 113–25.
10. Cole JH. The student selection process in three countries. *Austral J Physiother* 1978; **24**: 187–93.
11. Cole JH. *The Role of the Australian Physiotherapy Association in the Education of Physiotherapists in Australia.* A position paper. North Fitzroy, Victoria, 1988.

12. *Calculation of Physiotherapy Staffing Levels.* A position paper. Australian Physiotherapy Association (Victoria Branch). Fitzroy, Victoria,1985.
13. Jones AYM, Hutchinson RC, Oh TE. Chest physiotherapy in intensive care units in Australia, the UK and Hong Kong. *Physiother Theory Practice* 1992; **8**: 39–47.
14. Ntoumenopoulos G, Greenwood KM. Variation in the provision of cardiothoracic physiotherapy in Australian hospitals. *Austral J Physiother* 1991; **37**: 29–36.

Physiotherapy EC/UK

BERNADETTE HENDERSON, DIANA DAVIS

Physiotherapy is defined by the Chartered Society of Physiotherapy (CSP) as 'a health care profession which emphasises the use of physical approaches in the prevention and treatment of disease and disability'.[1] The Society goes on to state that this definition

distinguishes physiotherapy from other health care professions which either put greater emphasis on the bio-molecular or psychological functioning of the body, particular organ systems, or particular aspects of health or disease such as activities, nutrition and imaging'.

The core skills of movement, massage and manipulative therapy and electrotherapy offer physiotherapists a wide range of treatment modalities enabling an holistic approach to patient management.

The role of the chartered physiotherapist as an active member of the critical care multidisciplinary team is well established in both adult and pediatric units (Figs 15.4, 15.5). In the United Kingdom (UK), the majority of physiotherapists working with critically ill patients will be specialists in the assessment and management of patients with disorders of the cardiovascular and respiratory systems.

Governing and professional bodies in the UK

The Chartered Society of Physiotherapy, founded in 1894, is the professional, educational and trade union body for all chartered physiotherapists in the UK. Representing approximately 24 000 members, it is responsible for improving training, education, professional status and standards, and for fostering and developing the use of the core skills and associated forms of treatment.[2]

The Council for Professions Supplementary to Medi-

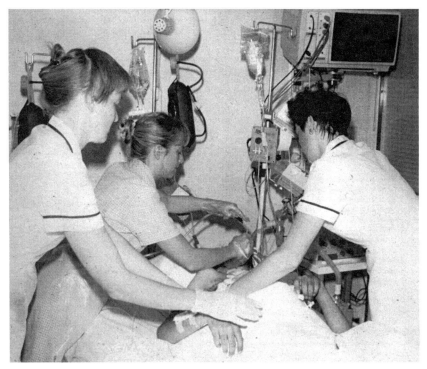

Fig. 15.4   Physiotherapists as part of the multidisciplinary critical care team in an adult unit.

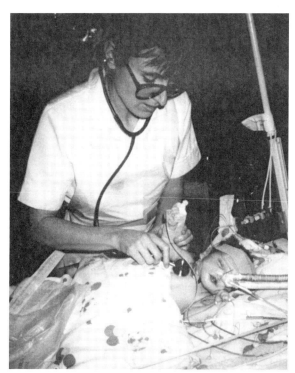

Fig. 15.5 Physiotherapy in a pediatric critical care setting. Reproduced by kind permission of the Chartered Society of Physiotherapy.

cine (CPSM) maintain the State Register of Physiotherapists. The provisions of the Professions Supplementary to Medicine Act (1960), which came into force in 1964, require all physiotherapists employed in the National Health Service (NHS) to be State Registered. The Physiotherapists Board of the CPSM recommends the approval of courses, examinations, qualifications and institutions under the Professions Supplementary to Medicine Act.

Education

UNDERGRADUATE EDUCATION

Undergraduate physiotherapy education is regarded as 'the first stage in a process of continuing professional education and development'.[3] The Royal Charter (1920) states the CSP will 'promote a curriculum and a standard or standards of qualification and institute and conduct examinations'.[2] Currently, a tripartite system to approve courses exists which involves the CSP, CPSM and the educational institution. The Joint Validation and Recognition Panel (JV&R), which consists of members of the Chartered Society of Physiotherapy and the Physiotherapists Board of the Council for Professions Supplementary to Medicine, was set up to consider validation of preregistration physiotherapy courses.[4]

Preregistration physiotherapy education has developed from an assessed 2-week training period (1895) to an all graduate profession (1992). Following the curriculum review of 1945–47, the training period was extended to 3 years and 2 months, leading to Membership of the Chartered Society of Physiotherapy.[5] In subsequent years the syllabus has undergone further revision, most recently with the development of the Curriculum of Study (1991)[1] upon which the present 3- or 4-year degree courses are based. In 1987, the Society's qualification was separated from membership to allow the new UK degree courses and overseas qualifications to be recognized, giving more physiotherapists membership eligibility. In line with this development, the CSP awarded a Graduate Diploma in Physiotherapy to those chartered physiotherapists who had qualified prior to the dissolution of the national exam system.

The Curriculum of Study of the CSP provides a broad base upon which undergraduate education is established. The curriculum is neither detailed or prescriptive and the interpretation of it is at the discretion of the educational establishment concerned. Each course is then submitted for the approval of the JV&R and successful completion of an approved course will lead to full membership of the CSP and inclusion on the CPSM State Register.

Undergraduate physiotherapy courses include both academic and clinical education components. The extent of the academic component of the curriculum relating to critical care varies from course to course but will include relevant anatomy, physiology, pathology and physiotherapy practice relating to this subject area. The clinical education element of undergraduate physiotherapy is viewed as essential and indispensable providing 'the focus for the integration of the knowledge and skills learnt at the college base'.[1] The curriculum of study stipulates that a minimum of 1000 hours must be spent in a clinical environment. Education and evaluation will be undertaken by clinical and professional educators. The number of hours spent in each specialist area and the academic year in which the component occurs are not dictated. However, although the experience gained will depend upon the course undertaken, the majority of newly graduated physiotherapists will have participated in some form of clinical education relating to critically ill patients.

Detailed standards for the clinical component of undergraduate education have been developed by the CSP Quality Assurance Working Party (QAWP), to assist with monitoring and evaluating students' experience in the clinical placement.[6] The standards help to ensure adequate provision of an environment conducive to learning, in which students can develop clinical competence and reasoning skills. Responsibility for this is shared equally between the educational institution, the clinical education provider and the student.

POSTGRADUATE EDUCATION OF CARDIORESPIRATORY PHYSIOTHERAPISTS

The involvement of physiotherapists in respiratory care originated in 1934 with the work of Miss Winifred Linton and Miss Jocelyn Reed at the Brompton Hospital, London. With the increasing body of knowledge in physiology, pathology and biomedical engineering, the associated advances in the care of critically ill patients and research-based physiotherapy practice, physiotherapy for this client group has become a specialist area (Figs 15.6, 15.7).

The definition of a cardiorespiratory physiotherapist is a Chartered Physiotherapist with a special interest in and a greater depth of theoretical and practical knowledge of the management of patients with cardiorespiratory problems. The majority of physiotherapists working in the critical care field will be cardiorespiratory specialists. In units dedicated to the management of particular client groups, e.g. neurologically impaired or burns patients, the physiotherapists employed will have additional specialist skills. The profession recognizes that individual

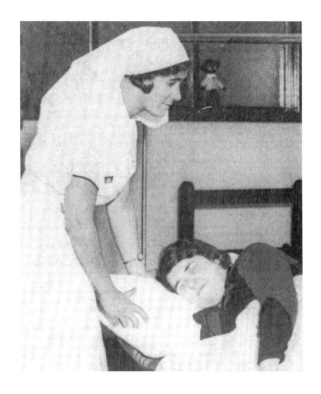

Fig. 15.6 Respiratory physiotherapy – past. Reproduced by kind permission of the Chartered Society of Physiotherapy.

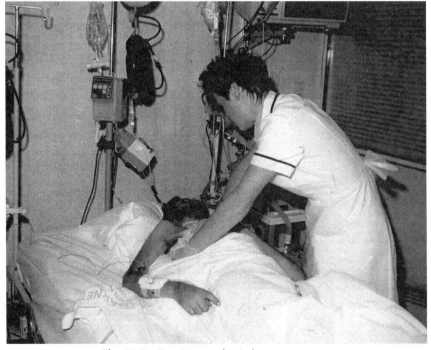

Fig. 15.7 Respiratory physiotherapy – present.

members can be specialists in their own field of practice.

The importance of formal postgraduate education in specialist areas of clinical practice is acknowledged by the profession. The Standing Liaison Committee of Physiotherapists states that 'physiotherapists should have the opportunity to study at higher academic levels in order to further develop their critical and evaluative skills'.[3] There is a wealth of critical care courses available of varying content and detail but currently few are accredited by the CSP. The content and duration of courses range from a 1-day overview of a specific area of interest to those, involving research projects, lasting a number of years. The opportunity to progress to recognized specialist status through an identified pathway of learning is in its infancy. Recently, some courses have attracted formal academic recognition at tertiary education level in the form of the Credit Accumulation and Transfer Scheme (CATS) and, in 1991, the CSP launched its Physiotherapy Access to Continuing Education (PACE). For details of recognized courses, see Table 15.10.

Clinical practice

FIRST TWO YEARS POSTQUALIFICATION

Following graduation, newly qualified physiotherapists usually seek employment as a junior physiotherapist in a hospital environment. These posts normally involve working in differing clinical specialties and with different client groups for periods of up to 6 months each. During these rotations newly qualified staff can consolidate and build upon the knowledge gained at undergraduate level. The graduate will be under the supervision of a senior member of staff whose responsibility it will be to educate, support and motivate the new member. At the end of each rotation, the junior staff member should be able to demonstrate increased clinical knowledge and skill. The majority of UK junior physiotherapists employed within the NHS will rotate through at least one placement specific to the care of critically ill patients. They will also participate in emergency duty rotas providing physiotherapy to acutely ill patients outside normal working hours. A substantial proportion of patients managed during these duties will be critically ill. The competency of the staff involved in these rotas is monitored at a local level by the senior clinician.

The CSP recognizes that the provision of a quality service requires well-trained and motivated staff. The importance of the first 2 years postqualification experience is acknowledged by the profession and, as a result, the 'Standards for Physiotherapists' First Two Years Post-Qualification' were published in 1991.[7] This includes standards for orientation and induction, rotational schemes, evaluation of practice, and education and training. In addition to these, many service providers have locally agreed learning objectives for junior staff rotating into the field of critical care. An example of the learning objectives for a junior grade physiotherapist in a critical care setting is given in Table 15.11.

The experience gained in clinical environments is often supplemented by in-service training programs available to all grades of physiotherapy staff. Despite the lack of formal funding, many physiotherapy departments organize and run their own in-service training programs. These can vary in frequency, level and format, from regular informal sessions to formal courses. The critical care component of in-service training will be organized locally. Certain training will be

Table 15.10 Details of recognized critical care related courses

Past courses	Present courses	Future courses
CSP Validated First Level Respiratory Care Course	CSP Accredited Respiratory Care Course – London	Master of Science – specific to critical care
CSP Validated Advanced Respiratory Care	Physiotherapy in Intensive Respiratory Care – Sheffield	
CSP Accredited Advanced Respiratory Care	Physiotherapy Management of the Acutely Ill Patient – Sheffield	
	Diploma in Advanced Physiotherapy Studies	
	Bachelor of Science in Physiotherapy	
	Master of Science	

Table 15.11   An example of the learning objectives for a junior grade physiotherapist in a critical care setting

AIM
The aim of the ICU placement is to familiarize staff with the routine in ICU, enabling them to carry out the assessment and appropriate effective management of the critically ill patient, especially when undertaking 'on call' duties.

OBJECTIVES
On completion of the rotation the member of staff should be able to:

1. Assess a critically ill patient
2. Draw up a problem list and plan appropriate course of treatment
3. Carry out the treatment according to the agreed treatment plan
4. Monitor the patient's condition and modify the treatment plan accordingly.

ACTION
1. Carry out a subjective and objective assessment of a critically ill patient including the interpretation of:

	Date achieved
The medical records	....
The ICU charts	....
Chest X-rays	....
Arterial blood gas analysis	....
Lung sounds	....

2. Interpret the assessment findings and devise a relevant problem list and treatment plan, demonstrating an ability to prioritize the treatment requirements of the critically ill, multiple pathology patient.

Date achieved
....

3. Be proficient in the theory and practice of the following treatment modalities:

	Date achieved:			
	Adult		Child	
	Theory	Practice	Theory	Practice
3.1 Positioning for maximizing V/Q, demonstrating a knowledge of the effect of artificial ventilation	....	....	....	....
3.2 Positioning for the drainage of bronchopulmonary secretions	....	....	....	....
3.3 Humidification	....	....	....	....
3.4 Saline instillation	....	....	....	....
3.5 Manual hyperinflation	....	....	....	....
3.6 Manual techniques	....	....	....	....
3.7 Suction	....	....	....	....
3.8 Ventilator management	....	....	....	....
3.9 Use of adjuncts to physiotherapy:				
IPPB	....	....	....	....
CPAP	....	....	....	....
BiPAP	....	....	....	....

mandatory for all staff, for example cardiopulmonary resuscitation and the assessment and treatment of the critically ill patient. In addition, senior and junior staff working in critical care related areas will be involved in updating peers by presenting research and case studies, reporting on courses attended and critical peer review.

CLINICAL INTEREST GROUPS

With the evolvement of specialisms within physio-therapy, physiotherapists have formed Clinical Interest Groups. These national groups attract the membership of physiotherapists with different levels of expertise but a shared clinical interest. The groups are formally recognized by the CSP if they fulfill certain criteria. The criteria include identification of a distinct clinical area or client group with a clear and valid relationship between the area of expertise/specialism and the physiotherapy core skills. The Association of Chartered Physiotherapists in Respiratory Care (ACPRC) was formed in 1980, and membership is now in excess of 600. The group is committed to developing this area of expertise by education, practice and research. In 1992, cardiorespiratory physiotherapists became eligible for associate membership of the British Thoracic Society (BTS). Subsequently, a member of the ACPRC committee was co-opted onto the BTS education subcommittee demonstrating a recognition of the physiotherapist's role in cardiorespiratory therapy.

STANDARDS OF PRACTICE

Development and formalization of audit and quality assurance mechanisms within the Health Service has led to an increasing demand from physiotherapists and service managers for nationally accepted standards of physiotherapy practice. This prompted the creation of the joint CSP and Association of District and Superintendent Chartered Physiotherapists (ADSCP) (now the Association of Chartered Physiotherapists in Management ACPM) Quality Assurance Working Party, in 1989. In conjunction with the clinical interest, occupational and client groups of the CSP the *Standards of Physiotherapy Practice* booklet was published in 1990.[8] The document is used by clinicians and managers as a basis to set local standards and to assess the quality of

their service. Subsequent to the publication of these standards, the majority of Clinical Interest Groups have produced standards of clinical practice for their particular field of activity. The *Guidelines Toward Good Practice in Respiratory Physiotherapy* were first published by the ACPRC in 1989.[9] A subgroup of the ACPRC is working on specific standards in the respiratory and critical care field. These Standards of Repiratory Care suggest methods of measurement by which clinical practice can be monitored.[10]

SCOPE OF PRACTICE

Rule One of the Rules of Professional Conduct for Chartered Physiotherapists states that 'Chartered physiotherapists shall confine themselves to clinical diagnosis and practice in those fields of physiotherapy in which they have been trained and which are recognized by the profession to be beneficial'.[11] This rule, however, does not exclude the extension of practice through innovation and research. It allows for

Table 15.12 An example of a problem list and options for the progression of the treatment

Problem	Treatment option	
	Spontaneous breathing/nonintubated patients	Intubated/ventilated patients
Sputum retention	Instigate humidification and in the presence of tenacious secretions ensure adequate oral fluid intake	Instillation of sodium chloride solution 0.9%
	Gravity assisted positioning appropriate to pathology	Gravity assisted positioning appropriate to pathology
	Active cycle of breathing techniques.[14]	Manual hyperinflation with inspiratory pause.
	Perform manual airway clearance techniques (e.g. shaking)	Perform manual airway clearance techniques (e.g. shaking)
	Ensure effective airway clearance techniques (cough, forced expiration technique).	Encourage coughing if patient is conscious
	Suction – if appropriate – with pre and post oxygenation	Suction – if appropriate – with pre and post oxygenation
	Educate patient and/or carers in airway management	Educate patient and/or carers in airway management
	Encourage patient mobility	
Decreased mobility exercise tolerance	Passive movement to all limbs	Passive movement to all limbs
	Active assisted bed exercises	Active assisted bed exercises
	Active bed exercises	Active bed exercises
	Resisted bed exercises	Resisted bed exercises
	Sit out in chair	Sit out in chair
	Mobilize – with supplementary oxygen if required (use pulse oximeter to monitor oxygen saturation if SaO_2 is <90%)	Mobilize – with hand ventilation and oxygen (use pulse oximeter to monitor oxygen saturation if SaO_2 is <90%)
	Increase distance walked	Increase distance walked
	Climb stairs – if appropriate	
	Motivated patients who demonstrate breathlessness on exercise or activities of daily living, should be assessed for exercise training program, i.e. 6MWD or shuttle test.[15]	
	Commence exercise training program.	

MWD = minute walking distance

the exploration and expansion of practice within the confines of the core skills detailed in the Charter. Before individual members seek to extend the scope of their practice, they must ensure that they have received the appropriate training, the modality is encompassed within the core skills and is recognized by the profession to be of benefit to the patient. The opinion of 'a responsible body' within the profession is sought when considering the inclusion of innovative physiotherapy modalities and philosophies. In the field of critical care, the views of members of the ACPRC are invited. A recent example is the inclusion of nasal intermittent positive pressure ventilation into the repertoire of adjuncts available to physiotherapists.[12]

The chartered physiotherapist in the UK is an acknowledged autonomous practitioner.[13] Current physiotherapy practice in critical care setting is based upon a problem solving approach. Each patient is individually assessed. Following assessment the physiotherapist, in conjunction with the patient/carer and the members of the multidisciplinary team, will identify a list of problems which may indicate or influence treatment. A treatment plan will be devised appropriate to the problems identified. An example of a problem list and options for the progression of treatment can be seen in Table 15.12. In some units locally agreed protocols

for basic procedures e.g. suction and manual hyperinflation exist.

PERSONNEL

Historically, there are no nationally agreed physiotherapy staffing levels for critical care services. Physiotherapy services in most critical care units will be provided by a highly skilled and specialized senior physiotherapist supported by additional physiotherapy staff. Locally agreed staffing levels will be based upon a variety of factors including bed occupancy, relative dependency of the patients and the other staff commitments. The senior physiotherapist is expected to train staff and students, evaluate practice, implement appropriate research and ensure effective communication with, and participate in, the multidisciplinary team.

As the role of the physiotherapist in the critical care arena has developed, requiring highly skilled and competent practitioners, so too have the expectations of employers. The attributes required by cardiorespiratory physiotherapists can be identified and an example of a role specification for a senior clinician working within this specialty can be found in Table 15.13.

Table 15.13   An example of a role specification for a senior physiotherapist working in a critical care setting (adapted by kind permission of the Physiotherapy Department, Royal Brompton National Heart and Lung Hospital, London)

	Essential	Desired
Qualifications	Inclusion on the register of the Physiotherapists Board of the Council for Professions Supplementary to Medicine (State Registered Practitioner).	Member of the Chartered Society of Physiotherapy (MCSP). Member of the Association of Chartered Physiotherapists in Respiratory Care. Postgraduate courses.
Experience	Minimum of 2 years postregistration cardiorespiratory experience. Supervision of staff and students.	
Skills	Clinical skills relating to critical care Communication. Organizational. Observational. Time management. Problem solving. Stress management.	
Specialized knowledge	Aspects of physiotherapy practice relating to critical care.	Research. Pediatrics. Quality assurance/standards setting.
Ability to meet special requirements of the job	Interest in research. Ability to recognize boundaries of own responsibilities. Ability to present information. Teaching skills.	Ability to monitor standards of service. Ability to critically evaluate own performance. Ability to assess level and ability of staff and students.

Future of critical care physiotherapy in the UK

Physiotherapy in critical care will be influenced by the inception of an all graduate profession and the development of accredited postgraduate education. It is anticipated that most postgraduate courses will attract both academic and professional recognition, ensuring that physiotherapists specializing in the critical care field can plan postgraduate training on a more formal basis. The advent of the PACE scheme and the increasing number of senior physiotherapists achieving masters degrees and doctorates in critical care related subjects is a stage in this process.

Advances in health care technology relating to both patient monitoring and intervention and the financial constraints within the National Health Service have influenced health care provision and physiotherapy practice. The importance of evaluating clinical practice and monitoring patient and treatment outcomes is being addressed; the trend is towards research-based physiotherapy. Long-term patient outcomes including assessments of quality of life, following critical care intervention, will influence the selection of potential patients. Future developments will include progress on a multidisciplinary approach to agreed protocols, procedures, competencies and collaborative care planning. This will facilitate the development of a comprehensive multidisciplinary framework for monitoring the quality of service provision and practice.

Multidisciplinary clinical practice requires continual evaluation. Currently, issues emerging from skillmix and reprofiling exercises will encourage close scrutiny of the physiotherapist's role in conjunction with that of the critical care nurse and respiratory nurse specialist. In the authors' opinion the way forward must be to promote multidisciplinary critical care teams where each professional member provides a distinct area of clinical expertise. With cooperation and recognition of interdependency within the team, the effectiveness of therapeutic interventions will be maximized in the interests of sensitive and high-quality patient care.

Physiotherapy in the European Community (EC)

PREREGISTRATION EDUCATION

In 1987, in the light of the impending European Directive 89/48/EEC, the Standing Liaison Committee of Physiotherapists within the European Community (SLCP) formed a working party to survey the provision of physiotherapy education in the EC member states. The countries included in the study were Belgium, Denmark, France, Greece, Ireland, Luxembourg, the Netherlands, Portugal, Spain, the UK and West Germany. Luxembourg was omitted from the final report as there are no physiotherapy establishments in this member state. All information regarding preregistration education in Europe detailed below has been derived from the findings of the SLCP reported in 1990.[3] Table 15.14 summarizes the physiotherapy education provision in the member states and the approximate number of students graduating per year are given.

The curriculum of study taught in each establishment was reviewed. Main academic subjects identified within the curricula are detailed in Table 15.15. The clinical education component of the courses was found to be predetermined by the health care system in each

Table 15.14 A summary of the physiotherapy education provision in the EC member states identified by the Standing Liaison Committee of Physiotherapists within the EC

Country	Number of inhabitants (millions)	Years of education required before entry	Length of studies (years)	Minimum total contact hours (hours)	Number of educational establishments	Number of graduates per year
Belgium	9.9	12	3 or 4	3450	25	1000
Denmark	5.1	12	4	3600	8	280
France	56	12	3 or 4	3330–3620	35	1465
Greece	10.1	12	3.5	4272	2	100
Ireland	3.6	13	4	3101	2	60
Italy	57.4	13	3	3500	72	1500
Netherlands	14.5	13–14	4	4200	10	1200
Portugal	10.3	12	3	3370	4	100
Spain	40	12	3	3600	11	456
UK	57.3	13–14	3 or 4	2625	30	922
West Germany[a]	61.5	10	3	5480	85	2500–2800

[a] Data preunification.

Table 15.15   The main academic subjects identified in the curricula by the Standing Liaison Committee of Physiotherapists within the EC

Foundation subjects	Physiotherapy theory and practice
Anatomy including kinesiology and ergonomics	Movement and mechanics
Physiology	Biomechanics
Psychology	Ergonomics
Statistics and research methodology	Manual therapies
Pedagogics	Massage
Sociology	Electrotherapy and thermotherapy
Physical sciences	Physical education and sports for the disabled
	Orthotics, prosthetics and aids for the handicapped
	Patient examination and assessment methodology
	Physiotherapy in medical, surgical and psychiatric conditions
	Hydrotherapy

Table 15.16   The components of physiotherapy undergraduate education identified by the Standing Liaison Committee of Physiotherapists within the EC

Country	Foundation subjects (hours)	Physiotherapy theory and practice (hours)	Observational clinical education (% of clinical education)	Responsibility for single element of patient management (% of clinical education)	Responsibility for total patient management (% of clinical education)
Belgium	720	1200	5	45	50
Denmark	700	1770	18	12	70
France	459	723	5	75	20
Greece	864	1168	19	37	44
Ireland	575	963	5	30	65
Italy	480	225	0	30	70
Netherlands	762	1276	4	21	94
Portugal	590	1100	2.5	18	79.5
Spain	690	1280	3.5	44	52.5
UK	520	422	7	18	75
West Germany[a]	264	1894	20	60	20

[a] Data preunification.

country. Location of the experience and the time spent in each placement/specialty varied between courses and member states. Table 15.16 details the number of taught hours for the foundation subjects and the physiotherapy theory and practice. In addition, clinical education, expressed as a percentage of the total clinical hours undertaken, is given.

In all countries studied physiotherapists, academic tutors and members of other professions including doctors of medicine were involved to some degree in the education program. Only France identified professions other than physiotherapy as participating in their clinical education. Clinical evaluation of students' work occurred in all countries although there was no official/formal link with the physiotherapy establishment in Belgium and the Netherlands. All countries assessed both theoretical and clinical elements of their education programs with involvement of both internal and external examiners. In the majority of the countries, the government was responsible for regulation of

physiotherapy education, although Ireland identified the university faculty as being the responsible body. In the UK, the tripartite system detailed previously was highlighted. Inspection visits from regulating authorities occurred in all countries except Italy.

The report went on to state that future SLCP policy would be to 'facilitate free migration of physiotherapists within the EC' and commonalty between the educational programs should be established. The following recommendations were made to equate the curricula. The educational programs should:

• incorporate statistics and research methodology;
• ensure a wide knowledge base for the development of professional practice;
• improve the integration of theoretical and clinical elements of the course;
• ensure a wide range of clinical experience offered with the opportunity for students to gain experience in other EC member states.[3]

Table 15.17 Recognized European physiotherapy qualifications (adapted from the report of the Standing Liaison Committee of Physiotherapists within the EC)

Country	Recognized qualification	
Belgium	Gradué en Kinesitherapie (Gegradueerde in de Kinesitherapie)	
	Licencié en Kinesitherapie (Licentiaat in de Kinesitherapie)	
Denmark	Masseuse/massøse (until 1953)	
	Physiotherapist/fysioterapeut (1953 onwards)	
France	Diplòme d'Etat de Masseur Kinésitherapeute (1946 onwards)	
	Certificat d'aptiude aux fonctions d'Aide-Dermatologiste (until 1960)	
	Certificat de Masseur Kinésithérapeute Moniteur (until 1976)	
	Certificat de Moniteur-Cadre en Masso-Kinésithérapie (1977 onwards)	
Greece	ΠΤΥΧΙΟ ΦΥΣΙΚΟΘΡΑΠΕΙΑΣ	
Ireland	Diploma MCSP	MICSP
	Bachelor of Science in Physiotherapy	B.Physiotherapy
	Bachelor of Science	BSc
Italy	Attestato di Terapista Della Riabilitazione	DTDR
Netherlands	Bewijs van bevoegdheid van fysiotherapeut	
Portugal	Diploma (Fisioterapeuta)	
Spain	Diplomado en Fisioterapia	TDF
UK	Diploma MCSP	MCSP
	Graduate Diploma in Physiotherapy	GradDipPhys
	Bachelor of Science	BSc
	Bachelor of Science in Physiotherapy	BSc (Phys)
	Bachelor of Science (Honors) Physiotherapy	BSc (Hons) Phys
West Germany[a]	Erlaubnis zur Führung der Berufsbezeichnung Krankengymnast/Krankengymnastin	

a Data preunification.

(The European Community Action Scheme for the Mobility of University Students (ERASMUS) initiative has assisted in the facilitation of this recommendation.)

The SLCP concluded that physiotherapy education should reflect the move to primary care and prevention to meet the changing demands of society. Emphasis should also be placed on cost-effectiveness and the introduction of quality assurance policies as it is essential for physiotherapists to possess skills for the evaluation of cost effectiveness.

EUROPEAN POSTGRADUATE EDUCATION

The European Directive 89/48/EEC aims to establish 'a general system for the recognition of higher education diplomas awarded on completion of professional education and training of at least three years duration' within the European Community (EC). This means that physiotherapists educated within the EC can seek employment in another member state under the same conditions that apply to its own nationals. Physiotherapy professional qualifications within the EC are therefore viewed as equivalent. Article five of the European Directive states that an applicant should be allowed, 'on the basis of equivalence', an adaptation

period to undertake the part of his professional education and training which he has not already undergone. The recognized European physiotherapy qualifications are detailed in Table 15.17.

Investigation of the provision of postgraduate physiotherapy education in Europe is at present being undertaken by the SLCP. Postgraduate cardiorespiratory physiotherapy courses are available in some European countries but the content and detail are not standardized. In 1989, an attempt was made by the French members of the European Society of Cardiovascular and Respiratory Physiotherapists to review the state of postregistration training in cardiorespiratory physiotherapy in Europe. Presentations from representatives of some of the member states highlighted a diversity in the provision of postgraduate education.

Currently, specialist interest groups similar to the ACPRC do exist in some member states, e.g. France and, more recently, Ireland. However, many European countries do not have formal interest group recognition. The European Society of Cardiovascular and Respiratory Physiotherapists has now disbanded. The recent formation of the European Respiratory Society, of which physiotherapists are active members, demonstrates a commitment to the sharing of knowledge and mutual development in this field of activity.

With regard to clinical practice, in many European countries specific respiratory and cardiovascular treatments are prescribed. Practitioner autonomy within each member state varies and physiotherapist scope of practice is determined by state legislation and the professional education of the individual.

The impending report from the SLCP postgraduate working group in 1993 aims to identify present trends and opportunities existing in postgraduate education for recognized specializations in Europe. The report will allow comparison of existing postgraduate qualifications. Harmonization of postgraduate specialist training within the EC will then be attainable and free migration of postgraduate physiotherapists within the critical care environment facilitated.

Acknowledgments

We wish to acknowledge the following officers at the Chartered Society of Physiotherapy for their support in the preparation of this chapter: Pat Allchurch, International Affairs Officer; Thelma Harvey, Continuing Education Officer; Maureen Muir, Information Officer; Stuart Skyte, Director of Public Relations and Jenny Carey, Preregistration Education Officer. We would also wish to thank Julia Botteley, General Secretary of the SLCP and Barbara Webber, Superintendent Physiotherapist at the Royal Brompton National Heart and Lung Hospital, London.

References

1. Chartered Society of Physiotherapy. *Curriculum of Study*. London: CSP, 1991.
2. Chartered Society of Physiotherapy. *Royal Charter*. London: CSP, 1920.
3. Standing Liaison Committee of Physiotherapists within the European Community. *Physiotherapy Education in the European Community*. Henley in Arden: SLCP, 1990.
4. Chartered Society of Physiotherapy. *Validation Guidelines*. London: CSP, 1991.
5. Stewart MA. A question of education – education for what? *Physiotherapy* 1985; **71**: 34–9.
6. Chartered Society of Physiotherapy. *Standards for Clinical Education Placements*. London: CSP, 1991.
7. Chartered Society of Physiotherapy. *Standards for Physiotherapists' First Two Years Post-Qualification*. London: CSP, 1991.
8. Chartered Society of Physiotherapy. *Standards of Physiotherapy Practice*. London: CSP, 1990.
9. Association of Chartered Physiotherapists in Respiratory Care. *Guidelines Toward Good Practice in Respiratory Physiotherapy*. London: ACPRC, 1989.
10. Association of Chartered Physiotherapists in Respiratory Care. *Standards for Respiratory Care*. London: ACPRC, 1994.
11. Chartered Society of Physiotherapy. *Rules One – Scope of Practice*. London: CSP, 1992.
12. Bott J, Carroll M, Conway JH et al. The effect of nasal intermittent positive pressure ventilation on acute exacerbations of chronic obstructive pulmonary disease (COPD). *Am Rev Respir Dis* 1991; **143**: A472.
13. Department of Health and Social Security. Relationship between the medical and remedial professions. *HC(77)33*. London: DHSS, 1977.
14. Webber BA, Hofmeyr JL, Morgan MDL, Hodson ME. Effects of postural drainage, incorporating the forced expiration technique, on pulmonary function in cystic fibrosis. *Br J Dis Chest* 1986; **80**: 353–9.
15. Singh SJ, Morgan MDL, Scott S, Walters D, Hardman AE. Development of a shuttle walking test of disability in patients with chronic airways obstruction. *Thorax* 1992; **47**: 1019–24.

CHAPTER 16

Education, Training and Role of the Clinical Engineer and the Clinical Scientist in Patient Care

SHYAM VS RITHALIA

Introduction   255
Historical background   256
Education and training   257
Certification and registration   258
Management of technology   258
Safety, standards and ethics   259
Clinical measurements   259
User training and education   260
Future directions   260
References   261

Introduction

From an engineering point of view, health care is one of the most interesting working environments. A modern hospital, which has great dependence on complex equipment and techniques, cannot function satisfactorily without technical assistance.[1,2] Several dozen medical devices may be in use around a single bed position at the high point of patient care (Fig. 16.1). Furthermore, the equipment plays an important part in the hospital's effort to maximize the efficiency and effectiveness of patient care. It is the responsibility of a clinical engineer/clinical scientist to provide safe, reliable and cost-effective medical technology. The concept of clinical engineering has existed in the UK and North America for many years.[3,4] In its early days the engineers and technicians in the hospital were primarily concerned with equipment repair and maintenance, and not directly involved with patient care.

Although there is still some controversy about the terminology, according to the American College of Clinical Engineers (ACCE), a clinical engineer is a professional who supports and advances patient care by applying engineering and management skills to health care technology. It is now generally accepted that s/he should have significant patient contact during his/her education and training as well as in day-to-day work.[5,6] A review of available literature on medical engineering indicates that typical academic qualifications for clinical engineers in the UK are either a master of science (MSc) or a doctor of philosophy (PhD), with an electrical or mechanical background, while technologists hold a certificate or diploma.[7-9] Organizational structures and policies differ throughout the world due to wide variations in political and health care systems. Many problems faced by the technologists are not of a purely technical nature and the best use of their expertise can be achieved only when they are closely integrated within the network of other hospital staff.

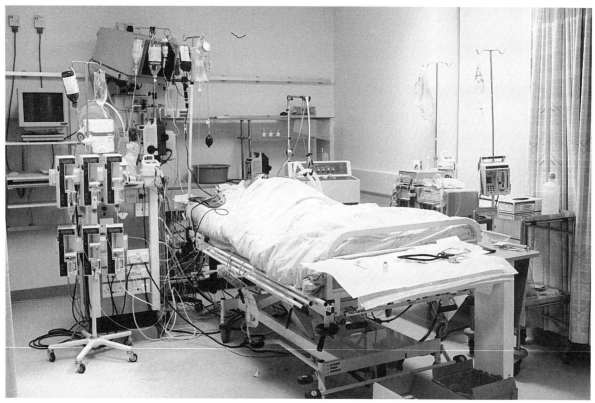

Fig. 16.1   Technical equipment in an intensive care area around a single bed position.

Historical background

There is a long history of informal collaboration between clinicians and technologists. For many years narrowly specialized technical personnel working outside the clinical environment were used to solve medical problems.[10] These people had no formal bioengineering education or training. The 1960s saw the introduction of the first graduate studies in medical engineering.[11] These early educational programs were options mainly based in electrical or mechanical engineering departments. Within a short time many universities in developed as well as in developing countries started to produce academically qualified biomedical engineers and scientists, mostly at PhD or MSc level, with very little or no practical experience of patient contact.[4,7] These scientists usually called themselves medical scientists or bioengineers and in most cases worked as full-time lecturers or researchers, which were already well established professions. However, with the merging of basic research and applied science, they brought fresh ideas and advanced techniques in the field of biomedical engineering.

During the late 1960s and early 1970s new areas of activity for technologists began to emerge, as medical practice became increasingly dependent on electro-medical instrumentation. At this stage technologists became directly involved in patient care but their primary concerns were physiological measurement, equipment repair and electrical safety.[12,13] Over the past two decades, with the rapid growth in engineering in medicine, clinical engineers and technologists working in hospitals began to take an interest in equipment evaluation, acquisition, preventive maintenance, user training and developmental research. These varied functions needed close patient contact and a highly planned technical approach, known as clinical engineering. It has now been recognized as having developed an identity distinct from other engineering disciplines.

The concept of clinical engineering has existed for some time in the USA, Canada and the UK, but its organization as a centralized department in health care establishments is relatively new. However, many departments of medical physics have recently included clinical or bioengineering in their title. The majority of these departments exist as separate entities. There are however some significant national differences in the organizational structure and services offered by them and there are variations between hospitals even within the same country.[5,14] In recent years, the issue of medical malpractice and liability related to equipment has been a powerful element for firmly establishing clinical engineering as a specialty in its own right. Now more and more engineers and technicians are employed all over the world in medical research institutions, clinics and hospitals.

Education and training

A fully qualified clinical scientist or engineer should have a combination of recognized academic qualifications and professional competency. This requires thorough understanding of engineering principles as well as a knowledge of biology, anatomy and physiology. Significant patient contact during training is also essential.[7-9] It is however difficult to establish a universally uniform standard of education for a field that has such a broad base. Except for some elective course options during general engineering degrees, formal education of medical engineers in most countries is at postgraduate level. After graduating in a traditional area of engineering, the master of science (MSc) degree has come to dominate the field of clinical engineering. An increasing range of courses with titles such as bioelectronics, biomaterials, biomechanics and system physiology are now available. Recently, there has been a lively debate in published literature on this subject and a move towards teaching it as a separate discipline at undergraduate level.[8,15] In intensive care the clinical scientists may not have exclusively an engineering background but are drawn from a number of disciplines.

It is not easy to prepare clinical engineers with the appropriate mix of high-quality engineering and life science skills to allow them to function in the diverse and sophisticated medical technology environment. Apart from technical capability the engineers must learn to speak the same language as physicians. They may also require significant management and communication skills. With comparable academic achievement they have at least as much management potential as other professional groups. In addition, they need a firm understanding of the economic aspects, technical standards and ethical issues concerning their profession (Fig. 16.2). As researchers and managers of technology, they have to face many issues raised by conflicts of interest due to patient confidentiality and defective or inadequate equipment. It is their responsibility to ensure the safety of both patients and users by taking an active part in electromedical equipment standardization work. They should also know the legal requirements, or where to get the pertinent information, which govern equipment safety.

By itself, academic education does not make a good clinical engineer. Therefore, in a successful educational program students are taught via a combination of formal instruction and in-service attachment or internship. The basic role of the engineer in the health care team is seen as a problem solver. All too often clinicians who identify and specify the problem have little understanding of the engineering approach. For accurate specification, which is the key to good engineering

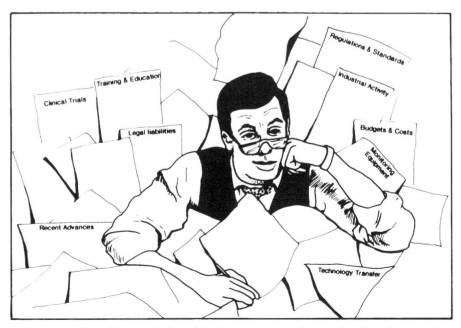

Fig. 16.2 A clinical engineer/clinical scientist must stay abreast of technical, economic, legal and ethical issues concerning patient care.

practice, the engineer must have patient contact in the clinical environment. Without this practical experience the students would have no idea of the routine work in hospitals, where day-to-day clinical engineering is practiced.

Unfortunately, the gap between academic education and training, and its application is nowhere wider than in developing countries. The culture and attitude of the people is such that education is seen as a means of escaping from any form of manual work. This results in large amounts of imported or donated equipment lying unused.[5, 16]

Certification and registration

In many cases, lives of patients depend on the availability and performance of medical equipment in a hospital. A clinical engineer has direct responsibility concerning the safe and effective use of technology. S/he is considered an important member of the health care team. Generally it is not known and appreciated that his/her work demands a high level of responsibility and intellect. Furthermore, unlike other health care professionals such as medical doctors, nurses, radiologists and physiotherapists, the clinical engineers have no universally recognized requirements for academic education, training, certification and registration.[7, 17] This is probably responsible for their unequal status. It must change if a genuine relationship between different members of the team is to be established. The partnership has to be real one, with full disclosure of each member's difficulties and limitations as well as attendant responsibilities for patient care. There is also a need for the creation of an appropriate mechanism for raising standards of professional competence, profile and recognition.

In the UK, clinical engineering certification is carried out by the Biological Engineering Society (BES). In addition to necessary academic qualifications the candidate must be able to demonstrate the s/he spends at least 50% of his/her time dealing directly with patients. Recently, the BES has published a formal register of clinical engineers which has been sent to the Department of Health (DoH). There has already been a strong recommendation from the DoH that all applicants for rehabilitation engineering posts in the National Health Service (NHS) should be certified clinical engineers. Certification by various societies representing the profession and licensure by state governments are becoming more and more common in North America. Although certified engineers in the USA earn more than noncertified individuals, there is no indication at present that certification or registration will become a legal requirement throughout all the states.[18] So far, Japan

seems to be the only country where technologists who want to work in the clinical field need a licence which is certified by the Ministry of Health and Welfare.[19]

In the UK clinical scientists, specialising in intensive care, may have qualified from a variety of scientific backgrounds. An additional higher degree in applied physiology, bioengineering or other life science is considered to be one of the requirements for recognition and registration as a National Health Service (NHS) Clinical Scientist.

Management of technology

The complexity, quantity and range of medical equipment is now so extensive that hospitals are being forced to pay close attention to the management of technology. With the reliability of electromedical instrumentation there has been a substantial shift of emphasis away from simple repair work towards a more comprehensive approach to equipment management. This includes many aspects, such as evaluation, specification preparation, procurement, acceptance testing, installing, optimum utilization and user training.[4, 20, 21] Successful analysis and implementation of all these processes requires technical competence as well as an insight into clinical needs (Fig. 16.3). Although hospital administrators and clinicians are experts in their own field, they do not have the technical resources or the versatility of a competent clinical engineer or clinical scientist. Therefore, his/her advice and involvement has become crucially important in the acquisition of medical equipment. The clinical engineer is uniquely prepared by education and training to effectively lead the management of health care technology.

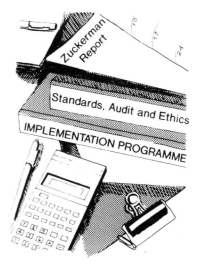

Fig. 16.3 Reports, plans and strategies are of little value until they are properly implemented.

In recent years the cost of health care has become a major issue in most technologically advanced countries. By using strict quality control, regular audit of the available technology, and the clinical engineering expertise at the point of purchase the engineer can save a significant amount of time, effort and money. The engineer should be involved during the planning, implementation and use of equipment. Performance and safety inspections are necessary on all devices whether newly purchased, leased, loaned or donated before releasing for usage. The users must be able to assume that the devices will function as expected when used on patients. Scheduled preventive maintenance programs are among the most important requirement for equipment management. The majority of so-called repair calls or user complaints and many reported patient injuries in a hospital involve operator error rather than equipment malfunction. In this context, close contact between the users on the wards and the clinical engineer is an integral part of the management. There is also evidence in the literature that in-house repair and maintenance is the most cost effective service.[21] Because of the quick response rate such a service is highly appreciated by the medical and nursing staff.

Safety, standards and ethics

The safety of the patients and users of medical devices is the paramount concern of a clinical engineer. This is achieved by keeping proper records of equipment-related incidents and by establishing a risk management program.[6] As a qualified and competent person, the engineer is able to propose and implement an effective in-service user training on the safe application of the technology, thus minimizing human error in the use of equipment. Periodic inspections and reviews of maintenance schedules, policies and documents concerning safety procedures must be carried out. All medical equipment for patients, whether in hospital or at home, should be tested for its proper function and safety before being released for use. Apart from taking more and more interest and responsibility in technical matters, clinical engineers should be representing moral issues

in the clinical care of patients. It must be remembered that as a professional and socially responsible people, they are personally liable for injuries resulting from their services. Clinical engineers also have a clear responsibility of their own to patients and cannot view their role as merely assisting clinicians.

National as well as international laws and standards regulate many aspects of equipment safety.[22–24] In order to make sure that up-to-date standards are maintained medical technologists should take an active part in product standardization work. They can offer their expertise to designers, manufacturers and hospital administrators in advising on the special and technical needs of the patients (Fig. 16.4). In this way, their wealth of professional knowledge can make a valuable contribution to patient health care. Product liability law makes a great demand not only on manufacturers and suppliers but also on maintainers of equipment.[25, 26] This is the most difficult area for clinical engineers, because they frequently make, assemble or modify electro-medical devices which are supplied to patients. But they have little to fear about this piece of legislation as long as they apply a good standard of quality control and professionalism to their work. Documents play an important part in the liability case, therefore engineers should make sure that up-to-date records are kept of all the technical items in their care. It is important to ensure that there is a written document retention policy and a responsible person in charge of enforcing compliance with it. Their legal and ethical duty is clear in managing of medical technology properly and efficiently. It has been said that inefficiency is unethical, as it deprives potential patients on the hospital's waiting list from getting health car benefits.[27, 28]

Clinical measurements

The responsibility of a clinical engineer/clinical scientist extends to most measurements and investigations carried out in the high-dependency wards, ICUs, theaters and various laboratories. S/he is also responsible for the work undertaken by technologists in calibrating and setting up the equipment for procedures such as

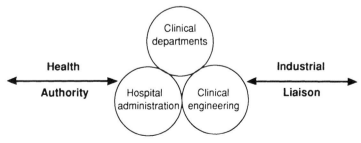

Fig. 16.4 Interaction of clinical engineers with the health authority and industry.

hemodialysis, hemofiltration, cardiac catheterization, pulmonary dynamics and respiratory function tests. It is essential that s/he, together with both the end users and technologists, is involved in preparing specifications for equipment used in the measurement of blood pressure, cardiac output, temperature, electrolytes, blood gases, ECG and EEG. It is not possible for a high-technology critical care facility to function properly without the services of clinical scientists, engineers and technologists.[6, 29] Their education, training and experience enables them to match the clinical needs of the patients and clinicians with the right technology.

During the last decade, major strides have been made by engineers in the design and fabrication of portable equipment for physiological measurements and diagnostic imaging techniques. Now most measurements and investigations of vital parameters are performed and immediately analyzed on the ward by a clinical engineer or a technologist.[6, 29] The acquisition and analysis of the data at the bedside provides an important and accurate feedback to the physician. By providing an early warning system, this enables closer control of the treatment and increases the safety factor to the patient. However, it is important that the clinical staff who work in the critical care areas should be appropriately trained in the proper use of technology.

User training and education

One of the functions of a clinical engineer is to provide user education and training. It is important to develop a closer relationship with nurses, physicians and other hospital workers to identify their equipment-related educational needs and coordinate engineering in service participation. The clinical engineer is responsible for providing safe and effective use of technology in the clinical environment.[4, 27, 30] The users must know the limitations, hazards and proper operation of the medical equipment (Fig. 16.5), and they should be kept informed thoroughly and comprehensively. Whenever new devices are purchased, it is essential for the clinical staff to understand how to use them properly. There is a need for the creation of an appropriate mechanism for sharing information.

Promoting interaction between equipment users and clinical engineers is extremely important. This may be achieved by regular 'teach-ins,' seminars and symposia. Perhaps the best way of achieving a successful in-service education program is for clinical engineers to join in medical ward rounds with the clinical staff and to establish a routine schedule of visits to the various theaters and laboratories. In this way, the engineer is available to answer any equipment-related questions immediately and can make sure that there are no potentially hazardous conditions in the workplace.

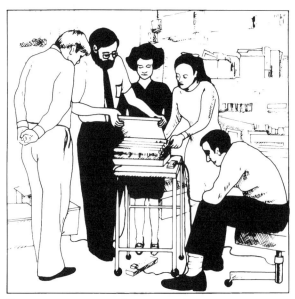

Fig. 16.5 In-service education and training is provided by the engineer.

Clinical scientists and engineers are also responsible for spreading knowledge of their profession to students, nurses, medical doctors and hospital administrators. Keeping the general public and nonmedical administrators informed on the management of technology in the health care system is also very important, since these people need to be reassured that they are getting good value for money by employing clinical scientists, engineers and technologists. Publicizing their role will also help in raising their professional profile and in attracting more resources for medical technology in patient care.

Future directions

With the introduction of modular electromedical equipment, the amount of technician's time required for carrying out repair and replacement of various components has decreased over the past decade. On the other hand, sophisticated instrumentation and complex technology management is demanding a more highly qualified person, or clinical engineer, with managerial skills, who can organize preventive maintenance schedules and be proficient in computing and budgeting. The engineer should also be a willing partner in assisting medical and nursing staff during various research projects, clinical trials and procedures (Fig. 16.6). Therefore, a lower ratio of engineers to technologists is expected in the future.[14] Many problems that are faced by the engineer may not be purely of a technical nature. As a member of the team, the engineer has to assume

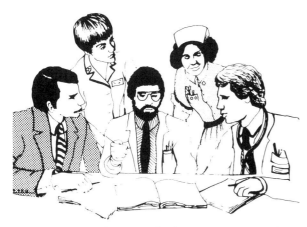

Fig. 16.6 Consultation with the engineer is vital on technical matters concerning a research project.

legal and ethical responsibility of his or her own to patients.

Health care technology is one of the most complex and demanding environments. But so far there is no worldwide recognized requirement for academic qualifications, training, certification or registration. This has adversely affected the professional profile and status of clinical scientists, engineers and technologists. There is a need to resolve these issues, as they are useful pointers for gaining resources and in determining the direction of a discipline. The status can be achieved only by a proper career structure integrating clinical scientists, technologists and engineers, and the recognition as well as acceptance of the profession by the hospital authorities and the general public at large. In recent years, most aspects of medicine have been affected by technology and the technological advances have been faster than the growth of medical knowledge. It important that medical and nursing students and staff should have some exposure to engineering. There is no one better suited than a clinical engineer to provide or coordinate teaching and training on the effective use of technology.

References

1. Rushmer RF. Technologies and health care in the 21st century. *IEEE Eng Medicine Biol* 1990; **4**: 50–2.
2. Gessner U. The role of the medical engineer in today's hospital. *Hospimedica* 1992; **10**: 30–3.
3. Ostrander LE. Presentation of the clinical engineering role to hospital administrator. *J Clin Eng* 1979; **4**: 11–19.
4. Frize M. The clinical engineer: a full member of the health care team? *Med Biol Eng Comput*, 1988; **26**: 461–5.
5. Machado GAS. Health care technical service in developing countries: Brazil. *IEEE Eng Med Biol* 1992; **11**: 44–54.
6. Rithalia SVS. Role of the clinical engineer in patient monitoring services. *J Med Eng Technol* 1991; **15**: 239–41.
7. Cook AM, Katona PG, Plonsey R. Biomedical engineering education: its current status. *Eng Ed* 1979; **69**: 787–93.
8. Bronzino JD. Education of clinical engineers in the 1990's. *J Clin Eng* 1990; **15**: 185–9.
9. Majercik SM. The BMET career: academic curricula, hospital needs, and employee perception. *J Clin Eng* 1991; **16**: 393–403.
10. Dowson D. Medical engineering – the multi-disciplinary challenge. *Proc Inst Mech Eng* 1991; **205**: 1–10.
11. Gowen RJ. Biomedical engineering education in perception. *Eng Ed* 1973; **64**: 175–6.
12. Hewer AJH. The role of a department of physiological (clinical) measurement in the UK National Health Service. *Biomed Eng* 1975; **10**: 59–62.
13. Selman AC. Systems for the maintenance of medical equipment. *Br J Clin Equip* 1978; **3**: 17–23.
14. Frize M. Results of an international survey of clinical engineering departments. *Med Biol Eng Comput* 1990; **28**: 153–65.
15. Baker RJ, Colvin JB. The future of biomedical engineering. *J Biomed Eng* 1991; **13**: 267–8.
16. McKie J. Management of medical technology in developing countries. *J Biomed Eng* 1990; **12**: 259–61.
17. Scott RN. Education and certification of biomedical engineers in Canada. *J Med Eng Technol* 1979; **3**: 180–3.
18. Pacela AF. 1992 Survey of salaries and responsibilities for hospital biomedical/clinical engineering and technology personnel. *J Clin Eng* 1992; **17**: 215–30.
19. Kanai H. Clinical engineering in Japan and the bill for the clinical engineering technician law. *Frontiers Med Biol Eng* 1989; **1**: 177–82.
20. Jarzembski WB. A global view of engineering in the hospital. *IEEE Eng Med Biol* 1985; **9**: 13–16.
21. Whelpton D. Equipment management: the Cinderella of bio-engineering. *J Biomed Eng* 1988; **10**: 499–505.
22. Simendinger EA, Natale D, Lee D. Contribution and Consequences of clinical engineering. *Eng Med* 1982; **11**: 163–7.
23. Staewen WS. Biomedical standards: what do they offer clinical engineering? *Biomed Instrum Technol* 1990; **24**: 51–3.
24. Garrett JA, Smithson PH. Meeting the international standard ISO 9002/BS5750. *J Biomed Eng* 1990; **12**: 253–8.
25. Grant LJ. Product liability aspects of bioengineering. *J Biomed Eng* 1990; **12**: 262–6.
26. Price JM. The liabilities and consequences of medical device development. *J Biomed Mater Res: Appl Biomater* 1987; **21**: 35–58.
27. Saha P, Saha S. Ethical responsibilities of the clinical engineer. *J Clin Eng* 1986; **11**: 17–25.
28. Maynard A. Is high technology medicine cost effective? *Phys Med Biol* 1989; **34**: 407–18.
29. Cox D. Intensive care technology and technologists. *Care Crit Ill* 1985; **1**: 28–30.
30. Shaffer M. Clinical engineering education in the high technology hospital. *Med Instrum* 1984; **18**: 280–2.

PART III

Audit

CHAPTER 17

The Process of Clinical Audit: with Special Reference to Critical Care

ROBERT J BYRICK

Introduction   265
The audit cycle principles   266
The audit cycle adapted for critical care   269
Summary   273
Future directions for critical care audit   274
References   275

Introduction

Clinical audit can be defined as 'a systematic critical analysis of the quality of medical care, including procedures used in diagnosis and treatment, use of resources and the resulting outcome for the patient.'[1] Recently, a more formalized audit process has been encouraged. It is this formal process of data collection and evaluation with special reference to critical care that is described as a cyclic process. The ultimate aim of an audit system is the formal identification of a plan of action and verification of effectiveness with accountability for change.

Clinical audit can cover any aspect of patient care, including nursing and paramedical services, as well as physician practice.[2] The purpose of a clinical audit[1] is the provision of 'the necessary reassurance to doctors, patients and managers that the best quality of service is being achieved within the limits imposed by the resources available.' If the focus of audit on quality care is to be maintained while diagnostic and therapeutic advancements are made, physicians and other health care professionals will have to be intimately involved in the design and control of the audit system.

Hopkins[2] has emphasized that no generally accepted

view exists regarding what data set or system best reflects quality of clinical care. The success of the process may depend on the adequacy of communication and a commitment to change, developed during the implementation phase. To understand the process of audit, it is important to clarify some differences between audit and related activities.

DIFFERENCE BETWEEN CLINICAL AUDIT AND RESEARCH

An audit system, as distinct from research, does not propose or test new hypotheses. The audit process is focused on ensuring that current knowledge is appropriately and completely used in the care of patients. For this reason, a current understanding of changes in both the process of care and the pathophysiology of disease is essential. More than data collection is involved. Audit involves an element of judgment, not dissimilar to research. This judgment is best made by comparing the results of data collected with accepted standards which reflect quality of health care delivery. However, for many aspects of practice, recognized standards of care have not been explicitly defined in the literature.

DIFFERENCES BETWEEN CLINICAL AUDIT AND RESOURCE MANAGEMENT

A common concern of physicians and other health care providers is that audit is equivalent to resource management. There can be no doubt that a major impetus to the collection and analysis of patient data has been cost-containment as well as a desire to improve the quality of care delivered while recognizing resource limitations.[1] In utilization management the use of resources is the priority issue, whereas quality of care is of secondary importance.[3] Similarities between clinical audit and resource management include the need for complete, accurate clinical data and a collaborative approach to data analysis and problem solving. Differences include the accountability for change in clinical audit, which is primarily a medical responsibility whereas, in most systems, accountability for resource utilization is an administrative responsibility. If an audit system is designed and controlled by health care professionals with a specialized knowledge base in the current practice of critical care, then an effective focus on the assessment of quality can be achieved. Audit for critical care is important not only because the costs are great, but also because of unanswered questions concerning the efficacy of this technologically based care and its impact on outcome. The challenge facing clinicians is not whether they should become involved, but rather to familiarize themselves with techniques used in industry and management in order to focus change on quality of patient care. This will prevent resource utilization from becoming the primary impetus to change.

AUDIT AND CASE REVIEW

A formalized audit process is distinguishable[4] from traditional chart review. The use of explicit audit criteria for assessing quality of care is different from implicit judgments, used in case review discussions. The lack of formal comparative criteria and numerical data comparing observed practice patterns with criteria established among peers are essential parts of a systematic audit as opposed to descriptive case reviews.[5]

The audit cycle principles

A SYSTEMATIC APPROACH

The general activities and stages (Fig. 17.1) of an audit[6,7] emphasize the need to adapt to local circumstances and needs (e.g. critical care). Whether a commercialized system, such as that proposed by Apache Medical Systems Inc.[8] can serve the dual purposes of utilization review and clinical audit better than a unit-based system remains unresolved. For the purposes of this discussion, a process used to develop a unit-based system will be outlined.

Crombie and Davies[7] have emphasized 'thinking through' the design of the audit system prior to embarking on data collection. Their approach[7] is similar to that used in industry to maintain quality and satisfy customer demands.[9,10] Deming's experience[9] suggested that 85% of problems were related to the system and 15% to the performance of individuals. In many

THE CYCLIC PROCESS OF AUDIT

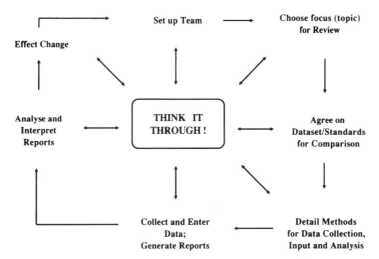

Fig. 17.1   A schematic (adapted from Crombie and Davies[7]) describing the steps for clinical audit emphasizing that each step must be thoughtfully developed, recognizing its relationships to other parts of the cyclic process.

instances, where the individual provider's judgment and skills were found deficient, the adverse event resulted from the interaction of judgment with facilities available. In critical care, a coordination of input from many health care providers interact to influence the outcome. Knaus *et al.*[11] have suggested that the process by which critical care is delivered can influence the survival of patients treated in different critical care units. Audit focuses on the 'system' and the process of delivering a product, not necessarily on individual workers. Such systems have been the basis of Continuous Quality Improvement activities in medical specialties such as anesthesia.[10]

COMPONENTS OF THE AUDIT CYCLE (Fig. 17.1)

The audit team

The key for audit team selection is the inclusion of individuals who understand the process of patient care. The personnel, expertise and facilities available may vary; however, a group of individuals who have a shared commitment to quality care can use their knowledge of local circumstances to conduct an audit. These unit-based personnel will, as a first priority, establish whether other individuals with specific expertise should (or could) be involved at any stage of the process. The ability of the audit team to perform each stage should be reviewed objectively. If specific expertise is needed, there should be no hesitation in identifying the need and proposing extra members.

Choosing the topic for audit

Perhaps the most important step in the process is the choice of audit focus or topic. Priority should be given to issues perceived as problems by unit-based personnel. Topics identified by users will lead to optimal data collection, realistic interpretation of results and a commitment to change. The discussion of topic should be multidisciplinary and potential topics should be recorded in writing for future reference. Cost may play an important role in selection of audit focus as high-cost patients or procedures may serve as markers. However, the focus of the process must remain on 'quality of care' issues. Whenever a clinical disagreement or controversy over appropriate medical therapy exists, the audit team should consider this topic as an appropriate focus. The occurrence of 'sentinel events,' such as unit readmission, can serve as a screening procedure for a given audit.

An audit is more likely to change clinical practice patterns if the activity chosen occurs commonly, so that a large data set can be collected and analyzed before practitioners sense that the experience is outdated. The topic identified should be well defined so there will be no disagreement that data collected reflect true practice patterns which can be compared to an accepted standard.[12] The most important aspects of choosing an appropriate topic are that it be perceived as important and be amenable to change.

If difficulties arise in agreeing on a topic for audit, Williamson[13,14] has suggested the use of a 'nominal group' procedure. This entails at least two group meetings of the audit team. Each person puts forward one suggestion for audit topic. These suggestions are then weighted as to the likely impact on improving quality of patient care. By listing topics by priority for improving quality care, the focus of audit on quality is emphasized and topic selection is facilitated.

Setting standards for comparison

In critical care, ICU policies and procedures, consensus statements in the literature or data from multicenter databases can form the basis for setting standard of quality care. Policies and procedures should be reviewed, defined and evaluated in the light of current medical knowledge, prior to setting explicit criteria for the audit. From critical care research, examples of standards that can be used for comparison include outcome from cardiac arrest in hospital,[15] prognosis using APACHE II severity of illness,[16] or prognosis in nontraumatic coma.[17] If the audit team is to reach agreement on which comparative standards to use, it is essential to develop a consensus. The standards applied should be realistic, given local conditions and circumstances.

The team may opt for a 'minimum acceptable standard,' then compare the clinical performance recorded to this predetermined standard. However, if quality care delivery is the goal of audit, the team should avoid 'minimalist standards of care' as they imply minimal thresholds of structure, process or outcome above which care is acceptable. Such floors frequently become ceilings.[18] The team could also elect to use the 'norm' as a standard for comparison. It has been emphasized that the objective of audit is to effect change and deviations from a 'norm' could be viewed as reflecting changes secondary to other factors (e.g. severity of illness, co-morbid conditions).

Specific statements[18] of purpose and/or algorithms for the clinical process studied can be useful in defining standards. These statements specify rules for procedures or interventions that are believed appropriate. Obviously, these are subject to ongoing reassessment, but they can form the basis for establishing standards. Use of an algorithm to duplicate the clinical decision making process can assist in defining these rules.

Selection of data set

The audit team must reach agreement regarding the details of the data set needed to answer the question(s) posed and the timing of data collection. The influence of potential confounding factors should be considered and included as part of the data collected. Confounding variables that change with time or that are different from data sets on which standards were established need careful attention. Outcome measures used in evaluation need to be discussed. These issues must be determined prior to initiating data collection. By detailing a data set, the audit team can accomplish several goals. First, all participants will understand why each piece of information is collected. This will enhance the effectiveness of data collection. Second, the members of the audit team will develop a framework for the future analysis of data. Third, it is important for efficient data collection and analysis, that 'orphan data' collection be minimized.[19] 'Orphan data' refers to the collection of data that are not required for the audit being performed, and are collected only because they are available.

In determining the data set, a table can be completed (Table 17.1) which organizes the data set (both content

Table 17.1 An outline which is used to develop a potential data set for an audit. When completed, this assists the audit team in examining the source of each element in the data set as well as the usefulness and validity of each piece of information

Population	Content of data collected			
	Patient demographics	Services provided	Resources used	Outcomes
Entire population				
Population sub group				

and source). This type of table can be completed for any audit topic and includes elements of structure, process and outcome. It is important that the cause of any variation in outcome should be easily established. In recording process or outcome, an empirical judgment as to their relationship must often be made. The acceptability of a variation in clinical practice from an accepted standard is a value judgment that should be discussed prior to the analysis of data.

Methods of data collection and analysis

Depending on the choice of topic and personnel available, the methods used to observe clinical practice

will vary. Although general techniques can be described, these must be adapted to specific circumstances. There must be agreement concerning the role of all participants in both data collection and analysis. This discussion should include such issues as the details of who will collect information, when this can be done and what format will be used, as well as support for data collection, data entry and analysis. It is imperative that all data collected are perceived to be meaningful; the audit team should therefore ensure that all participants understand why specific items in the data set are being collected and minimize wasteful 'orphan data' collection.[19]

A most destructive force, which can unwittingly divert the process of audit and antagonize participants, is to force data collection responsibilities onto one group (e.g. nursing staff) without adequate support. In our experience, these problems can be minimized by organizing data collection in tandem with current professional responsibilities (see below).

The role of computers will be detailed when considering data management for critical care audit, however, it should be emphasized that the process of data collection and data entry will determine the accuracy of reports. The methods of statistical analysis should be discussed before data collection begins[7] and the audit team should be involved in the design of reports which are generated from the data. Data used for report generation should be verified by the audit team before analysis. This verification process will ensure that no unexpected errors in data collection or entry have occurred which would create a lack of confidence in the reports.

Interpreting reports and effecting change

In practice, the most difficult aspect of clinical audit is the evaluation of reports such that change can occur. If the audit demonstrates that the topic or focus of audit is done well and no change in the process of care is warranted, this fact should also be communicated to the participants. There are few studies which analyze the effect of audit on outcome of patient care.

This cyclic audit process (Fig. 17.1) is intended to emphasize and promote an understanding of critical care delivery and create an organized, disciplined process for improvement. The participants should be reassured by the manner in which an audit is implemented that the aim of the process is to improve the quality of care delivered, minimizing any fear of reprisal.[10] Understanding that the focus of the process is patient-centered and multidisciplinary serves to reinforce the principle and promotes an innovative team approach.

The audit cycle adapted for critical care

The knowledge base in critical care crosses all conventional medical specialties such as nursing, pharmacy, respiratory therapy and physiotherapy, among other disciplines. It is clear that, because of the multidisciplinary nature of critical care, data collection, management and analysis must also cross these conventional boundaries if audit is to be successful. In adapting the 'thoughtful audit cycle' (Fig. 17.1) for use in critical care, we consider three components or functions (Fig. 17.2).[20] Each of the three components, the patient care function, the database function and the decision function, appear to be equally important in achieving a successful audit.

PATIENT CARE FUNCTION

Selecting audit team and system

A team is formed of individuals who are primarily involved in patient care. A multidisciplinary critical care committee can serve this purpose. Policies and procedures detail specific aspects of care and set the standards against which activity can be compared. If the team perceives a problem that is not covered by existing policies or procedures, an audit may be developed to assess the need for new guidelines, policies or procedures. The advantage of a unit-based system remains the locally controlled focus on quality of care issues. The advantage of a commercial package would be the availability of comparative data from a wide range of units and access to sophisticated epidemiologic tools and expertise.

Choosing the focus and data set

Many audit systems that have been developed collect a standard data set for all purposes. However, the process may be more effective if the data set is focused on information relevant to a specific problem over a specified period of time. This does not suggest that ongoing data collection systems which are often used for utilization review will not be valuable audit tools, but rather that these data sets may need to be tailored for specific topics of audit. This emphasizes that utilization review and audit overlap in many of the data elements that need to be collected, but these reflect different aspects of care.

The data-rich critical care environment provides a large potential data set that includes information on

AUDIT SYSTEM FOR CRITICAL CARE

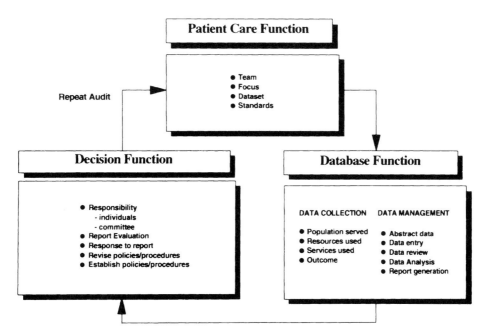

Fig. 17.2   A schematic showing an example of a clinical audit system used for critical care. Adapted from ref. 20 with permission.

patient population and unit structure (input), procedures and complications (process) as well as results (outcome). Examples of audit topics identified for evaluation are shown in Table 17.2. Tables 17.1 and 17.3 provide a partial guide to data set selection and potential data elements. In few other areas of medicine is there a validated severity of illness measure[21] to use in audit. The APACHE II(III) methodology has provided a very powerful tool for audit which has been used in teaching as well as nonteaching centers.[11] Another advantage of critical care is that interventions are well defined and relatively easy to document. The Therapeutic Intervention Scoring System (TISS) is a tool which can be modified by individual units to record use of specific technologic interventions.[22] The TISS methodology is more a reflection of interventions ordered and provided than a measure of nursing workload.

Specific problem areas related to choosing a data set for critical care should be mentioned. The 'process' of critical care is often difficult to record. One example is

Table 17.2 Examples of audits performed in a multidisciplinary critical care unit, listing a general description of the process used to conduct each audit

Audit process	Topic
1. Screening criteria	Admission criteria (need for specific resources)
	Readmissions to ICU (re-evaluation of discharge critera)
2. Preadmission review	Cardiovascular surgical services (selection criteria)
3. Concurrent review	Discharge criteria of patients kept in ICU
	Consent to treatment protocols
4. High-cost management	Long-stay patients – diagnoses/admission criteria/outcome
5. Organizational changes	Intermediate care areas – impact on patient outcome
6. Use of technology	Use of blood components
	Invasive monitoring techniques
7. Identified complications	Renal failure
	Nosocomial sepsis

Table 17.3 Information used in a critical care audit system emphasizing the input (patient descriptors and resources used), the process of care delivered and the outcome assessed

Input	Process	Outcome
Diagnosis (es)	Procedures	Complications
Severity of illness	Technologic intervention	Length of stay
Nursing workload	Nursing intervention	Mortality
Interventions used	Communication	Morbidity
	Transportation	
	Protocols	

nursing workload assessment. A validated nursing workload tool has not been described.[23, 24] Similarly, the diagnostic coding for critically ill patients poses a problem for accurate recording. It is important to establish definitions for all data elements prior to collection. We have used the International Classification of Diseases (ICD-9–CM) as one method of categorizing diagnoses and procedures,[25] but found that this became too detailed for meaningful analysis. Knaus and colleagues[8, 11] have developed a useful list of common critical care diagnoses included in the APACHE II(III) system. We find that this list is a more practical way of auditing admission diagnoses and provides clinically relevant information, especially when coupled with severity of illness. Another limitation is the recording of pathophysiological responses to interventions. Recent reports[26] of computer-assisted management of information in an intensive care unit which integrates a relational database with a text editor may further improve our ability to study the process of care.

Outcome assessment is problematic for all forms of audit as the concepts and definitions used to describe quality vary.[27] Mortality is the traditional outcome measure used in critical care but for many legitimate topics of audit this will be an insensitive outcome measure. Aspects of care that can be audited include accessibility, patient-centered decision making, effectiveness of therapy, efficiency and timing of interventions and coordination of care. The level of physical morbidity, psychological distress, patient satisfaction and 'quality of life' after discharge are outcome measures that can be used. Little work has been reported on the sensitivity of non-mortality-based measures of outcome in critical care. For this reason the choice of indicator depends on the experience and intuition of the audit team and their assessment of which outcomes will best reflect the quality of care delivered.

DATABASE FUNCTION

The database function of the audit system includes data collection and entry, data management, and analysis as well as report generation (Fig. 17.2). It is important to include two key support individuals, the data entry clerk and the computer programmer, in all aspects of the design, development and management of the database function.

Data collection

The sources of data may range from routinely collected information in the health record (e.g. physiologic data) or hospital statistics (e.g. length of stay) to special *ad hoc* data collected specifically for an audit. We have chosen to incorporate data collection into the daily routine of ICU staff without adding unduly to the burden of information management in the unit.

The clinical record is an incomplete description of the 'process' of care. A structured 24-hour flow sheet specifically designed for audit assists in recording data that can be retrieved by a trained health records technician (HRT). An aspect of instituting a clinical audit that must be considered is the need to have practitioners (nurses or physicians or others) complete a form that is not part of routine practice. This may independently alter or disrupt the process being audited. Outcome data (not related to length of stay or mortality) may require an *ad hoc* survey instrument (e.g. interview or questionnaire) to obtain information for quality of care assessment. If an audit is to be adequate for decision making, data collection should ensure a complete data set.

Physicians, in particular, must be sensitive to the additional workload required for data collection. In our system,[20] data collection, primarily by nursing staff, is integrated into the 24-hour worksheet for every patient. With few exceptions, this has minimized the additional time required for data collection at the bedside. Physician notes are written daily and specific issues for audit can be integrated into the daily note. This has minimized missing data elements from the data set. Areas in which we have had difficulty maintaining complete records include the listing of interventions and nursing workload and the relationship of interventions with complications. Computerized systems for automatic 'extraction' of data and interventions from a critical care flowsheet have been described.[28, 29]

We opted to have a single data entry clerk who is a trained HRT in our medical records department to perform all data entry. She has integrated data entry into routine chart abstraction for hospital purposes.[20] The disadvantage of this approach is that data cannot be abstracted from patient charts and entered into the database until after the patient has been discharged from hospital. Data collection is limited by information available from the chart. There is a delay of several months between the time that data are generated and their analysis. This disadvantage could be partially overcome by assigning a data entry clerk for the ICU. One advantage of this system is the establishment of a formal systematic data collection process that has minimal impact on the ICU routine. The audit team can focus on quality of care issues and need not be concerned with data collection, abstraction and data entry. The experience and training of the HRT with audit tools, such as APACHE and TISS methodologies, was important during program design and development.[30] Regular feedback from the HRT provided useful information that assisted the programmer in designing an effective user interface and improving data validation and input error trapping.

Data management

A relational database management system (dBase IV, Borland, Scotts Valley, CA, USA) was used to develop the application program (CareBase) for the audit system. The program is menu driven and consists of the main program and several major modules which control the operations of adding, editing and updating records, as well as report generation and routine database maintenance. The current version of the program has seven custom-designed data input screens accessing eight databases with a total of 388 nonredundant fields. The data input screens have extensive data validation and error-checking features to minimize data entry errors and facilitate the process of data entry. Periodically, refinements and improvements are made based on feedback from the HRT. Problems encountered during data analysis and report generation are discussed and resolved through procedural or program changes.

A simplified schematic of the critical care data model is shown in Fig. 17.3. This is a logical data model which defines the way that data are generated in the ICU setting and the relationships between various data subsets. Once this model is defined, it is used as the basis for the construction of the physical database system. This model was arrived at by analyzing the total patient data set and identifying entities such as 'diagnosis data' which name a class of information within the data set. Each entity is then analyzed to determine the attributes, such as diagnosis type, that relate to it. Finally, a relationship between entities is established. The diagram (Fig. 17.3) shows how data are generated when a patient is admitted to the hospital. For simplicity, only the most important relationships are shown. Patient-hospital data are primarily demographic and personal data. This is the primary database in the sense that it contains data generated during the patient's first contact with the hospital. The patient is then admitted to the ICU where unit specific data, such as unit admission/discharge dates, length of stay in the unit, and duration of ventilation, are generated. Since a patient may be admitted to the ICU more than once during a single hospital stay, this is shown as a one-to-many $(1:m)$ relationship. The remaining boxes represent data entities which are generated while the patient is in the unit. The boxes on the left side of the diagram are all indicated as one-to-many relationships relative to patient-unit data. This means that for a specific unit admission, a patient can have more than one diagnosis, or more than one procedure, etc. The boxes on the right are shown as one-to-one relationships. Strictly speaking these can be considered part of patient-unit data and could be physically merged with no loss of functionality. They are maintained as separate entities primarily

SMH CRITICAL CARE DATA MODEL

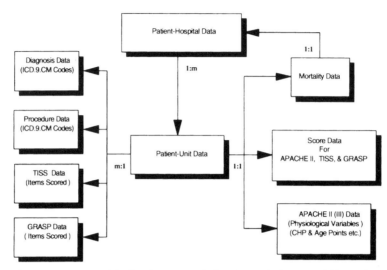

Fig. 17.3 A simplified schematic of the 'logical data model' used to develop the physical database structure. This reflects how data are generated after each patient is admitted to hospital. The one-to-many $(1:m)$ relationships indicate that more than one instance of an entity (defined in each box) can occur for each instance of a relating entity (e.g. patient admission to unit). Adapted from ref. 20 with permission.

to keep the physical databases smaller and easier to manage.

Factors related to the selection of hardware include the requirement for fast efficient data entry, minimum processing delays, and adequate hard disk storage and memory. Data input is labor-intensive and it is important that screen updates, data validation, input processing, and interactive editing proceed without unnecessary delays during the data entry process. The hardware and software chosen for an audit system will depend on specific needs and the resources and expertise available. A lack of computer support may encourage the use of commercial audit software, but this approach may lack the flexibility to customize for specific requirements. Although less powerful systems will serve the purpose, a recommended configuration would include a 33 MHz 486-based computer, a 200 Mb hard drive, 8 Mh of RAM (memory) and a tape backup system.

Report generation and primary analysis

The reports need to be developed by the audit team in conjunction with the programmer, who understands both the structure of the database system and the methods required to retrieve and analyze data prior to report generation. As in any research proposal, the methods of analysis should be discussed prior to data collection. One of the advantages of using a relational database program such as dBase is that files can be exported to powerful statistical programs such as SAS™ (SAS Institute Inc., Cary, NC, USA) for analysis.

The primary data analysis and report generation is done by specific audit team members with the programmer. The purpose of the primary analysis phase is strictly to ensure that the data is reported in a format that the full audit team will find useful. At this stage, we have frequently been able to identify unanticipated areas of weakness in the audit or missing data that may clarify some of the differences noted. The report(s) are given to the audit team for analysis and the decision making process proceeds.

DECISION FUNCTION

Important aspects of the decision function (Fig. 17.2) include responsibility for evaluation of reports and implementation of change. A written response is required, including any recommended revisions to unit policies or procedures. A structured audit system recognizes the need for continued re-evaluation of the impact of change on quality of patient care. Deficiencies in critical care delivery which are identified by audit may relate to either needed changes in administrative organization or improvements in the process of care. Three methods of implementing change in critical care (education, concurrent review of practice, and use of protocols) are outlined.

Education

The audit report may direct voluntary educational activities at specific individuals or groups identified as impacting on quality care. Discrepancies identified between observed practice and predicted standards create an atmosphere conducive to change. Feedback on personal performance can be a key component of the educational process.[29, 30] Simply providing feedback on deviations from established standards may not be adequate to effect change.[31] Lomas and Haynes[32] have suggested that continuing feedback is desirable to prevent a relapse into past practice patterns and continuing evaluation should be a routine part of the process.

Concurrent practice review

This technique for implementing change is based on feedback concerning clinical management decisions during the same ICU admission. One example is the use of surveillance criteria for blood transfusions. When a blood product is ordered without adherence to predetermined criteria being met, a hematologist contacts the critical care physician to discuss appropriate management. This form of concurrent review can result in an educational experience and reduced misapplication of blood component therapy. Similar concurrent review strategies have been applied to test ordering by staff. If this strategy is to be successfully applied to critical care, rapid and effective transfer of information is needed.

Protocols

The use of guidelines, checklists or algorithms can be used as protocols to implement change in clinical practice. Guidelines are flexible summaries of current information applicable to a clinical situation that are needed by both clinician and patient in order to make a fully informed decision. Guidelines summarize collective experience as determined scientifically at consensus conferences and in the literature. An example of guidelines is the use of low-osmolar contrast media for investigative techniques. The comparative risks involved between high- and low-osmolar agents have been reported and widely discussed.[33, 34] Because of resource limitations, decisions have been made to limit the use of low-osmolar contrast media to high-risk patients. The recognition of limited resources is an integral part of the definition of audit[1] and collaboration is needed between administrators and clinicians to enhance the hospital's abilities to care adequately for all patients. The publication of guidelines does not always effect change in physician practice patterns[35] Hopkins[2]

has emphasized that establishing guidelines does not solve problems unless 'guideline statements can be audited.' In critical care, there is likely to be an increasing emphasis on the use of guidelines as new, expensive technologies such as monoclonal antibody therapy become widely available. Checklists can be applied in critical care to ensure that specified actions (e.g. daily checking of the cardiac arrest equipment and respiratory therapy supplies) have been carried out. These checklists are often implemented by paramedical personnel.

Algorithms, in the form of 'decision trees,' can be used to direct diagnostic or therapeutic decisions. A branching flowchart for the use of gastric acid prophylaxis developed by our critical care committee is shown in Fig. 17.4. Such an algorithm can provide a basis for an audit which evaluates the use of prophylactic regimes.

The choice of method or methods used to implement change will depend on a variety of factors, including the attitudes of the audit team, facilities available, the adequacy of communication with multidisciplinary health care workers involved and the issue being discussed. It has been our experience that some form of protocol-based instrument is a valuable adjunct to educational activities alone. The final stage of audit that closes the 'audit cycle' is the reobservation of practice. Similar methodology should be used as in the original observational study so that any improvement or deterioration cannot be attributed to altered methods of assessment.

Summary

After an audit has been completed, the effect of change on other aspects of practice should be assessed. This 'audit of the audit' recognizes that increased efficiencies in one aspect of medical care can result in altered performance elsewhere. For example, if nursing staff implement a protocol that requires 2 hours per day checking equipment standards, then other nursing care functions may be ignored. Another consideration is the disturbance of the clinical routine for medical and paramedical staff in the ICU which may result from data gathering. This could adversely affect the time available for patient care. A thoughtful audit design can minimize this disruption if data collection is incorporated into the daily routine.

The cost of audit is important to assess. If patient care records are organized with a consideration towards audit, then routine data collection does not need to be duplicated for audit purposes. This avoidance of duplication will minimize both the cost of data collection and maintain the focus of unit personnel on patient care. It is

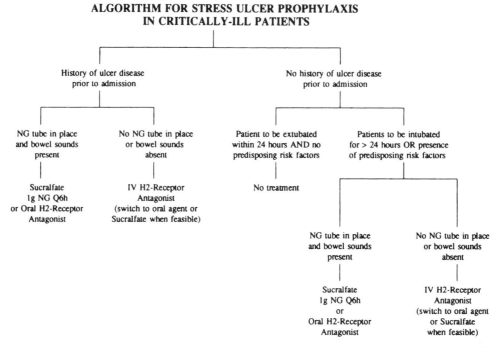

**ALGORITHM FOR STRESS ULCER PROPHYLAXIS
IN CRITICALLY-ILL PATIENTS**

Fig. 17.4   An algorithm outlining one clinical approach to stress ulcer prophylaxis in critically ill patients. This algorithm can be used to develop an audit of specific drug therapy used and the concurrence with the protocol.

vital to the success of the audit process that data collection and management which is intended to improve quality of care, does not impede patient care at the bedside. The audit system described incorporates data collection, data entry and analysis into the existing workload of hospital personnel. Whether such a unit-based system is more effective in ensuring quality of care as compared to a commercial system that includes clinical audit, nursing workload management and utilization management features has not been resolved. Whether one elects to use a commercial package or develop a unit-based system, the fundamentals remain the same and critical care personnel need to understand the limitations and problems of their audit system which could impede the successful achievement of change.

One aspect of audit that warrants emphasis is the need for confidentiality; this is equally important for any patient data management system (PDMS). In this respect the remote location from the intensive care unit of data storage and management can be a problem. Security capabilities on such computerized systems are required and the audit team and the programmer must be vigilant and aware of this issue.

Haynes and Walker[31] have emphasized that many claims for computerized medical information systems have exceeded documented effectiveness. Progress will only be made when known relationships between medical care process and outcome are established, and

this will necessitate computer-based information management systems. It is clear that the audit process itself needs to be considered as a new technology and evaluated thoroughly.

Future directions for critical care audit

Increasingly, computerized PDMS have been implemented in critical care units.[26, 28, 29] Such systems show promise for integrating information from a variety of sources (e.g. hospital record, laboratories, physician notes, etc.) for audit purposes. The limitations of such systems have been described[36–38] and little experience is available on the use of PDMS information for audit purposes. There is little doubt that this trend towards computerized PDMS will continue. Unless the basic principles of the audit process (Fig. 17.1) can be integrated with computerized PDMS, the impact of this technology on quality of care may be limited. The challenge for clinicians will be to organize and develop an audit process that makes use of this sophisticated and available technology to effect improvements in the quality of care delivered.

References

1. Department of Health, UK. *Working for Patients (White Paper)*. London: HMSO, 1989.
2. Hopkins A. Approaches to Medical Audit. *J Epidemiol Commun Health* 1991; **45**: 1–3.
3. Gumpert R, Lyons C. Setting up a district audit program. *Br Med J* 1990; **301**: 162–5.
4. Shaw CD, Costain DW. Guidelines for Medical Audit: seven principles. *Br Med J* 1989; **299**: 498–9.
5. Shaw CD. Criterion based audit. *Br Med J* 1990; **300**: 649–51.
6. Fowkes FGR. Medical audit cycle. *Med Ed* 1982; **16**: 228–38.
7. Crombie IK, Davies HTO. Computers in audit; servants or sirens. *Br Med J* 1991; **303**: 403–4.
8. Knaus WA, Wagner DP, Draper EA *et al.* The APACHE III prognostic system. *Chest* 1991; **100**: 1619–36.
9. Deming WE. *Out of the Crisis*. Cambridge, MA: Massachusetts Institute of Technology, 1986: 23–4.
10. Deasy TL. Quality improvement: the gurus and their approaches. *Int Anesthesiol Clin* 1992; **30**: 1–13.
11. Knaus WA, Draper EA, Wagner DP, Zimmerman JE. An evaluation of outcome from intensive care in major medical centers. *Ann Intern Med* 1986; **104**: 410–18.
12. Brook RH, Davies-Avery A, Greenfield S *et al.* Assessing quality of medical care using outcome measures: an overview of the method. *Med Care* 1977; **15** (Suppl. 9): 1.
13. Williamson JW. Formulating priorities for quality assurance activity. Description of a method and its application. *J Am Med Assoc* 1978; **239**: 631.
14. Williamson JW, Braswell HR, Horn SD. Validity of medical staff judgement in establishing quality assurance priorities. *Med Care* 1979; **281**: 1610.
15. Bedell SE, Delbosco TL, Cook EF *et al.* Survival after cardiopulmonary arrest in hospital. *New Engl J Med* 1983; **309**: 569–76.
16. Knaus WA, Draper EA, Wagner DP, Zimmerman JE. Prognosis in acute organ-system failure. *Ann Surg* 1985; **202**: 685–93.
17. Levy DE, Caronna JJ, Singer BJ, Lapinski RH, Frydman H, Plum F. Predicting outcome from hypoxic-ischemic coma. *J Am Med Assoc* 1985; **253**: 1420–5.
18. Berwick DM. Continuous improvement as an ideal in health care. *New Engl J Med* 1989; **320**: 53–6.
19. Nelson AR. Orphan data and the unclosed loop: a dilemma in PSRO and medical audit. *New Engl J Med* 1976; **295**: 617–19.
20. Byrick RJ, Caskennette G. Audit in critical care: aims, uses and limitations of a Canadian system. *Can J Anaesth* 1992; **39**: 260–9.
21. Wagner DP, Knaus WA, Draper EA. Statistical validation of a severity of illness measure. *Am J Public Health* 1983; **73**: 878–84.
22. Keene AE, Cullen DJ. Therapeutic Intervention Scoring System update 1983. *Crit Care Med* 1983; **11**: 1–3.
23. O'Brien-Pallas L, Leatt P, Deber R, Till J. A comparison of workload estimates using three methods of patient classification. *Can J Nursing Admin* 1989; **2**: 16–23.
24. Hjortso E, Buch T, Ryding J *et al.* The nursing care recording system. A preliminary study of a system for assessment of nursing care demands in the ICU. *Acta Anaesthesiol Scand* 1992; **36**: 610–14.
25. *International Classification of Diseases*, 9th edn, clinical modification. Washington DC, USA: US Government Printing Office, 1980; US Dept of Health and Human Services (publication number 80–1260) (PHS) vols 1,2.
26. Cereijo E. Computer assisted management of information in an intensive care unit. *Int J Clin Monitor Comput* 1992; **9**: 159–63.
27. Health Services Research Group, Clinical Epidemiology Unit, Sunnybrook Medical Centre, Toronto. Quality of Care: 1. What is it and how can it be measured? *Can Med Assoc J* 1992; **146**: 2153–8.
28. Shabot MM, Leyerle BJ, LoBue M. Automatic extraction of intensity-intervention scores from a computerized surgical intensive care unit flowsheet. *Am J Surg* 1987; **154**: 72–8.
29. Höltermann W, Knoch M, Pfeiffer H, Müller EE, Lennartz H. Marburger concept for computer-aided acquisition, processing and documentation of patient data in the intensive care unit. *Int J Clin Monitor Comput* 1990; **7**: 7–13.
30. Caskennette G, Byrick RJ, Mechetuk C. A critical care database management system for utilization management: the use interface and data input. *Can J Anaesth* 1992; **39**: A33.
31. Haynes RB, Walker CJ. Computer-aided quality assurance – a critical appraisal. *Arch Intern Med* 1987; **147**: 1297–1301.
32. Lomas J, Haynes RB. A taxonomy and critical review of tested strategies for the application of clinical practice recommendations: from 'official' to 'individual' clinical policy. *Am J Preventive Med* 1988; **4** (Suppl.): 77–94.
33. Steinberg EP, Moore RD, Powe NR *et al.* Safety and cost-effectiveness of high-osmolality contrast media as compared with low-osmolality contrast material in patients undergoing cardiac angiography. *New Engl J Med* 1992; **326**: 425–30.
34. Roy DJ, Dickens BM, McGregor M. The choice of contrast media: medical, ethical and legal considerations. *Can Med Assoc J* 1992; **147**: 1321–4.
35. Lomas J, Anderson GM, Domnick-Pierre K *et al.* Do practice guidelines guide practice? The effect of a consensus statement on the practice of physicians. *New Engl J Med* 1989; **321**: 136–11.
36. Gardner RM, Shabot MM. Computerized ICU data management: pitfalls and promises. *Int J Clin Monitor Comput* 1990; **7**: 99–105.
37. Green CA, Gilhooly KJ, Logie R, Ross DG. Human factors and computerisation in intensive care units: a review. *Int J Clin Monitor Comput* 1991; **8**: 167–78.
38. Avila LS, Shabot MM. Keys to the successful implementation of an ICU patient data management system. *Int J Clin Monitor Comput* 1988; **5**: 15–25.

CHAPTER 18

Quantifying Critical Illness

JF BION

Principles of severity measurement   276
Current methods   279
Applications   282
Future developments   285
References   285

A disease which I will treat
A disease with which I will contend
A disease not to be treated

This diagnostic classification of severity of disease – mostly injuries – was used by the surgeon-physician who wrote the Egyptian medical text known as the Edwin Smith Surgical Papyrus. The information which it contains probably dates from around 3000 BC, but the system of classification is still relevant today, and as a form of implicit prognosis constitutes part of every assessment which we make of patients referred for intensive care. Missing from it perhaps are those patients too well to need treatment, a phenomenon which has been examined in North American intensive care,[1] but fee-for-service presumably discouraged their separate identification. The Edwin Smith papyrus presents each clinical case in a highly structured form which relates diagnosis to prognosis and treatment, and it is clear from the text that decisions not to treat a particular condition are based on the severity of the disease process and therapeutic limitation. Some five millennia later we now find that medical technology can interfere with the relationship between disease and outcome by interposing organ system support. This ability to defer death even when we may not be able to deny it presents us with new ethical dilemmas; to quote Bertrand Russell: 'One of the troubles of our age ... is that as skill increases, wisdom fades.' However, knowing who to treat, and when to stop, is not only an ethical problem: it also requires predictive skills; and predic-

tion – the reduction of clinical uncertainty – requires systems of measurement.

The emotive aspects of prediction have complicated much of the discussion about the measurement of severity of illness. Systems of measurement used in a predictive mode enforce explicit decision making while at the same time arousing fears about the power of numbers replacing individual judgment. The problem is that any method of measurement must have some standard or outcome against which it can be validated, and in the case of critical illness this usually means death or survival: prediction then becomes an integral part of the system of measurement. Prediction is, however, only one of several uses to which such measures could be put. Of equal importance are stratification for clinical trials, quality of care issues, resource management, and service provision. These applications will be discussed, together with principles for measuring critical illness.

Principles of severity measurement

WHY DO WE NEED TO MEASURE SEVERITY OF ILLNESS?

Much of clinical medicine involves the assessment of risk. This is often a subconscious activity, or one that is poorly formalized and based on limited personal experience. We want to know what chance we, or our relatives, or our patients, may have of benefiting from a particular therapy, and what consequences may result from selecting one course of action rather than another. This cannot be done with any degree of accuracy unless the severity of the disease process is known and measurable. Prognostic uncertainty has an impact on clinical practice, as Detsky and colleagues showed in a study[2] of intensive and coronary care patients in which they compared expected and actual outcomes with costs of care. The highest costs were attracted by the patients with the least expected outcomes; that is, the survivors who were expected to die and the nonsurvivors who were expected to survive. One assumes that the former were correctly identified as being seriously ill and required considerable support to survive, while the latter were presumably treated to 'the bitter end.' Indeed, it costs more to die in intensive care than to survive, both in financial as well as emotional terms. If measures of severity of illness can reduce the duration of useless treatment by providing better prognostic information on which to base difficult decisions, then they should be employed as one would any other form of clinical test, with due regard for inherent inaccuracies and as an aid, not a substitute, for clinical judgment. When seen in this light, the concept that doctors do not need measures of severity of illness to tell them how ill their patients are is no more logical than dispensing with the need for chest X-rays. Moreover, the fear of applying severity scoring systems is often based on the withdrawal of treatment, whereas in reality severity scores might equally well be used to encourage its continuance; as Knaus has said, a predicted risk of mortality of 50% implies maximum uncertainty about the outcome. Comparisons of the predictive ability of medical staff versus scoring systems have tended to favor the latter,[3–5] and even if such systems are not used for clinical decision making, they may well become increasingly important as summary measures of activity to determine resource allocation for intensive care. Health expenditure is now a matter of concern to all governments, and subjective assessments of casemix will not be accepted when balancing competing demands.

HOW IS CRITICAL ILLNESS QUANTIFIED?

Critical illness means the potentially lethal acute failure of one or more organ systems. The extent to which acute disease determines outcome depends on a variety of factors. These include the severity of the acute illness, the type of disease process (diagnosis), the degree of physiological reserve, and the specificity and timing of therapy. A mechanical analogy for these four variables would be the applied load, the name (and hence durability) of the manufacturer, the engine capacity, and the skill of the operator.

Severity of acute illness

Severity of acute illness can be assessed in physiological, anatomical or functional terms, or a combination, and is the most important determinant of outcome. However, the degree to which acute illness affects physiological or functional variables depends on the balance between the illness itself and the patients' premorbid state of health – that is, their physiological reserve. Identifying the relative contributions of the two may not be necessary to predict death or survival, but it becomes more important when examining the potential quality of survival,[6] or when predicting risk in patients undergoing interventions such as major surgery. Physiological disturbance is one of the most important components of measuring severity of acute illness because health and homeostasis are closely linked, if not synonymous, phenomena. Living organisms preserve their integrity by maintaining cellular and systemic functions within a narrow range of physiological values, which Claude Bernard[7] referred to as the '*milieu interieur,*' and to which Walter Cannon[8] gave the name 'homeostasis.' We can define severity of illness in these terms as 'the extent to which a disease process has affected homeostatic mechanisms.' The assumption is that severity means physiological derangement, and that normal physiological values imply health. This view has been questioned by Shoemaker and his colleagues, because in certain acute disease states such as the sepsis syndrome 'normal' cardiorespiratory measurements may be inadequate to meet the increased requirements of the tissues for oxygen; supranormal physiological values have been proposed as appropriate for this population.[9, 10] Whether such values represent a different 'homeostat' (the therapeutic goal approach) or whether they are used to reflect severity of disease, is to some extent a semantic issue.

Physiological reserve

Physiological reserve is more difficult to measure than severity of acute illness. Examples include the limited value of serum creatinine as a measure of renal reserve and the need to employ time-consuming measures of clearance; angiography, radioisotope scans or treadmill tests to assess myocardial function; the absence of satisfactory markers of nutritional status and muscle power; or occult cirrhosis. One approach to this is to record only gross and simple measures of limitation, such as cancer, long-term steroids, biopsy-proven cirrhosis with varices, and age; the APACHE II[11] and III[12] systems do this, and the method seems to be as effective as earlier methods using more detailed grading.[13] Of interest is the fact that the impact of limited physiological reserve on mortality is diminished for elective postoperative admissions, and only fully expressed for emergency, unanticipated admissions, supporting the concept that, when there is time to provide it, prophylactic supportive therapy can be seen as a form of artificial reserve. Other methods of measurement have employed co-morbidities, but this requires an estimate of the relative importance of each additional diagnosis: those with a significant impact on the immune system appear to be the most important.[12] The difficulty is that reserve is often quantifiable only in the presence of a suitable stress, such as the treadmill referred to above. The treadmill principle is not easily transferable to other organ systems, which is in part why life-threatening complications of disease or therapy so often come as a surprise to attending clinicians. In addition, as described above, the fact that limited reserve is often expressed as more severe acute physiological disturbance complicates its independent measurement. The most commonly used surrogate measure of reserve is chronological age, but the relationship between the two is nonlinear, and in any case it is biological age which is important. We estimate biological age almost subconsciously, but quantifying it is much more difficult. It is of interest in this respect that the APACHE II age weighting underestimates the impact of age on mortality in Glasgow,[14] which is known to have a particularly unhealthy population, but overestimates it in Scandinavia,[15] where the reverse is true. An American study of outcome from intensive care for an elderly population has also suggested that chronological age has less impact on outcome when corrected for severity of illness.[16] This could be important when comparing outcomes between different groups, particularly on an international basis, in which instance perhaps some index of population health should be incorporated in the age weighting.

Diagnosis

Diagnosis contains implicit prognostic information, and the extent to which it does so is a reflection of therapeutic specificity and pathophysiological reversibility. The best example of this was provided by Knaus *et al.*[17] who showed that survival rates at similar levels of acute physiological disturbance varied between patients with sepsis, heart failure and diabetic ketoacidotic coma. Mortality at any given degree of severity was higher for sepsis than heart failure, while for diabetic coma there was no apparent relationship between the two. This shows that therapeutic specificity is greatest for diabetes, intermediate for heart failure, and least for sepsis. The problem about attaching prognostic weights to diagnosis is that they need revision depending on local factors and therapeutic advances; moreover, diagnostic labelling is complex,

and systems of coding and classification are still being designed and tested. An alternative approach has been to examine change in physiology with treatment, and systems which do this[4,18] perform as well for groups of patients as those which apply diagnostic weighting. In the new APACHE III system[12] change in score with time is stated by the authors to provide additional prognostic power. Can we then dispense with diagnosis when devising systems of measurement? There are three problems with this approach. First, common standards of care would be required to differentiate therapeutic incompetence from pathophysiological irreversibility. Second, diagnosis is often needed to explain why patients with end-stage failure of a single organ system die without necessarily suffering extensive physiological derangement. Finally, observing change in score with time makes preadmission assessment impossible because the patient must be subject to full intensive care for a defined period, an approach which might be considered inappropriate for certain diagnoses. It is likely that diagnosis will come to be used in broad categories (such as trauma, sepsis, autoimmune disease) in conjunction with specific definitions of organ system failures to explain physiology-based scores and change in score with therapy.

HOW IS THE ACCURACY OF SEVERITY MEASUREMENT DETERMINED?

All systems of measurement require some external and independent standard or outcome event with which they can be compared. Measures of critical illness tend to use mortality as the outcome marker because this is relevant to the underlying concept of 'severity' and is sufficiently common (8–40% of all admissions)[19] to be useful. Hospital, not unit, mortality is the endpoint used by most studies; though for audit purposes a comparison between the two may shed light on the quality of ward care or the timing of ICU discharge. Mortality is only one possible outcome however, and morbidity, functional disability and quality of life should be considered as well. Once an appropriate outcome has been chosen, the next step is to identify those variables which influence it, and attribute weights to them in order to generate a score. This can be performed either by clinical consensus or by multivariate statistical techniques, or most appropriately by a combination of the two whereby experienced clinical judgment undergoes statistical refinement. The system is then validated by testing it in an independent population. If the data set is large enough it can undergo internal validation first by using statistical techniques such as 'jack-knifing,'[20] which involves splitting the original data set into two parts, and then treating them as independent populations by testing the data derived from one group on the other while simultaneously subtracting one patient record at a time. The relationship between a summary score and the outcome frequency is presented as a probability using multiple logistic regression to generate a model, and this model can then be subject to goodness-of-fit analysis[21] as a test of its performance.

The process of validation involves calculating true-positive (sensitivity) and true-negative (specificity) rates at different cutoff points. In laboratory terms the cutoff point is the value at which the test becomes 'positive.' For a perfect test there would be no overlap (or 'gray area') of values. For severity scoring systems however, there is extensive overlap because increasing score means increasing risk: there is no single value above which all patients will die and below which all will survive, and for this reason single cutoff points should not be used to compare the predictive power of different scoring systems. The sensitivity and specificity should be calculated for a range of cutoff points to produce a graph known as a receiver–operator characteristic (ROC) curve,[22] a term derived from the wartime assessment of the accuracy of radar operators. The area under the curve is an index of the overall predictive power of the system. The sensitivity and specificity of the system at different cutoff points can be calculated using a standard two-by-two table of predicted vs actual outcomes; sensitivity (predicting death) is calculated as the number of correctly predicted nonsurvivors divided by the total number of deaths, and specificity (predicting survival) as the number of correctly predicted survivors divided by the total number of survivors. From these simple calculations one can obtain false-positive and false-negative rates, and positive and negative predictive values. Predictive values are measures of utility: the positive predictive value is the proportion of correct predictions of death, and the negative predictive value the proportion of correct predictions of survival. The positive predictive value will be reduced if the system were to be applied to a new population containing many more survivors, whereas sensitivity and specificity would be unchanged.

Current methods

The more commonly used measures of severity of illness, their acronyms, and their theoretical bases are given in Table 18.1. I will examine those that demonstrate particular principles.

ACUTE PHYSIOLOGY AND CHRONIC HEALTH EVALUATION (APACHE) II AND III

This is now one of the most widely used of all scoring systems for intensive care. The 34 variables and weights in the original version[13] were selected by clinical consensus, and then refined by statistical techniques to 12 physiological variables, with additional weighting for pre-existing chronic disease related to urgency of admission and age.[11] This has now undergone further development in another multicenter study in the USA, to produce version III.[12] APACHE III uses 17 physiological variables, a revised version of the Glasgow Coma Scale (GCS) based on eye opening, and is slightly more complex than APACHE II, though the principle is the same: the greater the extent of physiological derangement, the higher the score. The only chronic diseases or co-morbidities to have an impact on outcome are those which affect directly or indirectly the patient's immune status; and chronic health status only appears to be important for emergency, not elective, admissions. The authors continue to use the worst physiological values during the first 24 hours of intensive care, but do not explain in this context how the effect of sedative drugs on neurological function is distinguished from the effect of disease; careful reading of their paper suggests that admission values may be a satisfactory alternative to worst values, and that neurological assessment should reflect neurological disease and not some transient or secondary effect on cerebral function. Others[4, 18] recommend the use of the best neurological assessment rather than the worst, which compensates for this problem. The sum of the weighted values provides a score which can be used to stratify patients by severity *group*. Mortality risk assessment for *individual patients* requires the use of a predictive equation which employs additional weights for diagnostic category, and for treatment location before admission to account for the extent of earlier therapy on physiological abnormalities: this predictive equation is not in the public domain. Despite the considerable additional effort used to develop APACHE III, the improvement over version II in predictive power is modest (ROC curve area 0.9, vs 0.85 for APACHE II), perhaps because it is already very good. Both systems work well for risk estimation for groups of patients, and it remains to be seen whether APACHE III performs better than APACHE II or clinical judgment for predicting individual outcome.

APACHE-RELATED SYSTEMS

Three systems have been developed which are based on the APACHE II score. These are the Simplified Acute Physiology Score (SAPS),[23] the Sickness Severity Score (SSS),[4] and the Riyadh Intensive care Programme (RIP);[18] the latter two use change in score over time as a substitute for diagnostic weighting. None of these methods uses diagnostic weights.

SAPS has undergone revision to SAPS II.[24] The first version incorporated 14 variables, and excluded chronic health data, diagnoses, and measures of oxygenation; two variables which it did include (mechanical respiratory support and urine output) are sensitive to therapy rather than severity of illness. It did not provide probabilities of survival. SAPS II has been developed together with the new Mortality Probability Model (MPM) in a recently completed international multicenter study of around 15 000 patients. SAPS II[24] now includes 12 physiological variables with additional

weights for age, type of admission, and three underlying diseases – AIDS, metastatic malignancies or hematological malignancy. Urine output appears to have better predictive power than creatinine, and creatinine has therefore been excluded. The ratio of the arterial to inspired oxygen concentration (PaO_2/FiO_2) is used for ventilated patients as it is for the SSS, rather than the alveolar-arterial oxygen difference ($AaDO_2$) of the APACHE score or weights for mechanical ventilation

Table 18.1 Selected scoring and classification systems

Title and clinical area	Acronym	Theoretical basis	Reference
Intensive care			
Acute physiology and chronic health evaluation	APACHE	Physiological	13
APACHE second version	APACHE II	Physiological	11
APACHE third version	APACHE III	Physiological	12
Simplified acute physiology score	SAPS	Physiol + therapy	23
Organ system failures	OSF	Physiol + therapy	17
Sickness score	-	Dynamic APACHE II	4
Riyadh intensive care program	RIP	APACHE II + OSF	18
Mortality prediction model	MPM	Binary variables	24
Physiologic stability index	PSI	Physiological	75
Pediatric risk of mortality	PRISM	Derived from PSI	93
Hypoxic-ischemic coma outcome	-	Clinical neurology	35
Therapeutic intervention scoring system	TISS	Workload/costs	36
Time oriented score system	TOSS	Workload	63
Weighted hospital days	WHDs	Cost	64
Trauma			
Glasgow coma scale	GCS	Clinical neurology	27
Pediatric GCS	-	Clinical neurology	30
Abbreviated injury scale	AIS	Anatomical	38
Injury severity score	ISS	Anatomical	39
Triage index	TI	Physiological	94
Trauma score	TS	Physiological	33
Trauma score (revised)	rTS	Coded TS	40
Injury severity score + revised trauma score	TRISS	Combined	40
Pediatric trauma score	PTS	Physiological	95
DEFinitive methodology	DEF	MTOS TRISS statistics	96
Burns			
The burn index	-	Burn area + age	97
Cardiology			
Coronary prognostic index	CPI	Clinical + lab tests	98
Parsonnet score	-	Clinical + lab	42
Anesthesia			
Goldman cardiac risk index	CRI	Clinical	99
American Society of Anesthesiologists status	ASA	Clinical grading	100
Critical incident analysis	-	Error reporting	101
Functional quality			
Sickness impact profile	SIP	Functional ability	102
Uniscale	-	Subjective reporting	103
Karnofsky index	-	Physical activity	104
Others			
Sepsis score	SS	Clinical/physiological	105
Severity of illness index	-	Casemix	106
Physiological and operative severity score	POSSUM	Physiol + operative	43

from the earlier version of SAPS. Probability of survival is obtained from a graph which plots score against probability using logistic regression, as for the SSS. SAPS II performs well as a predictor of outcome for groups of patients (ROC curve area 0.86) and has the advantage of being easy to use. It is now being evaluated as a dynamic system recording change in score and risk over time.

RIP uses trend analysis of APACHE II scores in association with weighting for organ-system failures. The analysis takes into account both the absolute score and the rate of change to produce predictions of outcome – either death, or outcome uncertain. There were no false predictions of death in the test group, and the method is now undergoing further validation.

MORTALITY PREDICTION MODELLING (MPM)

This system has also undergone multicenter revision with SAPS. The first version[25] employed 11 binary variables (requiring yes/no responses) including emergency or previous ICU admission, age, coma, previous cardiorespiratory arrest, chronic renal failure, cancer, infection, systolic blood pressure, heart rate and surgery. It differs from physiologically based systems in that the variables were selected not by clinical consensus but by multiple logistic regression, and it provides a direct estimate of risk of death. It was initially validated in over 2000 patients and functions well in comparison with the physiological component of APACHE II and with SAPS.[26] The new version (the Mortality Probability Model)[27] has been developed from a cohort of over 19 000 patients and provides direct estimates of mortality risk on admission and at 24 hours using a larger number of binary variables. Like SAPS, SSS and RIP, it does not require specific diagnostic information. The MPM II has similar prognostic power to SAPS, with ROC curve areas around 0.83. It provides useful prognostic data at the time of ICU admission and is treatment-independent, but because it is a static measure this may limit its usefulness in time-based research. Binary systems of this type may be more useful for triage decisions than physiologically based methods.

ORGAN SYSTEM FAILURES (OSFs)

Organ system failures are attractive as a method of stratification because of their apparent simplicity, their ease of application, and because a large part of intensive care activities involve organ system support. Defining OSFs is more difficult, however. If defined in terms of supportive therapy (e.g. renal failure requiring dialysis, cardiovascular failure requiring vasoactive drugs), the

system becomes subject to the variability of clinical practice. Physiological definitions (e.g. serum creatinine, blood pressure) are more rigorous, but demand single cutoff points which offer less flexibility than systems like the APACHE score. One approach to this problem would be to develop some form of consensus about grading the degree of failure and hence the level of support required. Knaus and colleagues[17] applied strict definitions which were independent of therapy except for mechanical ventilation; they showed that the number and duration of failures were closely related to outcome, as have others.[28] OSFs with modified definitions also form part of the RIP system.

GLASGOW COMA SCALE (GCS)

This well-known scale[29,30] is a form of stratification applied to patients who have been in coma for 6 hours or more from the time of head injury. Pediatric versions have also been developed.[31,32] Its original function was to provide a common descriptive language, and indeed the system performs well between different observers.[33] There is now an international data bank of several thousand patients relating quality of survival to predicted outcome based on the GCS.[34] Weights were subsequently attached to the various components of the scale suggesting an equivalence which may not be valid, because the data are nonparametric and cannot be handled in the same way as continuous data. This may be a potential weakness of systems which incorporate the GCS. In the APACHE III score the GCS component has now been reordered according to eye opening and the verbal responses excluded, and the trauma score[35] appropriately employs a categorized version of the GCS. It should be remembered that the GCS was designed for assessing coma following trauma, and not for functional metabolic deficits. Recursive partitioning[36] has been employed to predict outcome from hypoxic-ischemic coma, and simple classification trees have been produced[37] using pupillary light reflexes and motor responses.

THERAPEUTIC INTERVENTION SCORING SYSTEM (TISS)

The basis of this system[38,39] is that therapeutic intensity defines severity of illness. A score of one to four points is awarded to each of 70 nursing and medical procedures. The system does not take into account the variability in clinical practice which may occur between ICUs and between different countries. It is however a useful system for assessing expenditure, and has been extensively used for this purpose. Studies in progress in the UK are said to show good predictive power in terms of forecasting expenditure.

INJURY SEVERITY SCORE (ISS), Trauma Score (TS) and TRISS

The Abbreviated Injury Scale (AIS),[40] like the GCS, was developed as an ordinal ranking system which attached values to injuries of increasing severity affecting each of six anatomical areas. The relationship between the summed ranked values and outcome is quadratic, but can be made linear by summing the squared values for each area: this is known as the ISS.[41] It can be calculated at death or discharge, in order to improve accuracy. The TS[35] in its revised form[42] is a simple physiological system designed for field use, which sums coded values for three intervals of the GCS, and five intervals of systolic blood pressure and respiratory rate. Both systems predict outcome accurately for groups of patients. Combining the ISS and the TS gives an anatomical and physiological index of severity of injury, the TRISS system,[42, 43] which is being used as the comparative index in the multiple trauma outcome study in the USA and the UK to determine casemix and mortality ratio differences.

PREOPERATIVE SCORING SYSTEMS: PARSONNET; POSSUM

With increasing emphasis on audit and risk stratification, various systems are being developed specifically for patients undergoing major surgery. Known or presumed risk factors are recorded, and then relative weights assigned to each on the basis of their ability to predict mortality or morbidity. Parsonnet's scoring system[44] is designed for patients undergoing cardiac surgery, and POSSUM[45] for general surgical patients. Such systems are potentially useful because they facilitate a common descriptive language, clarify the assessment of risk for the patient and potential costs of care for the hospital before intervention, and permit subsequent analysis of quality of care. It is likely that medical practice will increasingly be judged using this type of approach, and it is important that such systems are simple to use, are subject to extensive validation, and are introduced willingly by the medical profession rather than being imposed by others.

Applications

Scoring systems can be used for stratification for research, for the assessment of quality of care, for analysis of costs, and for clinical decision analysis related to the prediction of outcome. These applications are not mutually exclusive, but depend in part on the perspective of the user.

RESEARCH STRATIFICATION

An early example of the value of severity scoring is provided by the circumstances surrounding the use of etomidate in intensive care. This hypnotic agent was licenced for intravenous anesthesia during surgery, but clinicians then started using it for long-term sedation of critically ill patients undergoing mechanical ventilation. In 1983, the medical staff of an intensive care unit in Glasgow noted an increase in mortality rates in their patients admitted with multiple trauma. By using the ISS they were able to show that the excess mortality could not be attributed to an increase in severity of injury;[46] this unexpected negative finding led them to look for an alternative cause. Attention was directed to etomidate infusions as the only change in clinical practice.[47] Subsequent investigation identified the potent adrenocortical suppressant effect of etomidate,[48] hitherto unsuspected despite the concurrent interest in surgical stress reduction.

Research projects which use survival rates for comparing different treatments must ensure that the major factors which influence outcome have been identified and controlled. The conventional approach to this problem is the randomized, controlled trial in a specific patient population with a single diagnosis. However, disease severity may vary widely between patients with the same diagnosis, and to deal with this problem a sufficiently large number of randomized patients must be recruited to each group. This presents problems for intensive care where the number of patients in specific diagnostic categories are small, many have multiple diagnoses, and disease severity varies very considerably. Prior stratification for severity of illness is essential under these circumstances, and will help to reduce bias.[49-51] Most intensive care studies now incorporate such measures, and while they do not necessarily guarantee scientific purity (particularly when applied *post hoc*), they do help to relate differences in outcome to patient population, as recent antiendotoxin studies suggest.[52] Risk of death is a more appropriate form of stratification rather than using the score itself. Historical survival data are not acceptable for this purpose, and the value of studies which use this approach[53, 54] is limited.

AUDIT OF QUALITY OF CARE

Severity scoring can explain differences in survival rates between intensive care units with different management structures. In a study[19] of 13 hospitals, the ICU with the highest observed : expected mortality ratio had no defined policies for patient care, poor communication and working relationships between staff, and no clinical or nursing direction, in marked contrast to the units in hospitals with a better performance. Similar methods have been used to demonstrate that employing an intensivist can improve the efficiency and efficacy of pediatric intensive care,[55] and a retrospective study using APACHE II scoring has shown similar results for adult intensive care.[56] TRISS (the combination of the TS and ISS) allows the graphical presentation of the 50% rule for predicted mortality rates at different values of the TS and ISS, and this enables unexpected outcomes (nonsurvivors predicted to live, and vice versa) to be identified for further examination.[42,57] The Coronary Prognostic Index has recently been used to show that outcome following myocardial infarction has improved between 1969 and 1983 despite the absence of any reduction in severity of illness;[58] while new treatment modalities may explain this improvement, the index does not include measures of chronic health status, which may well have improved concurrently during the intervening years. APACHE II scoring has been used to examine the process of care given to critically ill patients undergoing secondary transport to a centralized intensive care unit. Such patients can be transported without physiological deterioration between hospitals provided that they are attended by experienced medical staff.[59] A separate study showed that complications during nonspecialist transport are related to the inexperience of the attendants and not the severity of illness of the patients.[60]

The principle which underlies comparisons between different ICUs is the calculation of the standardized mortality ratio (observed vs expected death rate). The expected death rate for each severity of disease level is determined from the data for the group as a whole; this is then calculated for each participating ICU and compared with their observed mortality rate. A ratio in excess of 1.0 suggests a performance worse than average, and lower than 1.0 better than average. Such ratios are themselves likely to be normally distributed, and judgments should not be passed on the data unless related to the standard deviation for the group. In addition, the mean for the group now represents the standard for comparison, and this may not be representative of all ICUs.

RESOURCE UTILIZATION

It is not enough only to know how much medical activities cost – the size of the resource. One also needs information about the way that resource is used. Collecting detailed information about expenditure is not complicated, but it is laborious, and surrogate measures are preferable. Salaries are the largest component of hospital budgets,[61] and nursing salaries account for over 50% of intensive care costs; measures of cost must therefore incorporate information about nursing and therapeutic dependence. Nursing dependency scores

can demonstrate differences in perceived severity of illness and the distribution of nursing staff,[62,63] but such systems have not been developed to the same scientific standard as other severity scores. A model relating SAPS to TISS proposes three levels of severity and the associated nursing ratios required,[64] but this assumes a linearity between severity of illness and the level of therapeutic support which may be entirely false: a conscious but confused patient may be much more work for the nurse than one with multiple organ failure who is sedated and paralyzed. An Italian group has developed a scoring system[65] which relates specific tasks to the time taken for their performance; the results correspond well with TISS, but the system is more complex than TISS, and it is difficult to imagine it being widely accepted by nurses who would presumably have to collect the data. At the other extreme is 'weighted hospital days,'[66] a method which describes ICU bed-days in terms of multiples of ordinary hospital bed-days; by this measure the first ICU day for a medical patient is worth three hospital bed-days, and two for each subsequent day in the unit. Surgical patients receive a slightly higher weighting. The method appears to correlate well with hospital charges in the USA. However, the TISS system for all its limitations seems to be a reasonable compromise between excessive simplicity and undue complexity.

Without scoring systems it is difficult to predict which patients will cost the most,[67] and scoring systems have been proposed as a method of reducing expenditure on patients who cannot benefit from intensive care.[68,69] For neonatal intensive care, birthweight is an excellent index of cost,[70] but matters are not so simple for adults. The highest costs in adult intensive care are attracted by emergency admissions who subsequently die, and it is these patients who have the highest APACHE II and TISS scores; these differences are not apparent for elective admissions.[6] The relationship between severity of illness and costs is nonlinear,[66] and is likely to reflect at least in part attitudes to monitoring and the level of care. For this reason it is more appropriate to compare standardized mortality ratios to cost, as this will give a better index of the efficiency of clinical performance. Most studies however use severity scores alone, without determining accompanying risk. The number of laboratory tests ordered in a pediatric intensive care unit has been shown to be related to the patients' severity of illness measured by the Physiological Stability Index (PSI).[71] The same scoring system has been used to reveal differences in clinical practice and therapeutic procedures in pediatric intensive care in the USA and France, despite similar admission severity scores and outcomes.[72] Diagnostic Related Groups (DRGs) are used in the USA for reimbursement, and have been shown to underestimate significantly the true costs of caring for critically ill patients.[73,74] Length of ICU and hospital stay will influence costs[66, 67] and the use of an index of severity of illness for all hospitalized patients can explain much of the variability in costs and length of stay between diagnostic groups.[75] The cost of the first day of intensive care can be predicted from the first 24-hour APACHE II score,[76] and this study also confirms the continuing high daily cost of supporting patients who ultimately die, as previously shown by Cullen,[38] who used TISS to demonstrate that survivors need less therapy as time passes, while the nonsurvivors require continuing high levels of support. Similar results have been obtained for critically ill children.[77]

CLINICAL DECISION ANALYSIS AND OUTCOME PREDICTION

Can measures of severity of illness be used to determine the extent of therapy for individual patients? The assumption behind this question is that scoring systems would substitute for, rather than assist, clinical judgment. The answer can be obtained by considering the following points. First, the type of patient for whom such an approach might possibly be considered would be one for whom the outcome was uncertain, not someone who was obviously too well or too sick to benefit from intensive care. What does clinical uncertainty mean in this context? It means that the predicted risk of death lies between 0 and 1, with the point of maximal uncertainty at 0.5 (or a predicted risk of dying of 50%). A predicted risk of 50% means that 50 of 100 patients in this risk band are likely to die, but it does not tell us which *individual* patient of the 100 patients will do so. Nor does it mean that all patients in risk bands above 0.5 will die. Even the 100% mortality band does not tell us the outcome for the next patient; all it does is to tell us that, given current therapy, survival of patients this sick is unprecedented. It is for this reason that scoring systems cannot determine therapy for individual patients, though they may well be used as guides as one would any other diagnostic test.

A number of studies have shown that scoring systems can predict outcome from critical illness as accurately as[3] or better than clinicians.[4, 5] It seems reasonable then to suggest that such methods should form part of clinical assessment. Opponents of this view should remember that scoring systems need not necessarily be used to favor withdrawal of treatment: they may also provide better than expected prognoses and thereby encourage continuing treatment. It is essential though that the weaknesses of scoring systems are understood. They provide information about groups of patients, not specific individuals;[78] they do not perform well outside the clinical context in which they were developed; systems of general applicability may appear to perform poorly when applied to single organ system dis-

eases;[79, 80] and the timing of data collection will have an impact on physiologically based systems because data collected after treatment has started will increase the number of patients incorrectly predicted to survive by lowering the scores, an effect known as lead-time bias.[81] Finally, the very nature of critical illness means that decisions to withdraw treatment based on an adverse prediction will guarantee the accuracy of that prediction – the self-fulfilling prophecy.

Triage

Given the limitations of scoring systems for predicting outcome for individual patients, do they have a role in determining access to intensive care? A study from the USA applied diagnosis-adjusted APACHE II scoring to 2419 adult patients referred for consideration for admission to a medical ICU; there was considerable overlap in scores between those admitted and those cared for in the ordinary wards.[82] This suggests either that factors other than severity of illness were influencing admission policy (not stated in the article), or that the APACHE II score does not distinguish reliably between patients with moderate levels of severity of illness in terms of their need for therapeutic support. Birthweight has been used in neonatal intensive care practice to show that neonates refused admission to intensive care because of resource limitations had a higher than predicted severity-adjusted mortality rate.[83] A similar study has shown that regional intensive care has a beneficial effect on survival rates of neonates of very low birthweight; but postnatal transfer of infants weighing more than 1.5 kg was associated with a higher mortality.[84] This is probably because low birthweight is a measure of limited physiological reserve rather than severity of illness, and above a certain weight other factors have a dominant effect on outcome. The Glasgow study[59] which severity-scored 50 critically ill adult patients undergoing transport to a centralized ICU suggested that high scores might be used prospectively for triage; but in a subsequent study of 112 patients, delay in referral of more than 24 hours was associated with an adverse outcome independently of severity of illness, with a progressively worse outcome the longer the delay.[85] Taken together, these two papers could be used as an argument for expediting the transfer of the patients with the higher scores rather than deferring them. What is missing of course is a measure of the potential for reversing physiological disturbance, as this approach requires the prior application of intensive care. Static, therapy-independent, and nonphysiological measures of risk such as the MPM could be useful in clarifying these issues when combined with APACHE-based methods: this is the principle of the TRISS system for trauma, but in practice the ISS cannot always be determined with confidence before hospital admission and investigation.

Treatment limitation

There has only been one study to date[86] which has examined the effect of severity scoring on clinical decision making in intensive care: following a period of observation and data collection in a number of French ICUs, clinicians were provided with individual prognostic estimates based on APACHE II scores. There was a small but significant increase in the number of treatment-withdrawals during this second period. However, there were some methodological difficulties with this study, as might be expected with any observational research which intends to influence clinical practice. In general, other researchers have tended to use severity scores to show that if clinicians had been given access to individual scores, and had acted on them, clinical practice might have been improved. Examples include the wasteful use of parental nutrition,[87] the useless treatment of severely ill patients with hematological malignancy,[88] the expensive treatment of trauma patients who subsequently die,[69] the variability of decisions to withdraw therapy,[89] and the unnecessary admission to intensive care of low-risk patients.[1, 68, 90] Differences have also been identified between hospitals in the use made of intensive care, suggesting inconsistencies in the selection of patients by clinicians.[91]

Quality of survival, rather than mortality, is a much less secure outcome measure. There is of course the added problem – and this is not intended facetiously – that one cannot obtain information about the quality of death from the patients who died. The Sickness Impact Profile (SIP) and Uniscale have been used as measures of function and life quality respectively, in a questionnaire study of 140 of 254 survivors from intensive care.[6] The worst outcomes were associated significantly with the highest TISS scores and total costs of hospital stay, and to a lesser extent with APACHE II score. Chronic health status before admission also predicted life quality and survival following discharge. Current evidence shows that impaired physiological reserve places constraints on the extent to which recovery is possible, while the severity of acute physiological disturbance determines the quality of survival only when extreme and prolonged. The implication is that predictions about potential quality of life should be based on careful history taking rather than the assistance of scoring systems.

Future developments

Existing measures of critical illness are relatively crude devices which are dependent for their development on improvements in investigative and diagnostic skills. Why is it that of two patients with the same predicted

risk of death, one may survive and the other die? Obviously there are variables which we either do not understand or which we cannot measure. Gastric tonometry, for example, may provide information about the adequacy of splanchnic oxygenation which cannot be derived from standard physiological indices,[92, 93] and techniques such as these may help to explain discrepancies in predicted and actual outcomes. Physiological reserve is another important area for development, particularly in the context of identifying patients at high risk of catastrophic deterioration,[94] as preventive intensive care almost certainly represents a better use of resources than trying to recover established organ system failures.

Given the current state of development, it is clear that scoring systems have a role in audit and the assessment of medical therapy, and could also be used to inform medical judgment. Dynamic systems and trend analysis will become important in the latter context, as a guide to the adequacy of therapy, but a balance must be found between identifying all the important variables and avoiding excessive complexity. One approach is to use relatively static measures such as the MPM or organ system failures, in conjunction with dynamic physiological scoring. Chang and his colleagues[18] employ OSFs with the APACHE II score, and use computer-assisted trend analysis to predict death. Bion et al.[4] have calculated the proportionate change in modified APACHE II score from admission to day 4 of intensive care, and showed that survival of the most severely ill patients was associated with a reduction in score of around 40%, and for patients with intermediate degrees of severity of illness, of 18%; failure to produce a reduction in score was associated with a worse outcome. The advantage of dynamic scoring methods is that they provide an alternative to diagnostic weights and contain an inbuilt assessment of the sensitivity of the underlying condition to medical therapy; the advantage of static systems is that they are therapy independent. The challenge is to find the best method of combining the two. This approach will receive considerable attention over the next few years.

References

1. Wagner DP, Knaus WA, Draper EA. Identification of low-risk monitor admissions to medical-surgical ICUs. *Chest* 1987; *92*: 423–8.
2. Detsky AS, Stricker SC, Mulley AG, Thibault GE. Prognosis, survival, and the expenditure of hospital resources for patients in an intensive-care unit. *New Engl J Med* 1981; *305*: 667–72.
3. Kruse JA, Thill-Baharozian MC, Carlson RW. Comparison of clinical assessment with APACHE II for

predicting mortality risk in patients admitted to a medical intensive care unit. *J Am Med Assoc* 1988; **260**: 1739–42.

4. Bion JF, Aitchison TC, Edlin SA, Ledingham IMcA. Sickness scoring and response to treatment as predictors of outcome from critical illness. *Intensive Care Med* 1988; **14**: 167–72.

5. Chang RWS, Lee B, Jacobs S, Lee B. Accuracy of decisions to withdraw therapy in critically ill patients: clinical judgement versus a computer model. *Crit Care Med* 1989; **17**: 1091–7.

6. Sage WM, Rosenthal MH, Silverman JF. Is intensive care worth it? An assessment of input and outcome for the critically ill. *Crit Care Med* 1986; **14**: 777–82.

7. Bernard C. *Leçons sur les Phenomenes de la Vie Commune aux Animaux et aux Vegetaux*. Paris, 1878.

8. Cannon WB. Organization for physiological homeostasis. *Physiol Rev* 1929; **9**: 399–431.

9. Shoemaker WC, Appel PL, Waxman K. Clinical trial of survivors' cardiorespiratory patterns as therapeutic goals in critically ill postoperative patients. *Crit Care Med* 1982; **10**: 398–402.

10. Bland RD, Shoemaker WC. Probability of survival as a prognostic and severity of illness score in critically ill surgical patients. *Crit Care Med* 1985; **13**: 91–5.

11. Knaus WA, Draper EA, Wagner DP, Zimmerman JE. APACHE II: a severity of disease classification system. *Crit Care Med* 1985; **10**: 818–29.

12. Knaus WA, Wagner DP, Draper EA *et al*. The APACHE III prognostic system. Risk prediction of hospital mortality for critically ill hospitalized adults. *Chest* 1991; **100**: 1619–36.

13. Knaus WA, Zimmerman JE, Wagner DP, Draper EA, Lawrence DE. APACHE – acute physiology and chronic health evaluation: a physiologically based classification system. *Crit Care Med* 1981; **9**: 591–603.

14. Ridley S, Jackson R, Findlay J, Wallace P. Long term survival after intensive care. *Br Med J* 1990; **301**: 1127–30.

15. Zaren B, Bergstrom R. Survival compared to the general population and changes in health status among intensive care patients. *Acta Anaesthesiol Scand* 1989; **33**: 6–12.

16. Wu AW, Rubin HR, Rosen MJ. Are elderly people less responsive to intensive care? *J Am Geriatric Soc* 1990; **38**: 621–7.

17. Knaus WA, Draper EA, Wagner DP, Zimmerman JE. Prognosis in acute organ-system failure. *Ann Surg* 1985; **202**: 685–93.

18. Chang RWS, Jacobs S, Lee B. Predicting outcome among intensive care unit patients using computerised trend analysis of daily APACHE II scores corrected for organ system failure. *Intensive Care Med* 1988; **14**: 558–66.

19. Knaus WA, Draper EA, Wagner DP, Zimmerman JE. An evaluation of outcome from intensive care in major medical centers. *Ann Intern Med* 1986; **104**: 410–18.

20. Efron B. *The Jackknife, the Bootstrap, and Other Resampling Plans*. Philadelphia, PA: Society for Industrial and Applied Mathematics, 1982.

21. Hosmer DW, Lemeshow S. *Applied Logistic Regression*. New York: John Wiley & Sons, 1990.

22. Weinstein MC, Fineberg HV. *Clinical Decision Analysis*. Philadelphia: WB Saunders, 1980.

23. Le Gall JR, Loirat P, Alperovitch A *et al*. A simplified acute physiology score for ICU patients. *Crit Care Med* 1984; **12**: 975–7.

24. LeGall J-R, Lemeshow S, Saulnier F. A new simplified acute physiology score (SAPS II) Based on a European/North American mulicenter study. *JAMA* 1993; **270**: 2957–63.

25. Lemeshow S, Teres D, Avrunin JS, Gage RW. Refining intensive care unit outcome prediction by using changing probabilities of mortality. *Crit Care Med* 1988; **16**: 470–7.

26. Lemeshow S, Teres D, Avrunin JS, Pastides H. A comparison of methods to predict mortality of intensive care unit patients. *Crit Care Med* 1987; **15**: 715–22.

27. Lemeshow S, Teres D, Klar J, Avrunin JS *et al*. Mortality probability models (MPM II) based on an international cohort of intensive care unit patients. *JAMA* 1993; **270**: 2478–86.

28. Pine RW, Wertz, Lennard ES, Dellinger EP, Carrico CJ, Minshew BH. Determinants of organ malfunction or death in patients with intra-abdominal sepsis. *Arch Surg* 1983; **118**: 242–9.

29. Teasdale G, Jennett B. Assessment of coma and impaired consciousness. A practical scale. *Lancet* 1974; **ii**; 81–4.

30. Jennett B, Teasdale G, Braakman R, Minderhoud J, Knill-Jones R. Predicting outcome in individual patients after severe head injury. *Lancet* 1976; **i**: 1031–4.

31. Morray JP, Tyler DC, Jones TK, Stuntz JT, Lemire RJ. Coma scale for use in brain-injured children. *Crit Care Med* 1984; **12**: 1018–20.

32. Reilly PL, Simpson DA, Thomas L. Assessing the conscious level in infants and young children: a paediatric version of the Glasgow Coma Scale. *Child's Nerv Syst* 1988; **4**: 30–3.

33. Teasdale G, Knill-Jones R, van der Sande J. Observer variability in assessing impaired consciousness and coma. *J Neurol Neurosurg Psychiat* 1978; **41**: 603–10.

34. Murray GD. Use of an international data Bank to compare outcome following severe head injury in different centres. *Statis Med* 1986; **5**: 103–12.

35. Champion HR, Sacco WJ, Carnazzo AJ, Copes W, Fouty WJ. Trauma score. *Crit Care Med* 1981; **9**: 672–6.

36. Friedman JH. A recursive partitioning decision rule for non-parametric classification. *IEEE Trans Comput* 1977; **16**: 404–8.

37. Levy DE, Caronna J, Singer BH, Lapinski RH, Frydman H, Plum F. Predicting outcome from hypoxic-ischemic coma. *J Am Med Assoc* 1985; **253**: 1420–6.

38. Cullen DJ, Civetta JM, Briggs BA, Ferrara LC. Therapeutic intervention scoring system: a method for quantitative comparison of patient care. *Crit Care Med* 1974; **2**: 57–60.

39. Cullen DJ. Results and costs of intensive care. *Anesthesiology* 1977; **47**: 203–16.

40. American Association for Automotive Medicine. *The Abbreviated Injury Scale (AIS) – 1985 Revision*. Des Plaines, IL, 1985.

41. Baker SP, O'Neil B, Haddon W, Long W. The injury

severity score: A method for describing patients with multiple injuries and evaluating emergency care. *J Trauma* 1974; **14**: 187–96.

42. Boyd CR, Tolson MA, Copes WS. Evaluating trauma care: the TRISS method. *J Trauma* 1987; **27**: 370–8.

43. Yates DW, Woodford M, Hollis. Preliminary analysis of the care of injured patients in 33 British hospitals: first report of the United Kingdom major trauma outcome study. *Br Med J* 1992; **305**: 737–40.

44. Parsonnet V, Dean D, Bernstein AD. A method of uniform stratification of risk for evaluating the results of surgery in acquired adult heart disease. *Circulation* 1989; **701** (Suppl.): 103–12.

45. Copeland GP, Jones D, Walters M. POSSUM: a scoring system for surgical audit. *Br J Surg* 1991; **78**: 356–60.

46. Watt I, Ledingham IMcA. Mortality amongst multiple trauma patients admitted to an intensive therapy unit. *Anesthesia* 1984; **39**: 973–81.

47. Ledingham IMcA, Watt I. Influence of sedation on mortality in critically ill multiple trauma patients. *Lancet* 1983; **i**: 1270.

48. Lambert A, Mitchell R, Frost J *et al.* Direct *in vitro* inhibition of adrenal steroidogenesis by etomidate. *Lancet* 1983; **ii**: 1085–1086.

49. Knaus WA, Wagner DP, Draper EA. The value of measuring severity of disease in clinical research on critically ill patients. *J Chronic Dis* 1984; **37**: 455–63.

50. Feinstein AR. An additional basic science for clinical medicine: III. The challenges of comparison and measurement. *Ann Intern Med* 1983; **99**: 705–12.

51. Green J, Wintfeld N, Sharkey P, Passman LJ. The importance of severity of illness in assessing hospital mortality. *J Am Med Assoc* 1990; **263**: 241–6.

52. Bone RC. A critical evaluation of new agents for the treatment of sepsis. *J Am Med Assoc* 1991; **266**: 1686–91.

53. Hook EW, Horton CA, Schaberg DR. Failure of intensive care unit support to influence mortality from pneumococcal bacteremia. *J Am Med Assoc* 1983; **249**: 1055–7.

54. Rogers RM, Weiler C, Ruppenthal B. Impact of the respiratory intensive care unit on survival of patients with acute respiratory failure. *Chest* 1972; **62**: 94–7.

55. Pollack MM, Katz RW, Ruttimann UE, Getson PR. Improving the outcome and efficiency of intensive care: The impact of an intensivist. *Crit Care Med* 1988; **16**: 11–17.

56. Brown JJ, Sullivan G. Effect on ICU mortality of a full-time critical care specialist. *Chest* 1989; **96**: 127–9.

57. Spence MT, Redmond AD, Edwards JD. Trauma audit – the use of TRISS. *Health Trends* 1988; **20**: 94–7.

58. Hopper JL, Pathik B, Hunt D, Chan WW. Improved prognosis since 1969 of myocardial infarction treated in a coronary care unit: lack of relationship with changes in severity. *Br Med J* 1989; **299**: 892–6.

59. Bion JF, Edlin SA, Ramsay G, McCabe S, Ledingham IMcA. Validation of a prognostic score in critically ill patients undergoing transport. *Br Med J* 1985; **291**: 432–4.

60. Bion JF, Wilson IH, Taylor PA. Transporting critically ill patients by ambulance: audit by sickness scoring. *Br Med J* 1988; **296**: 170.

61. Wilson L, Prescott PA, Aleksandrowicz L. Nursing: a major hospital cost component. *Health Serv Res* 1988; **22**: 773.

62. Lee TH, Cook F, Fendrick AM *et al.* Impact of initial triage decisions on nursing intensity for patients with acute chest pain. *Medical Care* 1990; **28**: 737–45.

63. Thompson JD. The measurement of nursing intensity. *Health Care Financing Rev* 1984; **6S**: 47.

64. Miranda DR, Langrehr D. National and regional organisation. In: Miranda DR *et al.* (eds) *Management of Intensive Care. Guidelines for Better use of Resources.* Amsterdam: Kluwer Academic Publishers, 1990.

65. Italian Multicentre Group of ICU Research. Time oriented score system (TOSS): a method for direct and quantitative assessment of nursing workload for ICU patients. *Intensive Care Med* 1991; **17**: 340–5.

66. Rapoport J, Teres D, Lemeshow S, Avrunin JS, Haber R. Explaining variability of cost using a severity-of-illness measure for ICU patients. *Medical Care* 1990; **28**: 338–48.

67. Chassin MR. Costs and outcomes of medical intensive care. *Medical Care* 1982; **20**: 165–79.

68. Henning RJ, McClish D, Daly B *et al.* Clinical characteristics and resource utilisation of ICU patients: Implications for organization of intensive care. *Crit Care Med* 1987; **15**: 264.

69. Fischer RP, Flynn TC, Miller PW, Rowlands BJ. The economics of fatal injury: dollars and sense. *J Trauma* 1985; **25** 746–50.

70. Tudehope DI, Lee W, Harris F, Addison C. Cost-analysis of neonatal intensive and special care. *Aust Paediatr J* 1989; **25**: 61–5.

71. Klern SA, Pollack MM, Getson PR. Cost, resource utilization, and severity of illness in intensive care. *J Pediatr* 1990; **116**: 231–7.

72. Davis AL, Pollack MM, Cloup M, Cloup I, Wilkinson JD. Comparisons of French and USA pediatric intensive care units. *Resuscitation* 1989; **17**: 143–52.

73. Bekes C, Fleming S, Scott WE. Reimbursement for intensive care services under diagnosis-related groups. *Crit Care Med* 1988; **16**: 478–81.

74. Kreis DJ, Augenstein D, Civetta JM, Gomez GA, Vopal JJ, Byers PM. Diagnosis related groups and the critically injured. *Surg Gynaecol Obstet* 1987; **165**: 317–22.

75. Horn SD, Bulkley G, Sharkey PD, Chambers AF, Horn RA, Schramm CJ. Interhospital differences in severity of illness: Problems for prospective payment based on diagnosis-related groups (DRGS). *New Engl J Med* 1985; **313**: 20–4.

76. Ridley S, Biggam M, Stone P. A cost-benefit analysis of intensive therapy. *Anaesthesia* 1993; **48**: 14–19.

77. Yeh TS, Pollack MM, Ruttimann UE *et al.* Validation of a physiologic stability index for use in critically ill infants and children. *Pediatr Res* 1984; **18**: 445.

78. Hopefl AW, Taafe C, Stephenson GC. Failure of APACHE II lone as a predictor of mortality in patients receiving total parenteral nutrition. *Crit Care Med* 1989; **17**: 414–17.

79. Fedullo AJ, Swinburne AJ, Wahl GW, Bixby KR. APACHE II score and mortality in respiratory failure due to cardiogenic pulmonary failure. *Crit Care Med* 1988; **16**: 1218–21.

80. Schaefer J-H, Jochimsen F, Keller F, Wegscheider K, Distler A. Outcome prediction of acute renal failure in medical intensive care. *Intensive Care Med* 1991; **17**: 19–24.

81. Dragsted L, Jorgensen J, Jensen N-H, Bonsing E, Jacobsen E, Knaus WA, Qvist J. Interhospital comparisons of patient outcome from intensive care: importance of lead-time bias. *Crit Care Med* 1989; **17**: 418–22.

82. Franklin C, Rackow EC, Mamdani B, Burke G, Weil MH. Triage considerations in medical intensive care. *Arch Intern Med* 1990; **150**: 1455–9.

83. Sidhu H, Heasley RN, Patterson CC, Halliday HL, Thompson W. Short term outcome in babies refused perinatal intensive care. *Br Med J* 1989; **299**: 647–9.

84. Powell TG, Pharoah POD. Regional neonatal intensive care: bias and benefit. *Br Med J* 1987; **295**: 690–2.

85. Purdie JAM, Ridley SA, Wallace PGM. Effective use of regional intensive care units. *Br Med J* 1990; **300**: 79–81.

86. Knaus WA, Rauss A, Alperovitch A, Le-Gall JR, Loirat P, Patois E, Marcus SE. Do objective estimates of chances for survival influence decisions to withhold or withdraw treatment? *Med Decis Making* 1990; **10**: 163–71.

87. Chang RWS, Jacobs S, Lee B. Use of APACHE II severity of disease classification to identify intensive-care-unit patients who would not benefit from total parenteral nutrition. *Lancet* 1986; **i**: 1483–7.

88. Lloyd-Thomas AR, Wright I, Lister TA, Hinds CJ. Prognosis of patients receiving intensive care for life-threatening medical complications of haematological malignancy. *Br Med J* 1988; **296**: 1025–1029.

89. Zimmerman JE, Knaus WA, Sharpe SM, Anderson AS, Draper EA, Wagner DP. The use and implications of Do Not Resuscitate orders in intensive care units. *J Am Med Assoc* 1986; **255**: 351–6.

90. Wager DP, Knaus WA, Draper EA *et al*. Identification of low-risk monitor patients within a medical-surgical intensive care unit. *Medical Care* 1983; **21**: 425–34.

91. Zimmerman JE, Knaus WA, Judson JAB, Havill JH, Trubuhovich RV, Draper EA. Patient selection for intensive care: a comparison of New Zealand and United States hospitals. *Crit Care Med* 1988; **16**: 318–26.

92. Gutierrez G, Palizas F, Doglio G *et al*. Gastric intramucosal pH as a therapeutic index of tissue oxygenation in critically ill patients. *Lancet* 1992; **339**: 195–99.

93. Schlichting E, Lyberg T. Letter. *Lancet* 1993; **341**: 692.

94. Sax FL, Charlson ME. Medical patients at high risk for catastrophic deterioration. *Crit Care Med* 1987; **15**: 510–15.

95. Pollack MM, Ruttimann UE, Getson PR. Pediatric risk of mortality (PRISM) score. *Crit Care Med* 1988; **16**: 1110–16.

96. Champion HR, Sacco WJ, Hannan DS. Assessment of injury severity: the triage index. *Crit Care Med* 1980; **8**: 201–8.

97. Tepas JJ, Ramenofsky ML, Mollitt Dl *et al*. The pediatric trauma score as a predictor of injury severity: an objective assessment. *J Trauma* 1988; **28**: 425–9.

98. Champion HR, Sacco WJ, Hunt TK. Trauma severity scoring to predict mortality. *World J Surg* 1983; **7**: 4–11.

99. Feller I, Tholen D, Cornell RG. Improvements in burn care, 1965 to 1979. *J Am Med Assoc* 1980; **244**: 2074–7.

100. Norris RM, Brandt PWT, Lee AJ. Mortality in a coronary-care unit analysed by a new coronary prognostic index. *Lancet* 1969; **i**: 278–81.

101. Goldman L, Caldera DL, Nussbaum SR *et al*. Multifactorial index on cardiac risk in noncardiac surgical procedures. *New Eng J Med* 1977; **297**: 845.

102. Dripps RD, Lamont A, Eckenhoff JE. The role of anesthesia in surgical mortality. *J Am Med Assoc* 1961; **178**: 261.

103. Cooper JB, Newbower RS, Kitz RJ. An analysis of major errors and equipment failures in anesthesia management: considerations for prevention and detection. *Anesthesiology* 1984; **60**: 34.

104. Bergner M, Bobbitt RA, Carter WB *et al*. The sickness impact profile: development and final revision of a health status measure. *Medical Care* 1981; **19**: 787.

105. Spitzer WO, Dobson AJ, Hall J *et al*. Measuring the quality of life of cancer patients: a concise QL index for use by physicians. *J Chron Dis* 1981; **34**: 585.

106. Hutchinson TA, Boyd NF, Feinstein AR *et al*. Scientific problems in clinical scales, as demonstrated by the Karnofsky index of performance status. *J Chron Dis* 1979; **32**: 661–6.

107. Elebute EA, Stonor HB. The grading of sepsis. *Br J Surg* 1983; **70**: 29–31.

108. Horn SD, Horn RA. Reliability and validity of the severity of illness index. *Medical Care* 1986; **24**: 159–78.

109. Wagner DP, Knaus WA, Draper EA. Physiologic abnormalities and outcome from acute disease. Evidence for a predictable relationship. *Arch Intern Med* 1986; **146**: 1389–96.

CHAPTER 19

Selection of Patients for Intensive Care

ALASDAIR IK SHORT

Definitions 289
Introduction 289
Selection criteria 290
References 294
Elective intensive care 291
Monitoring 291
Emergency admissions 291
Trauma 292
Who makes and polices the selection policy? 293
Summary 294
References 294

Definitions

INTENSIVE CARE UNIT

Intensive care is normally reserved for patients with potential or established organ failure. An intensive care unit (ICU) should provide the facilities for diagnosis, prevention and treatment of multiple organ failure. The most commonly supported organ is the lung but an intensive care unit should offer a wide range of facilities for organ support. This will require a multidisciplinary team approach and the highest possible standards of nursing and medical care. A nurse to patient ratio of 1 : 1 should be the minimum and the services of a full-time medical resident are essential.[1]

HIGH DEPENDENCY UNIT

A high dependency unit (HDU) is an area offering a standard of care intermediate between the general ward and full intensive care. The HDU should not manage patients with multiple organ failure but should provide monitoring and support to patients at risk of developing organ system failure. An HDU should be able to undertake short-term resuscitative measures and might provide ventilator support for a short time (less than 24 hours) prior to transfer of the patient to an ICU.

The HDU does not need and should not provide a full range of services. It would normally function with a nurse to patient ratio of 1 : 2 and does not require the exclusive services of a full-time resident doctor.[1]

Introduction

The ability to support patients through periods of major organ dysfunction or failure has been developed over the past 40 years. There have been many advances in the understanding of the pathophysiology of acute life-threatening disease, in drug therapies and in the technologies of monitoring and organ support. The public now have a preconceived idea of curative power of intensive care derived from the media and it is expected that all critically ill patients should receive intensive care as a natural course of events by right.

The assessment of the effectiveness of intensive care and therapeutic 'advances' on patient outcome has received somewhat less attention.[2,3] It is only within the past 20 years that serious systematic examination of long-term patient outcome following intensive care has been initiated.[4–11] This increase in interest has been primarily driven by the high cost of provision of intensive care, particularly for those patients who do not survive to leave hospital. These patients consume a very high proportion of the available resources.[12]

The hard reality of current economic difficulties in the face of increasing demand is forcing the intensive care community to reassess how and to whom intensive care is offered. The fact that treatment (of proven value or not) is possible is not in itself justification for proceeding to implement that therapy regardless of other factors operating in a particular patient's case. Appropriate management is desirable not only from the economic point of view, but more importantly for the proper care of the patient. Intensive care therapies and invasive monitoring techniques have complications[13,14] and inappropriate admission of low-risk patients wastes resources and exposes the patient to unnecessary risk. Proper selection of patients to receive intensive care is therefore essential to ensure proper management of both patient and scarce resources.[14] The difficulty is in identifying those patients for whom intensive care is of likely value (the cutoff points for this value using, for example probability of survival/mortality, have also to be determined) and denying admission to those whose condition does not warrant admission on the grounds of being unnecessary or futile. These decisions may have to be taken in the face of considerable pressure from referring physicians and patient's relatives, often with the added stress of limited bed availability.

This chapter attempts to cover the criteria available for patient selection, describing those patients who clearly select themselves and those who fall into a much more difficult category to assess. This will be followed by a discussion of some of the practical problems and solutions that might be applied to achieve the appropriate admission of patients to intensive care facilities.

Selection criteria

PATIENT OUTCOME DATA

The absolute minimum favorable outcome for the patient must be discharge from hospital alive. Therefore studies relating purely to survival to leave the intensive care unit will not be considered in detail.

Data on outcome had been slowly accumulating in generally small series of patients until the early 1980s. With few exceptions these were specialized disease, retrospective studies from individual tertiary referral centers. Extrapolation to general intensive care provision was difficult, to say the least.

Within the past 15 years the Acute Physiology and Chronic Health Evaluation (APACHE),[16–18] Mortality Prediction Model (MPM),[19,20] Pediatric Risk of Mortality (PRISM),[21] Simplified Acute Physiology Score (SAPS)[22,23] and other systems of patient outcome prediction and assessment have been developed. All, apart from MPM, require the collection of data for 24 hours following admission to intensive care. They are designed to adjust for casemix and currently are being developed and validated in many countries. Publication of large series of patients from the USA, the UK and continental Europe comparing the different methods are imminent.[23–25] There are still considerable problems to be overcome when using these methods to generate and compare observed with expected probability of death or survival. The difficulties of uniform physiological data collection and the effects on these data of lead-time bias and patient treatment immediately prior to and during the period of data collection are yet to be resolved.[20,26–28] These studies have prospectively examined patient outcome in intensive care units of different size, hospital status (teaching/university or not) and patient diagnosis. Despite these broader-based series the number of patients entered and analyzed is still inadequate to allow highly accurate individual prognostic assessment and selection in even relatively common conditions. There are also relatively few data available on long-term survival and quality of life following discharge from hospital.[6,11,29] Similarly the optimum facilities, staffing and organization of intensive care facilities required to produce the best patient outcome are still far from clear, although certain general principles have been suggested.[30] A national data collection system is currently being set up by the Intensive Care Society within the UK to allow the development of a database and prognostic system to try to resolve these problems.

As yet these methods are not proposed as a means of selection for admission to intensive care units. Only MPM is based on admission data and the developers of this method have cautioned against using any score alone to determine admission policy for any given patient.[19,22]

Given the current lack of definitive guidance available based upon robust studies for most clinical situations, what recommendations can be made?

AGE

From the data available from the APACHE studies only some 7–8% of the predictive power of the system is related to age. There is no evidence to justify the use of chronological age as a single absolute determinant of whether or not to admit to an intensive care unit. Although it was found in a comparative study between the USA and New Zealand that there was a clear policy of not admitting older patients in New Zealand,[31] there are several reports showing that age alone is not a valid criterion for selection for intensive care.[9, 32, 33]

UNDERLYING DISEASE PROCESS

Certain disorders have a very poor prognosis regardless of the intercurrent complication and one would question the use of expensive resources to prolong a patient's death, e.g. septic shock and respiratory failure in a neutropenic patient with acute myeloid leukemia in relapse or a patient with advanced solid organ malignancy.[34, 35] Patients suffering from acquired immunodeficiency syndrome (AIDS) form another group about which there is much discussion. Treatment of the first episode of pneumocystis pneumonia is often followed by worthwhile survival, although to date the ultimate outcome is inevitably death within 2–3 years.[36]

ACUTE PHYSIOLOGICAL DERANGEMENT

Systems such as APACHE, MPM, PRISM, SAPS, etc. show, for grouped data, a clear relationship between the component of the score measuring severity of physiological derangement and the probability of hospital survival. Only the MPM system claims to be able to provide a mortality prediction on the basis of admission data, but it does not claim to be able to predict outcome with high sensitivity for individual patients.[20] The APACHE and SAPS systems base their outcome prediction on physiological data gathered over the first 24 hours of intensive care. Most studies of scoring systems have been assessments of mortality/survival probabilities but an attempt has been made to adapt the APACHE system to produce a means of triage for emergency medical intensive care unit admissions. The conclusion was that current systems were not adequately sensitive or specific but specific diagnosis coupled with associated physiological and laboratory data might be used in the future.[37] It would take a brave person to advocate patient acceptance or denial for intensive care purely on the basis of admission physiology scores.

Elective intensive care

One group of patients that can be easily identified as likely to benefit from intensive care are those patients undergoing major elective surgery which produces severe short-term physiological disturbance, e.g. com-plicated cardiothoracic, vascular, neurological or transplant surgery. Provided these patients have been appropriately selected for their primary procedure, a period of intensive care will be part of their normal management with a very high expectation of good outcome and short ICU stay.[38, 39] Physiological oxygen transport goals have been suggested by Shoemaker's group for these high-risk patients with consequent improvement in survival[40] and to achieve these goals a period of intensive care will be required prior to as well as following surgery. There are studies showing benefit[41] from preoperative 'goal-directed' intensive care and lack of benefit from postoperative attempts to achieve these physiological goals,[42] but as yet no consensus has been reached. Whether or not goal-directed therapy is effective, there is little doubt that careful pre-, inter- and postoperative management is valuable for these high-risk patients. Specific intensive care areas are commonly set aside for these patients and admission is part of the normal management protocol. In the situation of mixed acute and elective units difficulty may be encountered in prevailing upon surgical colleagues to postpone elective operations when there are no available intensive care beds, rather than proceed in the hope that there will be no post-operative problems.[43] This results in bed crises when events do not go to plan, creating considerable disruption, acrimony and less than optimum patient care.

Monitoring

Monitoring is often given as a reason for admission to an intensive care bed. What evidence is there that monitoring in an intensive care area improves outcome? The one obvious situation is that of the coronary care unit (CCU), where the rapid detection and correction of early postmyocardial infarct ventricular fibrillation, complete heart block and other malignant dysrhythmias is essential for the best possible patient outcome and is highly effective. It is questionable as to how many of these patients truly require the facilities of an intensive care unit as defined at the beginning of the chapter. Local provision of facilities both structural (presence of CCU, HDU, etc.) and staffing (primarily nursing) will determine the extent to which patients may require ICU admission as opposed to an HDU. A major finding of the UK APACHE II study in comparing the UK and US data was the far greater number of patients with low risk of mortality admitted for monitoring to intensive care units in the USA.[29] Several explanations are possible including those mentioned above but the increased revenue to the hospital from patients admitted to intensive care areas in the USA cannot be discounted. The use of expensive and, at least in the UK, scarce intensive care resources for the monitoring of low-risk patients is as indefensible as inappropriate initiation or prolongation of intensive care in those with no prospect of satisfactory outcome.

Emergency admissions

This group of patients may be divided into those patients with single organ failure of short-lived, self-correcting type and the complex multiple organ failure complicating a primary disease process that may or may not be survivable even in the short term.

SINGLE ORGAN FAILURE

Clear benefit has been shown for the provision of intensive care to these patients. An early example of intensive care provision in the 1950s falls into this category, that of neuromuscular failure secondary to poliomyelitis.[44] Other common conditions are drug overdose producing central respiratory failure, uncomplicated respiratory distress syndrome of the newborn and Landry-Guillain-Barré syndrome. All of these conditions have an excellent prognosis which has come about following the introduction of intensive care.

COMPLEX MULTIPLE ORGAN DYSFUNCTION

Within this extremely heterogeneous group, sweeping statements are difficult to make. The picture is colored by the primary underlying condition and its prognosis, the superadded complication(s) and the severity of the physiological insult the patient has suffered at the time of referral (e.g. cardiorespiratory arrest).

However, in the emergency situation where no clear prior decision not to treat has been made or the patient does not have a well-established diagnosis of terminal disease (e.g. disseminated carcinomatosis, terminal chronic respiratory, cardiac or liver disease), admission should be the rule. There should be the clear understanding by all concerned that intensive care may be withdrawn once all relevant information has been obtained and the patient's condition followed over the next 24–72 hours. The APACHE III[19] and Chang's Riyadh[45] system are currently being developed to assess the response of patients scores to therapeutic intervention over the initial days following admission. From the change in score over the first 3–4 days an individual probability of mortality is calculated which may be used as a guide as to when withdrawal of intensive care

might be contemplated. This of course does not help with admission selection.

POST CARDIAC ARREST

There is now an extensive literature on the prospect of worthwhile survival following cardiorespiratory arrest.[46-48] The miserable results obtained in the situation of patient with unwitnessed, out of hospital arrest who arrive asystolic, would convince many that provision of prolonged resuscitation followed by prolonged and futile intensive care is not justifiable. Following successful prolonged cardiopulmonary resuscitation in the case of witnessed cardiac arrest in a patient with nonterminal disease, admission to an ICU is advisable as these patients commonly require ventilatory and cardiovascular support. Admission criteria may therefore be created following cardiorespiratory arrest and decisions should be made to withhold cardiopulmonary resuscitation in those patients not to be considered for intensive care.[15, 48]

POTENTIAL ORGAN DONORS

Brain stem dead, beating heart donors will normally be cared for in an intensive care unit as by definition they require artificial ventilation. Proper management of the organ donor once brain death has been declared requires intensive care facilities and the question of admission should not arise.[49]

However Feest *et al.*[50] in the UK have raised the issue of admitting patients to intensive care units for ventilatory and other support in the expectation of their proceeding to become brain stem dead and thus organ donors. The difficulties caused by the occupation of scarce intensive care resources and the possibility of producing patients in a persistent vegetative state have been raised by the authors. A larger study is awaited to verify or refute the value of this approach and the legal aspects of providing treatment to individuals which is arguably not for their benefit has yet to be resolved.

Trauma

The proper management of major trauma will require intensive care in most situations with multiple organ injury affecting head, chest and abdomen. The intensive care phase attempts to minimize the third peak of trauma death and the intensive care service should have close links and good communication with the trauma service.

Children

There has been considerable discussion as to the requirement for special facilities to be available for children. There is no question that for neonates special facilities are required. There would also be little debate that children with congenital abnormalities requiring complex surgery and intensive care require specialized intensive care. In the UK some 25% of admissions to intensive care units under the age of 16 years are admitted to mixed adult and pediatric units. In the USA Pollack *et al.*[51] have published a comparison of the outcome of patients under the age of 18 years and showed a more favorable outcome for children admitted to large teaching hospital pediatric intensive care units. There are methodological problems with this study[52] and as yet the issue as to which conditions require transfer to large centralized units is not at all clear. The other vexed issue is, when does a child become an adult? The acceptance of any particular age cutoff, for example 18 years as in Pollack's study, would be contested by many.

What is required is an accepted policy within any geographical area as to the way critically ill children should be managed. If this involves patient transfer, then adequate facilities for safe and rapid transportation must be provided.

Who makes and polices the selection policy?

As in all areas of medicine, cooperation and clear delineation of responsibility are necessary. Simple clear guidelines for admission are required and these should follow negotiation between the consultants responsible for providing intensive care and those referring their patients to the ICU. There is a requirement for experienced critical care clinicians to direct and staff the intensive care unit.[30,53–55] The local arrangement as to who retains overall responsibility for the patient in the ICU will obviously influence the practice in any particular institution. However this contentious issue is resolved, it is essential that only one service, the intensive care unit staff, coordinates therapy changes, otherwise a chaotic situation may result that is to the patient's detriment.[30]

Guidelines are however not sufficient to cover every individual emergency situation where the underlying diagnosis is often in doubt. Dialogue is required at senior (consultant) level to determine what is possible and necessary for the management of the underlying condition and what is possible in the way of intensive care support and outcome. There is often an unrealistic expectation of the time that will be required to successfully support a patient through their period of intensive care. It must be clearly understood by the referring specialty as well as by the patient's relatives, the considerable time that may be required to get the patient fit for discharge to the ward. The mistaken view that unless the patient is extubated within a day or two of admission that they are doomed is still encountered.

If guidelines are well structured, referrals and initiation of intensive care may become more timely. There is often significant delay between the onset of the early signs of impending major physiological decompensation, the calling for senior help and appropriate intervention. There may be a natural reluctance to accept that things are getting out of control and a tendency to feel that asking for help from the intensive care service is an admission of inadequacy with consequent loss of face. This can be a problem among medical staff of all seniority and is not helped by insensitive and deprecating comments in the heat of the moment from ICU staff.

The aim should be to intervene as early as possible and not when the patient has had a cardiac or more commonly respiratory arrest which, with the exception of early ventricular fibrillation after myocardial infarction, pulmonary embolism or sudden catastrophic hemorrhage, occurs relatively late in the process of deterioration. It is obvious that a superimposed global anoxic/ischemic insult will not increase the chance of a patient's recovery.

In the UK there seems to be a generally poor level of understanding of the pathophysiology of critical illness and the body's compensatory responses, coupled with poor performance in terms of patient resuscitation. This appears to be a major defect in medical education, both undergraduate and postgraduate. There is a clear need to expose clinicians in training in any of the acute specialties to intensive care experience. The aim is not to turn them into intensive care specialists, but into clinicians who can recognize the high-risk patient, the early signs of decompensation and the appropriate response to institute correct management. Timely referral to the intensive care service might well improve the lot of many patients and in any referral system stress must be put on the need for early consultation when a patient is at high risk of decompensation. This not only serves the patients' best interests but allows for the orderly preparation of a bed within the intensive care unit if and when needed. Ideally it is possible to avoid the precipitation of a crisis requiring movement of patients at short notice often in the middle of the night with all the attendant problems. The point can be illustrated with a common scenario: a patient is rushed to the operating theater by the surgeons with presumed perforation of the bowel (usually out of normal working hours); fluid resuscitation is somewhat inadequate and the patient's perfusion is poor throughout the procedure; fecal peritonitis is found due to perforated diverticular disease; surgery is completed and the patient will not tolerate extubation, has a marked acidemia and is hypotensive. The ICU is then contacted and at short notice has to galvanize a response that could have been better prepared at an orderly pace had the patient been referred prior to surgery, with a better result for all concerned.

The same rules should hold for patient transfers between ICUs and hospitals. Those ICUs accepting patients transferred from distant hospitals with conditions requiring the services of other specialties within the hospital have a responsibility to inform those specialties prior to the transfer. This will allow them to be prewarned and organize their plans accordingly. The same holds for specialist services admitting from other hospitals patients requiring or likely to require admission to intensive care.

All new emergency referrals should be seen by the ICU consultant early (within an hour) after admission and only the consultant on call for the ICU can deny admission. This allows for a definitive plan of management to be established with the minimum delay and communication with other involved specialties at a consultant level makes patient management speedier and more effective. Detailed patient management by telephone is difficult. It is surprising how often the impression of a patient's condition received over the telephone turns out to be quite different from that found when examining the patient in person. At present there is no direct evidence that early input from senior experienced clinicians alters outcome and hopefully this will appear as the process of audit and outcome evaluation gathers pace, but the evidence from the National Confidential Enquiry into Perioperative Death (NCEPOD)[56,57] is highly suggestive that this is the case.

Summary

Admission to intensive care facilities requires careful control. The availability of a trained, experienced critical care clinician 24 hours a day to provide advice and care is essential. At present the data are unavailable for many conditions to be able to make definitive decisions when patients are referred. The more widespread use of written prior decisions regarding intensive care provision in the event of deterioration would allow easier decision making in the acute situation. There is a need to collect national databases of intensive care patients and their outcome. In the future the information gathered on patient outcome extending into the post-hospitalization period may make admission decisions somewhat easier.

The only problem will be in deciding the probability of survival cutoff for withholding treatment. Currently, emergency referrals will generally require admission with further decisions being made on the basis of the underlying condition and the patient's response to treatment. At present there is no place for admission decisions being made purely on the basis of any single score using any of the currently available systems.

Policies regarding admission must be set in conjunction with the referring physicians and surgeons but individual patient decisions must be taken at consultant level to ensure rapid and definitive plans to be made for management.

Education is required at the undergraduate and postgraduate level:

1. to improve the speed with which patients are referred, by recognition of the conditions likely to proceed to major organ failure and the signs of early decompensation;
2. to understand what is and what is not possible with modern intensive care; and
3. to reinforce the fact that referral to the intensive care service is not an admission of failure.

We are as yet still a long way from fulfilling the aim of 'Selection for intensive care should be based on broad concepts of prognosis derived from statistical analysis of comparable cohorts of patients backed up by sound clinical trials' which was produced by a consensus panel in the UK in 1988.[3]

References

1. Intensive Care Society. *The Intensive Care Service in the UK*. London: The Intensive Care Society, 1990.
2. Linton AL, Naylor CD. Organised medicine and the assessment of technology. *New Engl J Med* 1990; **323**: 1463–7.
3. Intensive care in the United Kingdom: report from the King's Fund Panel. *Anaesthesia* 1989; **44**: 428–31.
4. Searle JF. The outcome of mechanical ventilation: report of a five year study. *Ann Royal Coll Surg Engl* 1985; **67**: 187–9.
5. Goldstein RL, Edward WC, Thibault GE, Mulley AG, Skinner E. Functional outcomes following medical intensive care. *Crit Care Med* 1986; **14**: 783–8.
6. Ridley S, Jackson R, Findlay J, Wallace P. Long term survival after intensive care. *Br Med J* 1990; **301**: 1127–30.
7. Mundt DJ, Gage RW, Lemeshow S, Pastides H *et al.* Intensive care unit patient follow up. Mortality, functional status and return to work at six months. *Arch Intern Med* 1989; **149**: 68–72.

8. Butt W, Shann F, Tibballs J, Williams J *et al*. Long term outcome of children after intensive care. *Crit Care Med* 1990; **18**: 961–5.

9. Chelluri L, Pinsky MR, Donahoe MP, Grenvik A. Long-term outcome of critically ill elderly patients requiring intensive care. *J Am Med Assoc* 1993; **269**: 3119–23.

10. Dragsted L. Outcome from intensive care: a five year study of 1,308 patients. *Danish Med Bull* 1991; **38**: 365–74.

11. Sage W, Rosenthal MH, Silverman JF. Is intensive care worth it? An assessment of input and outcome for the critically ill. *Crit Care Med* 1986; **14**: 777–82.

12. Detsky AS, Stricker SC, Mulley AG *et al*. Prognosis of survival and the expenditure of hospital resources for patients in an intensive care unit. *New Engl J Med* 1981; **305**: 670.

13. Abramson NS, Wald KS, Grenvik ANA *et al*. Adverse occurrences in intensive care units. *J Am Med Assoc* 1984; **252**: 2023–7.

14. Ferraris VA, Propp MA. Outcome in critical care patients: a multivariate study. *Crit Care Med* 1992; **20**: 967–76.

15. Jennett B. Inappropriate use of intensive care. *Br Med J* 1984; **289**: 1709–11.

16. Knaus WA, Zimmerman JE, Wagner DP, Draper E, Lawrence DE. APACHE – acute physiology and chronic health evaluation: a physiologically based classification system. *Crit Care Med* 1981; **9**: 591–7.

17. Knaus WA, Draper E, Wagner DP, Zimmerman JE. APACHE II: A severity of disease classification system. *Crit Care Med* 1985; **13**: 818–29.

18. Knaus WA, Wagner DP, Draper EA, Zimmerman JE *et al*. The APACHE III prognostic system. Risk prediction of hospital mortality for critically ill hospitalised adults. *Chest* 1991; **100**: 1619–36.

19. Lemeshow S, Teres D, Pastides H, Spitz Avrunin J, Steingrub JS. A method for predicting survival and mortality of ICU patients using objectively derived weights. *Crit Care Med* 1985; **13**: 519–25.

20. Lemeshow S, Teres D, Spitz Avrunin J, Pastides H. A comparison of methods to predict mortality of intensive care unit patients. *Crit Care Med* 1987; **15**: 715–22.

21. Pollack MM, Ruttiman PR, Getson PR. The paediatric risk of mortality (PRISM) score. *Crit Care Med* 1988; **16**: 1110–16.

22. Le Gall JR, Loirat P, Alperovitch A. Simplified acute physiology score for intensive care patients. *Lancet* 1983; **ii**: 741.

23. Le Gall J-R, Lemeshow S, Saulnier F. A new simplified acute physiology score (SAPS II) based on a European/North American multicenter study. *JAMA* 1993; **270**: 2957–63.

24. Rowan KM, Kerr JH, Major E, McPherson K, Short AIK, Vessey M. Variations in the case mix of adult admissions to general intensive care units in the UK and their impact on outcome. *Br Med J* 1993; **307**: 972–7.

25. Rowan KM, Kerr JM, Major E, McPherson K, Short AIK, Vessey MP. Outcome comparisons of UK intensive care units using the US APACHE II method to adjust for case mix: The Intensive Care Society's UK APACHE II Study. *Br Med J* 1993; **307**: 977–81.

26. Dragsted L, Jorgenson J, Jenson NH *et al*. Interhospital comparisons of patient outcome from intensive care: importance of lead time bias. *Crit Care Med* 1990; **17**: 418–22.

27. Rapoport J, Teres, D, Lemeshow S, Harris D. Timing of intensive care unit admission in relation to ICU outcome. *Crit Care Med* 1990; **18**: 1231–5.

28. Boyd O, Grounds RM. Physiological scoring systems and audit. *Lancet* 1993; **341**: 1573–4.

29. Rowan K. Outcome comparisons of Intensive Care Units in Great Britain and Ireland using the APACHE II method. PhD thesis, Oxford University, 1992.

30. Knaus WA, Draper EA, Wagner DP, Zimmerman JE. An evaluation of outcome from intensive care in major medical centres. *Ann Intern Med* 1986; **104**: 410–18.

31. Zimmerman JE, Knaus WA, Judson JA *et al*. Patient selection for intensive care: a comparison of New Zealand and United States hospitals. *Crit Care Med* 1988; **16**: 318–26.

32. Pesau B, Falger S, Berger E *et al*. Influence of age on outcome of mechanically ventilated patients in an intensive care unit. *Crit Care Med* 1992; **20**: 489–92.

33. Kass JE, Castriotta RJ, Malakoff F. Intensive care unit outcome in the very elderly. *Crit Care Med* 1992; **20**: 1666–71.

34. Lloyd-Thomas AR, Wright I, Lister TA, Hinds CJ. Prognosis of patients receiving intensive care for life threatening medical complications of haematological malignancy. *Br Med J* 1988; **296**: 1025–9.

35. Schapira DV, Studnicki J, Bradham DD, Wolff P, Jarrett A. Intensive care, survival, and expense of treating critically ill cancer patients. *J Am Med Assoc* 1993; **269**: 783–7.

36. Wachter RM, Luce JM, Hopewell PC. Critical care of patients with AIDS. *J Am Med Assoc* 1992; **267**: 541–7.

37. Franklin C, Rackow EC, Mamdani B, Burke G, Weil MH. Triage considerations in medical intensive care. *Arch Intern Med* 1990; **150**: 1455–9.

38. Varon AJ, Hudson-Civetta JA, Civetta J, Yu M. Preoperative intensive care unit consultations: accurate and effective. *Crit Care Med* 1993; **21**: 234–9.

39. Teplick R, Caldera DL, Gilbert JP, Cullen DJ. Benefit of elective intensive care admission after certain operations. *Anesthesia Analgesia* 1983; **62**: 572–7.

40. Shoemaker WC, Appel PL, Kram HB *et al*. Prospective trial of supranormal values of survivors as therapeutic goals in high risk surgical patients. *Chest* 1988; **94**: 1176–87.

41. Boyd O, Grounds RM, Bennett ED. The beneficial effect of supranormalisation of oxygen delivery with Dopexamine hydrochloride on perioperative mortality. *Intensive Care Med* 1992; **18** (Suppl. 2): S73.

42. Hayes MA, Timmins AC, Yau E, Palazzo M, Hinds CJ, Watson JD. Evaluation of systemic oxygen delivery in the treatment of critically ill patients. *New Engl J Med* 1994; **330**: 1717–22.

43. Marshall MF, Schwenzer KJ, Orsina M *et al*. Influence of political power, medical provincialism, and economic incentives on the rationing of surgical intensive care unit beds. *Crit Care Med* 1992; **20**: 387–94.

44. Ibsen B. The anaesthetist's viewpoint on the treatment of respiratory complications in poliomyelitis during the

epidemic in Copenhagen in 1952. *Proc Roy Soc Med* 1954; **47**: 72–4.

45. Chang RWS, Jacobs S, Lee B. Predicting outcome among intensive care unit patients using computerised trend analysis of daily APACHE II scores corrected for organ system failure. *Intensive Care Med* 1988; **14**: 558–66.

46. Gray WA, Capone RJ, Most RJ. Unsuccessful emergency medical resuscitation – are continued efforts in the emergency department justified? *New Engl J Med* 1991; **325**: 1393–8.

47. Tunstall-Pedoe H, Bailey L, Chamberlain *et al.* Survey of 3765 cardiopulmonary resuscitations in British hospitals (the BRESUS study): methods and overall results. *Br Med J* 1992; **304**: 1347–51.

48. Blackhall LJ. Must we always use CPR? *New Engl J Med* 1987; **317**: 1281–5.

49. McKersie RC, Bronsther OL, Shackford SR. Organ procurement in patients with fatal head injuries: the fate of the potential donor. *Ann Surg* 1991; **213**: 143–50.

50. Feest TG, Riad HN, Collins CH *et al.* Protocol for increasing organ donation after cerebrovascular deaths in a District General Hospital. *Lancet* 1990; **335**: 1133–5.

51. Pollack MM, Alexander SR, Clarke N *et al.* Improved outcomes from tertiary center pediatric intensive care: a statewide comparison of tertiary and nontertiary care facilities. *Crit Care Med* 1991; **19**: 150–9.

52. Teres D, Lieberman. Are we ready to regionalize paediatric intensive care? *Crit Care Med* 1991; **19**: 139–40.

53. Brown JJ, Sullivan G. Effect on ICU mortality of a full time critical care specialist. *Chest* 1989; **96**: 127.

54. Reynolds HN, Haupt MT, Thill-Baharozian MC, Carlson RW. Impact of critical physician staffing on patients with septic shock in a university hospital medical intensive care unit. *J Am Med Assoc* 1988; **260**: 3446–50.

55. Pollack MM, Katz RW, Ruttiman UE, Getson PR. Improving the outcome and efficiency of intensive care; the impact of an intensivist. *Crit Care Med* 1988; **16**: 11–17.

56. Campling EA, Devlin HB, Lunn JN. *The Report of the National Confidential Enquiry into Perioperative Deaths 1989*. London: HMSO, 1990.

57. Campling EA. Devlin HB, Hoile RW, Lunn JN. *The Report of the National Confidential Enquiry into Perioperative Deaths 1990*. London: HMSO, 1992.

CHAPTER 20

Results of Critical Care and the Quality of Survival

MARVIN L BIRNBAUM, SALLY KRAFT

Introduction   297
The critical care process   298
Impact of critical care   298
Impact on patient care and survival   299
Prognostic scoring systems   301
Severity of illness   304
Mortality and survival as a measure of outcome   305
Quality of life as an outcome measure   309
Unmeasured ICU outcomes   311
Impact of critical care on costs of health care   312
Conclusions   312
References   313

Introduction

A great deal has been written about the development of critical care in many sectors of the world. However, throughout the development of critical care, little has been published concerning its impact upon the patients for whom it has been applied, the institution in which it resides, or the health care system of which it is a part. This chapter is a summary of what is known about the impact of critical care services upon these aspects of the society in which it is practiced.

Critical care evolved out of the need to provide support to postoperative patients requiring intensive titration of therapy and from the need to monitor and aggressively treat patients with an evolving myocardial infarction. Gradually, patients with other medical problems that seemingly could benefit from intensive monitoring, aggressive intervention, and careful titration of therapies were added to this 'intensive care' population. Thus, the casemix for which intensive care

seemingly provided substantial benefit expanded progressively, and the demand for more and more resources for this patient population became a driving force in the hospital environment.

Thus, the growth of critical care medicine has been explosive since the 1950s. Only 40 years ago, intensive care units were virtually unheard of; now they are a part of the vast majority of hospitals throughout the USA and Europe. The intensive care unit (ICU) has developed into a separate space within the hospital where monitoring and sophisticated diagnostic and therapeutic interventions are provided to patients who are critically ill or at risk for developing life-threatening complications. Larger hospitals may have more than one ICU, and some of these units provide care specialized for specific patient populations such as pediatric, renal, respiratory, cardiac, and postoperative surgical units. Thus, the spectrum of care is broad and the casemix varies from general to highly specific. Few units are similar, each is embedded within a structure specific to the institution, and has developed its own, unique culture. This heterogeneity makes the results of the care provided in the intensive care unit difficult to obtain and even more difficult to generalize to critical care medicine in general. Many of the studies of the results of the critical care process have very poor external validity, and hence the findings from one unit are difficult to apply elsewhere.

Critical care medicine has now become one of the most expensive fields of medicine. In the USA, ICUs account for 7–10% of all acute care hospital beds and 20–30% of hospital costs.[1] Approximately 1% of the US gross domestic product is spent on ICU services. Despite the exorbitant costs of critical care medicine, the demand for these services continues to increase.

The critical care process

The practice of critical care is the *process* by which numerous inputs are brought together to produce an improvement (benefit) in a given patient's health status

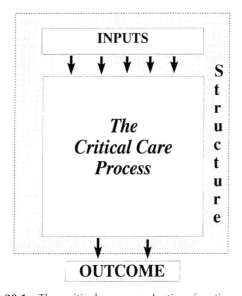

Fig. 20.1 The critical care production function. The critical care process is within the structure of the hospital and health care system and converts the inputs into the outcome(s).

(Fig. 20.1).[2] This process occurs within a *structure*. The *structure* consists of all of the elements that combine to produce the results (outcome). These elements include the physical structure in which critical care is practiced, the equipment used in the monitoring and care of the patient, and the system of which the critical care unit is a part. The structure enables the process to achieve its goals. This includes the structure of the health care system, the institution, and even the written policies and procedures that govern the practice of medicine and

nursing in the setting in which the care is delivered. The critical care process combines the elements of structure with other inputs to produce the benefits associated with the delivery of critical care.

The entire function associated with the production of the benefits attributed to critical care is described by the economists as a production function and has some mathematical equivalents. But, in order to define the production function associated with the delivery of critical care, one first must define the benefits. However, the benefits of these costly services generally remain unproved. There are no 'randomized, double-blinded' studies that demonstrate the efficacy of ICU care; and, indeed, it seems unthinkable to design a study that would deny ICU access to critically ill individuals in an attempt to 'prove' the benefits of ICU care. However, in this era of 'assessment and accountability,' the efficacy of critical care medicine must be examined.[3] This chapter will review what is known of the outcomes from the ICU process and will discuss the problems inherent in the conduct and analysis of such studies.

Impact of critical care

Thus far, the published results of the critical care process have focused exclusively on patient-oriented outcomes associated with application of the process. Moreover, almost all of the studies have focused on the *mortality rates* associated with the process. Perhaps, it would be more refreshing to think of the outcomes in a positive sense rather than in this negative one. Importantly, we believe the critical care process enhances the survival and well-being of the patients submitted to the process. When possible in this chapter, we will discuss these outcomes from the perspective of survival rather than death.

Thus, the rapid evolution of critical care has impacted many aspects of health care delivery other than the microcosm of individual patients. The entire orientation and structure of the health care systems in the developed world have changed as a result of this new stepchild. This has been true especially in the USA.

EFFECTS ON HOSPITAL STRUCTURE AND PROCESS

It is important to view this evolution from the perspective that prior to the implementation of critical care units, intensive care was provided on general care units or in a postoperative recovery unit. Care in these settings often was provided by 'special' nurses (sisters). Intensive care units were not initiated with the noble objective of enhancing the levels of monitoring and care. Instead, they evolved as a move towards accumulation of these patients into a single setting within the institution; it was an attempt to achieve *economy of scale* – it was more *efficient* to provide these services in a single area rather than to deliver them scattered throughout an institution. Therefore, there were no attempts to define the efficacy of this type of care. The accumulation of patients requiring intensive monitoring and care was economically and efficiency based. Clearly, the development of intensive care and critical care units has accomplished this goal of enhanced efficiency associated with the economies of scale and the concentration of patients.

Secondarily, this environment also proved ideal for the development of enhanced techniques for monitoring and treating patients. The centralization of patients who required such services, at least perceptually, fostered the development of special nursing skills as well as a new breed of medical expertise. Thus, the evolution of critical care nurses and physicians was gradual and arose from the needs specific to this special setting. These developments were patient-care based. Since it seemed apparent that some patients survived as a direct result of this special care, the units as well as the expertise and technology were allowed to expand in both scope and practice, always with the widely accepted assumption that provision of care in this special environment enhanced outcomes for many patients. Gradually, the utilization of such units became commonplace for most patients who required any level of care beyond the routine. Fear of the potential development of a complication became a criterion sufficient to merit admission to an intensive care area.

As a result, it has become increasingly difficult to provide adequate levels of care to patients with other than routine, minor problems anywhere in a hospital outside of an intensive care unit, and general care units gradually became unable to care for really sick people. Staffing levels for these general care units dwindled, and the capabilities of the rest of the hospital to care for 'sick' patients declined accordingly. Thus, the development and evolution of critical units have had a negative impact on the patient-care capabilities of the rest of the hospital.

In addition to the changes that have resulted in the non-special care areas of the hospitals, it is important to consider the impact such services have had on the development and use of other resources in the hospital. The provision of the intense monitoring and diagnostic services required in ICUs has had a profound impact on the ancillary services in the hospital. Patients in these units require substantial and immediate use of such services as laboratory, radiographic and imaging services, respiratory support services, physical therapy, pharmacy, and the like. It, therefore, is not possible to judge the impact of these ICUs, at least in economic terms, without considering their impact on the rest of the hospital.

EFFECTS ON HEALTH CARE STRUCTURE AND PROCESS

Similar changes to those that occurred within individual hospitals also have occurred in other parts of the health care systems. Various levels of critical care exist in the health care facilities comprising a given system. As the intensive care units in tertiary care centers flourished, they became dependent on smaller hospitals to refer patients for both practical (practice makes perfect) and economic reasons. Thus, the special capabilities housed in the tertiary care centers required the referral of patients from the surrounding region into their units. Sophisticated patient transport systems evolved in association with the development of these units. Major centers actively sought patients from smaller, 'less sophisticated' hospitals, and sent teams as well as equipment to the community hospitals to retrieve such patients. As a result, the ability to provide this special care to patients appeared to be enhanced, particularly at the regional hospitals. The community hospitals were both relieved and alarmed at the transfer of such patients, and a process of decreasing capabilities of the community hospitals has resulted. The development of critical care services in the tertiary care hospitals and the continued care provided by these facilities following completion of the critical care process have weakened the role and credibility of the community hospitals and many have failed financially.

Moreover, these major critical care facilities often are far from the home of the patient, and the patient and her/his loved ones are displaced, often having to travel long distances or find accommodation away from home. This results in the inability to maintain normal activities for the family and may significantly impact on the economic viability of the family unit.

Hence, the development of critical care has had far-reaching effects on the health care structure of which it is a part. Critical care is not an entity unto itself, but it impacts on all of health care.

Impact on patient care and survival

Almost all of the studies conducted on the results of critical care have focused on the survival of individual patients. The bulk of what follows concentrates on what is known about these effects and the ability of the critical care process to effect benefits to the patients, their families, and the staff who are components of the process. Although the results of critical care may seem quite obvious, they have been extremely difficult to document. Many of the benefits commonly associated with the delivery of critical care never will be proven. Yet, we will be called to account, as the process and outcome of critical care will be scrutinized in every health care system in which intensive care units exist. Suppose that we will be unable to define what we accomplish?

PROBLEMS IN DEFINITION OF IMPACT

The 'need' for intensive care has increased and the casemix has become more and more diverse. There neither was sufficient time nor were there sufficient resources available to allow the study of outcomes, and units evolved without evaluation of impact. By the time interest developed in defining the impact and efficacy of the provision of such special care, it was no longer possible to implement the controlled studies required to define the impact. From an ethical perspective, the concept of denying such care to a control group of patients for whom the critical care process potentially could provide some benefit, can no longer occur. Therefore, techniques other than randomized, controlled, prospective studies have had to be developed to study the impact of intensive care.

GOALS OF CRITICAL CARE

Despite the phenomenal proliferation of critical care and the widespread acceptance of the need for intensive care units and the critical care process, the goals of critical care medicine are not well defined. Raffin stated that the two goals of the critical care process are 'to save the salvageable or to help the dying have a peaceful and dignified death.'[4] However, most of the care provided in the ICU is not related to patients who are likely to die; it provides levels of care and monitoring not possible economically or practically in other units within the hospital setting. The definition of critical care used by the (US) National Institutes of Health Consensus Conference on Critical Care in 1983 was broader in concept than the limited goals stated by Raffin.

> Critical Care Medicine is a multidisciplinary and multiprofessional medical/nursing field concerned with patients who have sustained or are at risk of sustaining acutely, life-threatening disease or injury. These conditions necessitate prolonged, minute-to-minute therapy or observation in an intensive care unit (ICU) which is capable of providing high level of intensive therapy in terms of quality and immediacy.[5]

It has been estimated that many of the patients who are admitted to intensive care units are admitted only for monitoring purposes (they are believed to be at risk).

Some believe that such units have been overutilized for this purpose. The US General Accounting Office (GAO) reviewed a sample of Medicare ICU admissions from 1982 and 1983.[6] The GAO report concluded that 23% of Medicare patients admitted to ICUs were at very low risk of requiring any intensive care *therapy*, and therefore, could have been monitored and cared for adequately in an alternative, less costly setting. It seems to some, particularly persons not familiar with the dynamics of their respective health care system, that patients previously treated on general wards now may be admitted to the ICU simply because 'it is there.' Others believe the use of the critical care process for the monitoring and care of these patients is related to the belief that such patients cannot receive the attention needed to prevent some unfortunate complication elsewhere in the hospital where capabilities have declined progressively since the advent of critical care. Is the admission of these patients consistent with the goal for critical care?

It has been shown that as the demand for hospital beds increases, the number of beds increases. The same principle applies to the demand and supply for ICU beds. Strauss *et al.*[7] noted that the demand for critical care beds has continued to increase and the response has been to build more intensive care beds and units. Has the acuity of patients continued to increase? Or has a 'tradition' of caring for these patients in critical care units developed? Is there evidence that these ICU admissions are justified relative to the benefits likely to be accrued by the patient and/or the family and/or the operations of the rest of the hospital?

Until quite recently, the appropriate benefits to be achieved by admitting a given patient to an intensive care unit have not been defined. Hence, the goals are diffuse and without codified benefits to be attained, exclusion of a patient from admission to an ICU is difficult; certainly it is not objective. The Society for Critical Care Medicine Task Force on Cost-Containment has developed a list of such potential benefits,[8] but the list just now is being applied to the study of admissions to intensive care units. Thus, criteria for admission to an intensive care unit have not been codified and tested, and the process used for screening patients remains ambiguous.

These ambiguities in the definition of goals and benefits make outcome analyses of the critical care process problematic. Clearly, there are patients suffering from disease processes that unequivocally require the type and level of care provided in an ICU, but there are a larger number of patients who receive ICU care without definitive evidence that this level of care is necessary or appropriate.

The challenges then, are to assess the *efficacy* of the critical care process as it exists, and to study the effectiveness and efficacy of new assessment modalities, therapies, and interventions as they develop. A great deal of research effort has been directed towards the former of these goals; little has been accomplished towards the study of new modalities. Most of the studies available have used *mortality rates* as *the* measure of outcome. Mortality is an attractive endpoint because it is an objective finding and the data are easy to obtain. However, the use of mortality as the endpoint has many problems. Some researchers have focused on the *quality of life* of ICU survivors, but it is more difficult to obtain objective measures of quality. All of this is confounded further by the wide range of casemix found in most intensive care units, each patient with a different underlying disease process, problem set, severity of illness, likelihood of survival, and possibility of attaining a reasonable quality of life. Comparison of survival (mortality) rates between hospitals or intensive care units with diffuse patient populations provides little in the way of the answers to the efficacy of critical care.

CLASSIFICATION SCHEMES

Paramount to all of these investigations is a methodology that accurately classifies critically ill patients in order to analyze outcome for similar patient populations. Therefore, any measure of critical care efficacy must include a system to group patients together who are 'equally ill.' Outcome measurements are more meaningful when comparisons are made between groups of patients with similar underlying problems and with the same *severity of illness*. Substantial research has been directed towards the development of indicators of the probability of death as the outcome. However, there exists substantial confusion between assessments of the severity of illness and prognostic indicators. Often, these terms are used interchangeably. Prediction of the likelihood of survival for a given patient is one measure of the severity of illness, but it is not the only measure. Survival is not the only goal of the critical care process and additional severity scoring systems must be evolved to help classify patients correctly for the study of other benefits. For example, the location of a myocardial infarct is a predictor of the likelihood of significant residual incapacity, with the likelihood for the development of low cardiac output state being significantly greater in those with an anterior wall infarction than with those suffering an inferior wall infarction.[9] Severity scores must reflect these differences; even though the mortality rates may be different, the potential functional state of the survivors also may be quite different. Does the use of thrombolytic agents in the treatment of an acute myocardial injury, an intervention that is part of the critical care process, make a difference in the functional state of the survivor? Clearly, the severity scores relating these events must reflect the differences in functional status resulting from the treatment with thrombolytic agents and the defini-

tive care and support that accompany the use of these agents.

PREDICTION OF PROBABILITY OF DEATH

To date, researchers have concentrated on predicting the likelihood that a given patient will die while in the critical care process. The goal of these prognostic scoring systems is the ability to define futile care when a patient presents to the ICU, and to have an objective means to discuss the probable outcome of the process with the patient and/or family. In addition, use of these methods would allow comparison of the relative effectiveness of specific intensive care units by comparing actual mortality rates with the predicted mortality rate, for the comparison of the actual death rates for different intensive care units, or for judging the effectiveness of a given technology or group of technologies on the likelihood of death. The following discussion briefly reviews the essential elements of the best known prognostic scoring systems and severity scoring systems and the potential uses of these models.

Prognostic scoring systems

In the last 15 years, there has been substantial interest in the development of methods to predict the probability of death as early as possible in a patient's course in the intensive care unit. The principal goals of the methods devised have been noted above. Several distinct prognostic scoring systems have evolved. The sole purpose of these scoring systems is to predict a given patient's likelihood for survival. They provide the physician with the probability of a given patients survival, and as such move the likelihood of survival from a subjective judgment to an objective finding. This information, then can be used in decision making relative to the continued vigor of therapy. They also have utility in comparing an individual unit's mortality rate with the predicted probability for a given prognostic score. In this way, the relative effectiveness of an ICU can be compared with the average. This latter use is a valuable quality assessment tool. Table 20.1 is a list of the most popular prognostic scoring systems in use today.

Unfortunately, many have equated the scores obtained using these systems with the severity of a given patient's physiologic dysfunction and hence *severity of illness*. However, for the most part, the prognostic scoring systems were not designed for this purpose and the direct transfer of the score from these systems into an area of medicine for which they were not designed is a dangerous extrapolation.

Table 20.1 Prognostic scoring systems. These scoring systems are used to predict the probability for survival of a given patient in the ICU. They also have utility as a quality of care assessment tool

---

Cullen classification system[43]
Therapeutic intervention scoring system (TISS)[31, 32]
Acute physiology and chronic health evaluation (APACHE)[11, 12, 14]
Simplified acute physiology score (SAPS)[15, 16]
Mortality prediction model (MPM)[18, 19]
Pediatric risk mortality (PRISM)[17]

This is not to say that the probability of a patient dying is not one measure of how sick a patient is. Indeed, patients who have a high probability for death are very ill, by definition. Unfortunately, little work has been done to validate the use of these scoring systems as the index of severity. This is evident particularly with the recognition that regardless of the scoring system used, most of the patients who are admitted to an ICU have a relatively low probability for death, yet their outcomes need to be compared and the patients need to be meaningfully grouped for comparison of outcomes for a similar severity. It is for the patients that have a low to middle likelihood of death in the ICU that the critical care process probably makes its greatest impact and severity scoring systems that allow comparisons of outcomes for similar severity of illness will have their greatest application. It is in this group that accurate assessments and interventions will have the greatest consistent impact on the results of the critical care process. It is not tenable that the only function a critical care unit is to avert the arrival of the 'angel of death'.

Nonetheless, the prognostic indicators are an important tool in evaluating the results of critical care on a relatively small subset of patients admitted to the ICU. It is in this population that one attempts to identify those patients in whom additional therapy is futile.

Unfortunately, none of these prognostic scoring systems is perfect. They do not identify which patients are included in the 5% of the patients that have a computed probability of 0.95 for death, will survive. Given these limitations, it is important to have a firm grasp on the scoring systems available.

The first of the prognostic indicators that evolved was the clinical judgments of the staff providing care for the patient. As of yet, there has been no index that is consistently more reliable than is that of the experienced critical care physician.[10] However, these constitute subjective judgments and raise substantial questions as to their utility in discussing the issues with the patient and family or in making decisions whether to withhold or withdraw therapy. The prognostic indicators provide some objective measure of this probability upon which the judgments can rest. They serve to support the judgments and actions of the responsible medical staff.

Many of these prognostic scoring systems have undergone multiple revisions. Therefore, it is not possible to compare the probabilities derived with an earlier version of these systems with those obtained in a latter version of the same.

The first of the true physiologic scoring systems to define the statistical probability of a patient dying while in the hospital, the Acute Physiology and Chronic Health Evaluation (APACHE) system, was developed in 1981.[11] It has undergone significant and substantial revisions twice since its introduction. With each revision, its accuracy in predicting the probability for survival of a given patient improved. Each of these systems uses variables that define the degree of physiologic disturbance. Both the variables used and their relative weights have been modified with each successive modification of the scoring system. Each has been tested in numerous large scale studies in both the USA and Europe.

In the first version of APACHE, acute physiologic data were combined with the patient's age and chronic disease state to stratify patients according to their relative risk of death (likelihood of survival). Thirty-four physiologic variables were selected. The most abnormal measurement for each variable occurring within the initial 32 hours of the patient's stay was recorded. Chronic health was graded from A (excellent) to D (failing), and this letter grade was combined with the acute physiology score to classify patients according to their probability of survival/death.

There were several problems with APACHE I. The large number of variables made data collection difficult and subject to error. A data element that was not measured was assumed to be normal. The physiologic variables were selected by a panel of physicians rather than through statistical analysis. The system did not relate to the underlying disease process prompting the admission.

A revised version, APACHE II, was introduced in 1985.[12] The number of physiologic variables included in this model was reduced from 34 to 12, and modifications were made in several of the relative weights assigned to these variables. The most abnormal physiologic data point was collected in the initial 24 hours in the ICU as compared to the 32 hour collection time in the previous model. Chronological age, chronic health status, and underlying disease state were incorporated directly into the APACHE II score with increasing points assigned for greater age. Risk points were assigned if the patient suffered from severe organ system dysfunction. Patients were placed into specific diagnostic categories based on the diagnosis prompting the ICU admission.

In general, the predicted group mortality rate correlated well with the actual group mortality rate.

However, it was relatively inaccurate for some specific disease categories such as trauma, cardiac pulmonary edema, liver failure, and hematologic malignancy.[13] In addition, APACHE II tended to underestimate the mortality of patients transferred from other hospitals, ICUs, or other units within the same hospital. It was postulated that patients transferred from other wards already had received therapy and were transferred because they had not responded to the therapy, whereas those patients admitted directly to the ICU had not received a trial of therapy and had the opportunity to respond to these interventions.[13]

The most recent revisions of this scoring system, APACHE III, added five variables to increase the predictive accuracy for risk of death in the hospital.[14] The relative risks assigned to the physiologic variables were modified, but assignment of points for the presence of severe organ system failure was eliminated; in its place, a list of co-morbid conditions with associated risk points was added. The patient's location prior to the present ICU admission was included. The APACHE III demonstrated validity in its ability to provide continuous outcome predictions: it seems to have some validity in estimating the risk for death over subsequent ICU days.[12]

Potential sources of error still exist with the use of the APACHE III system.[13] As with the previous two APACHE scoring systems, inaccurate data collection is a possible source of error, although this error is minimized in APACHE III by direct entry of the data into the computer program. The number of physiologic variables used in the computation of the APACHE III score is increased as compared to APACHE II. Unmeasured variables again are assumed to be normal.

The ability to provide frequent repeat predictions of hospital mortality introduces the possibility that the predictions may influence the physician, and treatment decisions may be altered on the basis of the predicted mortality. For example, if the probability of death on the first ICU day was 0.70, and remains unchanged by the fifth ICU day, the patient or the patient's family may request that the physician limit the extent of ICU support, and subsequently the patient dies. Thus, predicted probability of death may affect decision making and the process may become self-serving.[13]

The APACHE scoring systems, especially when combined with logistic regression, comprise the most widely used prognostic scoring tool in critical care. Each of the versions has been validated with international studies. The accuracy has improved with each version. For the most part, each version is physiologically based. As such, each also has been used as a measure of severity of the physiologic disturbances.

The Simplified Acute Physiology Score (SAPS)[15] was developed in 1984 and recently has been revised as SAPS II.[16] This scoring system was developed independently of the APACHE system. Logistic regression modeling technique was used to select the 17 variables that are used to compute the SAPS II score. Twelve of these variables are physiologic measurements and, like the APACHE II and III systems, the most abnormal measurement for each variable in the initial 24 hours is recorded. The five non-physiologic variables include:

1. age;
2. type of admission (scheduled surgery vs medical or emergency surgery);
3. AIDS;
4. metastatic cancer; and
5. hematologic cancer.

An equation, based on the multiple logistic regression model, then converts the SAPS II score to a probability of hospital mortality. Unlike APACHE II, SAPS II is not disease specific. The authors felt that it was too difficult to assign a single diagnosis to the majority of the patients studied: in their patient sample, only 37% of the patients admitted to the ICU would fit into a single diagnostic category. The SAPS II scoring system is an effective model for estimating the probability of hospital death.

The Pediatric Risk of Mortality (PRISM)[17] is similar to the SAPS. It uses the same variables, but is the result of logistic regression and the use of subjective weights. The variables are entered at the end of the first 24 hours and thus, there is a delay, as with the APACHE systems, for at least 24 hours following admission.

The Mortality Prediction Model (MPM) was designed exclusively for the prediction of the probability for death. It is not also used as an index of severity of illness. It is not an index of physiologic dysfunction. The MPM was described first in 1985[18] and revised (MPM-II) in 1993.[19] The MPM-II system consists of two models; the MPM_0 which estimates the probability of hospital mortality at the time of ICU admission, and the MPM_{24} which estimates the probability of mortality at 24 hours in the ICU. The MPM_0 contains 15 variables which were selected and weighted using multiple logistic regression modeling; the MPM_{24} utilizes another eight variables that are combined with five variables from the MPM_0. The variables used in these models are obtained easily and require minimal laboratory determinations.

One advantage of the MPM_0 is its ability to predict hospital mortality at the time of admission to the ICU with variables that are readily available, minimizing data collection errors. This differs from the APACHE scoring system which requires 24 hours of data collection before a prognostic score can be generated. The data used in the MPM admission prediction equation are treatment independent; data obtained in the APACHE system may be affected by therapy given during the first 24 hours. The MPM is a general model that does not require the specification of a single admitting diagnosis.

In summary, each of these models was developed to predict the probability of death in the ICU. Models that accurately predict mortality in the ICU have numerous potential applications and provide some of the tools that are necessary to study one aspect of effectiveness and efficiency. The models reviewed are not perfect; each has strengths and weaknesses, but these models allow investigators to begin to critically review some of the benefits and costs of critical care medicine. It will be interesting to see whether any of these indices will tell us that the critical care process is becoming more effective in enhancing actual survival. For as the critical care process becomes more effective in enhancing survival of those considered not likely to survive today, these prognostic indices either should become increasingly inaccurate (underestimate the probability for survival), or revisions of the predictive models will be necessary to include different variables or to change the relative weights of the variables used. This latter manipulation will be a clear indication that the process is changing and that the methods used for prediction need to change to meet the demands for accuracy. Hopefully, the status of these indices will be in flux. However, such changes will make longitudinal comparisons invalid.

Models that accurately predict the probability of a patient's death allow the grouping of patients into cohorts with equal predicted probabilities of survival. This facilitates comparisons of the probabilities of death between groups of similar patients and between actual and predicted survival. The mortality predictive models allow patients to be stratified according to their calculated risk of death. Comparing actual mortality rates to those predicted by the model is one measure of quality assessment in an the individual intensive care.

Severity of illness

Severity is defined as 'the state of being severe; rigor; intensity'. *Severe* is defined as 'serious; grave; afflictive; distressing; extreme; intense'.[20] The severity of an illness is not necessarily synonymous with the probability of death. For example, a patient suffering ventilatory insufficiency is severely ill and would die promptly without the organ system support provided in the ICU. Given the ability of the staff and equipment available in an ICU, such a patient has a very low likelihood of death in the ICU. Severity scoring measures used also may have distinct prognostic implications. But, they have greater utility in identifying changes in patient conditions that result from the critical care process and

Table 20.2 Severity of illness scoring systems. These scoring systems are related to the severity of the physiologic dysfunction present in a given patient or are related to the intensity of the care being provided

---

Therapeutic intervention scoring system (TISS)[31, 32]
Acute physiology and chronic disease evaluation (APACHE)[11, 12, 14]
Wisconsin ischemic heart index (WIHD)[33, 42]
Dyspnea index
Peak expiratory flow rate (PEFR)[30]
Chest pain index
Glasgow coma scale (GCS)[21]
Trauma severity scoring systems
   Injury severity score (ISS)[22]
   Trauma score (TS)[23]
   Revised trauma score[24]
   Abbreviated injury acale (AIS)[25, 26]
   CRAMS Scale[27]
   TRISS methodology[28]
   Pediatric trauma score[29]
Septic severity score[29]
Physiology stability index
Rapid acute physiology score[62]

---

in measuring the impact (effectiveness and efficacy) of changes and additions to the critical care process.

There are a host of severity scoring systems that can be utilized to define what we do and how we do it. A partial list of the severity scoring systems available today is in Table 20.2. They include the Glasgow Coma Scale,[21] the multiple trauma scoring systems,[22–29] indices of dyspnea,[30] and even scoring systems for levels of intervention and support required.[31, 32] There also are indices that weigh the amount of care a patient requires.

An example of the results of one of the uses of these severity indices, the Wisconsin Ischemic Heart Index, is illustrated in Fig. 20.2.[33] From this study, it was possible to document that the efficacy of one aspect of the critical care process differs between rural, community hospitals and a tertiary care center. It provides evidence that the critical care process at the receiving facility was superior to that available in the rural community hospitals in enhancing survival for patients of the same severity of illness. This study finally documented what the referring physicians knew all along: they transferred patients to the tertiary care center because they believed the patient could get better care for her/his severe problems in the receiving facility. There are not practical differences in the actual survival rates for patients with ischemic heart disease at low level of severity. Studies such as this provide important information regarding the effects of critical care.

It is important to note that in this study, the use of the severity scoring process was used to compare actual survival rates in one institution compared to another.

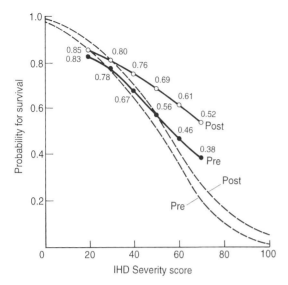

Fig. 20.2 Actual survival rates for persons with ischemic heart disease before and after an advanced cardiac life support course. Significant differences occurred only in the mid-severity range.[42]

Unlike the discussions relative to the use of the prognostic scoring systems noted earlier, the use of severity scores here compare actual survival rates, not actual survival rates versus those predicted using the prognostic scoring systems.

The first of the scoring systems to be used widely in the quantification of the severity of illness related severity to the amount and types of interventions being required by a given patient. This Therapeutic Intervention Scoring System (TISS) was developed by Cullen and his group in Boston in the early 1970s when critical care still was in its infancy.[31,32] This scoring system affixed a weight to many of the tasks and physiologic monitoring that constitute the critical care process. It is a measure of the quantity of resources being expended on a given patient and combined scores define the relative workloads required from the staff. It also was shown that the higher the TISS score, the more likely the patient was to succumb. However, it is not a good prognostic index. By following TISS scores, it is possible to define the hospital course taken by a given patient. As the score declined, the patient either was on the road to recovery or was having therapy withdrawn. The TISS remains a valuable tool for the quantification of illness severity and of the intensity of resource consumption required for the support and treatment of an individual patient in the ICU.

The Chest Pain and Dyspnea indices are subjective measures of the patient's perception of the severity of their dyspnea or pain compared to the worst pain or shortness of breath they ever have suffered. Usually a scale of 1 (minimal) to 10 (worst ever) is used. It is helpful to use an analog scale for these determinations when possible. These indices have utility in defining the patient's perception of the effectiveness of an intervention. Changes in these scores indicate whether or not the patient achieved benefit from the intervention. Measurement of a patient's perception of the effects of an intervention or a complex process such as critical care is an important element in the assessment of the results of critical care.

The remainder of the indices listed in Table 20.2 are measurements of the physiologic status of patients. They are objective measurements of organ system function. Changes in either direction constitute a change in the severity of a patient's dysfunction. For example, the improvement in Peak Expiratory Flow Rate (PEFR) following the administration of a bronchiolar dilating agent provides objective evidence for the effectiveness of the intervention.[34] They interrelate with the prognostic scoring systems that use many of the same variables and generally weights for each variable tend to be related to their contribution to the likelihood of death/survival. Each of these has advantages and shortcomings, but the use of the appropriate system provides valuable information relative to the efficacy of the critical care process.

Each of these measures of severity needs to be applied to answer the questions of, 'so what?' It is time to use them effectively and to carefully evaluate each system. Continuous changes in these indices will minimize their utility. The Glasgow Coma Scale[21] is an example of a stable severity index and its value increases steadily with the passage of time. The use of both the prognostic and severity indices will be used in the discussions of the impact of the critical care process that follows.

Mortality and survival as a measure of outcome

How can the benefits of ICU care be measured? There are *no* studies that compare mortality or survival rates between critically ill patients randomized to receive care either in the ICU or on the general ward. In most of the relatively few studies of outcome conducted so far, patient *mortality* has been the standard outcome measured. As mentioned earlier, mortality is an attractive endpoint to study because it is easy to define, the data can be obtained readily from review of hospital records or records of governmental agencies responsible for maintaining vital statistics, and there are no 'shades' of death. On the other hand, there are endless 'shades' of survival. Since one of the goals of the critical care process is to save the lives of critically ill or injured patients,[4] it is appropriate to utilize death as an outcome and survival as a benefit.

IN-HOSPITAL SURVIVAL

Most of the patients admitted to an intensive care unit with severe, often life-threatening illness or injury survive to discharge. In-hospital, ICU survival rates range from 60 to 94%.[35,36] However, mortality/survival rates alone do not provide useful information unless there is some description of the patient population examined. To know that patients in ICU-A have an overall survival rate of 90% as compared to the survival rate of 70% for the patients in ICU-B does not impart much information relative to the quality of care delivered in either unit. The value of this information is confounded by the respective casemix of patients in the each of the two ICUs. Survival/mortality rates are meaningful only when combined with a measure of stratification based on the predicted probability of death, or in comparison of the survival of patients with identical probabilities for death, or in comparison of actual mortality rates for a given severity of illness.

The need to stratify patients when interpreting survival/mortality rates is illustrated further by the work of Knaus *et al.*[35,36] In the first of these reports,[35] the overall ICU mortality rates for 13 hospitals ranged from 8.9 to 38.3%. It would be logical to conclude that the

hospital with the 8.9% mortality rate performed at a superior level compared to the hospital with the 38.3% mortality rate. In fact, the opposite was true. When the patients were stratified according to APACHE II scores, there were no statistical differences in performance for the 13 institutions.

In 1993, Knaus and associates published the results comparing the ICU performance of 42 different intensive care units located in 40 US hospitals.[36] Data were collected prospectively on 17 440 admissions with the APACHE III system used to estimate each patient's probability of death in the hospital. Mean predicted group death rates at each hospital were compared to the actual group death rates. Observed death rates in the 42 ICUs ranged from 6 to 40%; 90% of this variation was due to measured patient characteristics and hospital discharge practices. These observations demonstrate the importance of interpreting ICU mortality rates in conjunction with a method to stratify patients.

The relative effectiveness of two institutions in the treatment of specific patient populations can be compared using measures of mortality rates stratified by severity of their disease process. The data in Fig. 20.3 provide an example of the use of actual mortality rates for the comparison of the relative effectiveness of institutions in the treatment of patients with ischemic heart disease.[33] The data were collected on consecutive patients admitted to nine rural community hospitals and to a university hospital. The substantial differences in survival of patients at moderate to high levels of severity constitute justification for the transfer of

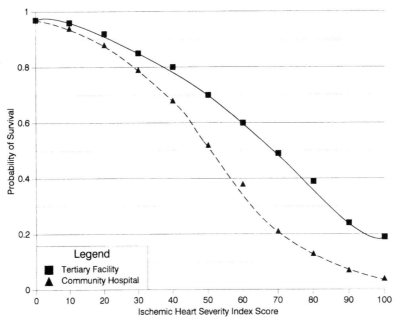

Fig. 20.3 Actual survival rates for a given severity of illness for patients with ischemic heart disease in a community hospital and a tertiary care center as determined using logistic regression.

patients with severity scores in this range from the community hospitals to the tertiary care centers.

By far, most of the patients admitted to an ICU survive regardless of the type of unit or hospital in which they receive care. For many of the patients that do survive the ICU process, their survival is the result of the critical care process. But, raw, short-term survival rates, even when corrected for the predicted probabilities for survival/death, offer little to the definition of the results of the critical care process. When viewed as a function of severity of illness, survival rates are useful for comparison of quality and for definition of the impact of specific monitoring techniques or interventions as they are introduced.

LONG-TERM SURVIVAL

The use of in-hospital mortality as an outcome measure provides some information on the immediate outcome of ICU intervention, but gives no information as to the length of survival following the stay in the ICU (application of the critical care process). Given the high costs of ICU medicine and concerns regarding the appropriate use of resources, the study of long-term survival following a stay in an ICU is essential. Survival rates at some period following hospital discharge are helpful in defining the results of the critical care process.[37]

Several studies have reported long-term survival after ICU care.[38-41] Three of these studies are summarized in Table 20.3. In these studies, 66–83% of the patients survived to hospital discharge. At 18–24 months following discharge, between 49 and 64% of the patients still were alive. This compares with 97% of non-ICU patients who survived to discharge, and 85% of whom still were alive 24 months following discharge. Of substantial importance is an observation in the study by Parno *et al.*[38] that following hospital discharge, both those patients who had been in an ICU and those not in an ICU during their hospitalization had the same survival rate: two years after discharge, 83% of the patients who survived hospitalization that included a stay in an ICU were alive compared to 89% of those who were not in an ICU during their respective hospitalization.

These results are encouraging. Clearly, more long-term studies of survival of ICU patients compared to non-ICU admitted patients are needed. In addition, the studies of survival as an independent variable of severity of illness need to be extended into the post-discharge phase. Much information about the results of critical care will come from such studies.

Lastly, the impact of the delivery of futile care upon the overall survival of patients will be interesting. When patients for whom futile care is not provided are excluded from these patient populations, the results in terms of actual survival following intensive care may come even closer to that of patients discharged without a stay in an ICU.

In summary, it is significant that patients sick enough to be admitted to a critical care unit, presumably because they were at risk for death, survive and most of those that do, survive at a rate equivalent to other patients who survive hospitalization. The mortality and survival rates defined so far indicate that patients provided care in the critical care process survive, but in general, it is not known whether patients with identical problems would have survived without the critical care process. The issues surrounding survival are complex and must be studied. Experimental design will be difficult, if not impossible. Increases in the probabilities of survival over time will indicate improvements in the critical care process.

CHANGES IN EFFECTIVENESS OVER TIME

Another measure of effectiveness would be the comparison of mortality rates in a given ICU over time. Is the critical care process improving? Is the survival rate increasing? The impact of an intervention can be defined by the comparison of survival rates before and after an intervention. Figure 20.2 illustrates this utility.

Table 20.3 Long-term survival of patients discharged alive from the hospital following care in an intensive care unit

Study	n	Hospital survival (%)		Time after discharge (months)	Postdischarge survival (%)	
		ICU	Non-ICU		ICU	Non-ICU
Parno[38]	458	83	97	24	64	85[a]
Ridley[41]	497	76		18–24	52	
Jacobs[40]	313	66		24	49	
Sage[57]	337	89		18–24	75	

[a] After discharge, survival rates were the same: ICU = 83%; non-ICU = 89%.

In this longitudinal comparison, the impact of Advanced Cardiac Life Support (ACLS) training on survival was assessed by comparing actual death rates for a given severity of ischemic heart disease.[42] The curves were generated through logistic regression techniques of the severity of the disease using the Wisconsin Ischemic Heart Index (IHD) and the actual survival rates. Thus, the ACLS training used in this study had little impact on the survival of those patients with a high degree of severity (e.g. asystole) or with a very low severity of illness (e.g. sinus tachycardia), but had a marked impact on those patients with a moderate severity of illness.

Progressive improvement in survival would constitute evidence that the critical care process is becoming more effective. But, there are very little data available regarding changes in mortality over time. In comparison of the survival and follow-up data in critically ill patients from 1972–1973[43] to 1977–1978, Cullen *et al.* observed a 1-year mortality rate of 73% in 1973 versus 69% in 1978 (differences not statistically significant). Does this mean there were no significant improvements in the ICU care of this patient population over the 5-year period?

Clearly, comparing mortality rates over time is problematic. Most of the prognostic indices still are in evolution and change is common. The identical patient classification scheme must be used for longitudinal studies, since even minor revisions may change the casemix of the populations studied and may render the comparison invalid. Even if the same method is used, changes in the ICU population may not be detected by the classification method selected, yet may be significant enough to make a difference in the mortality rates measured and thus make the comparison less meaningful. Although the patients in the above study were all categorized as Class IV, those patients who became critically ill after emergent major vascular surgery had a 31% survival compared to 67% for patients who became critically ill following elective major vascular surgery.[43] Thus, a new addition to the stratification methodology became apparent. It is important to note here that the classification scheme used for these patient groups was a *severity index* and not a prognostic index. The severity of the illness of patients categorized as Class IV was specific to their cardiac function. It needed to be refined by the addition of the precipitating event to the classification system. Again, measures of severity or some other stratification process must be used to gain sufficient insight into the effectiveness of the critical care process in enhancing survival across periods of time when changes in the critical care process are inevitable. Currently, we do not know whether the 'improvements' in the critical care process over the last 20 years really have had a significant impact on patient survival. Future longitudinal studies will reveal the impact of the changes on survival.

MORTALITY IN SPECIFIC PATIENT POPULATIONS

Several patient populations in the ICU have received a great deal of attention regarding the appropriateness of care. Most often, these groups have consisted of patients with a low probability of long-term survival. One such group consists of elderly patients admitted to the ICU. This patient population is of particular interest in the USA given the increasing age of the general population and the large percentage of health care dollars expended for the care of the aging population. Studies have noted increased ICU mortality associated with increasing age.[45] However, it seems that this difference is due largely to patients who die of an acute myocardial infarction or are admitted to an ICU following a cardiopulmonary arrest.[46,47] When these latter patients were excluded, Fedullo[47] could not identify any correlation between age and survival. Given consideration of these factors, it is not clear whether the generalization that age bears significantly on the results from critical care is true. It seems that all of the confounding variables associated with increasing age may impact substantially on survival, especially long-term survival, in the elderly.

Several studies have confirmed that long-term survival after ICU admission also is lower in the elderly population.[43,48,49] In patients >85 years of age, Kass reported a 30% ICU mortality rate (vs 9% for patients <65 years of age), and a 1-year mortality rate of 64%.[50] To be significant clinically, these mortality rates must be compared with the overall mortality rates for the age group being evaluated.

The challenge is to identify which patients will benefit from critical care interventions and live to enjoy long-term survival. This challenge also applies to a number of other patient populations that face low probabilities of long-term survivals. Studies of intensive care outcome have been done in patients with cancer, AIDS,[51] following bone marrow transplant,[52,53] and other diseases associated with high mortality rates. Each of these studies indicates a lower degree of efficacy for the critical care process when judged by survival. Other factors bear heavily on the potential benefits that may be associated with bringing patients in these groups into an ICU. Hopefully, these and future studies will help clinicians direct these limited resources to those patients who will benefit from them and prevent suffering as well as preserve the dignity of patients in whom the rigors of critical care provide no positive effects.

In summary, mortality/survival rates frequently are used to assess ICU effectiveness, but there are many problems with using these data for this purpose. First, the patient population being studied must be well defined. The stratification method used will depend on the intent of the research for which the data are being collected. However, the use of multiple different classification methods makes it nearly impossible to reach conclusions regarding the efficacy of the critical care process using ICU mortality rates. Even studies performed at the same institution over time have theoretical problems. The current data available on ICU mortality are not able to answer the question, 'Does the critical care unit make a difference?'

One other major problem exists relative to the use of the prognostic indices for evaluating the results of the critical care process: the use of these indices misses the outcome for the *majority* of patients who are admitted to an intensive care unit. This is illustrated in Fig. 20.4 which provides an example of the distribution of patients in the intensive care units of one tertiary care hospital as a function of their acute physiology score. The probability for death/survival using the APACHE scoring system also is shown. Several observations are important. The most important is the observation that in all instances, the majority of patients in this sample fall into the categories for which the probability of death is quite low. For all of the 634 patients admitted to intensive care units in this sample, 64% have a greater than 0.45 probability for survival and more than one-third of the patients have more than a 75% likelihood of survival using the APACHE scoring system. Furthermore, this probability differs by casemix within the individual units. For example, almost 80% of the

patients admitted to the surgical intensive care unit had a high probability for survival while 54% of the patients in the multidisciplinary critical care unit (TLC) had an excellent chance for survival. Thus, using the prognostic scoring systems for evaluation of the efficacy of the critical care process misses the outcome analysis for the majority of patients. It would not be expected that changes in the critical care process would affect the probabilities for survival/death that were weighted heavily toward the survival side. It certainly would apply to those patients who had a predicted zero probability for survival today, if the critical care process used began to result in survival. Most of the patients entering the critical care process survive. Thus, other measures of the results of critical care are vital to any analysis of the results of the critical care process.

Quality of life as an outcome measure

To survive in the ICU, but never to regain a meaningful quality of life, is not a desirable goal of the critical care process. Although some would say that there is no quality of life if a person is dead, 'survival' in some cases appears to be worse than death.

It is much more difficult to measure the quality of life

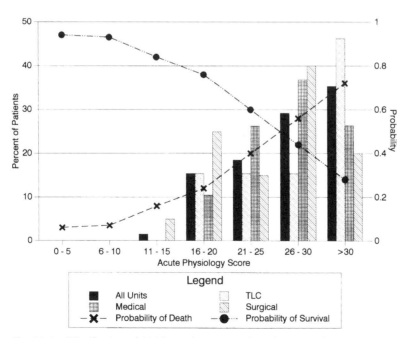

Fig. 20.4 Distribution of 634 intensive care patients in one tertiary care center with three ICUs and the probabilities of death/survival from APACHE. Distinct differences in the distribution of patients according to the ICU are present. TLC in a multidisciplinary, critical care unit with full-time critical care physicians in attendance.

than it is to measure mortality. Unlike the objectivity of mortality, the quality of life is subjective: there are many shades of survival. Each person has an individual concept of what defines a meaningful existence. A frail 80-year-old person will have a different view of what constitutes a good quality of life as compared to a robust 25-year-old. The patient may have a different concept of a quality and meaningful life than does her/his family, or than does the health care professional or the staff providing the care in an intensive care unit. Although it is very difficult to measure satisfaction with life, it may be the most important measure of the benefits associated with the process of critical care medicine. Several studies focus on quality of life after surviving an ICU admission and offer some insight into the long-term benefits (positive and negative) of the critical care process.

The Task Force on Cost-Containment of the Society of Critical Care Medicine defined the return of a patient to her/his normative health status for her/his age as a goal of critical care, indeed for all of therapeutic medical science.[8] The normative health status was defined as that state of health appropriate for most individuals in a given culture for their respective ages. It defined 100% health status as that held by a normal infant at birth, and zero health status as death. Expectations to return an ill person to a health status above the normative line was considered unrealistic. The normal individual at age 20 years should possess a state of health that is very different than that expected at age 80 years. It is important that quality of life measures be judged in relation to normative expectations.

Several studies have evaluated the functional status of survivors following discharge from the hospital in which they received some care in an intensive care unit.[20, 54–56] These results, in terms of functional status following an ICU admission, are summarized in Table 20.4. Remarkably, between 79 and 97% of the patients reported that they had regained the functional level they had prior to the hospitalization. Thus, only 3–21% of the patients had not returned to their previous functional state. In one of these studies, 60% had returned to full-time employment.[44] Although for the most part, these studies were dependent upon the patients' recall of their functional status prior to hospitalization, the results still provide substantial insight into the level of recovery afforded most patients by the critical care process. This is coordinate with one of the objectives of critical care process noted above: returning patients to their normative health status following a serious illness or injury.

Other more objective assessment tools have been used to assess the health status of persons discharged alive following treatment in an intensive care unit. Sage *et al.*[57] and Patrick *et al.*[58] used an instrument called the Sickness Impact Profile (SIP) to assess the patients' perception of the health following their ICU stay. The SIP is used to assess perceived dysfunction for multiple different aspects of daily life. In addition, Sage *et al.* used the Uniscale assessment tool in which patients rated their respective health status from worst to best on an analog scale. Using these two tools, Sage *et al.* concluded that patients' perceptions of their health status was better than was their actual health status.

Patrick *et al.*[58] combined the Sickness Impact Profile with a newly devised tool, the Perceived Quality of Life Scale (PQOL), in which the patient rates their level of satisfaction for 11 different aspects of life:

1. health;
2. thinking;
3. happiness;
4. family;
5. help;
6. community;
7. leisure;
8. income;
9. respect;
10. meaning; and
11. work.

Overall, the affective status of the patients in this study was positive although 59% of patients interviewed rated their health as only fair to poor. This poor health rating compares to 30% in persons 65 years or older in the general population. The PQOL scores indicated that most patients were moderately to highly satisfied with their quality of life: the mean score was not significantly different than that of a group of healthy, elderly individuals. Interestingly, the authors noted that a patient's health-related dysfunction was only moderately correlated with her/his perceptions of her/his quality of life. Thus, health status was not a good

Table 20.4   Functional status of patients surviving hospitalization with stay in an ICU as assessed 8–24 months following discharge

Study	*n*	Time after discharge (months)	Change in status (%)		
			Better	Unchanged	Worse
Cullen Class IV[43, 44]	12			79	21
Jacobs[40]	118	24	2	77	21
Goldstein[56]	2213	8	71	26	3
Bams[55]	238			87	13

predictor of self-perceived life quality. A number of factors may explain this discrepancy. What is perceived as a good quality of life may change after being in an intensive care unit for any period of time. Past experiences will influence and change preferences and perceptions. Future studies will need to address these issues.

OTHER FACTORS IMPACTING QUALITY OF LIFE

Jacobs *et al.*[40] noted that other factors seem to impact upon the level of recovery following an intensive care stay. Principal among these were age and severity of illness. It seems logical that the more severe the illness while the patient is confined to the ICU, the less would be the extent of the recovery. It is not known whether the bulk of the patients who achieve a high functional level following discharge is comprised of patients brought to the ICU only for monitoring purposes. Clearly, this important research must be continued, but with better descriptions of the casemix of patients for whom quality of life measures are being assessed. Collaboration with researchers in the social sciences will be essential in the definition of this aspect of the results of the critical care process. Much more work needs to be done in this area.

QUALITY OF LIFE AS A FUNCTION OF AGE

Although both short-term and long-term mortality rates in the elderly population are quite high, survivors appear to enjoy a relatively good quality of life. In a small follow-up on patients >75 years of age, 12–24 months after admission to a respiratory ICU,[48] McLean reported that the majority of these patients believed their quality of life was 'worthwhile' and would undergo treatment in the ICU again. Among the very elderly patient group (≥85 years) in the article by Kass,[50] only 23% of ICU survivors reported a decrease in functional status as compared to their preadmission status. Mahul reported that 88% of elderly patients were living at home 1 year following ICU admission and 70% were able to live independently.[49] Thus, the studies of the elderly following intensive care show that this group of patients has high short- and long-term mortality, but the quality of life of the survivors appears 'acceptable'.

Despite the difficulties inherent in studying the quality of life of ICU survivors, the importance of these studies cannot be overlooked. To simply 'survive' is not enough; patients should be able to survive and then rehabilitate to achieve a level of health that allows them to have a meaningful life. Measures need to be developed to allow researchers to more adequately study satisfaction with life. Future research needs to explore how the critical care process changes patients' perspectives regarding life quality.

Unmeasured ICU outcomes

The number of lives saved and the quality of life of survivors only are two measures of ICU outcome that merit further study. After nearly 2 years of deliberation, the Task Force on Cost-Containment in Critical Care of the Society of Critical Care Medicine defined a list of benefits associated with the critical care process.[8] As deliberations progressed, it became clear that most of the benefits identified had both positive and negative aspects. The Task Force suggested that this list of benefits could be used as an admission tool to define the benefits expected for each patient at the time of ICU admission. Inability of the admitting physician to identify any positive benefits that are sought for the individual being admitted would make the ICU admission inappropriate.

Acquisition of this information would provide a list of the reasons why persons are admitted to the critical care process. The benefits actually achieved would be documented on discharge from the ICU. This would define the results of the critical care process. Some of the benefits associated with the critical care process are patient- and family-oriented, while others are benefits to the care-givers and/or to the healthcare system.

Some of the more than 20 positive benefits of critical care identified by the Task Force are listed in Table 20.5. Although stated in a slightly different manner, the first two of these benefits have been discussed in detail above and continue to be studied. However, for some patients, the inverse of these two elements may be

Table 20.5 Positive benefits to patients afforded by the critical care process[8]

1. Increases longevity
2. Minimizes impact of critical disease on quality of life
3. Buys time for diagnosis
4. Buys time for treatment to take effect
5. Allows additional diagnoses to be developed
6. Allows early detection of complications
7. Allows early initiation of therapy
8. Shortens overall length of hospital stay
9. Allows biological support for organ donation
10. Stimulates development of medical ethics
11. Provides satisfaction for patients, family, and staff
12. Initiates the grieving process

achieved. For example, the ICU process may shorten the life of some patients: confinement to an intensive care unit may result in the development of complications that are inherent in the delivery of the process. Sudden death related to instrumentation of the patient is an example of how the process may result in shortening the lifespan of a patient. Similarly, the process may result in previously unachievable survival, but with a dismal quality of life associated with the survival. Thus, as discussed earlier, each of these benefits has a flip or down side. These latter outcomes may be referred to as 'negative benefits'.

The remaining elements listed in Table 20.5 are as important as the first two, but are even more difficult to measure than is the quality of life. Yet, it seems that each of these constitutes a potential benefit associated with the critical care process and merits study. It is known, but not quantified, that the organ system support provided as part of the critical care process often sustains patients for the period of time necessary to develop an accurate diagnosis of the underlying condition, and that appropriate treatment of this underlying problem promotes the survival of the patient and may result in an enhanced quality of life. Similar logic applies to the provision of organ system support providing sufficient time for the definition of the most appropriate therapy and for that therapy to become effective. These benefits are important and the measurement of them is essential in evaluating the results and hence efficacy of the critical care process.

As noted earlier, the General Accounting Office studied the nature of the population admitted to the critical care process and determined that 23% of the patients admitted stood little risk for developing the complications for which they were being observed.[6] However, early detection of such complications that may be life- or morbidity-threatening and prompt initiation of appropriate treatment may far outweigh the costs of the resources consumed in this process. The long-term consequences of this early detection and treatment on mortality, morbidity, and economic and human costs were not considered in this report. This analysis of the critical care process may be more important than those previously discussed. Appropriate tools for the study of these benefits need to be developed and their impact defined.

Does the critical care process shorten the length of hospital stay for some patients? Intuitively, we know it does, but how does one go about documenting it? Randomized, controlled studies corrected for severity of illness can no longer be conducted from an ethical perspective. What are the benefits associated with the biological support provided to a potential organ donor? What is the value to the patient and the family of providing comfort during the dying process and assisting with the initiation of the grieving process? These benefits may seem soft, but are real and measurable.

Impact of critical care on costs of health care

The results of the critical care process cannot be discussed without parallel discussions on costs. As noted in the beginning of this chapter, the costs of intensive care have added substantially to the costs of health care.[1,2] Health care costs now threaten the economic security of the developed countries regardless of their respective health care delivery system. The high costs of the critical care process are certain to come under greater scrutiny as the problems of financing the entire health care industry receive increasing attention.[2] Mortality rates will be reviewed in conjunction with costs and the costs of survival will be examined.

New technologies are introduced into the ICU and accepted as 'standard of care' before studies are performed demonstrating the utility (benefit) of these technologies in the ICU. But, to measure ICU effectiveness, the goal of the intervention must be defined. Resources utilized in the ICU are resources that can be used for other goods and services. During this era of cost awareness, the 'amount of health' purchased for US $100 spent in the ICU will be compared with the 'amount' purchased if US $100 were spent on a preventive vaccination program or a blood pressure screening program or another alternative use. These opportunity costs associated with the delivery of critical care will be judged as to their worth. We must be prepared to answer the question: 'Is it worth it?'

Conclusions

The goals of critical care medicine include saving the salvageable and allowing the dying to die with peace and dignity.[4] How do you measure the quality of death? At what point in the patient's ICU course is it appropriate to limit or withdraw support? How do you ensure that death will come without suffering? These are questions that every intensivist deals with regularly: indeed, half of the deaths in the ICU occur after the decision has been made to limit care.[59] Attention needs to be directed to the goal of ensuring a peaceful and dignified death.

To come full circle from the beginning of this discussion several pages ago, many of the benefits associated with the critical care process are related to its impact on the providers of the care, the structure of the institution in which the process is practiced, and the health care system of which it is a part. Critical care is not practiced in isolation; it impacts on the entire health care system no matter where it is practiced. It has become an essential part of the health care system. The results of the use of this critical care process perhaps have been studied in greater detail than have most of the other processes of medicine. Others can learn from us. We are coming to know what we do and why we do it and what it is worth. But, the job is far from finished. In this time of careful scrutiny of health care, the answers are at hand. We must pursue outcome research in this expensive part of the health care system, no matter where it is practiced.

References

1. Knaus WA, Wagner DP, Zimmerman JE, Draper EA. Variations in mortality and length of stay in intensive care units. *Ann Intern Med* 1993; **118**: 753–61.
2. Birnbaum ML. Cost-containment in critical care. In: Rippe JM, Irwin RS, Alpert JS, Fink MP (eds) *Intensive Care Medicine*. Boston: Little, Brown and Co., 1991: 1977–97.
3. Relman AS. Assessment and accountability: the third revolution in medical care. *New Engl J Med* 1988; **319**: 1220–2.
4. Raffin ARRD 1989; **140**: s28–s35.
5. NIH Consensus Development Conference Statement on Critical Care Medicine. In: Parrillo JE, Ayers SM (eds) *Major Issues in Critical Care Medicine*. Baltimore: Williams & Wilkins, 1984: 277.
6. Medicare: past overuse of intensive care services inflates hospital payments. Report to the Secretary of Health and Human Services, United States General Accounting Office, Washington, DC, GAO/HRD 86-25, March 1986.
7. Strauss *et al*. *J Am Med Assoc* 1986; **225**: 1143–6.
8. Task Force on Cost-Containment, Society of Critical Care Medicine, Report to Council, 1993.
9. Gersh BJ, Clements IP, Chesebro JH. Acute myocardial infarction: A. Diagnosis and prognosis. In: Brandenburg RO, Giuliani ER, McGoon DC (eds) *Cardiology: Fundamentals and Practice*, vol. 2. Chicago: Year Book Medical Publishers, 1987: 1116–52.
10. Kruse JA, Thill-Baharozian MC, Carlson RW. Comparison of clinical assessment with APACHE II for predicting mortality risk in patients admitted to a medical intensive care unit. *J Am Med Assoc* 1988; **260**: 1739–42.
11. Knaus WA, Zimmerman JE, Wagner DP *et al*. APACHE – acute physiology and chronic health evaluation: a physiologically based classification system. *Crit Care Med* 1981; **9**: 591–7.
12. Knaus WA, Draper EA, Wagner DP, Zimmerman JE. APACHE II: a severity of disease classification system. *Crit Care Med* 1985; **13**: 818–29.
13. Cowen JS, Kelley MA. Error and bias in using predictive scoring systems. *Crit Care Clin* 1994; **1**: 53–72.
14. Knaus WA, Wagner DP, Draper EA *et al*. The APACHE III prognostic system: risk prediction of hospital mortality for critically ill hospitalized adults. *Chest* 1991; **100**: 1619–36.
15. Le Gall JR, Loirat P, Alperovitch A *et al*. A simplified acute physiology score for ICU patients. *Crit Care Med* 1984; **12**: 975.
16. Le Gall JR, Lemeshow S, Saulnier F. A new simplified acute physiology score (SAPS II) based on a European/ North American multicenter study. *J Am Med Assoc* 1993; **270**: 2957–963.
17. Pollack MM, Ruttiman UE, Getson PR. Pediatric risk of mortality (PRISM) score. *Crit Care Med* 1986; **16**: 1110.
18. Lemeshow S, Teres D, Pastides H *et al*. A method for predicting survival and mortality of ICU patients using objectively derived weights. *Crit Care Med* 1985; **13**: 519–25.
19. Lemeshow S, Teres D, Klar J *et al*. Mortality probability models (MPM II) based on an international cohort of intensive care patients. *J Am Med Assoc* 1993; **270**: 2478–86.
20. Thatcher VS *et al*. *The New Webster Dictionary of the English Language*. Chicago: Consolidated Book Publishers, 1971: 669–70.
21. Teasdale G, Jennett B. Assessment of coma and impaired consciousness practical scale. *Lancet* 1974; **ii**: 81.
22. Baker SP, O'Neill B, Haddon W *et al*. The injury severity score: a method for describing patients with multiple injuries an evaluating emergency care. *J Trauma* 1974; **14**: 187.
23. Chamion HR, Sacco WJ, Carnazzo AJ *et al*. Trauma score. *Crit Care Med* 1981; **9**: 672.
24. Deane SA, Gaudry PL, Roberts RF *et al*. Trauma triage: a comparison of the trauma score and the vital signs score. *Aust NZ J Surg* 1986; **156**: 19.
25. American Medical Association Committee on the Medical Aspects of Automotive Safety. Rating the severity of tissue damage: the abbreviated scale. *J Am Med Assoc* 1971; **215**: 277.
26. Civil ID, Schwab CW. The abbreviated injury scale, 1985 revision: a condensed chart for clinical use. *J Trauma* 1988; **28**: 87.
27. Gormican SP. CRAMS scale: field triage of trauma victims. *Ann Emergency Med* 1982; **11**: 132.
28. Boyd CR, Tolson MA, Copes WS. Evaluating trauma care: the TRISS method. *J Trauma* 1987; **27**: 370.
29. University of South Alabama, College of Medicine, Division of Pediatric Surgery. Pediatric trauma score: a rapid assessment and triage tool for the injured child. 1986.
30. Wright BM, McKerrow CG. Maximum forced expiratory flow rates as a measure of ventilatory capacity. *Br Med J* 1959; **228**: 221.
31. Cullen DJ, Civetta JM, Briggs BA *et al*. Therapeutic intervention scoring system: a method of quantitative comparison of patient care. *Crit Care Med* 1974; **2**: 57.
32. Keene AR, Cullen DJ. Therapeutic intervention scoring system: update 1983. *Crit Care Med* 1983; **11**: 1.
33. Birnbaum ML, Hunter-Handler D, Robinson NE *et al*. Comparison of populations and outcomes for patients with ischemic heart disease in rural community hospitals and a tertiary care center. Abstract. *Circulation* 1984; **70**: 164.

34. Wright BM, McKerrow CG. Maximum forced expiratory flow rates as a measure of ventilatory capacity. *Br Med J* 1959; **228**: 221.

35. Knaus WA, Draper EA, Wagner DP, Zimmerman JE. An evaluation of outcomes from intensive care in major medical centers. *Ann Intern Med* 1986; **104**: 410–18.

36. Knaus WA, Wagner DP, Zimmerman JE, Draper EA. Variations in mortality and length of stay in intensive care units. *Ann Intern Med* 1993; **118**: 753–61.

37. Miranda DR. Critically examining intensive care. *Int J Technol Assess Health Care* 1992; **8**: 444–56.

38. Parno JR, Teres D, Lemeshow S, Brown RB. Hospital charges and long-term survival of ICU versus non-ICU patients. *Crit Care Med* 1982; **10**: 569–74.

39. Ridley S, Jackson R, Findlay J, Wallace P. Long term survival after intensive care. *Br Med J* 1990; **30**: 1127–30.

40. Jacobs CJ, van der Vliet JA, Roozendaal MT, van der Linen CJ. Mortality and quality of life after intensive care for critical illness. *Intensive Care Med* 1988; **14**: 217–20.

41. Ridley S, Jackson R, Findlay J, Wallace P. Long term survival after intensive care. *Br Med J* 1990; **30**: 1127–30.

42. Birnbaum ML, Robinson NE, Kuska BM *et al.* Effect of advanced cardiac life-support training in rural, community hospitals. *Crit Care Med* 1994; **22**: 741–9.

43. Cullen DJ, Ferrara LC, Briggs BA *et al.* Survival, hospitalization charges and follow-up results in critically ill patients. *New Engl J Med* 1976; **294**: 982–7.

44. Cullen DJ, Keene R, Waternaux C *et al.* Results, charges, and benefits of intensive care for critically ill patients: Update 1983. *Crit Care Med* 1984; **12**: 102–6.

45. Nicolas F, LeGall JR, Alperovitch A *et al.* Influence of patients' age on survival, level of therapy and length of stay in intensive care units. *Intensive Care Med* 1987; **13**: 9–13.

46. Campion EW, Mulley AG, Goldstein RL, Barnett GO, Thibault GE. Medical intensive care for the elderly: A study of current use, costs, and outcomes. *J Am Med Assoc* 1981; **246**: 2052–6.

47. Fedullo, *Crit Care Med* 1983; **11**.

48. McLean RF, McIntosh JD, Kung GY *et al.* Outcome of respiratory intensive care for the elderly. *Crit Care Med* 1985; **13**: 625–9.

49. Mahul PH, Perrot D, Tempelhoff G *et al.* Short- and long-term prognosiss, functional outcome following ICU for elderly. *Intensive Care Med* 19[49] Champion HR, Sacco WJ, Carnazzo AJ *et al*: Trauma score. *Crit Care Med* 1981; **9**: 672.

50. Kass JE, Castriotta RJ, Malakoff F. Intensive care unit outcome in the very elderly. *Crit Care Med* 1992; **21**: 1666–71.

51. Rosen MJ, DePalo VA. Outcome of intensive care for patients with AIDS. *Crit Care Clin* 1993; **9**: 107–14.

52. Denardo SJ, Oye RK, Bellamy PE. Efficacy of intensive care for bone marrow transplant patients with respiratory failure. *Crit Care Med* 1989; **17**: 4–6.

53. Afessa B, Tefferi A, Hoagland HC *et al.* Outcome of recipients of bone marrow transplants who require intensive-care unit support. *Mayo Clin Proc* 1992; **67**: 117–22.

54. Chasin. *Medical Care* 1982; Vol. XX: 165–79.

55. Bams JL, Miranda DR. Outcome and costs of intensive care: a follow-up study of 238 ICU patients. *Intensive Care Med* 1985; **11**: 234–41.

56. Goldstein RL, Campion EW, Thibault GE *et al.* Functional outcomes following medical intensive care. *Crit Care Med* 1986; **14**: 783–88.

57. Sage WM, Rosenthal MH, Silverman JF. Is intensive care worth it? An assessment of input and outcome for the critically ill. *Crit Care Med* 1986; **14**: 777–82.

58. Patrick DL, Danis M, Southerland LI, Hong Guiyoung. *J Gen Intern Med* 1988; **3**: 218–23.

59. Zimmerman JE, Knaus WA, Sharpe MD *et al.* The use and implications of do not resuscitate orders in intensive care units. *J Am Med Assoc* 1986; **255**: 351–6.

60. Skau T, Nystrom P-O, Calsson C. Severity of illness in intra-abdominal infection. *Arch Surg* 1985; **120**: 152.

61. Yeh TS, Pollack MM, Ruttimann UE *et al.* Validation of a physiology stability index for use in critically ill infants and children. *Pediatr Res* 1984; **18**: 445.

62. Rhee KJ, Fisher CJ, Willitis NH. The rapid acute physiology score. *Am J Emergency Med* 1987; **5**: 278.

CHAPTER 21

Evaluating the Costs and Consequences of Critical Care: Critical Appraisal of Health Technology

KEVIN J INMAN, WILLIAM J SIBBALD

Introduction   315
Evaluating evidence of benefit   317
Establishing costs   321
Combining costs and consequences   322
Costs, consequences and the individual practitioner   325
Conclusions   327
References   327

Introduction

A US National Institutes of Health consensus conference has defined critical care as:

> a multidisciplinary field concerned with patients who have sustained or are at risk of sustaining, acutely life threatening, single or multiple organ system failures due to disease or injury. Critical Care seeks to provide for the needs of these patients through immediate and continuous observation and intervention so as to restore health and prevent complications.[1]

From a modest beginning, the intensive care unit (ICU) has grown into a substantial hospital service, with a concomitant and dramatic increase in both utilization and cost. This growth has been facilitated by a number of factors, including an aging population, the development of life-sustaining technologies and increasing expectations amongst both patients and health professionals. Some critics however argue that the modern ICU, including most of its technology, has evolved without objective evidence of benefit to either the patient or society. An increasing imbalance between the *demand* for health care services and the *supply* of health care resources will mean that this relatively unrestrained expansion of ICU services in the previous two decades is impossible to sustain.

The financial impact of providing critical care services cannot be overemphasized. Crude estimates have placed the daily cost of ICU care from two to five times that required for care at the general ward level.[2] As much as one-third of a hospital's resources may be devoted to caring for critically ill or injured patients.[3] Despite its resource intensity, few attempts have been made to evaluate the ICU, that is to systematically link these costs with patient outcomes. 'Thus, it is time for a rigorous effort to establish what procedures produce beneficial outcomes under what conditions – and to eliminate stark instances of "over-utilization". Physicians and hospital administrators should put establishing quality standards at the top of their agendas'.[4]

To deal with the imbalance between the supply and demand for critical care services, three approaches are possible:

1. strategies which aim to reduce *demand*;
2. strategies which limit the *supply* (i.e. rationing);
3. strategies which attempt to improve the *efficiency* of existing services.

Health technology assessment deals with the last of these. It is our objective to provide the reader with an overview of the methods for technology assessment in general, and the means of evaluating the efficiency of different critical care alternatives in particular. We will not provide a 'cookbook' approach to the subject, rather, we will highlight specific areas from which the reader might infer local applicability. This chapter will begin by defining terms commonly used in the lexicon of health care technology assessment. A brief discussion of methods used to evaluate the beneficial effects of technology will follow. Estimating the costs of ICU services will comprise the next section, followed by a discussion of methods used in an economic evaluation of health care alternatives. We will conclude with a discussion as to how critical care practitioners can incorporate this knowledge to improve efficiency in their ICU services.

DEFINITIONS

Assessing health care technologies prior to their widespread use is increasingly required by both funding and regulatory agencies. However, the assessment process remains both confusing and controversial to many critical care practitioners! In part, confusion arises because of concern over the lexicon of terms used to describe the assessment process.

Health care technology has been defined (Table 21.1)

as all of the instruments, equipment, drugs and procedures used in health care delivery, as well as the organizations supporting delivery of such care.[5] Key to this definition is its scope. Not only are agents and devices considered technology, but also the programs we implement. Thus, a hospital's critical care services can be viewed as a distinct health care technology just as easily as a new drug or diagnostic test.

Technology assessment is the process of designing and conducting investigations to evaluate and render judgment on the technology being assessed.[6] The goal of health care technology assessments is to establish the criteria for efficacious, effective and efficient care of the patient. *Efficacy* studies are investigations which examine the probability of benefit to patients in a defined population from a medical technology applied for a given, correctly diagnosed, medical problem under ideal conditions of use.[7] These studies address the question of whether the technology can produce clinical improvements. *Effectiveness* evaluations examine the probability of benefit to individuals in a defined population from a medical technology applied for a given medical problem under average conditions of use.[7] These investigations are far more pragmatic, asking whether the implementation of the technology does indeed result in clinical improvements.

Two recently conducted multicenter randomized controlled trials[8, 9] which examined monoclonal antibodies to endotoxin as an adjunct to standard therapy for patients with sepsis illustrate that differences between efficacy and effectiveness studies are far more than just semantics! Neither study demonstrated that monoclonal antibody to endotoxin reduced mortality in the overall study population. In subsets of patients with Gram-negative infection, however, both studies demon-

Table 21.1   Definitions associated with health care technology assessment

Health care technology	That which encompasses all of the instruments, equipment, drugs and procedures used in health care delivery, as well as the organizations supporting delivery of such care.
Technology assessment	Process of designing and conducting investigations to evaluate and render judgement on the efficacy, effectiveness, and efficiency of the technologies being assessed.
Efficacy	The ability of a technology to achieve its intended clinical benefits when implemented under ideal conditions.
Effectiveness	The ability of a technology to achieve its intended clinical benefits when implemented under average conditions.
Efficiency	The relationship between the costs and consequences, or inputs and outputs of implementing differing health care alternatives.
Technical efficiency	The production of health care goods and services at the lowest possible cost.
Allocative efficiency	Health care goods and services are produced and distributed so as to maximize the welfare of the community.

strated a significant reduction in mortality. From the efficacy standpoint these studies showed that in patients presenting with the signs and symptoms of sepsis, monoclonal antibodies to endotoxin as an adjunct to standard therapy can reduce mortality. Under average conditions of use, however, where over 60% of septic patients did not have documented Gram-negative infection, monoclonal antibody did not achieve its intended benefits.

If a particular technology is found to be either efficacious or effective, the question then becomes, at what cost are these benefits achieved? *Efficiency* investigations address this question by simultaneously examining both the costs and consequences, or inputs and outputs, of implementing different health care technologies. Economists conceive of efficiency in terms of *technical efficiency*, ensuring that goods and services are produced at the lowest possible cost, and *allocative efficiency*, ensuring that goods and services are allocated so as to maximize the welfare of the community. The latter definition is the one most applicable to health care since the primary goal for the economic evaluation of health care alternatives is to maximize health rather than to minimize costs. Efficiency studies therefore provide information regarding whether the technology should be implemented under the conditions examined.

Evaluating evidence of benefit

All studies examining the efficiency of different health care alternatives are predicated on the generation of evidence regarding the consequences, outputs or benefits of the alternatives in question. This section will provide the reader with the fundamental principles for critically appraising the evidence of benefit for therapeutic agents and diagnostic and monitoring technologies.

THERAPEUTIC TECHNOLOGIES

Therapeutic technologies are those agents and programs, which directly impact on patient outcome. Figure 21.1 shows the various methods used to examine the benefit, if any, of these technologies. Lacking in the use of any controls (i.e. nontreated patients), the *case series* is the least valid. Its major deficiencies include the potential for the placebo effect to explain clinical improvement, the lack of blindness to treatment assignment for both patient and clinician, and the potential for the lack of interinstitutional applicability. An example of the drawbacks of the case series approach is the previous use of mammary artery ligation to treat angina pectoris. While initial case series reports were positive,[10] a subsequent randomized controlled trial[11] showed no benefit of mammary artery ligation in the management of angina pectoris. Despite its limitations, the case series approach does have a role in establishing primary evidence of efficacy and effectiveness. Where a patient's prognosis is very poor, any therapy which demonstrates evidence of improvement may be considered worth adopting. Examples include the use of dialysis to treat oliguric renal failure and ventilatory therapy to treat acute respiratory failure due to respiratory center depression.

The *case control* design is another method used to establish primary evidence of benefit. Conducted retrospectively, this method selects and groups individuals in terms of their status regarding the outcome of interest. Cases, those with the outcome of interest, are compared with controls, those who do not have the outcome of interest. Where possible, cases and controls are matched on potentially confounding variables such as age, sex, diagnosis and severity of illness. The investigator then determines whether or not each

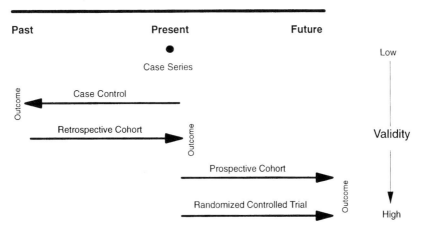

Fig. 21.1 Summary of the study designs examining the clinical benefit of therapeutic agents.

individual was exposed to the agent of interest. The association, if any, between polyneuropathies in the critically ill and exposure to neruomuscular blocking agents or high-dose corticosteroids would lend itself well to this method. In this model, cases, those with a polyneuropathy, would be matched with controls, those without a polyneuropathy. The two groups would then be compared on their frequency of exposure to the agents of interest. As data are examined retrospectively, however, the chance of obtaining biased results in the case control design can never be ruled out. If significant associations are detected, there is no guarantee that they are causal in nature. Even so, there remains a role for case control studies in the ICU since they are relatively inexpensive, easy to carry out, and for rare diseases and late adverse effects they are the only feasible method by which associations can be detected.[12] Overall, the case control method may be considered particularly valuable as a hypothesis generating rather than hypothesis testing tool.

Cohort studies, whether assembled retrospectively or prospectively, are investigations in which a group of individuals (the cohort) who have been exposed to a particular technology are followed over time and their outcome(s) are compared with a second group of individuals who were not exposed. Unlike the case control method, groups are assembled based on exposure, and followed to determine their outcome(s). Charlson and Sax used the cohort approach to assess the efficacy of a critical care unit.[13] A cohort of more than 600 admissions was assembled, some of whom were directly admitted to the ICU (those exposed), and some of whom were not (those not exposed). When comparing the mortality experience of the cohort, the major finding was that direct admission to the ICU was efficacious for the moderately ill, unstable patient. No differences in mortality between direct admission to the ICU and admission to the ward were found for the unstable severely ill patient, nor for stable (mildly or moderately ill) patients. Again, results based on cohort studies are also to be interpreted with caution! For example, without random assignment to receive direct ICU admission or ward admission, there is no guarantee that direct admissions and nondirect admissions were comparable on other, potentially confounding variables. Suppose, for example, that those admitted directly to the ICU were both older and had more concomitant morbidity than those admitted directly to the ward, would the same results have been obtained?

The *randomized controlled trial* (RCT) represents the most valid, and commonly used method for obtaining primary evidence. A RCT is a prospective study that compares the effect and value of an intervention(s) against a control procedure (Fig. 21.2). While RCTs have traditionally been used to examine whether new drug therapies have their proposed benefit, they are equally applicable to the evaluation of other medical

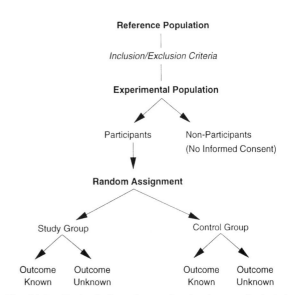

Fig. 21.2   Basic design of a randomized controlled trial.

technologies. The primary advantage of random assignment to treatment groups is that both known and unknown confounding factors are balanced between the study groups, thereby lending maximal internal validity to the study. While validity is highest, one must be cautious as to how generalizable the study's results are to the reference population.

Consider the two multicenter RCTs which examined the effect of antiendotoxin monoclonal antibody in patients with sepsis.[9,10] Both investigations wanted to establish conclusions regarding treatment in the reference population, septic patients. However, the experimental populations differed in each study because of subtle differences in the selection criteria. Additionally, it should be noted that the resulting study populations were self-selected, as informed consent was provided to participate in the investigation. It should therefore come as no surprise that results from the two studies were not consistent. Finally, it must be remembered that RCTs also have their drawbacks, including their expense and length of time until results are available.

DIAGNOSTIC AND MONITORING TECHNOLOGY

Although diagnostic and monitoring technology are the cornerstone of the modern ICU, few of these technologies are native to this setting. In fact, the majority have diffused into the ICU setting without formal evaluations of their efficacy or effectiveness, let alone their economic impact.

A diagnostic test is evaluated based on the indices of sensitivity, specificity, positive and negative predictive-

**Disease Status as Judged
by Gold Standard**

		Present	Absent	Total
Test Result	Positive	A	B	A+B
	Negative	C	D	C+D
	Total	A+C	B+D	N

Stable Properties:
Sensitivity = A/A+C
Specificity = D/B+D

Prevalence (A+C/N) Dependent Properties:
Positive Preditive Value = A/A+B
Negative Predictive Value = D/C+D
Accuracy = A+D/N

Fig. 21.3 Important indices in diagnostic technology assessment.

ness, accuracy and prevalence (Fig. 21.3). *Sensitivity* is defined as the number of diseased individuals with a positive test divided by the total number of diseased individuals. Conversely, *specificity* is defined as the number of nondiseased individuals divided by the total number of nondiseased individuals. Thus, sensitivity identifies how well the test performs in *ruling in* the disease, while specificity indicates how well the test is at *ruling out* disease. While a high sensitivity and specificity are desirable for any diagnostic test, of greater concern to the critical care professional are the test's predictive values since the patient's true disease status (as determined by the gold standard of diagnosis) is usually not known at the time the diagnostic test is administered. The *positive predictive value* of a diagnostic test is the probability that the disease is present if a positive test is achieved. Conversely, the *negative predictive value* is the probability that the disease is absent given a negative test result.

While the application in clinical practice of these four indices appears straightforward, problems and biases can influence results.[14] In the diseased and nondiseased populations, variations in the extent, location, or cell type (pathologic), the chronicity and severity (clinical) or the amount and type of coexisting ailments (comorbid) may all affect sensitivity and specificity, respectively. Work-up bias can affect the assessment if patients exhibiting a positive test go on to further confirmatory testing, while those exhibiting a negative test do not. Diagnostic review bias is possible when test results affect the subjective review needed to establish the true diagnosis. Test review bias can occur when the diagnostic test of interest is run after the true diagnosis is known. In the latter two cases, blinding the assessment of the test of interest from the true diagnosis is essential.

Once the aforementioned indices are known, a diagnostic test is further evaluated by examining its likelihood ratios. Briefly, likelihood ratios express the odds that a given diagnostic test result would be expected in a patient with (as opposed to one without) the target disorder. They are calculated as the sensitivity (the true-positive rate) divided by the false-positive rate ($b/b + d$). For a further discussion of likelihood ratios, their calculation interpretation, and pre- and post-test probabilities of disease an excellent reference can be found in the *Canadian Medical Association Journal*.[15]

As is the case with diagnostic technologies in the ICU, monitoring technologies have received little formal assessment prior to widespread diffusion to the ICU. The vast majority of monitors estimate physiologic parameters, and initial evaluations should therefore attempt to ascertain the degree to which the two methods (the monitored and physiologic measures) agree. Unfortunately, many evaluations have been conducted by calculating the degree to which the two methods of measurement are correlated. While this does confer some information, the correlation coefficient is not the appropriate index to examine. At least three reasons highlight why this is the case.[16] First, correlation measures the strength of relation between two variables, not the agreement between them. Perfect agreement occurs only if all points lie along the line of equality, but perfect correlation exists if all points lie along any straight line. Second, it would be surprising if two methods of measuring the same index did not agree. Thus, the test of significance (a high correlation coefficient and low *p* value) is irrelevant to the measure of agreement. Finally, data which are in poor agreement can show a high degree of correlation.

Given the pitfalls of using correlation, how should the degree of agreement between a monitored value and a physiologic parameter be assessed? First, the bias and precision of the monitored values must be calculated.

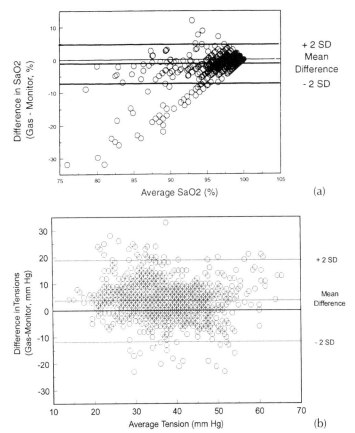

Fig. 21.4 Assessing the degree of agreement between pulse oximetry (a), end-tidal capnography (b) and arterial blood gas values.

Bias is simply the average difference between the monitored and measured values, and precision is the standard deviation of this difference. While these indices confer 'global' properties of the monitor, they do not illustrate how the monitor functions over a range of physiologic values. Bland and Altman[16] present a simple visual method for assessing the degree of agreement between two methods of clinical measurement. A simple plot is constructed of the difference between the two measures (the bias) against the average of the two measures. Excellent agreement therefore exists when all points lie on, or near zero over all ranges. Both pulse oximtery[17] and capnography[18] have been examined in this manner. The former shows good agreement over the normal oxygen saturation range, while the latter does not.

If a diagnostic test is accurate and a monitor is shown to be in good agreement with its physiologic measure, should monitoring be implemented on this information alone? The answer is an unconditional no! Just because these technologies provide valid data does not mean they are an efficient use of scarce health care resources. Technologies which have little or no impact on subsequent decisions should not be implemented! Even technologies which have a positive impact on decision

making may not represent an efficient use of resources. If treatment decisions are not, or cannot, be altered as a result of the diagnostic or monitored information, the technology is also not worth adopting. Thus, once the accuracy of diagnostic and monitoring technology has been established, the questions then revolve around the impact the data have on the provider of care. While it may be somewhat unfair to expect a diagnostic or monitoring technology to be associated with improved patient outcomes, ultimately these technologies will have to be proved to be an efficient use of resources before their widespread adoption can be justified. One need look no further than the controversy and concern surrounding the pulmonary artery catheter to see the reasons for a more comprehensive assessment approach.

In summary, various methods exist for establishing if either therapeutic or diagnostic and monitoring technologies achieve their proposed benefit. While these methods exist, they have not traditionally been applied in the critical care setting with any consistency. The critical care practitioner who can critically appraise the evidence of benefit will be able to make better, and more informed decisions regarding the implementation of new technology in the ICU.

Establishing costs

The identification, measurement and valuation of costs is required by all forms of economic evaluation. Since there are more beneficial health care technologies than there are resources to provide them, cost represents, in economic terms, an alternative opportunity foregone. For example, suppose that the decision has been made to purchase new ventilators for the ICU. Resources expended on this purchase may limit resources to implement other potentially useful technologies. Given finite resources there will always be more good programs than there is money to provide them.

It seems intuitive that since most hospitals are run on a not-for-profit basis, charges, the rate the patient pays, would be a good proxy for cost, the price the hospital pays. How costs are calculated highlights the reasons why costs and charges should be discerned. Costs can be fixed or variable, and either direct or indirect (Figure 21.5). Fixed costs are those that do not vary with the quantity of output in the short term such as equipment lease payments and some salaries. In contrast, variable costs are those which do vary with the level of output. For example, nurse staffing, physician fees and supplies will vary depending on the number of patients seen. Direct costs include the operating and organizing costs within the health sector, as well as those costs borne by the patient (or patient's family). Similarly, but harder to identify and measure, are direct benefits. These take the form of future health care resources not consumed, for example medical and surgical therapy avoided as a result of implementing the new technology. The imple-

mentation of technologies such as coronary angioplasty are an example of this concept since the intent of the technology is, in part, designed to avoid future surgery. Direct costs can be thought of as production losses and include lost time from employment and travel costs. Indirect benefits are viewed as future gains in production, such as early return to work after laprascopic versus traditional surgical techniques.

Identifying the components of cost in this manner allows for the calculation of a number of summary indices regarding cost. The *total cost* to produce a given level of health output is the sum of fixed and variable costs. *Average cost* is the mean cost per unit. However, the most important expression of cost in economic evaluations is that of *marginal cost*, the cost of producing one extra unit. Given how costs are calculated and expressed, the importance of distinguishing between the two is highlighted by the following example.

Assume we have two ICUs, each providing treatment to patients with sepsis, and each is governed by the same reimbursement mechanism. In ICU-A, 200 septic patients with Gram-negative bacteremia are seen in each year, while in ICU-B, only 100 septic patients with Gram-negative bacteremia are seen in the same interval. Now, presume that a new diagnostic technology becomes available which enables rapid identification of septic patients with a Gram-negative infection and its cost is Can $1 000 000. Both hospitals wish to purchase the technology. Since both hospitals receive reimbursement in the same manner, charges for the treatment of septic patients should be similar at both institutions. However, purchasing the new technology at the smaller of the two ICUs will result in larger increases in both

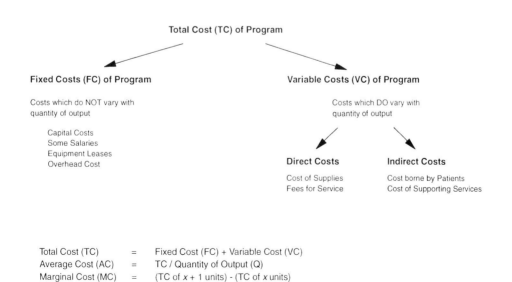

Fig. 21.5 Components of health care program cost.

Are Both Costs and Consequences Examined?

		NO		YES
		Examines Only Consequences	Examines Only Costs	
Is There Comparison of Two or More Alternatives?	**NO**	Outcome Description	Cost Description	Cost-Outcome Description
	YES	**Efficacy** or **Effectiveness** Analyses	Cost Analysis	**Cost-Minimization Cost-Effectiveness Cost-Benefit Cost-Utility** Analyses

Fig. 21.6   Characteristics of health care evaluations.

their average and marginal costs since there are fewer patients per year over which to spread the fixed cost of buying the diagnostic technology.

Combining costs and consequences

As evident in the preceding sections, the examination of costs or consequences alone does not give a complete picture regarding the impact of introducing new health care technologies. Economic evaluations simultaneously examine both costs and consequences, and thus they are needed to fully address the economic impact of implementation.

Evaluations of health care alternatives can be viewed as partial or full, depending on their scope (Fig. 21.6). Cost or outcome descriptions are considered partial evaluations since they examine only one health care

alternative, the first in terms of resources consumed, the latter in terms of potential patient benefits. While examining both costs and consequences, cost–outcome descriptions are considered partial evaluations since only one alternative is evaluated. Establishing the clinical benefits of new technologies is an integral part of full evaluations. However, since costs are ignored in efficacy and effectiveness evaluations, the economic impact of the technologies in question remains unknown. Similarly, cost analyses are partial evaluations since no consideration is given to potential differences to which outcomes may differ. While these studies do not allow the question of efficiency to be addressed, they serve as an important and essential step in examining the true impact of introducing new technology.

Full economic evaluations include: cost-minimization, cost-effectiveness, cost-benefit, and cost-utility analyses (Table 21.2). While the identification, valuation, and measurement of the costs of providing the

Table 21.2   Types of economic evaluations

Types of analysis	Measurement of costs	Identification of consequences	Valuation of consequences
Cost-minimization	Dollars	Identical in all relevant respects	None
Cost-effectiveness	Dollars	Single effect of interest, common to both alternatives, but achieved to different degrees	Natural units (e.g. life-years gained)
Cost-benefit	Dollars	Single or multiple effects of interest, not necessarily common to both alternatives, and common effects may be achieved to different degrees	Dollars
Cost-utility	Dollars	Single or multiple effects of interest, not necessarily common to both alternatives, and common effects may be achieved to different degrees	Quality adjusted life years (QALY) Healthy years equivalent (HYE)

Adapted from ref. 26.

alternatives of interest is inherent to all these methods, the nature of the consequence side of the equation differs substantially. Similarly, the viewpoint from which the analysis is undertaken also differs. Ultimately society pays for all of the goods and services it receives, and thus all of the direct and indirect costs and benefits should be included. However, for the critical care practitioner forced to make a choice between two technologies, this viewpoint may be too broad and include costs and benefits far removed from the ICU or hospital. As a result, a more focused viewpoint such as the hospital or third-party payer may be more applicable. While it is possible to compare more than two health care alternatives simultaneously, we will restrict our discussion to the case where a new technology is being considered for implementation. Unless otherwise stated, its comparator is the existing technology. Each type of analysis, as it relates to this scenario, is discussed in turn.

COST-MINIMIZATION ANALYSIS

Cost-minimization analyses are a subset of cost-effectiveness analyses. In the former, all patient outcomes are equivalent between the two technologies of interest and the more favorable technology is the one with the lower costs. The use of pulse oximetry versus serial arterial blood gas analysis to monitor oxygen saturations while weaning ventilated patients provides an example of this type of analysis. Pulse oximetry was originally introduced to reduce the incidence of clinically undetected hypoxemia, with the premise that patient safety would be improved. While pulse oximetry has been shown to detect significant episodes of hypoxemia before the appearance of clinical signs, there is no conclusive evidence that patient outcomes have improved as a result of applying this technology.[19] However, given that it is a relatively precise and unbiased means of estimating arterial oxygen saturations,[17] implementing pulse oximetry can result in substantially fewer arterial blood gas analyses, without compromising the patient's care.[20] Given that no differences in outcomes exist between patients weaned using serial arterial blood gas analyses and a pulse oximetry guided weaning protocol, it is possible to conduct a cost-minimization analysis of pulse oximetry guided weaning.

COST-EFFECTIVENESS ANALYSIS

Determining the cost-effectiveness of medical technologies is becoming increasingly important as health care costs continue to rise. As shown in Table 21.2, cost-effectiveness analyses examine a single, naturally occurring health outcome, common to both technolo-

gies, as the consequence of interest. In these analyses the comparison of interest is the ratio of the net increase in health care costs to the net effectiveness in terms of increased patient benefits. Using this criteria, some authors[21] have advocated that new technologies be considered cost-effective when one of three conditions is met:

1. the new technology is at least as effective as the current technology and less costly;
2. the new technology is more effective and more costly than the current technology, but the added benefits are considered worth their added cost;
3. the new technology is less effective and less costly than the current standard and the added benefits of the current standard are not worth its added costs.

In a recent study, we determined the clinical benefits and cost-effectiveness of an air suspension bed in the prevention of pressure ulcers in the 'at risk' critically ill patient.[22] Using an RCT to determine effectiveness (i.e. few entry criteria), we found that the use of an air suspension bed resulted in significantly fewer patients developing single, multiple or severe pressure ulcers. The viewpoint taken for the economic evaluation was that of the third-party payer, and costs were broken down into prophylactic, diagnostic and hospital treatment. Further, costs were stratified by the severity of the pressure ulcer. Examining the incremental change in costs and outcomes, a cost-effectiveness ratio of less than zero was obtained. This meant that when compared to the standard ICU bed and frequent rotation of the patient, air suspension therapy was a dominant technology, providing increased benefit for less cost than the technology.

A second example of cost-effectiveness analysis in critical care is that of the use of monoclonal antibodies as an adjunct to therapy for the treatment of sepsis.[23] The intent of this study was to provide the information required to guide the implementation of this new (and expensive) therapy on a national and hospital-specific basis by examining the incremental change in costs for each life year saved. Since monoclonal antibody to endotoxin is most effective in patients with sepsis as a result of Gram-negative bacteremia, and since only approximately 35% of the patients ultimately had this diagnosis, the authors also varied the proportion of correctly identified cases using two strategies; the *treat strategy*, in which all patients receive therapy, and the *test strategy*, which was based on a hypothetical new diagnostic aid which would improve the identification of those patients with a Gram-negative infection. Under the treat strategy, the use of monoclonal antibody would result in a cost-effectiveness ratio of Can $24 100 per life year saved. Under the test strategy, with fewer false-positives, this ratio declined to Can $14 900 per life year saved. The authors then conducted a sensitivity analysis in which the cost of different input variables was varied as well as the proportion of correctly identified cases. The cost-effectiveness ratios were influenced relatively little by changes in the cost of therapy or acute care hospitalization; the ratios never exceeded Can $29 500 per life year saved in the treat strategy and Can $19 000 in the test strategy. However, if the assumption that patients would gain an average of 4.33 discounted years of life as a result of therapy was overly optimistic, the cost of implementing a monoclonal antibody program rises sharply. If only one life year is gained, the ratios rise to Can $110 000 and Can $67 900 per year of life saved in the treat and test strategies, respectively. The current example highlights the need to evaluate critically the assumptions used in models of cost-effectiveness. This is especially true in this example given that relatively little is known regarding the long-term survival for patients with sepsis.

COST-BENEFIT ANALYSIS

Cost-benefit studies are based on the Paretian principle in economics which states that optimum efficiency is reached when resources cannot be reallocated to make one person better of without making at least one other person worse off.[24] While these analyses were applied to many kinds of non-health care studies such as transportation and environmental projects, they are recently enjoying renewed interest in the health care setting. As seen in Table 21.2, cost-benefit analysis departs significantly from cost-effectiveness analysis in two ways. First, the consequences of each program are measured in monetary terms, where benefits are measured in terms of reduced direct costs of future care and reduced indirect costs of future mortality and morbidity. Second, and more importantly, while cost-effectiveness analyses were limited to those scenarios where there was a single health effect of interest common to both programs (and all other effects were shown or assumed to be equal), cost-benefit analysis allows us to examine single or multiple effects of interest which may or may not be common to both programs.

While many studies in the critical care literature have claimed to examine the cost-benefit of different therapies, in fact, few sound studies have been conducted. Boyle *et al.*[25] have examined the cost-benefit of neonatal intensive care for very low birthweight infants. Using evidence based on a before/after neonatal intensive care evaluation, they examined the cost-benefit of intensive over non-intensive care for infants weighing less than 1000 grams and for infants weighing between 1000 and 1499 grams. For both birthweight groups, providing neonatal intensive care increased cost in excess of the increase in projected benefits. The net losses per live birth were Can $2 600 and Can $16 100

for infants weighing between 1000 and 1499 grams and less than 1000 grams, respectively. In this study, neonatal intensive care was therefore shown to represent increased net cost to society, consuming more resources than it saved or created.

The preceding example illustrates two fundamental points regarding the economic evaluation of health care technology. First, there are instances in which society chooses to deploy its resources in an inefficient manner. Many centers continue to treat infants in this weight range on a routine basis, due in part to the high value our society accords to the care of infants. Second, it must be remembered that this assessment was carried out at one point in time, and was not based on the results of a rigorous study design. There is no guarantee that if the aforementioned study could be replicated today different results would not be obtained, given the advances in medical knowledge. Thus, technology assessment must be a continuously evolving process, as single assessments rarely provide the definitive information upon which to base long-term policies.

COST-UTILITY ANALYSIS

Cost-utility analyses are an economic appraisal which are somewhat similar to cost-effectiveness analyses. While some authors consider them a subset of cost-effectiveness analysis, we contend that they are separate and distinct for two reasons. First, like the cost-benefit approach, cost-utility analysis provides a means of comparing alternatives with single or multiple outcomes which are not necessarily common to both programs or achieved to the same degree. This is not possible in cost-effectiveness analysis. Second, cost-utility analyses represent the first attempt to include *quality of life* as part of the evaluation criteria. In this case health improvements are most commonly measured in terms of the number of quality adjusted life years (QALYs) gained. Thus, while there are many similarities with cost-effectiveness evaluations, cost-utility analyses are sufficiently different so as to constitute a separate entity.

Cost-utility analyses are most applicable when one of the following situations is evident:[26] quality of life is *the* important outcome, quality of life is *an* important outcome, when the program has effects on both mortality and morbidity and such an outcome is needed that combines the two, and when the programs being compared have a wide range of outcomes necessitating a common unit of output. Quality of life is represented by a continuum of health states from death (worst case) to full health (best case). Utility measurement thus constitutes an approach which assigns preferences to different health states to produce a scale. Various approaches and methods exist to assign utility values to each of the health states, and interested readers are referred to Torrance[27] for a more thorough discussion. Briefly, medical scenarios depicting different health states are described to the respondents who are then asked to rate the desirability of these health states.

Once the utilities for each health state have been derived, they are applied to the results obtained for the study. As an example, suppose we were interested in the QALYs gained for patients treated in the ICU for severe polyneuropathies. Treatment in the ICU for this affliction is associated with 10 years of life extension. However, during this 10 years you are confined to a wheelchair, and have a very limited range of activity. Using one of the above three methods, a utility value for this health state is calculated. For example, suppose that a sample of respondents rated the above health state utility at 0.65. The QALYs gained from treating polyneuropathies in the ICU would then be (0.65) × (10 years) = 6.5 QALY gained.

Using QALYs, tentative guidelines for the adoption and utilization of new medical technologies in Ontario have been proposed as a means of becoming more efficient given the fiscal restraint current health care systems face.[28] Using graded evidence on patient benefits coupled with distinct increments for cost-effectiveness/utility, these authors have come up with a means of grading technologies from Grades A through E. Grade A technologies are those that are more effective and less costly and should be adopted. Grade E technologies are those that are more costly and less effective and should not be implemented. Grades B, C and D, evaluations which show the new technology to be either less effective and less costly or more effective and more costly, have been subdivided into components *a* and *b*. Cutoff points of Can $20 000 and Can $100 000 per QALY are used as a means of grading the recommendations into moderate and weak evidence for acceptance, respectively.

While the authors' intent was to provide a framework with which to interpret economic evaluations, and thus provide the necessary information to make sound decisions regarding the adoption and utilization of health services technology, their work has aroused much debate. Chief among its criticisms is the degree to which the QALY can be used as a common yardstick between programs, given the large differences in utility scores obtained using different methods[29] coupled with the fact that long-term survival years are seldom known.[30] This is especially true in the critical care setting as evidenced by the paucity of long-term follow-up data. Another criticism is the inherent assumption that 'a pool of under employed or inefficiently employed resources, although not identified, exists somewhere within the current health care system' and can be used to offset the increased cost of providing those technologies which increase patient benefits at increased cost.[31] Suffice it to say that the paucity of long-term follow-up data coupled with the lack of a

valid and sensitive instrument for measuring quality of life in the critically ill patient have resulted in few true cost-utility studies being undertaken in this setting.

Costs, consequences and the individual practitioner

Prior to concluding, the following section will establish a framework within which the individual practitioner can approach decisions regarding the implementation of new technologies in the ICU. We propose that a series of questions be posed as a guide (Table 21.3). The objectives of posing these questions are two-fold. First, it is hoped that readers will be able to critically appraise the results of existing technology assessments. Second, by structuring the evaluation process, it is hoped that more critical care practitioners will become involved in the technology assessment process, given that change is both imminent and more palatable if orchestrated by those within the system rather than imposed from outside the system.

First and foremost, is there any evidence that patient outcomes are improved as a result of implementing this technology? If so, is the evidence based on an evaluation in the critical care setting? If the answer to the former is no, an efficacy or effectiveness evaluation is warranted, preferably in the critical care setting. If the answer to the latter is no, the degree to which results are applicable to the critical care setting should be addressed before a decision is made regarding implementation. Ideally, these evaluations would include the appropriate measure of economic impact.

THERAPEUTIC AGENTS

For therapeutic agents where improved patient outcomes are claimed in critical care, were these claims based on a rigorous study design? As discussed previously, results based on nonrandomized studies must be interpreted with extreme caution. If claims of benefit are based on the results of a randomized controlled trial, were all patients accounted for at study completion? If not, the results of the trial are suspect. Similarly, if beneficial claims were based on a subset of those patients enrolled, caution should also be exercised.

Were results of the clinical trial not only statistically significant, but clinically meaningful? It must be remembered that small (and relatively meaningless) clinical differences can be detected with a large sample sizes, and thus the magnitude of improvement should be critically reviewed. Furthermore, are the significant results real outcomes? Many trials suffer from substituting an improvement in a risk factor for an improvement

Table 21.3   A guide to more informed technology implementation

1. Is there any evidence that patient outcomes are improved as a result of implementing this technology?
2. If so, does the evidence come from a critical care population?

    2.1 Therapeutic agents

    Was beneficial evidence based on a rigorous study design?
    Were all patients accounted for at study completion?
    Were results clinically significant?
    Were all relevant outcomes included?
    Were all patients comparable to your setting, and is the study maneuver feasible in your setting?

    2.2 Diagnostic tests

    Were all diagnostic indices reported?
    Were sufficient numbers of diseased and nondiseased patients included?
    Was there any evidence that bias entered into the evaluation of the test?
    Did tests results alter therapy?

    2.3 Monitoring technology

    Were both the precision and bias reported?
    Was the degree of agreement between the two measures assessed?

3. Has the economic impact of implementing the technology been addressed?

    Was a full economic evaluation conducted? If so, what type?
    Was the perspective of the analysis explicitly stated?
    Were all components of costs (direct and indirect) of the competing alternatives included?
    Were costs estimated from a variety of sources or derived directly from the patient population?
    When applicable, was quality of life addressed?
    Was a sensitivity analysis performed to examine different model assumptions?

in patient outcome. Consider coronary angioplasty, for example, where the intent is to obviate the need for surgery to correct myocardial ischemia. Beneficial claims should not be based on the ability to increase patency of the vessel (a risk factor), but rather on the decreased incidence of surgery (the appropriate patient outcome). Were all clinically relevant patient outcomes considered? If only selected outcomes were included in the analysis, further information is required.

Finally, were patients in the study sufficiently similar to those in your ICU to allow generalizability of the study's results to your practice, and was the study maneuver feasible in your setting? It must be remembered that the vast majority of clinical trials conducted in critical care are done so in large tertiary care centers, under intense internal scrutiny, and use patients in which compliance with the study protocol is virtually ensured. This can be very different from the community ICU where the infrastructure is simply not developed enough so as to allow efficient implementation of the therapeutic agent.

DIAGNOSTIC AND MONITORING TECHNOLOGY

Similar questions should also be posed when considering the implementation of new diagnostic technologies.

Of primary concern is the concise reporting of all diagnostic indices outlined in Fig. 21.3. Were sensitivity, specificity and the predictive indices reported and calculated correctly? Of concern to the critical care practitioner is the primary intent of the test, since these indices convey different meanings. If it is of paramount concern to rule out the disease, then a high specificity and negative predictive value are desired. Conversely, if ruling in the disease is of primary importance, then highly sensitive and positive predictive values are needed. Thus, the primary intent of the diagnostic test must be determined in order to critically evaluate the correct indices. This discussion must also be interpreted in the context of the type of patients studied and the manner in which the evaluation was conducted. The critical care practitioner must therefore ask if sufficient numbers of diseased and nondiseased patients were included in the evaluation? Was there any evidence that bias entered into the evaluation? Finally, will the results of the diagnostic test be incorporated into the treatment decisions? Unfortunately, many diagnostic tests employed in the critical care setting fail in these regards.

Monitoring technology can be evaluated in a relatively straightforward manner. First and foremost, how precise and/or biased is the monitor? A case can be made for the implementation of biased monitors providing the bias is unidirectional and they have a high level of precision. In theory, an example might be of a noninvasive blood pressure monitor that consistently overestimates the systolic blood pressure by 3–5 mm Hg in all patients. Has the degree of agreement between the two methods been assessed beyond simple correlation, and over a clinically meaningful range of values? Given the simple approach outlined previously, this should be considered a prerequisite before implementation is considered. Finally, how will the information from the monitor be used? Will it replace the need for some tests? Will it aid in titrating patient therapy? Clearly, like the case of pulse oximetry, the argument of enhanced patient safety will no longer be the primary cause for implementation.

Given that there is sufficient evidence of benefit, has the economic impact of implementing the new technology been addressed? If not, there should be compelling evidence regarding improved patient outcomes before widespread implementation is undertaken in the current climate of fiscal restraint.

If the economic impact has been addressed, was a full economic evaluation conducted? As mentioned, it should be readily discernible that at least two competing alternatives were compared in terms of both their costs and consequences. Further, was the perspective of the analysis explicitly stated or implied? As mentioned, perspective is crucially important when deciding which costs are to be included in the analysis. Given that the perspective of the analysis is evident, were all relevant components of cost included? Similarly, were costs estimated from a variety of sources or were they derived directly from the patient population? It cannot be overemphasized that these are extremely germane issues which require intense scrutiny when considering the implementation of a new technology. By taking a relatively short amount of time to assess these issues the pitfalls of implementing previous technologies such as the pulmonary artery catheter may be avoided. Was a sensitivity analysis undertaken? Without this, the individual practitioner is left with a point estimate of what in essence is a continuum of possible economic impact. Thus, a thorough sensitivity analysis should be considered a requisite before widespread implementation. Finally, where applicable, was quality of life addressed? Given the limitations of the methods used in calculating quality of life, this is not yet of paramount importance. However, in the future it most assuredly will be.

Conclusions

It has been the intent of this chapter to provide the individual practitioner some insight into the area of technology assessment in the hopes that a more comprehensive approach will be adopted in the critical care setting. While critical care has grown into a vital

hospital service, it has evolved with little emphasis on demonstrating which technologies result in improved patient outcomes. In conclusion, we recommend the following steps as one means of beginning to rectify this problem.

1. Critical care must improve its ability to evaluate critically the technologies it employs. Curricula for future critical care practitioners must be expanded to include teaching the methods of a comprehensive technology assessment process.
2. National and international critical care bodies with a specific mandate to evaluate medical technologies should be developed. These bodies should be multi-disciplinary in nature, composed of those health care professionals necessary for sound and thorough evaluations. An important early role for these bodies may be that of an information source. By collecting, rating, and storing information on the types, scope and merit of individual technology assessments, the critical care practitioner would have a valuable asset to assist in making decisions.
3. There exists a need to establish explicit funding sources for the evaluation of new (and existing) medical technologies. The assessment of new technologies is a relatively expensive undertaking, albeit with the potential to identify the magnitude of potential benefit and economic impact. Given its potential, guaranteed funding sources should be established.
4. Industry must be encouraged to develop stronger liaisons with the hospital sector. Traditionally, hospitals are consulted relatively late in the genesis of a new medical technology. Most hospitals are approached when a working version of the technology is at hand. Unfortunately, the development of many of these technologies has proceeded on the 'can we make this' premise rather than on the premise of 'will this help our patients'. This recommendation is not intended to chastise industry, but rather to encourage a more collaborative approach to new technology development.

In conclusion, the imbalance between the demand and supply of health care resources ensures that tough choices regarding the provision of services must and will be made. Given the disproportionate impact of ICU services on a hospital's budget, they are a logical point from which to start.

References

1. NIH Consensus Development Conference Statement on Critical Care Medicine. In: Parillo JE, Ayers SM (eds).

Major Issues in Critical Care Medicine. Baltimore: Williams & Wilkins, 1984: 277–89.

2. Berenson RA. *Intensive Care Units (ICUs): Clinical Outcomes, Costs and Decision Making*. Health Technology Case Study 28, prepared for the Office of Technology Assessment, 1984.

3. Sibbald WJ, Escaf M, Calvin JE. How can new technology be introduced, evaluated and financed in critical care? *Clin Chem* 1990; **36**: 1604–11.

4. Califano JA. The health care chaos. *New York Times Magazine* 1988; **44**: 44–8.

5. Battista RN. Innovation and diffusion of health-related technologies: a conceptual framework. *Int J Technol Assess Health Care* 1989; **5**: 227–43.

6. Sibbald WJ, Inman KJ. Problems in assessing the technology of critical care medicine. *Int J Technol Assess Health Care* 1992; **8**: 419–43.

7. Lasch K, Maltz A, Mosteller F, Tosteson T. A protocol approach to assessing medical technology. *Int J Technol Assess Health Care* 1987; **3**: 103–22.

8. Ziegler EJ, Fisher CJ Jr, Sprung CL *et al*. Treatment of Gram-negative bacteremia and septic shock with HA-1A human monoclonal antibody against endotoxin. *New Engl J Med* 1991; **324**: 429–36.

9. Greenman RL, Schein RMH, Martin MA *et al*. A controlled clinical trial of E5 murine monoclonal IgM antibody to endotoxin in the treatment of Gram-negative sepsis. *J Am Med Assoc* 1991; **266**: 1097–102.

10. Adams R. Internal mammary artery ligation for coronary insufficiency, evaluation. *New Engl J Med* 1958; **258**: 113–15.

11. Cobb LA, Thomas GI, Dillard DH *et al*. An evaluation of internal mammary artery ligation by a double blind technique. *New Engl J Med* 1959; **260**: 1115–18.

12. Mausner JS, Kramer S. *Epidemiology – An Introductory Text*. Toronto: WB Saunders Company 1985: 159–66.

13. Charlson ME, Sax FL. The therapeutic efficacy of critical care units from two perspectives: A traditional cohort approach vs a new case-control methodology. *J Chronic Dis* 1987; **40**: 31–9.

14. Ranoshoff DF, Feinstein AR. Problems of spectrum and bias in evaluating the efficacy of a diagnostic test. *New Engl J Med* 1978; **299**: 926–30.

15. Department of Clinical Epidemiology and Biostatistics, McMaster University. Interpretation of Diagnostic Data: 5. How to do it with simple maths. *Can Med Assoc J* 1983; **129**: 947–54.

16. Bland JM, Altman DG. Statistical methods for assessing agreement between two methods of clinical measurement. *Lancet* 1986: Feb 8: 307–10.

17. Inman KJ, Rutledge FS, Cunningham, DG, Sibbald WJ. A visual method of comparing saturations obtained by pulse oximetry and the arterial blood gas. *Crit Care Med* 1993; **21**: S215.

18. Inman KJ, Rutledge FS, Cunningham DG, Petti K, Sibbald WJ. Capnography and arterial blood gas carbon dioxide tensions: a visual method of comparison. *Crit Care Med* 1993; **21**: S215.

19. Severinghaus JW, Kelleher JF. Recent developments in pulse oximetry. *Anesthesiology* 1992; **76**: 1018–38.

20. Roberts D, Ostryzniuk P, Loewen E *et al*. Control of blood gas measurements in intensive care units. *Lancet* 1991; **337**: 1580–2.

21. Doubilet P, Weinstein, MC, McNeil BJ. Use and misuse of the term cost-effective in medicine. *New Engl J Med* 1986; **314**: 253–6.

22. Inman KJ, Sibbald WJ, Rutledge FS, Clark BJ. The clinical utility and cost-effectiveness of an air suspension bed in the prevention of pressure ulcers. *J Am Med Assoc* 1993; **269**: 1139–43.

23. Schulman KA, Glick HA, Rubin H, Eisenberg JM. Cost-effectiveness of HA-1A monoclonal antibody for Gram-negative sepsis. *J Am Med Assoc* 1991; **266**: 3466–71.

24. Drummond MF, Stoddart GL, Torrance GW. *Methods for the Economic Evaluation of Health Care Programmes*, Oxford Medical Publications. Oxford: Oxford University Press, 1990: 149–67.

25. Boyle MH, Torrance GW, Sinclair JC, Horwood SP. Economic evaluation of neonatal intensive care of very-low-birth-weight infants. *New Engl J Med* 1983; **308**: 1330–7.

26. Drummond MF, Stoddart GL, Torrance GW. *Methods for the Economic Evaluation of Health Care Programmes*, Oxford Medical Publications. Oxford: Oxford University Press, 1990: 112–48.

27. Torrance GW, Feeny D. Utilties and quality-adjusted life years. *Int J Technol Assess Health Care* 1989; **5**: 559–73.

28. Laupacis A, Feeny D, Detsky AS, Tugwell PX. How attractive does a new technology have to be to warrant adoption and utilization? Tentative guidelines for using clinical and economic evaluations. *Can Med Assoc J* 1992; **146**: 473–81.

29. Naylor CD, Williams JI, Basinski A, Goel V. Technology assessment and cost-effectiveness analysis: misguided guidelines? *Can Med Assoc J* 1993; **148**: 921–9.

30. Gafni A, Birch S. Guidelines for the adoption of new technologies: a prescription for uncontrolled growth in expenditures and how to avoid the problem. *Can Med Assoc J* 1993; **148**: 913–17.

PART IV

Ethics

CHAPTER 22

Establishing Health Care Priorities

JUNE DALES

The need for establishing priorities 332
Closing the gap between available and affordable care 332
Mechanisms for setting priorities 333
The role of economic analysis in setting priorities 334
Measuring costs and benefits 335
The development of intensive care 336
Costs and benefits of intensive care 336
Heterogeneity 337
Economic studies of intensive care 338
Conclusions 341
References 341

David M Eddy MD PhD: ... we must ask two questions. First, are the benefits and harms of a treatment worth whatever costs people will have to pay? Second, if there are many treatments to choose from and if there are not enough resources to do them all, which treatments should receive priority? Answering both these questions requires estimating not only the treatment's benefits (and harms) but also its costs.

Maxon H Eddy MD: That's pretty abstract. In actual practice we don't stop to ask those questions. It's pretty clear-cut what we must do and we do it.

DME: Oh, but I think you do address those questions. You just do it intuitively. Tell me, do you put all your patients in an intensive care unit (ICU) when they leave the recovery room after surgery?

MHE: All of them? No.

DME: Why not?

MHE: Because it isn't necessary.

DME: What do you mean by 'not necessary'? Isn't there some chance that the patient would have a myocardial infarction, an embolism, or some other emergency and that being in the ICU might save his or her life?

MHE: Well, I suppose there is *some* chance. But if you select your patients carefully, it's terribly small.

DME: You agree there would be some benefit. So why not put all your patients in the ICU?

MHE: Well, aside from the fact that it's not a very pleasant place to be, I wouldn't put all my patients there because the amount of benefit would be too small to justify it.

DME: To justify what? The cost? Taking up a bed that might be used by another patient at higher risk who would derive greater benefit?

MHE: I see where you're going.

DME: The fact is that we do not put all our post-operative patients in ICUs because we believe the benefits would be too small to justify the costs. Instead, we reserve the ICU for patients who have a sufficiently high risk of emergencies so that the expected benefits are believed to be worth the costs.

From Eddy. 47 Copyright 1992, American Medical Association.

The need for establishing priorities

The demand for health care is rising. As treatments have been found which dramatically improve quality of life and cures found for previously fatal diseases, life expectancies have increased and the consequent aging population presents a pattern of disease which is more demanding of health services. The expectations of health service users are constantly being redefined as the range of possible treatments expands and the willingness to accept death, illness and vulnerability as normal aspects of human life, declines. In addition, people increasingly know more about medical affairs and decide more readily to go to health care systems with their medical problems.

On the supply side, medical progress is intrinsically limitless. Science and technology stimulate medicine and attract funding and attention, resulting in increasingly sophisticated and expensive technologies and an ever growing range of possible methods of diagnosis and treatment. The supply of health care has to some extent generated its own demand. Developers of medical science and technology rarely consider costs and benefits at either the individual level or in terms of what societies are willing and able to afford. There is a tendency to apply existing methods of diagnosis and treatment more widely and effective and appropriate methods are often used for cases other than those for which they have been proved to be so.

Against the upward pressures of rising expectations of health service users, increasingly aging populations and the development and dissemination of new technology, there are limited funds, facilities and other resources available for health care and choices must be made about their deployment. The devotion of resources to a particular intervention or course of treatment means that those resources are not available to spend on other things. Thus there is an 'opportunity cost' of pursuing a particular activity, which is the value of benefits that could have been obtained by spending the resources elsewhere. The establishment of health care priorities reflects the relative desirability of alternative options for deploying resources and determines which patients are treated and which treatments are offered. In this sense priority setting can be viewed as a form of rationing, a term which is used technically to define any mechanism for allocating scarce resources amongst competing uses. If resources were not limited there would be no need for such rationing.

The rest of this chapter discusses priority setting in general before moving on to the specific issues relevant to intensive care. Towards the end of the chapter an attempt is made to establish the apparent priority of intensive care in relation to other possible uses of health care resources. The shortcomings in available evidence are described and the chapter finishes with some conclusions about the way forward.

Closing the gap between available and affordable care

Three possible mechanisms for closing the gap between the potential demand for health care and available resources are to make more resources available, to use existing resources more efficiently, and to make explicit choices about the care that will be funded.

MORE RESOURCES

The availability of resources for health care is determined largely on the basis of macroeconomic considerations in which a political choice is made between the social importance of health care and other social needs. Unless we are prepared to spend an unconscionable proportion of resources on health care, letting schools, roads, housing and manufacturing investments suffer in comparison, we cannot possibly afford every medical advance that might be of benefit.[1] Coupled with that is the policy aim of many governments to reduce the burden of taxation on individuals. The amount of resources that could be made available can be debated but it is clear that however many resources there are, they will not be enough to satisfy all demands.

EFFICIENCY

In discussions about choices in health care the question regularly arises whether it is possible to avoid them by improving efficiency either by delivering care more efficiently (i.e. for the lowest possible cost) or by delivering more efficient care (i.e. when appropriate and in the absence of cheaper alternatives).

Attempts have been made to build internal incentives into health care systems to improve efficiency. In a number of countries the commissioning and delivery of health care have been separated and commissioners given a budget with which to 'shop around' alternative providers to supply health care which meets the needs of the populations for which the commissioners are responsible. Funding has shifted from cost reimbursement to predetermined, fixed per-capita rates of remuneration. Suppliers compete on the basis of price, quality of service and outcome.

Some believe that a more efficient system coupled with the right incentives, would be enough to create long-term, sustainable moderation in demand, thus containing health service inflation to within affordable limits. Others point to the difficulties being experienced even in the most efficient systems and believe that upward pressures on demand will inevitably expand costs beyond available resources.[1] The autonomous growth of supply and demand are likely to contribute to a growing gap between necessary and available funding even when the effects of improved efficiency are taken into account. Increasing efficiency by reducing waste has its limits. At some point, it will only be possible to increase efficiency further by making explicit choices. Improving efficiency should be accorded a high priority and could probably delay the need to make choices in care, but it cannot avoid the necessity for choice.

CHOICES

Decisions to no longer provide a medical treatment with a low chance of success and a high cost or to replace a very expensive and effective treatment with a much cheaper one that is slightly less effective are examples of choices in health care. The financial resources liberated by such choices can then be spent on health services which were not previously available and which would produce more health benefits. Such choices are painful because they mean denying certain kinds of care to some people.

Numerous mechanisms already exist for rationing health care. Charges have been introduced for specific items, negative and positive lists have been compiled which dictate which treatments receive funding and which do not, treatment protocols have been drawn up to determine the method and circumstances under which certain treatments are delivered, and the use of new technologies has been explicitly limited. Certain sectors of the population have been excluded from receiving free care and some services are restricted in availability. These measures have varying effects on access and equity and have been introduced in a mainly piecemeal fashion, aimed at cost-containment rather than making explicit choices to improve the deployment of resources.

On another level, rationing is implicit. Decisions have been taken not to continue treatment of terminally ill people not only because it would be kinder to the patient, but also because it would be a waste of resources. Patients have regularly been denied admission to intensive care units; diabetic patients have been refused renal dialysis; alcohol misusers have been turned down for liver transplants.[2] This rationing is rarely publicized but can be detected by analyzing waiting lists and profiles of patient populations who do or do not receive certain, usually expensive, treatments. Such rationing of care is done by the most random of all processes, the decree of a single doctor or administrator,[3] and is an implicit result of the powers in the system and not of any explicit decision making process.

Implicit rationing has the advantage of being more politically expedient and flexible, but while it concentrates decision making in the hands of clinicians it also forces them to set the limits.[4] This type of decision making often solves the practical situation faced by individual clinicians, but offers no means of checking the implicit ranking of alternatives that has been made. The consequences of such decision making are undesirable both from the point of view of social justice and that of public health.[5]

Mechanisms for setting priorities

In many sectors of the economy resource allocation decisions are made through market mechanisms. However, distortions in markets for health care mean that prices are unlikely to very closely reflect the true value of health services to society. Distortions arise from imperfect information (e.g. consumers of health care often have limited information about the nature and quality of care being provided and its likely effectiveness); imperfect competition (e.g. geographical, regulatory and other barriers to entry mean that there is often little real competition between suppliers); and externalities (e.g. an individual's health care consumption decisions may confer uncompensated costs or benefits on other members of society).[6] Because a free market is neither desirable nor feasible in health care, there is a case for involving the public in guiding the commissioners about which services to buy, how much of them and where.[4]

The process that should be employed in setting priorities depends on the purpose in setting them, the medical care system and economic and cultural circumstances. The most basic criteria for determining priorities are that care should be necessary, effective and appropriate. There is a cultural and ethical dimension to the question of choice because demand and supply of health care are deeply influenced by the culture and values of society. People do not need everything they want and not all needs for health care are equally important. A report by a government committee on choices in health care in the Netherlands describes health from three perspectives.[5] For an individual, health is linked to self-determination and autonomy and means different things to different people. Thus patient satisfaction with health care is an important measure of effectiveness of health care received. The medical perspective of health is the absence of disease and effectiveness of care is measured objectively with the most important criteria being danger to life and extent of normal biological functioning. From a community perspective, health is seen as the possibility for every member of society to function normally. Individual preferences and needs are not given priority here, but society's values and norms are important. A hierarchy exists amongst the three approaches, although they are not mutually exclusive. The community approach rules decision making at a macro-level, the professional approach rules within the limits of the community approach, and the individual approach within the limits of the professional approach.

If health care is viewed as a community responsibility then funders, the public, patient organizations and others should be involved in setting the standards of appropriate care as well as health care professionals. Funders must encourage the appropriate use of care within financial constraints, for example, by limiting payment for unnecessarily expensive items or limiting the length of time over which a given treatment will be funded. Responsibility for setting standards and making protocols for the appropriate use of facilities lies in the first place with health care professions. Together with patient organizations and funders they must reduce and restrict defensive medicine and marginal practices. It is important that this occurs openly so that consensus can be reached as far as possible. Arbitrariness must be avoided. Funders should not take sole responsibility for this because of the danger of solely financial limits being used to determine standards of care.

By specifying quality, volume, price and efficiency of care, the commissioners of health care could offer effective and efficient care to individuals through agreements with health care providers. Commissioners could delegate assessment and decision making partly or completely to health care providers. Patient/consumer organizations should evaluate policies from the user's point of view and develop information networks to facilitate commissioner's choices. Consumer protection is extremely important in making responsible choices among policies, but it requires objective and critical information.

The role of economic analysis in setting priorities

Priority setting requires consideration of both the costs and benefits of alternatives. Priorities set solely on the basis of cost militate towards cost-minimization at the expense of medical considerations. Priorities which refer only to outcomes will tend to lead to resources being spent on treatments that achieve dramatic improvements in health, probably at relatively high cost, at the expense of delivering a small amount of health gain to greater numbers of people. In both cases, opportunities to redistribute resources in a way that achieves greater overall improvement in the health of the population may be missed.

Economic analysis provides a framework for systematically and explicitly measuring and comparing combinations of expenditure and outcomes and assessing the mix of services that will generate the best outcome for the available resources. Types of care which generate relatively low benefits at high cost can be identified as being of lower priority. It is worth noting that a procedure cannot be cost-effective if it is not clinically effective.

Economic analysis can play a useful role in resource allocation at the macro, professional and individual level. It can help to determine the amount, frequency and setting of treatment that generates the greatest benefit within available resources; help in deciding which patients are treated in circumstances where resources may not allow for them all to be treated; and where one option is clearly more cost-effective than others and other criteria are satisfied it may allow clinicians to develop protocols which avoid wasting resources.

The most common forms of economic analysis used in evaluating health care options are cost-effectiveness and cost-utility analysis. One intervention is more cost-effective than another if it yields a bigger improvement in health for the same cost or the same improvement in health for a lower cost. Outcomes are measured in natural units such the number of lives saved or proportion of patients who return to full health. Unfortunately this means that comparisons across treatment categories in which outcomes are measured in different units is precluded. It would be difficult to weigh up for example, the relative priority of true positives detected in a screening program against lives saved through intensive care treatment. Cost-effectiveness analysis does not attempt to place any values on the outcomes and therefore cannot shed light on issues such as the extent to which extended life is preferred over improved quality of life.

Cost-utility analysis places values on the benefits derived from health care interventions and can therefore be used to compare interventions in different fields of medicine. An example of such analysis is the quality adjusted life year (QALY). It combines mortality and various measures of morbidity, such as pain and disability, in a single index of health outcome and is derived by referring to a set of values or weights that reflect the relative desirability of different health states. Although used by researchers for some years, QALYs are still subject to continuing technical development and there are unresolved issues such as who should make the valuation of different health states and how the values should be incorporated into the analysis.

The role of cost-benefit analysis is worth a brief mention. It requires that both benefits and costs are enumerated in monetary terms and compared. The option with the largest net benefit is selected. The difficulty of expressing the more subjective and qualitative consequences of health care interventions in monetary terms has meant that cost-benefit analysis has not been used very frequently in evaluating health care options. It implicitly requires directly placing a monetary value on life, an idea which sits uneasily with medical ethics.

In making choices in health care on the basis of cost-effectiveness and cost-utility analysis it is important that the assessment is done in relation to a carefully defined set of indications. Types of care that are very cost-effective for one indication may be unnecessary for another indication. It is also important to remember that economic analysis simply provides an analytical framework on which to build. Other considerations such as access, equity and ethics are important in setting priorities and may imply different choices from those suggested by economic analysis.

Economic analysis cannot and should not replace clinical judgment in the assessment of individual patients. Clinicians are in the best position to assess the likely consequences of their decisions for individual patients. However, although decisions about individual patients are extraordinarily difficult, a more systematic approach would permit a more objective and less arbitrary basis for decision making.[7] Shortages in resources alter the doctor–patient relationship. The health care provider has to weigh the needs of one patient against another and against the community as a whole. He/she must therefore not only look after the interests of the patient, but also take responsibility for the distribution of care.[8] This suggests the need to reduce the differences in working methods and medical practices which are not justified, develop economic stimuli to promote types of care which deserve priority, and develop financial reward systems to ensure the maintenance of quality of care when financial budgeting is applied. As mentioned above, consumer protection is important and an individual's ability to depart from the standard should be encouraged, but be able to be justified.

Measuring costs and benefits

Comprehensive measures of costs and benefits should be incorporated into economic analysis. A reasonable assessment of costs should include three areas. First the organizational and operating costs within the health service should be measured, including inpatient, outpatient and day case costs, community care and care by primary physicians. Such costs should include both the direct costs of providing the service, e.g. staff and consumables, and the overheads such as depreciation of capital equipment and administration. Second, some costs are borne outside the health service, including those incurred by social services, voluntary agencies and local government agencies. Third, there are costs incurred by patients, families and carers such as travelling costs.

Economic analysis has the capacity to encompass benefits that are not simply of a physiological nature and can incorporate quality as well as quantity of life. Three types of benefits can be distinguished: direct benefits of saving health care resources; indirect benefits such as minimizing earnings lost due to premature death or disability or benefits accruing to furthering research; and intangible benefits such as minimizing discomfort and discontent or the benefit that society gains from the knowledge that health care resources are expended in a fair and equitable way. Economic analysis can incorporate the values that society places on outcomes.

Decision makers are frequently attempting to decide on the scale of treatment that should be provided, rather than whether it should be provided at all. Economic analysis can be helpful in this situation because it distinguishes between average and marginal costs. Thus economies of scale and the pattern of resource utilization can be taken into account. The cost of treating one more patient may well be far lower than the average cost per patient, because the equipment and staffing costs are to some extent fixed overheads that will be incurred whatever the level of activity.

Costs and benefits are unevenly distributed over time. Although an intervention's effects extend over a period of time, a decision to undertake it must be made at a prior point. The calculation of present value involves the calculation of future streams of costs and benefits into today's values. Discounting is used to do this, and reflects the fact that a sum of money today is worth more than the same sum of money at some point in the future. Another influence on the annual equivalent cost is the rate of depreciation, which depends on assumptions made about the length of life of equipment and buildings.

In the constantly evolving world of medical technology, unit costs may rise or fall as a result of new developments. It is therefore important to reappraise costs and benefits as more information becomes available. Risk and uncertainty are related to the lack of guarantee that events will turn out as planned. It is therefore important to conduct sensitivity analysis to identify the effects of changing the assumptions. The apparent cost-utilities of programs can vary considerably by changing the assumptions.

The development of intensive care

The growing experience of clinicians in the use of sophisticated monitoring systems and therapeutic regimes in intensive care means it is now possible to treat greater numbers of older, critically ill patients than ever before. Many patients who in the past were classified as the most severely ill are now classified as less severely ill, and many patients who would not have survived do so now. Lessons learned from the most critically ill patients are rapidly applied to the less ill, thereby reducing morbidity, shortening hospital stays and preventing the catastrophes that lead to critical impasses.[9] The various activities that are undertaken in intensive care are still being developed and are growing in number.

The high cost of intensive care means it is subject to particular scrutiny when priorities in health care are being considered. Resources are devoted to relatively few patients so the opportunity cost is the potential benefit of treating larger numbers of less seriously ill patients. Decisions to start, continue or terminate intensive care are often based on real and perceived need for beds and someone's 'best guess' of survival or death. They are made in conjunction with the patient whenever possible, or the family when the patient is not competent, and nursing and medical staff. However, society is clearly involved, because the enormous cost of intensive care depends on society's ability or willingness to pay for it.[7]

The priority given to intensive care should depend on the relative net benefits it yields compared to alternative uses of resources. It has been suggested that a randomized controlled trial would be the best way of establishing the therapeutic efficacy of intensive care.[10, 11] However, in any such trial the control group would have to receive conventional care. Such care is not designed to closely monitor and treat or prevent unpredictable, life-threatening changes in critically ill patients. Without life support and prophylactic monitoring, survival is unlikely. Therefore such a trial would not only be unethical but would fail.[7, 12] Nevertheless, within intensive care medicine, controlled trials are necessary to determine the limitation of different therapeutic modalities.

Several authors have pointed to the need for objective risk estimates, precise quality assurance programs and utilization management strategies in the provision of intensive care.[13, 14]

Costs and benefits of intensive care

Many studies have focused on whether or not the patient is discharged alive from the hospital.[15–17] Relatively few studies have examined long-term survival[18, 19] and still fewer have examined any outcome other than mortality.[9, 12, 20] Studies that have tried to incorporate an element of quality of life into their results are generally based on small samples, and appear to give conflicting results. Some studies report near normal recovery for the vast majority of patients,[21, 22] whilst others report residual disabilities in quite large proportions of survivors.[7, 9] These contradictions imply that the results are dependent on the type of patient treated in the intensive care unit and their prognosis as much as the care given to the patients whilst there. In general coronary care units and medical intensive care units have reported low mortality rates and surgical intensive care units have reported high rates. However, Bams and Miranda attribute the low mortality rates in their study of surgical admissions to the standard of care[23] and Knaus et al. concluded that the degree of coordination of intensive care significantly influences its effectiveness.[24] These examples point to the potential difficulty of transferring the results of studies between countries and hospitals. Admission and discharge policies and patient populations differ, treatment protocols vary widely and persistence in life support may reflect the ethical climate of the unit. It is therefore important to study the results from a variety of intensive care units to gain some understanding of the impact of these facilities on survival and the quality of life of critically ill patients.[22] As long ago as 1976 Cullen called for standardized terminology for critical illness so that patients from one intensive care unit could be compared with patients from another.[9]

The critically ill patient needs and receives enormous resources to progress towards successful recovery. Costs of intensive care units have been estimated to be three to five times greater than those incurred on general wards[11, 23, 25, 26] and the high levels of staffing and complex technology make them vulnerable to increases.[27] Several studies have found that intensive care patients incurred around 50% of their hospital costs in the intensive care unit, but spent around only 17% of their hospital stay there.[18, 21, 23] The costs of intensive care are likely to continue to escalate, due to inflation, continuing technical advances and demands of patients and clinicians. Although a single patient might benefit profoundly from a technological improvement that would also greatly lower the cost of care, the overall effect on intensive care units is that even sicker patients will be admitted and treated, and some of them will survive.[7]

Average costs derived from total expenditure and the number of patient days mask large cost differences between individual patients.[25] A small proportion of patients often account for a large share of the total expenditure, in common with other areas of medicine. Studies that have used a top down approach to calculate costs, starting with the total budget and working down to produce average costs per patient, are not very informative in intensive care units where patients do not conform to a similar pattern of severity of illness. Other studies have used nurse to patient ratios as a proxy for costs, but these may be influenced by staffing levels rather than patient requirements. Another difficulty is that some studies use charges as a proxy for costs, and these often do not reflect true treatment costs. It is therefore difficult to use the results of such analysis to allocate resources more effectively.

Many studies have restricted the measurement of costs to those incurred in the intensive care unit, ignoring repercussions for costs in other parts of the hospital or health care system, often because of the difficulty of measuring them. It has been claimed that intensive care leads to more expensive and long-term institutional care, the multiplier effect, although other studies contradict this. Few studies have explored the effects of economies of scale or the impact of changes in utilization volumes and casemix. Very few studies indeed have measured costs incurred outside the hospital setting.

Sophisticated analysis is required to explore the resource consequences of a change in policy, as the implications may not be straightforward. For example, earlier discharge from an intensive care unit may result in the requirement for more intensive nursing and monitoring on an ordinary ward than normal.

Expenditure incurred in intensive care units depends on the severity of illness, level of intervention and intensive care mortality.[25] The results of several studies support the contention that intensive care units generally do not benefit patients who are stable and not ill, i.e. those who do not require organ support and are simply there for intensive monitoring.[28–30] Patients who are less ill may be more appropriately cared for in a high dependency unit where staff costs are lower.[25] Costs can also be reduced by discontinuing care for patients who are unlikely to survive. Jennett lists five factors implying the inappropriate use of intensive care.[31] These are that the care is unnecessary (the condition is not bad enough); unsuccessful (the condition is too severe); unsafe (too many complications); unsound (the quality of life of the survivor is unacceptable); and unwise (diversion of resources).

Several studies have found an inverse relationship between costs and survival.[15, 25, 32, 33] The average cost per day of survivors was much lower than that of nonsurvivors because their expenditure was averaged over many more days before discharge, and because they spent a much shorter period in the intensive care unit, although the total costs of the two groups might be quite similar because the nonsurvivors spent more time in intensive care. These studies demonstrate the need for care in interpreting reported results. Several studies have shown that among survivors and nonsurvivors, expenditure was greatest for those with unexpected outcome.[15, 32] Often a lot of resources in intensive care units are devoted to patients with poor prognosis.[7, 12, 19, 20, 33]

Heterogeneity

A difficulty in establishing the net benefit of intensive care is that a range of heterogeneous activities are undertaken in intensive care units for a variety of reasons, rather than a specific intervention aimed at curing or alleviating a particular health problem. Intensive care is most often part of a package of treatment rather than the sole treatment and patients tend to be admitted to intensive care units according to the severity of their illness rather than the illness itself. Intensive care populations vary tremendously in their composition, depending on the type of hospital that patients have been selected from and the admission and discharge policies of intensive care units.

The heterogeneous range of patients means that in setting priorities it is inappropriate to view intensive care as a single, homogeneous treatment. The costs and benefits must be considered alongside the condition, disease and type of patient. Intensive care is undoubtedly of great benefit to some, but of more questionable benefit to other groups of patients, for example, those with very little chance of survival, irrespective of treatment, and those who are less severely ill and could be cared for in less intensive and less costly environments, with little or no impact on outcome. In setting priorities it is therefore important to distinguish between the different subgroups of patients who are treated in the intensive care unit. Comparisons between various studies of intensive care are often invalidated by differences in patient mix.

Methods have been developed to attempt to identify subgroups of patients who are characterized by particular costs and outcome probabilities, and who can be identified prior to treatment or early enough to enable more cost-effective use of resources. They provide an objective means of characterizing severity of illness in a diverse group of patients and can facilitate comparisons between intensive care units with different mixes of patients.

The Therapeutic Intervention Scoring System (TISS) categorizes patients into one of four groups, defined by quantifying of therapeutic interventions according to required nursing time and effort. The system uses the level of medical intervention as a proxy for severity of illness. However, it presumes the validity and appropriateness of interventions and that all clinicians can and do treat similar clinical problems in the same way. This is unrealistic and an unqualified use of TISS scores to indicate the severity of illness is misleading, as demonstrated when treatment is withdrawn. Byrick *et al.* found that TISS points could not distinguish between survivors and nonsurvivors in a group of respiratory failure patients.[20] However, some useful results have been found, for example, a positive relationship between intensive care costs and number of TISS points and that the ultimate outcome for patients who maintain high TISS points over several days is dismal.[7]

The Acute Physiology and Chronic Health Evaluation (APACHE) system uses information on risk factors of acute physiological disorders, chronic health status and age to categorize severity of illness. It is combined with information on diagnosis, indication for admission and surgical status to calculate the probability of survival using a multiple regression equation. A number of studies have shown a correlation between APACHE scores and outcomes,[13,32,34–37] although others have been unable to establish such a relationship for some groups of patients, for example a study by Civetta *et al.* of surgical patients.[38] Ridley *et al.* found that total costs could be predicted by APACHE score.[25] The APACHE system has been refined over a period of time.

The use of a generally accepted scoring system would facilitate comparison of the results of different studies.[39] TISS points and APACHE scores represent a step in this direction, but there is scope for further development of these methods. The combination of a system for judging severity of illness and individual variables, depending on the type of disease, may considerably enhance the possibility that the correct decisions are made early enough to ensure that intensive care is given appropriately. Estimates of the risk faced by a patient during the course of treatment can be useful in determining the optimal time for discharge or deciding how long to continue therapy.

There is reasonable correlation between APACHE and TISS scores, indicating that increasing physiological impairment requires increasing therapy. Studies have demonstrated varying usefulness of these scores depending on types of patients and standard of care. Scoring systems are insufficient for reliable individual prognostication in all cases. For example, in their study of surgical patients, Civetta *et al.* found a false-classification rate of scoring systems to be 15% and the expected mortality of nonsurvivors was only 20%.[38] Even small error rates are unacceptable where life and death decisions are being made.

Other variables have been found to be useful prognostic indicators. Several studies suggest that the underlying disease, age and renal function are important in determining the likely outcome of intensive care. To investigate the feasibility of identifying early those patients with the least chance of survival, Cullen *et al.* analyzed survivors and nonsurvivors of a group of severely critically ill patients to determine whether there were any discriminating factors in the outcomes.[7]

Age, sex, ASA risk, disease category, admission platelet count, admission creatinine and need for dialysis all affected the outcome. Patients with renal failure had a much higher mortality rate than those without renal failure. A study by Parno *et al.* found that the most important factors in determining longer-term survival were age, coma, cardiopulmonary resuscitation, renal failure infection, shock and white blood cell count.[22]

Many advantages accrue to patients in intensive care units which enhance the probability of a desirable outcome. Specially trained clinicians are available to care for patients and there is a concentration of highly skilled nurses who can react appropriately to subtle changes in the patient's condition, are familiar with the equipment, and can anticipate catastrophes, allowing medical intervention before such catastrophes occur. Sophisticated, expensive equipment is concentrated in one area and utilized more efficiently. Experience gained in caring for the most critically ill patients can be transferred to less severely ill patients. The impact of intensive care units on educational programs, clinical research and the function of nonintensive care wards have received little attention.[13] In a teaching hospital, improved patient care, education and clinical research are potential benefits of intensive care.

Most disadvantages of intensive care pertain only to the patient himself and relate to discomfort and stress caused by often unpleasant interventions. An additional disbenefit of intensive care units is that they may divert highly qualified nurses and anesthetists from caring for others who have a better prognosis.[7]

Ideally, these broader impacts should be considered in assessing the priority of intensive care. Although budget and time constraints never allow the assessment of all relevant costs and benefits, any important omissions should be accounted for in analysis.

Economic studies of intensive care

Few studies have examined the costs and benefits of intensive care in a way which enables its cost-utility or cost-benefit to be assessed. The studies that do exist appear to rank adult intensive care therapy among the most expensive interventions that have been evaluated, whereas neonatal intensive care ranks with some of the lowest cost per QALY estimates in health care. The lower costs of treatment and longer life expectancies, compared with adult intensive care patients, make the treatment of neonates much more cost effective. Averaging their hospitalization costs over their many more years of life expectancy favorably influences the cost-effectiveness of their critical care.

Table 22.1 shows some comparisons which draw on published studies and are just a few examples from a register of cost per QALY of different interventions that has been assembled from the literature by the UK Department of Health. Extreme caution must be exercised in interpreting the results. There are many health interventions for which there is no information available and these may be very much more expensive than the therapies that have been studied. The studies have been conducted at different times and comparisons between them may be misleading because technologies and the costs of technology change over time, resulting in either rises or falls in the unit cost of treatment. The studies have also been conducted in different countries and different settings and have used different measures of costs and benefits. The patient populations being studied may vary as the result of different admission and discharge policies. The studies may also have used different comparators against which to measure cost-

Table 22.1 Costs per QALY 1991

<£5000
Screening insulin-dependent diabetics for diabetic retinopathy
Coronary artery bypass graft for left main vessel, severe angina
Cholecystectomy
Drug treatment for ulcers
Lithotripsy for kidney stones
Intensive care for neonates >1000 g
Intensive care for drug overdosing
Streptokinase for acute myocardial infarction
Screening for prostate cancer
Surgery for inguinal hernia

£5000–£50 000
Bone marrow transplant for leukemia
Coronary artery bypass graft for two vessel disease for mild angina
Varicose vein surgery after a 1-year delay
Hospital dialysis for end-stage renal failure
Kidney transplant for end-stage renal failure
Home dialysis for end-stage renal failure
Intensive care for neonates 500–1000 g
Intensive care for multiple trauma
Drug treatment of HIV
Hysterectomy
Drug treatment for mild hypertension
Knee replacement

>£50 000
Coronary care unit
Intensive care for myocardial infarction
Intensive care of abdominal catastrophe
Intensive care of hepatorenal failure
Liver transplant
Intensive care of end-stage renal failure
Low dose subcutaneous erythropoetin for anemia
Cholesterol drug for coronary heart disease
Advice to exercise to prevent coronary heart disease in exercise-haters

effectiveness. In some cases the cost per QALY has been derived from the published material rather than quoted directly. For these reasons, Table 22.1 simply shows some broad categories of interventions to give a very general idea of the sort of priorities that appear to be emerging from the literature. For the purposes of comparison all costs per QALY have been recalculated to 1991 prices.

The studies of intensive care for neonates were conducted by Boyle *et al.*[40] These authors comprehensively evaluated the economic aspects of neonatal intensive care of very-low-birthweight infants, using outcomes and costs of care before and after the introduction of a regional intensive care program in Hamilton–Wentworth County, Canada. Cost-effectiveness analysis was used to investigate the additional costs and net economic cost per life saved and per life year gained; cost-utility analysis was used to investigate the additional cost and net economic cost per quality adjusted life year gained; and cost benefit analysis was used to appraise the net economic benefit in dollars of intensive neonatal care over non-intensive care. Analyses were done up to discharge from hospital, 15 years of age and death. A discount rate of 5% per annum was applied to costs, earnings and effects. All hospital and follow-up costs, transport costs and costs to other sectors were measured.

Anticipated lifetime earnings of survivors were subtracted from costs to yield a net economic cost. A classification of health states was developed to measure the health of survivors according to their physical function, role function, social and emotional functions and health problems. The relative values that members of society attach to the various possible health states of survivors was determined by asking a random sample of parents of schoolchildren to rate the desirability or otherwise of a health state relative to other health states. The utilities were used to adjust life years for quality. Forecasts of lifetime outcomes and costs were made independently by two developmental pediatricians using the health history that was available for each child.

Neonatal intensive care increased both survival rates and costs. By every evaluative measure that the authors undertook, it was more favorable to provide intensive care for infants weighing 1000–1499 g at birth than for those weighing 500–999 g. This finding was robust when tested by making changes in the assumptions about the discount rate, life expectancy, condition of children lost to follow-up and utility values. The authors point to the different conclusion that could result if clinical outcomes were the only consideration. For example, neonatal intensive care of infants weighing 750–999 g at birth resulted in the largest gain in survival rate of all the subgroups of patients that were studied, but produced the largest net economic loss.

The authors ascertained that factors that could influence birthweight-specific mortality risk at the time of birth did not make an important contribution to the difference in mortality between the groups of patients.

Possible difficulties in transferring the results of the study are mentioned by the authors: costs are a function of the level of intensity of the program and therefore may not be transferable; data relied partly on parental recall of costs and events, and their level of accuracy is unknown; intangible aspects of outcomes are not measured, for example, the emotional impact on families, outlook for future pregnancies, and improvements that may have occurred as the result of clinicians gaining more experience; changes that have occurred over the time period of the study (1964–1977) have not been accounted for.

The authors describe possible applications of the results of their study as giving priority to infants in the 1000–1400 g group where countries or regions have insufficient present capacity to provide intensive care for all very-low-birthweight infants, and developing facilities for 1000–1499 g birthweight infants first where there are no existing facilities.

The study suggests that new approaches to the prevention of extreme prematurity and to neonatal intensive care of infants weighing less than 1000 g at birth are needed. A report by the Office of Health Economics (OHE) concludes that spending on intensive care for neonates may be more effectively directed towards research into the causes and the prevention of preterm birth.[41] A system has been in operation in France since 1971, and it has been suggested that the preterm birth rate has fallen as a result, but there is no cost information so it is difficult to assess the cost-effectiveness. The OHE report also estimates that the average cost of a surviving preterm infant weighing 700–799 g is around £150 000 (1984 prices), but that this falls to about £8000 for a heavier infant weighing between 1400 and 1499 g.

The US Health Technology case study of intensive care reviews economic studies of intensive care units and is the source for the references to intensive care in Table 22.1 for drug overdosing, end-stage renal failure and myocardial infarction.[42] Among those studies, Mulley *et al.*[28] and Wagner *et al.*[43] have projected cost savings that would be generated by more selective admission and earlier discharge policies, but neither account for the possibility that earlier transfer from the unit might alter the rate of complications and thus affect costs or that average general ward costs might be raised because of the need for more intensive nursing and use of monitoring equipment. In a study reported in 1984, Fineberg *et al.* estimated that for patients with about a 5% possibility of having sustained a myocardial infarction, admission to a coronary care unit would cost US $139 000 per year of life saved, as compared to care in an intermediate care unit.[44]

A study by Bendixen *et al.* was used to derive the entries in Table 22.1 for intensive care for drug overdosing, multiple trauma, abdominal catastrophe and hepatorenal failure.[45] The study looked at cost per life year saved. This approach assumes that survival is a benefit and that the value of survival is directly related to its length. Bendixen's formula does not discount future costs and benefits into present values and therefore overstates the importance of predicted remaining lifespan. Acknowledging these difficulties, Bendixen estimated a cost per life year saved of US $84 for a barbiturate overdose and US $180 000 for hepatorenal failure at 1977 prices.

Another method of attempting to assess the cost: benefit ratio of intensive care has been used in some studies, by assessing the average charges necessary to achieve one survivor. Table 22.2 shows the results of a study by Parno *et al.* of hospital charges per survivor alive 2 years after discharge[21] and Table 22.3 shows the results of a similar study by Cullen of charges to achieve one survivor alive 1 year after hospital discharge.[7]

Table 22.2   Hospital charges per survivor alive 2 years after discharge

	US $'000s 1978
Surgical	
Peripheral-vascular	11
Neurological	13
Trauma	13
Gastrointestinal	19
Thoracic	19
Aortovascular	26
Medical	
Overdose	2
Neurological	6
Gastrointestinal	9
Cardiac	10
Pulmonary	18
Infection	35
Renal	46

From ref. 21.

Neither additional posthospital costs nor physician charges were included in these estimates and neither set of estimates allow for consideration of the quality of life. The differences in cost per survivor for the various subgroups of patients is of more interest than the absolute figures. If the differences are valid the figures imply that intensive care is much more cost-effective for some subgroups than others, although an important caveat must be that differences in quality of life and longer-term survival of patients should be taken into account in establishing the true differences.

Table 22.3 Hospital charges per survivor alive 1 year after discharge

	US $'000s 1977/78
Massive trauma	23
Elective major vascular surgery	24
Unexplained complication of elective surgery	28
Neurosurgery and head trauma	41
Emergency abdominal catastrophes, nonbleeding	60
Emergency major vascular surgery	88
Gastrointestinal bleeding, cirrhosis and portal hypertension	171
Elective operation for malignant disease	233

From ref. 7.

Conclusions

The demand for health care is growing but resources to devote to it are limited. Whilst the efficient delivery of health care is rightly pursued it does not obviate the need for setting priorities. Choices must be made and if health care is viewed as a community responsibility those choices must be made explicitly and on the basis of reliable information. Funders, the public, patient organizations and others must be involved as well as health care professionals.

One of the first attempts at making priority setting explicit was undertaken by the Oregon Health Services Commission. A cost-utility method was used to develop a ranked list of condition/treatment pairings, incorporating public values. The creation of the list showed that it is possible to involve a wider audience than just health care professionals in determining priorities. However, there were considerable difficulties in collecting reliable scientific evidence on the costs and effects of treatment and representative public values about different health states. It proved difficult to translate opinions about quality of life into weights to apply to outcome measures, and the rankings in the list were shown to be very sensitive to the methodology employed and assumptions made in the cost-utility analysis.

Producing a list of priorities will inevitably entail a process of argument, persuasion and consensus building. If the Oregon experience has shown anything it is that there is no technological fix: imputing values to statistics and decisions about methods to derive ranking are themselves political. Technical exercise may be a useful way of starting up the dialogue and providing statistical scaffolding that may subsequently be dismantled, but they cannot resolve conflicts of values or interests.[46]

Funders could use their own data to form a picture of effectiveness and efficiency of medical practices and compare these with the results of internal assessments by providers of health care. Inter-doctor variation could be reduced by identifying differences in efficiency and appropriateness of the use of interventions. Professionals should participate in the management of facilities and take a share of responsibility for expenditure. Patient and consumer organizations should contribute to the appropriate use of health care, but they must have access to objective and critical information to do so.

The development of auditing and prognostic systems have helped to improve the cost-effectiveness of the use of resources devoted to intensive care. Further research is required into the costs and benefits to replace anecdotal information with objective data. Attention should be paid to identifying which costs and benefits should be measured. It is important that the costs incurred outside the intensive care unit itself but incurred as a result of intensive therapy, and the long-term survival and quality of life of patients are included. Further work is required to establish how the values that are placed on outcomes should be incorporated. Research on all these issues should ideally be incorporated into clinical research where possible.

The literature implies that neonatal intensive care ranks as a high priority when compared to other uses of health care resources, but that adult intensive care is less cost-effective. The heterogeneity of patients and interventions means it is important to make appropriate distinctions between subgroups of patients. The importance of doing this is demonstrated by the sometimes conflicting results of studies, which have occurred because of differences in patient populations rather than in the effectiveness of treatment.

Finally, it is worth repeating that economic analysis cannot replace clinical decision making at individual patient level. It can merely provide a pointer and must be considered alongside many other factors including equity, access and ethics. However, there is much that can be done to improve the measurement of costs and benefits and to use the results of analysis to improve the use of available resources and establish priorities.

References

1. Callahan D. Rationing medical progress. *New Engl J Med* 1990; **322**: 1810–13.
2. Moss AH, Sigler M. Should alcoholics compete equally for liver transplantation? *J Med Assoc* 1991; **265**: 1295–8.
3. Kelly G. Rationing health care. *Br Med J* 1991; **302**: 288.
4. Dixon J, Welch HG. Priority setting: lessons from Oregon. *Lancet* 1991; **377**: 891–4.

5. *Choices in Health Care.* A Report by the Government Committee on Choices in Health Care, The Netherlands. Zoetermeer, The Netherlands, 1992.

6. Dixon S. *Cost Utility Analysis in Health Policy.* Victoria University of Wellington, Graduate School of Business and Government Management. Working paper series 2/91, September 1990.

7. Cullen DJ. Results and costs of intensive care. *Anaesthesiology* 1977; **47**: 203–16.

8. Mechanic D. *Politics, Medicine and Social Science.* New York: John Wiley & Sons Ltd, 1974.

9. Cullen DJ, Ferrara LC, Briggs BA, Walker PF, Gilbert J. Survival, hospitalization charges and follow-up results in critically ill patients. *New Engl J Med* 1976; **294**: 982–7.

10. Hiatt HH. Protecting the medical commons: who is responsible? *New Engl J Med* 1975; **293**: 235–41.

11. Griner PF. Medical intensive care in the teaching hospital: costs vs benefits: the need for assessment. *Ann Intern Med* 1973; **78**: 581–5.

12. Thibault GE, Mulley AG, Barnett GO *et al.* Medical intensive care: indications, interventions and outcomes. *New Engl J Med* 1980; **302**: 938–42.

13. Knaus WA, Wagner DP, Draper EA *et al.* The APACHE III prognostic system. Risk prediction of hospital mortality for critically ill hospitalized adults. *Chest* 1991; **100**: 1619–36.

14. Kalb PE, Miller DH. Utilization strategies for intensive care units. *N Med Assoc* 1989; **261**: 2389–95.

15. Detsky AS, Stricker SC, Mulley AG, Thibault GE. Prognosis, survival and the expenditure of hospital resources for patients in an intensive-care unit. *New Engl J Med* 1981; **305**: 667–72.

16. Spagnolo SV, Hershberg PI, Zimmerman JH. Medical intensive care unit: mortality experience in large teaching hospital. *New York State J Med* 1973; **73**: 754–7.

17. Turnbull AD, Carlon G, Baron R, Sichel W, Young C, Howland W. The inverse relationship between cost and survival in the critically ill cancer patient. *Crit Care Med* 1979; **7**: 20–3.

18. Chassin MR. Costs and outcomes of medical intensive care: implications for cost control. *Med Care* 1982; **20**: 165–79.

19. Nunn JF, Milledge JS, Singaraya J. Survival of patients ventilated in an intensive therapy unit. *Br Med J* 1979; **1**: 1525–7.

20. Byrick RJ, Mindorff C, McKee L, Mudge B. Cost effectiveness of intensive care for respiratory failure patients. *Crit Care Med* 1980; **8**: 332–7.

21. Parno JR, Teres D, Lemeshow S, Brown RB. Hospital charges and long-term survival of ICU versus non-ICU patients. *Crit Care Med* 1982; **10**: 569–74.

22. Parno JR, Teres D, Lemeshow S, Brown RB, Avrurin JS. Two-year outcome of adult intensive care patients. *Med Care* 1984; **22**: 167–76.

23. Bams JL, Miranda DR. Outcome and costs of intensive care. *Intensive Care Med* 1985; **11**: 234–41.

24. Knaus WA, Draper EA, Wagner DP, Zimmerman JE. An evaluation of outcome from intensive care in major medical centres. *Ann Int Med* 1986; **104**: 410–18.

25. Ridley S, Biggam M, Stone P. Cost of intensive therapy. *Anaesthesia* 1991; **46**: 523–30.

26. Shiell A, Griffiths RD, Macmillan RR, Atherton ST. Pilot assessment of the cost-effectiveness of a British intensive care unit. *Br Med J Hospital Med* 1989; **42**: 144–5.

27. Rippe JM, Howe JP. Public policy in intensive care medicine. In: Rippe KM, Irwin RS, Alpert JS, Dala JE (eds) *Intensive Care Medicine.* Boston: Little Brown & Co., 1989: 64–70.

28. Mulley AG, Thibault GE, Hughes RA, Barnett GO, Reder VA, Sherman EL. The course of patients with suspected myocardial infarction: the identification of low risk patients for early transfer from intensive care. *New Engl J Med* 1980; **302**: 943–8.

29. Singer DE, Carr PL, Mulley AG, Thibault GE. Rationing intensive care: physician responses to a resource shortage. *New Engl J Med* 1983; *309*: 1155–60.

30. Ron A, Aronne LJ, Kalb PE, Santini D, Charlson ME. The therapeutic efficacy of critical care units. Identifying subgroups of patients who benefit. *Arch Intern Med* 1989; **149**: 338–41.

31. Jennett B. Resource allocation for the severely brain damaged. *Arch Neurol* 1976; **33**: 595–9.

32. Gilbertson AA, Smith JM, Mostafa SM. The cost of an intensive care unit: a prospective study. *Intensive Care Med* 1991; **17**: 204–8.

33. Civetta JM. The inverse relationship between cost and survival. *J Surg Res* 1973; **14**: 265–9.

34. Knaus WA, Zimmerman JE, Wagner DP, Draper EA, Lawrence DE. APACHE-acute physiology and chronic health evaluation: a physiologically based classification system. *Crit Care Med* 1981; **9**: 591–7.

35. Knaus WA, Draper EA, Wagner DP *et al.* Evaluating outcome from intensive care: a preliminary multihospital comparison. *Crit Care Med* 1982; **10**: 491–6.

36. Wagner DP, Knaus WA, Draper EA. Statistical validation of a severity of illness measure. *Am J Public Health* 1983; **73**: 878–84.

37. Knaus WA, Wagner DP, Draper EA. The value of measuring severity of disease in clinical research on acutely ill patients. *J Chronic Dis* 1984; **37**: 455–63.

38. Civetta JM, Hudson-Civetta JA, Nelson LD. Evaluation of APACHE II for cost containment and quality assurance. *Ann Surg* 1990; **212**: 266–76.

39. Cullen DJ. The importance of comparative data in critical care analyses. *Crit Care Med* 1982; **10**: 618.

40. Boyle MH, Torrance GW, Sinclair JC, Horwood SP. Economic evaluation of neonatal intensive care of very-low-birthweight infants. *New Engl J Med* 1983; **308**: 1330–7.

41. Griffin J. *Born too Soon.* London: Office of Health Economics, 1993.

42. Congress of the United States, Office of Technology Assessment. Health Technology Case Study 28. *Intensive Care Units (ICUs). Clinical Outcomes, Costs, and Decision Making.* November 1984.

43. Wagner DP, Knaus WA, Draper EA. Identification of low-risk monitor patients within a medical-surgical intensive care unit. *Med Care* 1983; **21**: 425.

44. Fineberg HV, Scadden D, Goldman L. Care of patients with a low probability of acute myocardial infarction – cost effectiveness of alternatives to coronary care unit admission. *New Engl J Med* 1984; **310**: 1301.

45. Bendixen HH. The cost of intensive care. In: Bunker JP, Barnes BA, Mosteller F (eds) *Costs, Risks, and Benefits of Surgery*. New York: Oxford University Press, 1977: 372–84.

46. Klein R. On the Oregon trail: rationing health care. *Br Med J* 1991; **302**: 1–2.

47. Eddy DM. Cost-effectiveness analysis: a conversation with my father. *J Am Med Assoc* 1992; **267**: 1669–75.

Chapter 23

Withholding and Withdrawing

JEAN-LOUIS VINCENT————————————————————————————————————

Introduction   344
Withholding and withdrawing therapy are sometimes necessary   345
What is death after all?   346
Withholding or withdrawing treatment in a competent person with no terminal illness   347
Who should decide?   347
Differences between countries   348
References   349

Introduction

The developments in medicine in general and the technology of life-support in particular have provided the means of maintaining organ function for prolonged periods of time. It is clear that these forms of therapy should not be applied to every patient and there are at least three situations where treatment in an intensive care unit (ICU) or even admission to the ICU should be denied:

1. When death comes at its 'appropriate' time. Attempts to prolong life in a physiologically old patient could represent a stubborn fight against a natural process, although this has to be judged on the patient's previous level of health and the underlying disease.
2. When death becomes inevitable, as in the presence of a terminal disease such as disseminated malignancy.
3. When there is permanent and extensive brain damage so that no measurable quality of life can be restored. A possible exception to this is in the case of a brain dead patient who may be admitted prior to organ donation simply to preserve the function of the physiological systems.

In any of these three situations, treatment will not achieve any meaningful survival, and would thus be defined as futile. Another proposed definition of such 'futile' treatment is where there is either a less than 1% chance of success or where the treatment merely preserves a state of permanent unconsciousness or continuous dependence on intensive medical care.[1]

Such criteria should be used when making decisions about the selection of patients for admission to the ICU. Unfortunately, these guidelines are not always observed and a number of patients with terminal disease or severe and extensive brain damage are admitted to the ICU. A recent European enquiry revealed that two-thirds of ICU doctors admitted patients with no hope of surviving beyond a few weeks, but only half of these felt that it was right to do so.[2] These findings perhaps reflect the pressure exerted by primary physicians to have their patients admitted to the ICU. Nevertheless, even the correct application of the criteria described above would not abolish the problems of withholding or withdrawing treatment for two major reasons.

Firstly, the complete background information about a patient is not always available at the time of admission to the ICU, especially in the emergency situation. ICU admission should not be denied on the basis of advanced age alone because elderly patients with acute illnesses such as decompensated diabetes, acute infections, intoxications or acute cardiac problems may have a good chance of being restored to a meaningful life. Patients may be admitted with a previously undiagnosed terminal disease or alternatively they may present with a severe disease process for which the therapeutic possibilities have not been fully evaluated. For instance, it is sometimes difficult to assess the chance of recovery of viable brain function after severe head trauma or after cardiopulmonary resuscitation (CPR) for a cardiac arrest.

The second reason is that the ICU course may be less favorable than initially hoped. The physiological reserve of a patient may be less than initially assumed, complications may develop and then lead to a terminal situation. Anticipated recovery from brain damage may not occur. Therefore, the decision to withhold or withdraw therapy will have to be reconsidered in groups of patients where initially there might have been a degree of therapeutic optimism.

Withholding and withdrawing therapy are sometimes necessary

There are many circumstances in which therapy is withheld from patients outside the ICU. If this were not the case, many more patients would be admitted to the ICU without good reasons. The decision not to perform CPR in cases of cardiac arrest, the so-called 'Do not resuscitate' (DNR) orders, represents a typical situation where therapy would be futile in that particular patient. It is well recognized that these orders have to be applied to some patients in order to avoid the unwarranted use of life-support systems. Nevertheless, DNR orders have been criticized because they are often more broadly interpreted so that other forms of care become inadequate. An enquiry performed by the European Society of Intensive Care Medicine a few years ago revealed that not all ICU doctors routinely applied DNR orders.[2]

There have been attempts made to distinguish between 'ordinary' and 'extraordinary' forms of therapy, or between 'simple' and 'heroic' measures. Such distinctions are however largely artificial and should be avoided. Much of current technology has become 'ordinary,' for it would be difficult for instance to regard the use of mechanical ventilation, renal support or vasoactive therapy as 'extraordinary' by present-day standards. Some procedures, such as extracorporeal lung assistance or ventricular assist devices, might still justifiably be considered 'extraordinary,' but no consensus exists and for each form of therapy, the 'benefit versus burden' approach is more appropriate: any form of treatment should be considered provided the benefits outweigh the burdens.

It is now widely admitted that there are no ethical differences between withholding and withdrawing life support.[3] The reasons are the same as those given previously: the complete information might not have been available at the time of initiation of the life-support or the course might have been unfavorable despite therapy. Furthermore, establishing a distinction between withholding and withdrawing treatment could have deleterious consequences, as it could perhaps imply the premature withholding of potentially beneficial therapy for fear of providing prolonged life-support which would be futile if there was no chance of meaningful recovery. For example, the duration of efficient CPR might be curtailed for fear of there being permanent extensive brain damage. Permitting withdrawal of therapy in cases where failure of treatment is clearly demonstrated ensures the application of maximal therapy to the patient.

Although these principles might sound obvious, it is nevertheless very important to give them emphasis, since *psychologically* it is more difficult to discontinue treatment than not to start it in the first place.

Withholding or withdrawing treatment not only *may* be, but *must* be, applied in patients where the prolongation of intensive care would only represent prolonged suffering for the patient. It has been shown that many deaths in the ICU are related to the withholding and withdrawing of life-support.[4,5] However, a recent European enquiry revealed that 13% of ICU doctors claimed that they do not withhold therapy and 33% reported that they do not withdraw therapy.[2] These attitudes are indefensible. Clearly, the results of the enquiry reflect the values which, whilst important, have become incompatible with the progress and understanding of medicine. The 'defense of life at all costs' has become unrealistic in the era of sophisticated life-support systems.

Ethical decisions should not be influenced by financial considerations, as they are entirely different entities. An attempt to give a price to a human life may have dangerous consequences. Nevertheless, useless prolongation of care can lead to unnecessary costs for the patient's family in particular and for society as a whole. It may also deflect resources that would otherwise be available to others. The continuation of such useless therapy would then be in opposition to the ethical principle of the best allocation of limited resources.

There have been many recent discussions concerning the ethics of euthanasia.[6] Most of these extend to circumstances outside the ICU, as they concern the conscious and mentally competent patient who desires to die with dignity and without pain. This issue, which involves the oncologist and the neurologist more than the intensivist, remains complex and encompasses a number of situations. Indeed, the word 'euthanasia', which refers to the application of measures aimed at ending life, can have several other connotations,[7,8] so that the word must not be used imprudently. Many physicians are opposed in principle to any form of 'killing act' such as euthanasia or assisted suicide. It is argued that if the barriers against such killing are broken, liberties may be taken in cases which are not clear-cut and a dangerous precedent will be established with unpredictable consequences.

The distinction between 'killing' and 'letting die' ('active' and 'passive' euthanasia) becomes quite subtle in the ICU, where life-support systems are readily available. This concept is well illustrated by James Rachels, Professor of Philosophy at the University of Alabama, in his book *The End of Life*.[9] He took the example of a man whose intention was to kill a child by drowning him in a swimming pool, so as to simulate an accident. Before any murder was performed, the child unexpectedly slipped into the pool and fell unconscious. The man deliberately did not intervene, so that the child died. Is there a real ethical difference between killing or letting die in the particular circumstances where the adult could so easily intervene to prevent death?

In practice the difference between the withdrawal of life-support and the administration of sedative medications becomes tenuous. An example is that of the 'terminal weaning' of a patient with respiratory failure. Here, almost by definition, the patient will not be able to breathe without respiratory support, so that he or she will soon need sedation or analgesia to relieve discomfort before cardiac arrest ensues.[10–12] For the same end, it may therefore be more advisable to administer the medication whilst the patient is still mechanically ventilated, in order to avoid any anxiety, discomfort or suffering.

For these reasons, we prefer to refer to a general term of 'termination of care' that encompasses all forms of discontinuation of therapy in the ICU. Regardless of the methods used to terminate care, these are neither murder not assisted suicide. These attitudes are not criminal *because it is the medical condition rather than the medical act that is the cause of death*. The discontinuation of lifesupport basically allows a natural process to take place.

It is possible to envisage several practical situations other than the discontinuation of mechanical ventilation.[13] For instance in patients who require vasoactive support, termination of care is usually quite easy, as the discontinuation of the inotropic drugs is rapidly followed by a marked alteration in mental state and death. However, many patients do not require such vasoactive support at the time of termination of care. Discontinuation of hemodialysis or other forms of renal support is, for example, a more complex issue, as cardiac arrest does not immediately ensue. The question then arises whether prolongation of some form of palliative care is still indicated while awaiting a death which has become inevitable.

There are other situations where life is not supported by sophisticated forms of therapy but has nevertheless become meaningless as in the presence of a permanent vegetative state. In such patients, discontinuation of feeding has been seen in many US states as an accepted form of withdrawal of life-support.[14] Many Europeans are more hesitant towards this approach, not only because it is a long process that will undoubtedly lend to death, but because of some opposition to the concept of 'starving to death.' The principle of 'avoiding killing' must then be weighed against the one of 'avoiding starving to death.' In any case, the discontinuation of feeding is a form of terminal withdrawal which is used primarily outside the ICU for patients who do not require any form of life-support.

Once the decision for termination of treatment has been taken, prolongation of supportive care may only bring unnecessary suffering and useless expense. Further prolongation will be incompatible with the ethical principles of beneficience and nonmaleficence, and even social justice.[15]

What is death after all?

The definition of death has changed from ancient times when it was characterized by the cessation of respiration ('the breath of life') to more recent times when it was characterized by the absence of a heartbeat ('the pulse of life'). Recently, death has been defined by the cessation of brain function,[16] a concept that arose for four reasons:

1. Cardiopulmonary arrest is no longer always the end of life. Endotracheal intubation with mechanical ventilation may sustain gas exchange and CPR techniques may restore adequate cardiac activity.
2. Modern life-support techniques have enabled brain death to be recognized as an entity (originally described as 'coma dépassé') where cerebral cortical function is totally and irreversibly lost while the function of the other organs can be maintained artificially.
3. The public have become increasingly aware of the futility of 'existence' in the absence of cognitive brain function. The *Quinlan* case in the USA was illustrative of the drama of the persistent vegetative state; a young patient remained alive after discontinuation of life-support systems but 'without realistic possibility of returning to any semblance of cognitive or sapient life' (cited in ref. 3).
4. Patients with extensive and irreversible brain damage may not meet the criteria of brain death, but nevertheless may be in an analogous situation in that no form of social relation can be recovered. In these patients, prolongation of care becomes futile, as it

does not prolong or restore any meaningful survival. The concept of 'quality of life' must here be weighed against the concept of 'preservation of life.'

Withholding or withdrawing treatment in a competent person with no terminal illness

Termination of care in the ICU usually concerns issues relating to terminal illness in patients who are also unconscious at the time of any decision. There are, however, situations where the patient is conscious and competent and the illness is not terminal. Outside the practice of the ICU there are many such examples of competent patients who refuse therapy.

In the ICU, two noteworthy situations can be encountered. One is the patient who refuses blood transfusions on religious grounds. It has been widely accepted in the USA that the patient has the right to refuse blood transfusion even in life-threatening situations, but the situation is ambiguous in Europe. A recent European enquiry revealed that many doctors would, in critical situations, still transfuse despite the patient's refusal.[17]

The second situation is illustrated by a patient who has profound neurological damage but has preservation of a degree of brain function. A typical example is that of the quadriplegic patient where the application of life-support measures is a common ethical problem. Once it is certain that the quadriplegia is complete and irreversible, should one intervene further and treat a serious complication when it occurs? In the acute conditions following the accident, the patient rarely expresses any desire to die, but rather remains silent. Such a desire to die may be expressed once the situation is stabilized, and discontinuance of life-support has sometimes been allowed in the patients who request it.

Who should decide?

Many recent publications have emphasized the public concern toward the use of life-support technology and insistence on the patient's right to decide. These elements are directly related to the ethical principle of autonomy. It is a fundamental right for anyone to refuse treatment, a right that also applies to life-support treatment.

In the USA, the principle of autonomy is strictly applied and any patient who is capable of making a decision and is appropriately informed has the right to refuse any form of therapy, life-sustaining or not.[18, 19]

Since the decision in the *Cuzan* case, it has become clear that any patient (terminally ill or not) is entitled to refuse any form of treatment.[20] The situation is not so clear-cut in many European countries, where the physician is usually more involved in the decision making process, supposedly representing the best interests of his or her patient.[21]

Concerns about the patient being depressed will often prevent a physician accepting a patient's request. In many conditions, it is unclear whether the patient wants the treatment to be continued or discontinued. For the ICU patient, the ability to decide is often impaired by the advanced degree of illness, the unfamiliar environment and frequently the effects of sedative drugs needed to manage the illness. Often the full information is not given for fear it will distress the patient. As a consequence, the patient is no longer able to understand the information provided and is therefore unable to make a rational decision. The implications are that there is no indication for the termination of life-support in a competent patient who expresses no desire to die, but the opposite is not necessarily true, in that therapy should not always be withdrawn at the request of a competent patient. This situation may become analogous to that of the patient who refuses a life-supporting measure following an attempted suicide; termination of life-support must be clearly distinguished from assisted suicide.

However, if the patient is competent and expresses the desire to die, termination of life-support may be permissible when the treatment has become futile or when the patient shows no clinical evidence of depression.

In all circumstances, it is always advisable to communicate with the family, keeping them informed and discussing future plans concerning the patient's care. Reliance on the opinion of relatives to guide therapeutic plans is limited by several factors. First, the relatives are also involved in a complex psychological reaction that can affect their ability to make rational decisions. Second, even close relatives might not always act in the patient's best interests; financial issues or other practical considerations may influence a decision. Third, family members may express different opinions. In particular, this may occur in the case of marital separation or complex 'relationships.' Fourth, there might not be any close relative, and then there will be concern as to whether a more distant relative or a close friend can reflect the patient's best interest.

The relatives may know the opinion of the patient if he or she has been in a position to express it. Such information can then be very valuable towards making a decision, especially in difficult cases. It is also a valuable alternative to written advance directives, i.e. a 'living will.' Advance directives have major limitations, first because it is difficult for someone to anticipate their own decision in a situation that he or she has not experienced. Second, the individual might have changed their mind since having written the advance directive, but might not have documented the changes. Third and most importantly, the real implications are doubtful; if the treatment has not become futile, then the request for withholding or withdrawing would be a request for murder, which obviously cannot be complied with. If the treatment has become futile, it has to be discontinued regardless of the previous request of the patient. 'Advance directives' might help to forego life-support in the case of permanent vegetative states, but this could be discussed with the family and the physician without the need for any written statement.

In the USA, if the patient is incompetent, because of the illness and/or its treatment, the opinion of a surrogate should be sought about the continuation or termination of care. The surrogate's decision should be based either on 'objective' standards (the best interests of the patient) or on 'substituted judgment' standards, in which the surrogate presents the opinion that the patient would probably have expressed if he or she were capable. Courts can even nominate a guardian to defend a patient's rights. Advance directives are encouraged perhaps more for legal ends than for ethical purposes.[22]

Figure 23.1 shows a possible algorithm based on the decision of the patient and the patient's family. In all cases, it is clear that the severity of the illness and the likelihood of success of the therapy play the major role.

Even though 'medical paternalism' must be avoided, such decisions are primarily of a medical nature, as they are based on the facts detailing the nature of the illness, its degree of severity and the possibilities of treatment. Whenever possible, these decisions should be corporate, involving not only a number of doctors, but also nurses and other allied health personnel; this will maximize the objectivity of the decision and help to avoid incompatible feelings and disquiet by any member of the ICU team.

Differences between countries

There are important differences in the recommended attitudes and practices of different countries. Although the legal pressure is stronger in Europe today than previously, there is a much stronger legal influence on these decisions in North America than in most European countries. In North America, the fear of malpractice suits can be an important determinant in the decision making process,[3,23] with more direct application of the decisions of the patient and his or her surrogate. The practice in the USA is based more on a

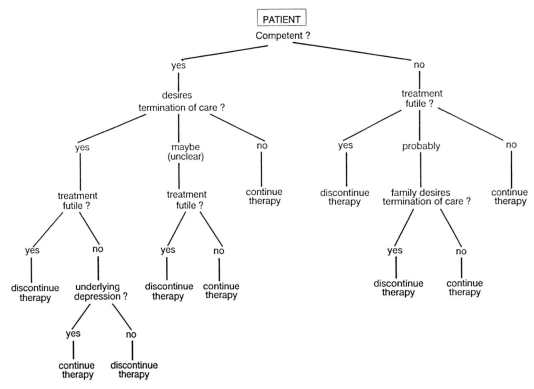

Fig. 23.1 A possible algorithm based on the decisions of the patient and the patient's family.

contract between the patient and the physician, who will have to withdraw from caring for the patient in the case of any disagreement with the patient and/or the family.

In Europe, decisions related to withholding or withdrawing therapy remain largely the doctor's province. Doctors are seen as defenders of the patient's benefits, so that the privilege of therapeutic choice is still left largely to them.

In Europe, a physician's duty to support the patient when there are reasonable chances of improvement remains important, so that the opinions of the patient and the family are not always followed. However, the physician, and in particular the family physician, usually has established strong links with the patient and his or her family, so that the physician is considered to act in their best interests. There is usually an empathetic relationship between the patient, the patient's family and the doctor. In addition, the condemnation of futile therapy is a general principle, while the practical issues of termination of care remain 'in a no man's land.'[21] Many are concerned that legalization of some form of euthanasia would officially recognize the right to provoke death, although in the Netherlands there is evidence of a more permissive attitude.

Regardless of these differences, dying is part of life and should be respected as such. Fears of malpractice suits should never lead to useless prolongation of life-support or to lack of sensitivity to the need to relieve suffering.[24] One must accept that many deaths in the ICU are associated with the withholding and withdrawing of life-support.[4,5] It is fortunate that the scientific and technologic advances in medicine have allowed us to develop strong weapons against illness and injury, but they must not be abused to prolong an agonal process. Dying should remain a natural process.

References

1. Jecker JS, Schneiderman LJ. Futility and rationing. *Am J Med* 1992; **92**: 189–96.
2. Vincent JL. European attitudes towards ethical problems in intensive care medicine: results of an ethical questionnaire. *Intensive Care Med* 1990; **16**: 256–64.
3. Meisel A. Legal myths about terminating life support. *Arch Internal Med* 1991; **151**: 1497–1502.
4. Vincent JL, Parquier JN, Preiser JC, Brimioulle S, Kahn RJ. Terminal events in the intensive care unit: review of 258 fatal cases in one year. *Crit Care Med* 1989; **17**: 530–3.
5. Smedira NG, Evans BH, Grais LS *et al.* Withholding and withdrawal of life support from the critically ill. *New Eng J Med* 1990; **322**: 309–15.
6. Benrubi GI. Euthanasia – the need for procedural safeguards. *New Eng J Med* 1992; **326**: 197–8.
7. Brewin TB. Voluntary euthanasia. *Lancet* 1986; 1085–6.
8. Reichel W, Dyck AJ. Euthanasia: a contemporary moral quandary. *Lancet* 1989; 1321–3.
9. Rachels, J. *The End of Life*. New York: Oxford University Press, 1986.
10. Edwards MJ, Tolle SW. Disconnecting a ventilator at the request of a patient who knows he will then die: the doctor's anguish. *Ann Intern Med* 1992; **117**: 254–6.
11. Crippen D. Terminally weaning awake patients from life-sustaining mechanical ventilation: the critical care physician's role in comfort measures during the dying process. *Clin Intensive Care* 1992; **3**: 206–12.
12. Wilson WC, Smedira NG, Fink C, McDowell JA, Luce JM. Ordering and administration of sedatives and analgesics during the withholding and withdrawal of life support from critically ill patients. *J Am Med Assoc* 1992; **267**: 949–53.
13. Crippen D. Practical aspects of life support withdrawal: a critical care physician's opinion. *Clin Intensive Care* 1991; **2**: 260–5.
14. Council on Scientific Affairs and Council on Ethical and Judicial Affairs. Persistent vegetative state and the decision to withdraw or withhold life support. *J Am Med Assoc* 1990; **263**: 426–30.
15. Luce JM. Conflicts over ethical principles in the intensive care unit. *Crit Care Med* 1992; **20**: 313–15.
16. Bernat JL, Culver CM, Bernat G. On the definition and criterion of death. *Ann Emergency Med* 1981; **94**: 389–94.
17. Vincent JL. Transfusion in the exsanguinating Jehovah's witness patient: the attitude of intensive-care doctors. *Eur J Anaesthesiol* 1991; **8**: 297–300.
18. Bone RC, Rackow E, Weg JG, Members of the ACCP/SCCM Consensus Panel. Ethical and moral guidelines for the initiation, continuation, and withdrawal of intensive care. *Chest* 1990; **97**: 949–58.
19. Task Force on Ethics of the Society of Critical Care Medicine. Consensus report on the ethics of foregoing life-sustaining treatments in the critically ill. *Crit Care Med* 1990; **18**: 1435–9.
20. Lo B, Rouse F, Dornbrand L. Family decision making on trial: who decides for incompetent patients? *New Eng J Med* 1990; **322**: 1228–32.
21. Euthanasia around the world. *Br Med J* 1992; **304**: 7–10.
22. Medical Section of the American Lung Association. Withholding and withdrawing life-sustaining therapy. *Am Rev Respir Dis* 1991; **144**: 726–31.
23. Goetzler RM, Moskowitz MA. Changes in physician attitudes toward limiting care of critically ill patients. *Arch Intern Med* 1991; **151**: 1537–40.
24. Misbin RI. Sounding board – physicians' aid in dying. *New Eng J Med* 1991; **325**: 1307–11.

Ethical Issues of Organ Donation

CJ HINDS, CH COLLINS

Cadaveric organ retrieval   351
Increasing the pool of brain stem dead potential donors   355
Alternative sources of organs for transplantation   357
Xenografts and artificial organs for permanent implantation   358
Allocation of donated organs   358
Payment for donated organs   358
Conclusion   359
References   359

> I know death has ten thousand several doors for men
> to take their exits
>
> John Webster ?1580–1625

The authors are practicing intensive care doctors, not ethicists, philosophers or lawyers. In this chapter we have highlighted some of the controversies and ethical issues related to organ donation from one perspective of the intensive care clinician.

The Oxford English Dictionary defines 'ethical behaviour' as 'that which follows a set of moral principles or guidelines.' In relation to medical practice it could perhaps be defined as 'clinical care of the patient which would be considered reasonable and sensible by the majority of one's peer group'; in the context of organ donation it is particularly important to extend this definition to encompass the care of the patient's relatives and next of kin. Ethical standards are, of course, not immutable; they have to be constantly adapted in response to changes in techniques and advances in therapy, whilst at the same time remaining in tune with the contemporary moral climate. Not so long ago some questioned whether it was ethical to operate on the heart, whereas it is now considered unethical to keep patients waiting for cardiac surgery. Similarly, the development and expansion of transplant techniques, particularly in the 1980s has increased the demand for donor organs and forced practicing clinicians to consider new ethical dilemmas. Over time attitudes have changed and ethical standards have been modified to accommodate new clinical practice.

The death of an otherwise fit, healthy and often relatively young patient due to failure of a single vital organ is a particularly tragic, wasteful and often unnecessary loss. Equally the sudden, unexpected death of a previously well individual who could have anticipated many years of useful life, for example as a result of a severe head injury or massive intracerebral hemorrhage is especially distressing. Transplant therapy enables at least some good to result from such a tragedy and can therefore be viewed as a desirable goal not only from the point of view of the recipients, but also that of the donor and their respective families and friends. The degree of consolation may be enhanced if more than one life can be saved, for example by multiple organ donation, when as many as seven recipients could in theory benefit. Nevertheless, for many, interference with a human corpse is distasteful and there is often a vague mistrust of those who seek to do so. As we shall see, this unease is shared by some of the members of the medical profession and can only be allayed by ensuring strict adherence to the highest ethical standards.

Cadaveric organ retrieval

The vast majority of organs are obtained from brain dead beating heart donors. This allows the transplant surgeon to receive organs in the best possible condition, whilst the planned nature of the procedure makes retrieval more acceptable to the donor's family, as well as the doctors and nurses. Beating heart donation is only possible when cardiorespiratory function can be maintained artificially until the time of organ retrieval and is therefore dependent on the concept of brain stem death.

DIAGNOSIS OF BRAIN STEM DEATH[1]

The means of establishing death with certainty has always been a cause for concern and for centuries people have been alarmed by the prospect of being declared dead when still alive. It is fundamental to the understanding of the difficulties encountered in diagnosing with certainty that a patient is dead to appreciate that death is a process, not an event, the problem being to define the moment in this process when death can be safely declared. The precise time at which different cells in various organs cease to function is therefore not as important as is the certainty that the process has become irreversible. The classical signs of death (permanent cessation of breathing and heartbeat) are major and easily detectable events following which the process of dying normally rapidly accelerates and passes the point of no return. It has, however, been recognized for many years that absence of heartbeat and respiration does not inevitably preclude recovery, particularly when cardiorespiratory arrest occurs as an acute event in a previously fit person. Many early papers, for example, concentrated on the victims of drowning, lightning strikes and other sudden events. In the eighteenth and nineteenth centuries members of the Royal Humane Society and others clearly appreciated the importance of defining the clinical signs whereby those who might be revived could be distinguished from those who were irretrievable, or, as James Curry put it in 1815 the difference between 'absolute' and 'apparent' death. He concluded that a 'beginning putrefaction of the body is perhaps the only unequivocal proof of death we are yet acquainted with in such cases.' The importance of at least one of the brain stem reflexes was, however, appreciated by Fothergill as long ago as 1795; he stated:

> 'If the eyes appear clear, the pupils not greatly dilated, nor totally void of contraction on being approached with a lighted taper ... there are still some hopes that recovery may be effected. On the other hand, if the eyes appear misty or suffused – the pupils destitute of contraction – the countenance livid – the body stiff, cold and insensible to stimuli, the case would seem desperate.

By the beginning of this century it was widely recognized that after cardiac arrest heart action could be restored by internal cardiac massage. Later expired air artificial respiration was described and finally the efficacy of external cardiac massage was established. As a result it is now common experience that cardiopulmonary resuscitation can interrupt, and sometimes reverse, the process of dying so that the context in which cardiorespiratory arrest occurs assumes considerable importance in determining whether cessation of breathing and heartbeat can be taken as representing death. It is also now routine practice to support critically ill patients with long-term mechanical ventilation. This is often life-saving when used to treat a patient with, for example, reversible respiratory failure but, when used to support a patient whose respiratory center has ceased to function as a result of irreversible brain damage, simply prolongs the process of dying as different organs in turn cease to function, culminating in asystole. Thus, cessation of heartbeat and/or respiration do not indicate that the process of death has become irreversible, but there are now other 'points of no return' which can precede cardiac arrest. A person should therefore not be considered dead unless their brain is dead; arrest of the heart and circulation indicate death only when they persist long enough for the brain to die.

Brain death was first described by two French physicians, Mollaret and Goulon in 1959[2] and termed 'coma dépassé' (a state beyond coma). As well as obvious signs indicating death of the nervous system, they described other features indicative of brain death including poikilothermia, diabetes insipidus, resistant hypotension and progressive acidosis. They differentiated 'coma dépassé' from 'coma prolonge', a condition now termed 'persistent vegetative state'. In 1968 the Ad Hoc Committee of the Harvard Medical School defined brain death as irreversible coma, the patient being totally unreceptive and unresponsive. The Harvard criteria also required that reflexes should be absent and that there should be no spontaneous respiratory effort during a 3-minute period of disconnection from the ventilator. The report unambiguously proposed that this clinical state should be accepted as death. Soon thereafter it was suggested that 'in patients with known but irreparable intracranial lesions' irreversible damage to the brain stem was 'the point of no return' and that the diagnosis 'could be based on clinical judgement.'[3] These authors introduced the concept of a purely clinical diagnosis with etiological preconditions, as well as emphasizing the importance of apnea and brain stem areflexia.

The next milestone, which profoundly influenced clinical practice with regard to brain death in the UK and elsewhere in the world, was the memorandum issued by the Conference of Medical Royal Colleges and their faculties in the UK in 1976.[4] This emphasized that 'permanent functional death of the brain stem constitutes brain death' and that this should only be diagnosed in the context of irremediable structural brain damage, after certain specified conditions have been excluded. It also described how the permanent loss of brain stem function could be established by simple clinical tests. A second memorandum in 1979 equated brain stem death with death itself.[5] Thus the evolution of the diagnosis of death has involved two important conceptual steps – from classical signs of death to the diagnosis of total brain death and from total brain death to establishing death of the brain stem. Human death, it has been suggested, can be conceived to be a state in which there is irreversible loss of the capacity for consciousness combined with irreversible loss of the capacity to breathe (and hence maintain a heartbeat). Alone neither would be sufficient. Both are essentially brain stem functions and death of the brain stem is the necessary and sufficient component of brain death.[1]

The concept of brain stem death is now almost universally accepted and, although they have never been tested in law, the recommendations of the Conference of Royal Colleges and their Faculties in the UK, or similar guidelines, are believed by most practicing doctors to be a correct and ethical means of diagnosing brain stem death. Death can therefore be declared once brain stem death has been confirmed (and not some time later when the heart stops or mechanical ventilation is discontinued) and most would argue that the ethically correct course of action is then to discontinue artificial ventilation as soon as possible. This should be viewed as ceasing a futile and useless intervention in a patient who is already dead rather than withdrawing support to allow a patient to die. The only situation in which it could be considered inappropriate to discontinue ventilating a brain stem dead patient is when they are pregnant. In some such cases it has been possible to support the mother, for up to 3 months, to permit growth of the fetus until delivery by cesarian section can be performed safely.

It is also important to appreciate that the concept of brain stem death was not developed in order to facilitate organ donation and that even if transplantation therapy did not exist it would still be necessary to make the diagnosis in order to practice intensive care humanely. To continue to ventilate a brain dead patient until asystole supervenes, as it inevitably will, is a grim experience which is unnecessarily distressing for the relatives and can have a devastating effect on staff morale. It is also an inappropriate use of limited resources. Most clinicians therefore find the decision to discontinue ventilating a brain dead patient relatively straightforward when compared to the more difficult ethical dilemmas involved in withdrawing or limiting

treatment for patients in a persistent vegetative state or critically ill patients in whom the prognosis is considered to be hopeless.

CONCERNS ABOUT BRAIN STEM DEATH AND BEATING HEART DONATION

There is, however, a small minority of practicing clinicians in the UK who still dispute the validity of brain stem death procedures. They claim that it is not a legal necessity to diagnose brain stem death in order to discontinue mechanical ventilation and that the concept is therefore only required to facilitate organ transplantation. They suggest[6] that the clinical brain stem tests in routine use are not exhaustive, that they cannot ensure the permanent absence of all brain stem function and that their satisfaction does not ensure that the brain has been destroyed or that higher brain function has ceased irreversibly. They are also uncomfortable with 'beating heart' donors and feel that 'informed consent' in such cases is not truly informed; it is, for example, still a common misconception that life support is withdrawn prior to organ retrieval. They suggest that if the public were fully aware of what was entailed in obtaining organs there would be much greater reluctance to agree to donation and that if more members of the medical profession had direct experience of organ retrieval they would be more hesitant about requesting consent for the procedure.

There is also some evidence to suggest that many operating theater staff are concerned that mechanically ventilated beating heart donors are not truly dead, an anxiety which may be fuelled by the hypertension and tachycardia often observed during organ retrieval.[7] These hemodynamic responses have been attributed to intact spinal reflex arcs between afferent pain fibers and efferent sympathetic nerves, humoral responses after adrenal stimulation or residual brain stem function. Although apparently a few anesthetists are more comfortable if volatile anesthetics are administered during organ retrieval, most consider the use of such agents, other than to control potentially harmful tachycardia and hypertension, illogical. It is also generally recommended that somatic motor reflexes, similarly mediated at a spinal level, should be controlled with a muscle relaxant both for esthetic reasons and to facilitate surgery.[8] The vast majority of clinicians accept that the presence of these reflex hemodynamic and motor responses to surgical stimulation, and the need to control them during organ retrieval, do not invalidate the current clinical criteria for diagnosing irreversible damage to the brain stem and thereby establishing that there is no prospect of recovery.

Finally, some have claimed that there has been no

satisfactory 'controlled trial' to assess the prognostic value of the clinical signs of brain stem death. There are, however, a total of over 1000 cases in the world literature who have been supported after brain stem death has been established clinically. The biggest single series was from three neurosurgical centers in the UK.[9] Asystole was the invariable outcome, usually within a few days.

Despite these minority views there is no real debate in the UK as to whether or not the current brain stem death and organ retrieval procedures are ethical. In order to avoid conflict it is, however, important that all the intensive care unit staff, and operating theater personnel, understand the concept of brain stem death, are comfortable with the implications of this diagnosis and are familiar with the procedures to be followed once the diagnosis has been established. Education and training for staff, and the institution of clear protocols are of paramount importance. The intensive care consultant should be closely involved throughout.

SECURING PERMISSION FOR ORGAN RETRIEVAL

The principle is that we seek to ascertain the previously stated wishes of the deceased. Should this not be possible then lack of objection to donation is sought from the next of kin. In some instances this raises the problem of deciding who is the next of kin. In Australia relatives are graded in order of seniority, authority to consent being vested in the most senior who can be contacted, and in the USA the Uniform Anatomical Gift Act determines the order of priority of the closest relatives to clarify who should be considered to be next of kin. In the UK there are no formal guidelines but it is clearly important to identify the nearest, or at least the most concerned relative, who can canvass views within the family and act as a spokesperson. In the event of disagreement amongst the relatives it might be considered reasonable to respond to the wishes of the nearest or most interested relative, or in a situation where there are several close relatives, the majority of their wishes provided they have been given sufficient time to consider the issue. In the event of a serious dispute amongst family members it may be wiser not to proceed to organ donation unless further discussion and explanation resolves the conflict. In general a caring, sympathetic and compassionate attitude amongst the intensive care unit staff will help the family to reach a decision which is correct for them. It is important that discussions with the relatives should specifically address the issue of multiple rather than limited organ retrieval.

Difficulties may also arise when the next of kin attempt to overrule the deceased's clearly stated wish to donate organs in the event of their death. This may arise, for example, when the patient was carrying a donor card or had registered their wishes on a computer database. Currently the generally accepted legal view in the UK is that the person lawfully in possession of the body is the hospital administrator and that the relatives do not therefore have the power of veto over the deceased's wishes. In practice this situation must be handled with considerable sensitivity in order to avoid causing unwarranted distress to family members and, once the issues have been fully discussed, it is almost always advisable to concur with the relatives' wishes. In the USA all organ procurement agencies routinely request consent to harvest organs from the next of kin, even when the potential donor has correctly signed an organ donation card.

All potential donors must be tested for human immunodeficiency virus (HIV) status and it is recommended that permission should first be obtained from the relatives, a task which requires considerable sensitivity and tact. A positive test must be revealed to those at risk of contracting the disease from the deceased (for example sexual partners, intravenous drug abusers with needle sharing); this requires care and consideration, combined with the provision of appropriate counselling and follow-up services.

MAXIMIZING THE SUPPLY OF CADAVERIC ORGANS

As a result of advances in immunosuppression, surgical technique and intensive care, transplantation of thoracic and abdominal organs is now a life-saving therapy for patients with end-stage organ failure. Survival of transplanted organs has improved to the extent that 1-year graft survival has been reported to be greater than 80% for heart transplants, approximately 75% for liver transplants and between 70 and 80% for renal transplants.[10] Unfortunately the increase in the numbers undergoing transplant surgery has failed to keep pace with the accumulation of patients with end-stage organ failure who might benefit from transplantation. In Britain more than 4000 patients are awaiting kidney transplants but the annual rate of kidney transplantations is less than half this number. The waiting list for heart and lung transplants is much smaller but this underestimates the need because up to a quarter of those awaiting thoracic organs die before transplantation.[11]

Causes of the shortfall of donor organs

Although at one time it was thought that the requirement for cadaveric organ donors could be satisfied if a higher proportion of brain stem dead patients became organ donors, recent surveys[12,13] suggest that brain stem death is a possible diagnosis in only about 14%

(between 1700 and 1800 cases) of the estimated 13 000 patients who die each year in intensive care units in England and is confirmed in only approximately 10% of these deaths (between 1200 and 1350 cases a year). These represent about one-half and one-third, respectively, of previous estimates and, even if the proportion of confirmed brain stem dead patients who become actual donors increased substantially, would yield far fewer than the projected number of kidneys needed in England every year. Moreover there is evidence from the USA that this shortage of organs may be compounded by a recent fall in donor numbers, possibly as a result of a reduction in deaths from motor vehicle accidents, improved trauma care and the exclusion of some potential donors by HIV screening[14] and there is reason to believe that there are similar trends in many other countries.

This shortfall of potential donors is compounded by patients confirmed as brain stem dead failing to become donors because of general medical contraindications to organ donation (approximately 18% of cases), relatives' refusal to consent to organ retrieval (30% of those asked refused) and failure to ask about organ donation (only 6% of potential donors). Nonperformance of brain stem tests when brain stem death is a possibility may also account for a significant number of missed donors. Finally, in some cases logistical difficulties prevent the procurement of offered, suitable organs. It is important, therefore to maximize organ retrieval rates from suitable brain stem dead patients.

Obtaining consent for organ donation

Opting in or opting out?

The 'opt in' system, in which members of the public are encouraged to indicate their willingness to become an organ donor by carrying a card or by registration is used in the UK. Because this system has failed to meet the demand for organs and because of the large proportion of families who refuse consent[12, 13] some have recommended that we should reconsider adopting opting out schemes.[13] A recent survey by the British Kidney Patient Association showed that 61% of the population were in favor of adopting an 'opt out' policy, or presumed consent,[15] whereas the Department of Health found that 54% were opposed, more than half of whom were 'very much opposed.' Moreover a poll of transplant coordinators in Britain found that only five were in favor of an opting out policy, with 34 opposed, many of whom were 'very opposed,'[11] whilst intensive care clinicians seem to be divided on the issue. In general it seems that there is no great mandate amongst the relevant organizations for a change to opting out and only limited enthusiasm amongst transplanters, nor is there an overwhelming majority amongst the general public in favor of opting out. It also seems unlikely that

any UK government would be prepared to undertake such a change of direction. It would seem, therefore that for the time being the best course of action is to concentrate on improving the operation of opting in, for example by establishing a comprehensive computer database and expanding the registers which have already been introduced locally. It also seems sensible that when an individual attends hospital for any reason their wishes regarding organ donation should whenever possible be recorded in the hospital notes.[11] Indeed, surveys of patients' attitudes indicate that they would be very willing both to be asked and to have their views recorded.

Increased publicity and education might reduce the number of relatives refusing consent, as well as the proportion of restricted offers by otherwise consenting families. It could also increase the numbers who 'opt in.' In a UK survey, for example, just under half of those questioned had not thought about organ donation; 15% suggested that they were concerned that the diagnosis of death might not be accurate, 47% of responders did not completely trust doctors to establish death after a serious accident and 30% were worried that doctors might be pressurized by their transplanter colleagues to remove organs before they were certain that the donor was dead.[16]

Required request or required discussion

In the USA it is the legal duty of every physician to request consent for organ donation from the relatives of brain stem dead potential donors – 'required request.' Although it has been suggested that a significant number of suitable donors are lost through the reluctance of doctors to approach the next of kin, several studies have demonstrated that in practice this is unusual and that required request would have little impact on the supply of donor organs.[12, 13, 17] It could also be argued that such a requirement infringes the clinical freedom of medical and nursing staff.

Instead it has been suggested that required discussion, where clinicians would be obliged to discuss all brain stem dead patients with their local transplant team or coordinator, particularly concerning general medical contraindications (see below), might increase the proportion of confirmed brain stem dead patients who become actual donors.[12] Certainly early referral is strongly recommended to allow time for discussions about donor care and agreement on medical suitability for donation of specific organs.[18]

General medical contraindications

General medical contraindications, such as infection, malignancy and age, may prevent as many as 18% of those confirmed as brain stem dead becoming organ donors. Moreover, it has been claimed that there may on occasions be serious disagreements between transplant coordinators, intensive care specialists and transplant surgeons regarding general and organ-specific contra-indications to donation.[19] This emphasizes the importance of early discussion with the transplant team or coordinator about every brain stem dead potential donor.

Multiple organ donation

This should now be the objective in all brain stem dead potential donors. Assiduous supportive treatment, based on a clear understanding of the physiological changes associated with brain stem death, is essential to prevent deterioration of initially suitable donors, as this will both increase the likelihood of successful donation and improve graft survival and function.[20]

Unused organs

Causes of failure to use offered, suitable organs include nonsuitability of the organs by the time of donor surgery, lack of suitable recipients, nonavailability of a transplant team, lack of theater time and shortage of intensive care beds for the recipient. Attention to these logistical difficulties and the allocation of organs might help to reduce the incidence of nonprocurement of offered suitable organs.[18] Prompt completion of brain stem testing should minimize the incidence of organs becoming unsuitable due to deterioration of the donor. In some studies refusal by the coroner to release the body has been a common cause of missed potential donors.[17] Home Office guidelines to the coroners state that permission for donation should be refused only when the organ might be required in evidence or might be of value to any further inquiry. Clearly it is essential to discuss the case with the coroner before death is certified but coroner's refusal should at worst be a declining impediment to donation.

Religious objections

Religious or moral objections to organ donation are rare[16] but do occasionally prevent procurement of suitable organs. At one extreme are the Christian Scientists who, because they believe in the reality of the spiritual realm and the ultimate unreality of the body, sickness and death, oppose not only the specific techniques of organ transplantation but also the entirety of traditional medical practice. In the Jewish faith there are now few who would dispute the rightfulness of kidney transplantation from a healthy living donor and opinion is moving towards acceptance of brain death as representing the termination of life, thereby removing a major obstacle to procurement of cadaveric organs. It has also been argued that secondary concerns, such as mutilation of the dead, gaining profit from their remains

and deferring burial, are immediately overruled where the life of a prospective recipient is at stake.[21] Nevertheless some very orthodox Jews (for example Hassidics) do not accept the concept of brain stem death and will not agree to discontinuation of mechanical ventilation, let alone organ donation. Although Islamic views on transplantation are based on the underlying principle of saving human life, and donation of organs from both the living and the dead is generally regarded as permissible, religious beliefs regarding bodily resurrection and cultural norms surrounding the treatment of the dead with respect and consideration make organ donation loathsome to some Muslims.[22] For Buddhists, on the other hand, realization of the oneness of human kind and the universe allows human beings to share in the suffering, as well as the happiness, of their fellows and organ donation can therefore be viewed as a noble act.[23]

Increasing the pool of brain stem dead potential donors

ELECTIVE VENTILATION

Elective ventilation has been advocated as a means of retrieving organs from the pool of potential donors who are known to die on general wards from cerebrovascular events without being mechanically ventilated[24–26] and has the potential almost to double the number of brain stem dead organ donors.[24] Whereas conventional brain stem dead organ donors are initially ventilated in the hope that they will recover, this former procedure involves instituting mechanical ventilation in the certain knowledge that the patient will die.

The ethical dilemma is that one is intervening before the point of death with invasive, 'extraordinary' measures which, although likely to benefit others cannot benefit the patient, whose death has been deemed inevitable. Proponents of elective ventilation argue that it involves no more than the management of an inevitable and rapid death in such a way as to maintain vital organs in a suitable condition for donation, intervention taking place as close as possible to the time of natural death (i.e. immediately before or at the point at which breathing ceases). Moreover, patients are only ventilated after the situation has been fully explained to the next of kin and permission has been obtained to proceed. Since surveys indicate that 75% of the public would wish to donate their organs in the event of sudden death, it can be argued that elective ventilation is justified because it ensures that the wishes of the majority of patients are fulfilled.

There is a discrete group of patients who suffer overwhelming intracerebral vascular events, usually subarachnoid hemorrhage, which inevitably progress rapidly to death. Some of these patients arrive in hospital with inadequate or absent breathing, undergo immediate resuscitation and are admitted to intensive care units where it soon becomes obvious that the prognosis is hopeless. Active efforts cease and the patient is declared brain stem dead. Others arrive in hospital slightly earlier in the course of events with adequate spontaneous respiration, the prognosis is assessed as hopeless and they are admitted to a general ward to die. In both cases the sequence of events is determined largely by the timing of the patient's arrival in hospital; this may be related as much to where they live as to any other factor. To deny one group of patients the opportunity of becoming organ donors, and to deny the recipients the possibility of receiving an organ, solely on the basis of geography, could be seen as arbitrary and wasteful.

Many have been concerned that elective ventilation could place unacceptable demands on limited facilities and might adversely effect staff morale. Perhaps more worrying is the suggestion that the procedure could produce significant numbers of patients in a persistent vegetative state. Were this to happen it would indeed be a tragedy and would considerably increase the ethical dilemmas posed by the procedure. The experience of the Exeter Group, however, is that, using their strict protocol for identifying potential donors, no such patients have been produced in the first 5 years and to date there have been no published instances of such an outcome. Clearly, more information will be required before the majority of the medical profession can form an opinion.

Not only might it be seen as unethical to artificially delay a patient's death in the interests of a third party, but some lawyers consider it illegal to intervene in a patient's demise without their express consent. They argue that at the time of intervention the patient, who is not a corpse, is incapable of giving informed consent and that any treatment undertaken must therefore clearly be seen to be in their best interests. It is, however, unlikely that the issue will be resolved on the basis of legal opinion alone. Provided elective ventilation became accepted as reasonable practice by the majority of clinicians it would probably be unnecessary to enact specific legislation. Furthermore, if it is considered that the doctor's responsibility is not just to a single patient but to patients in general, then the benefits of elective ventilation are clear. The recipients benefit because they otherwise would not receive organs and, in the majority of cases, the patient's wish to become an organ donor is fulfilled. The donor's family may also benefit since their grief may be lessened by knowing that some good has come out of an inevitable death. On balance therefore it would seem that, although the legality of elective ventilation will be difficult to establish, provided prior consent is obtained

from the next of kin, respect for the patient is maintained and brain stem death is established before organ retrieval, many practitioners would consider such behavior reasonable, morally right and, therefore, ethically correct. It is essential that carefully designed protocols, particularly regarding who should make the decision to institute elective ventilation, the identification of suitable patients and when to intervene, should be agreed by all interested parties.

Following publication of the Exeter experience in 1990 a combined working party of the Royal College of Surgeons and the Royal College of Anaesthetists produced a report. This working party took advice from the President of the British Transplantation Society and the Chairman of the Intensive Care Society. The report recommended that 'Elective ventilation should be looked at by other units and that consideration should be given to following the Exeter Protocol.' Subsequently the issue was discussed by the British Medical Association (BMA) Ethics Committee, which has a large membership of clinicians, nurses, lawyers, philosophers, ethicists and lay people. This group again gave their approval to the procedure of elective ventilation provided the relatives were fully informed and that a comprehensive protocol, common to all centers in the UK, was observed. Most recently elective ventilation was discussed by the Ethical Committee of the British Transplantation Society, who suggested that all transplant units in the UK should encourage such practice, utilizing the guidelines issued by the BMA. Finally, the Royal College of Physicians published a discussion document in 1993 which again supported the practice of elective ventilation according to the BMA guidelines for organ donation in this particular group of patients. Since 1990 the elective ventilation procedure has been widely discussed throughout the country and has been generally accepted by those involved in transplantation and by general physicians, as well as intensive care clinicians and nurses. It appears that the majority of medical practitioners consider elective ventilation for the purpose of organ retrieval responsible and reasonable behavior; it can therefore be considered ethically correct. The legal position remains unclear, however, and a few remain concerned that the acceptance of elective ventilation for organ donation, a procedure from which the patient cannot benefit, represents the first step along a particularly dangerous path.

NON HEART BEATING CADAVERIC DONORS

Because kidneys are relatively resistant to ischemia they can in theory be retrieved soon after cardiac arrest, provided prior consent has been obtained from the patient, or the relatives' consent immediately after the event. A large but as yet untapped source of potential donors includes victims of motor vehicle or other accidents who rapidly succumb to their injuries, with cardiorespiratory arrest supervening either immediately before or on arrival in hospital. Since kidneys tolerate no more than 30 minutes of warm ischemia this approach has so far been limited by the need to obtain consent before organ retrieval. Some now suggest immediate percutaneous cannulation and cold perfusion whilst the views of the next of kin are sought.[27] Provided this approach is tightly controlled, and well designed protocols are followed, it may become acceptable practice in the future. Currently, however, most would hold the view that the permission of relatives should be obtained before invasive procedures, designed solely for the purpose of salvaging organs, are instituted.

Alternative sources of organs for transplantation

LIVING DONORS

This source of organs for transplantation does not directly concern the intensive care doctor, and is used infrequently in the UK. It raises some important ethical considerations which involve balancing the risks to the donor against their altruistic desire to donate an organ to a sick relative and their right to dispose of their own body parts as they wish. Clearly live donation should only be considered when the immediate risks are minimal and longer-term donor survival is not seriously jeopardized; it is therefore confined to removal of one of a pair of organs (e.g. kidney), part of an organ (e.g. pancreas, liver) or a tissue such as bone marrow. Even under these circumstances the incidence of complications is sufficient to cause concern. In living related kidney donors, for example, major perioperative complications were seen in 7% of donors and included wound infections, splenic injury and pancreatitis. Major late complications occurred in 20% of those followed for 1–15 years and included hypertension, incisional hernia, bowel obstruction and nephrolithiasis.[28] Recently the ethics of transplanting a lobe of the liver from the recipient's parent[29] and of lung transplantation using a live donor,[30] have been addressed with regard to the balance between risks and benefits, selection and informed consent for both recipients and donor.

The decision of the donor must be informed and voluntary, and the risks of donor complications must be fully explained. It is particularly important to establish that the donor has not been pressurized to consent to the procedure, although it is often difficult to determine whether there has been coercion within the confines of a family. Incompetent persons (e.g. children and the mentally retarded) must be excluded because they cannot give informed consent.

The legality of live donation is not in question but there is no licence to consent to a practice in which the risk/benefit ratio would be manifestly to the consenter's disadvantage, and an individual could not, for example, consent to donate their heart. Equally it is unlawful to consent to accept an organ in the certainty or near-certainty that it would be fatal to do so. Finally, genetically unrelated live donation is illegal, although the Unrelated Live Transplant Regulatory Authority (ULTRA) can authorize such an operation provided it is satisfied that no payment is involved, the donor has been counselled and consents to the risks of the operation and that both the donor and recipient have been interviewed in such a way as to enable the counsellor to identify any difficulties in communication.

THE DONOR AS VENDOR[31]

Concerns about this practice were crystallized when it was discovered that kidneys were being purchased, mainly from Turkish donors, for use in private hospitals in London. Subsequently this practice was outlawed in the UK, the practitioners involved were either struck off or had their practices severely curtailed and the UK General Medical Council said that they would respond very strongly if such an event were to happen again. Some, however, wonder whether it is in fact reasonable to condemn all such transactions. They argue that individuals have an absolute right to dispose of their body parts as and when they wish. Clearly it is reprehensible that some people are so poor that they are forced to consider selling their organs (often their only asset), but some have suggested that it is equally indefensible to prevent them benefiting from such a process whilst doing nothing to alleviate their poverty. Can it be considered unethical for someone to sell their kidney in order, for example, to purchase medicines for their own child, when at the same time it is acceptable for that person to donate the same kidney to the same child. Many, however, feel that the purchase of organs is a fundamentally degrading process, which is likely to have adverse effects on society's values as a whole, and would expect the state to protect its most vulnerable citizens from such exploitation. In the current climate it is unlikely that attitudes to this practice will change, at any rate in the UK, and payment for organs from unrelated donors will almost certainly remain illegal.

ANENCEPHALIC DONORS[32]

Organ retrieval from anencephalic donors concerns practitioners in neonatal units rather than intensive care units but it raises some particularly difficult ethical issues. The only source of such potential donors are anencephalic fetuses born to women who object to termination under any circumstances or when a mother wishes to mature the fetus solely for the purpose of providing organs for transplantation. There are those who suggest that, since anencephalics are 'brain absent,' incapable of consciousness and have no ability to respond to the outside world other than by reflex action, they cannot be considered to be truly alive. Philosophers might contend that an anencephalic is not a person and lawyers might suggest that they are not 'a reasonable creature in being.' Others consider this argument to be a first step along a very dangerous slippery slope. It is the view of the Royal Colleges that 'Organs for transplantation can be removed from anencephalic infants when two doctors who are not members of the transplant team agree that spontaneous respiration has ceased.' This will almost certainly form the basis of accepted practice, although there are many who would not consider this to be ethical behavior.

It is disturbing that similar arguments have been applied to those in a persistent vegetative state, some philosophers describing them as 'socially dead.' The question of whether such patients should be considered as potential organ donors has therefore been raised. However the irreversibility of unresponsiveness in such cases can only be predicted with 95–98% accuracy, and death of the cortex with an intact brain stem cannot be sufficient to determine death. Although some[33] have in the past considered the possibility of organ retrieval from breathing 'cadavers' this practice is illegal, is likely to remain so, and is most unlikely to achieve wide acceptance. The vast majority of clinicians would consider this suggestion to be unethical.

THE FETUS AS DONOR

Following spontaneous or therapeutic abortion fetal tissue might be used for transplantation, subject to the informed consent of the mother. The therapeutic value of fetal tissue, for example implantation of cells from the substantia nigra into patients with Parkinson's disease, depends on the fact that the cells are actively proliferating. Because of concerns about the transplantation of parts of human brains the BMA have recommended that only isolated neurones or tissue fragments should be used.

Xenografts[34] and artificial organs for permanent implantation

There is reason to hope that in the future these techniques will be used to reduce the waiting lists for transplantation. There has been some success with developing transgenic pigs, for example. Intensive care clinicians are likely to be involved in the preoperative and postoperative care of the recipient but these techniques are unlikely to pose any serious ethical dilemmas, although some in the Animal Rights lobby object to what they consider to be unwarranted exploitation of animals.

Allocation of donated organs[35]

The allocation of organs is clearly not the responsibility of intensive care practitioners and is organized by the National Transplant Societies in various countries. Ethical dilemmas do arise and include such issues as whether liver transplants should be performed in those with alcoholic liver disease. Scoring systems for allocation of organs have been developed based on factors such as time spent on the waiting list, matching of tissue antigens, medical urgency and logistics. Unfortunately selection of recipients by scoring is time-consuming and such systems only work well for kidneys which tolerate a considerably longer preservation time with currently available techniques than do organs such as the heart and liver.

Payment for donated organs

Although in the UK any inducement to donate organs by payment is illegal, it is recognized that considerable costs are incurred by the donor hospital. This is a particular issue for hospitals without transplant units which derive no direct benefit from transplantation surgery, for example by reducing their waiting lists or taking patients off dialysis. In the UK an official reimbursement scheme which makes some contribution towards these costs has recently been introduced without any real debate about the ethics of such a policy, which could be seen as involving an element of inducement. The general public might also be uncomfortable with reimbursement. Most would agree, however, that provided they are strictly controlled, such payments are reasonable and ethical.

Conclusion

Continuing advances in all aspects of transplantation, for example the use of artificial hearts as a 'bridge' to transplantation, are certain to increase the demand for donor organs. Not only must new transplantation techniques be developed and organ retrieval maximized, but we must remain vigilant to ensure that the highest ethical standards are maintained.

References

1. Pallis C. ABC of brain stem death. *Bri Med J* 1983.
2. Mollaret, P, Goulon M. Le coma depasse (memoire preliminaire). *Rev Neurol* 1959; **101**: 3–15.
3. Mohandas A, Chou SN. Brain death – a clinical and pathological study. *J Neurosurg* 1971; **35**: 211–18.
4. Conference of Medical Royal Colleges and their Faculties in the U.K. Diagnosis of death. *Br Med J* 1976; **ii**: 1187–8.
5. Conference of Medical Royal Colleges and their Faculties in the U.K. Diagnosis of death. *Br Med J* 1979; **i**: 3320.
6. Hill DJ, Evans DW, Gresham GA. Availability of cadaver organs for transplantation (letter). *Br Med J* 1991; **303**: 312.
7. Gramm H-J, Zimmermann J, Meinhold H, Dennhardt R, Voigt K. Hemodynamic responses to noxious stimuli in brain-dead organ donors. *Intensive Care Med* 1992; **18**: 493–5.
8. Timmins AC, Hinds CJ. Availability of cadaver organs for transplantation (letter). *Br Med J* 1991; **303**: 583.
9. Jennett B, Gleave J, Wilson P. Brain death in three neurosurgical units. *Br Med J* 1981; **281**: 533–9.
10. [Editorial]. Organ donors in the UK – getting the numbers right. *Lancet* 1990; **335**: 80–2.
11. Taylor RMR. Opting in or out of organ donation. *Br Med J* 1992; **305**: 1380.
12. Gore SM, Hinds CJ, Rutherford AJ. Organ donation from intensive care units in England. *Br Med J* 1989; **299**: 1193–7.
13. Gore SM, Cable DJ, Holland AJ. Organ donation from intensive care units in England and Wales: two year confidential audit of death in intensive care. *Br Med J* 1992; **304**: 349–55.
14. Alexander JW. The cutting edge – a look to the future in transplantation. *Transplantation* 1990; **49**: 237–40.
15. Social Surveys (Gallup Poll). *Attitudes Towards Kidney Doning*. London: Gallup, 1992.
16. Wakeford RE, Stepney R. Obstacles to organ donation. *Br J Surg* 1989; **76**: 435–9.
17. Bodenham A, Berridge JC, Park GR. Brain stem death and organ donation. *Br Med J* 1989; **299**: 1009–10.
18. Gore SM, Taylor RMR, Wallwork J. Availability of transplantable organs from brain stem dead donors in intensive care units. *Br Med J* 1991; **302**: 149–53.
19. Gore SM, Armitage WJ, Briggs JD *et al*. Consensus on general medical contraindications to organ donation? *Br Med J* 1992; **305**: 406–9.
20. Timmins AC, Hinds CJ. Management of the multiple organ donor. *Curr Opin Anaesthesiol* 1991; **4**: 287–92.
21. Weiss DW. Organ transplantation, medical ethics and Jewish law. *Transplant Proc* 1988; **xx**: 1071–5.
22. Sachedina AA. Islamic views on organ transplantation. *Transplant Proc* 1988; **xx**: 1084–8.
23. Tsuji KT. The Buddist view of the body and organ transplantation. *Transplant Proc* 1988; **xx**: 1076–8.
24. Feest TG, Riad HN, Collins CH, Golby MGS, Nicholls AJ, Hamad SN. Protocol for increasing organ donation after cerebrovascular deaths in a district general hospital. *Lancet* 1990; **335**: 1133–5.
25. Salih MAM, Harvey I, Frankel S, Coupe DJ, Webb M, Cripps HA. Potential availability of cadaver organs for transplantation. *Br Med J* 1991; **302**: 1053–5.
26. Hibberd AD, Pearson IY, McCosker CJ *et al*. Potential for cadaveric organ retrieval in New South Wales. *Br Med J* 1992; **304**: 1339–43.
27. Anaise D, Smith R, Ishimaru M, Waltzer WC, Shabtai M, Hurley S, Rapaport FT. An approach to organ salvage from non-heartbeating cadaver donors under existing legal and ethical requirements for transplantation. *Transplantation* 1990; **49**: 290–4.
28. Dunn JF, Richie RE, MacDonnell RC, Nylander WA, Johnson MK, Sawyers JL. Living related kidney donors. A 14 year experience. *Ann Surg* 1986; **203**: 637–43.
29. Singer PA, Siegler M, Whitington PF *et al*. Ethics of liver transplantation with living donors. *New Engl J Med* 1989; **321**: 620–1.
30. Shaw LR, Miller JD, Slutsky AS *et al*. Ethics of lung transplantation with live donors. *Lancet* 1991; **338**: 678–81.
31. Wight JP. Ethics, commerce and kidneys. *Br Med J* 1991; **303**: 110.
32. Beller FK, Reeve J. Brain life and brain death – the anencephalic as an explanatory example. A contribution to transplantation. *Med Philos* 1986; **14**: 5–23.
33. Younger SJ, Bartlett ET. Human death and high technology: the failure of the whole brain formulations. *Ann Intern Med* 1983; **99**: 252–8.
34. Calne R. Organs from animals. *Br Med J* 1993; **307**: 637–8.
35. Starzl TE, Shapiro R, Teperman L. The point system for organ distribution. *Transplant Proc* 1989; **21**: 3432–6.

CHAPTER 25

Clinical Research in Intensive Care Medicine: Ethics in Clinical Research

BARA RICOU, PETER M SUTER

Necessity for research in intensive care medicine   360
Ethics committee   361
Requirements for good research   362
Complexity of research in the ICU   362
How to achieve good standards in research   365
References   366

Necessity for research in intensive care medicine

Human beings have always tried to resist death, and physicians working in an intensive care unit (ICU) are at the forefront of this fight. Because of the serious nature of the illnesses encountered in ICU patients, research in intensive care medicine has often been seen as difficult, although a scientific approach is clearly required. Scientific research is the only way to improve medical care since it leads to the understanding of disease phenomena and sound evaluation of new therapies. It is not an aim in itself, but a means of achieving progress. Experimental research and clinical investigation have made possible the tremendous advances seen in intensive care medicine during the last three decades. Patients now survive after severe trauma when in the past they would have died. The same is true for those undergoing major surgery, who are now submitted to intensive surveillance to minimize the risk of postoperative complications.

Clinical research also influences decisions concerning admission to the ICU; such research suggests which patients will derive the greatest benefit from intensive care, as well as the choice of treatment that will have the greatest effect on outcome. However, in many instances the technology has outstripped our capacity to judge the scientific value of modern therapeutics. There are numerous examples of so-called compassionate treatments where the physician, facing an extreme situation in a critically ill patient, feels motivated to try a new treatment before its complete evaluation (i.e. extracorporeal carbon dioxide removal, high-frequency jet ventilation, hemofiltration, cardiac assist devices, intravenous oxygenator, etc.). However, how do we know whether all these advanced technological therapeutics will really change the outcome in these patients? Do these interventions really change the patient's future in terms of mortality, morbidity or quality of life? Don't they only prolong illness and sustain life in ICU? Many recently developed techniques improve hemodynamics or respiratory variables on a short-term basis, without there being documented benefit on long-term outcome, cost:benefit ratio or patient comfort.

The progressive rise in medical costs is at least one of the consequences of the application of new technologies.[1] Intensive care medicine accounts for a substantial part of the hospital budget, while it treats only a small percentage of the whole population. Its elevated cost is not only due to the high technology used in ICU and the requirement for highly trained staff, but also to the prolonged stay of some patients who eventually die. An important effort in research has provided a number of scoring systems such as the Acute Physiology and Chronic Health Evaluation (APACHE), the Simplified Acute Physiology Score (SAPS) and the Mortality Prediction Model (MPM), allowing the estimation of hospital mortality for well-defined patient groups. However, none of these scoring systems can predict the outcome for an individual, and they are even less valid for other important outcome variables such as morbidity or quality of life. Thus, at the present stage of our knowledge, intensive care is applied to many patients who might not need it. More research is required to ascertain which treatment is useful or futile in which kind of patients.

Many areas and topics in intensive care medicine require more research. The Research Division of the Society of Critical Care Medicine (SCCM) has recently published a statement summarizing their view of the current and future status of research in critical medicine.[2] The fields of research identified in this statement are grouped into:

- natural history, risk and outcome research
- intensive care unit technology and therapeutic intervention
- optimal personnel and technical resources in the ICU
- disease entity research (Table 25.1).

The task of the intensive care physician intent on using the scientific approach will be difficult. He or she will have to collaborate with basic scientists in this research

Table 25.1   Priority disease entities for investigation in intensive care medicine

Multiple organ system failure
Nosocomial infections
Head injury and coma
Acute respiratory failure
Acute obstructive lung disease
Nutrition in the critically ill
Liver failure
Circulatory shock
Cardiogenic shock
Extracardiac obstructive shock
Distributive (low peripheral vascular) shock
Severe heart failure
Cardiopulmonary resuscitation
Serious arrythmias
Unstable ischemic heart disease syndromes
Malignant hypertension
Acute aortic dissection
Acute renal failure
Electrolyte and endocrine problems
Trauma management in the ICU
Burns and electrical injuries
Psychiatric problems in the critically ill
Ethical issues and brain death

and help to bridge the gap between the laboratory bench and the bedside care of patients.

If the answer to the question 'Is research in intensive care medicine useful?' is definitively yes, the next question is 'Is it ethical to undertake clinical investigations in ICU patients?'.[3] Those patients have life-threatening illnesses, and any procedure may trigger a complication which could be fatal. However, as stated before, well-designed studies on specific questions need to be conducted so that the treatment of patients can be based on solid scientific knowledge. Indeed, without research, we will never be sure of the validity, nor the hazards, of a specific treatment. We will not understand the mechanisms leading to disease, an understanding of which is essential if we are to apply the right treatment in the future. However, in addition to a sound scientific reasoning, the ethical feasibility has to be examined for every project. Typically, an ethical committee should be responsible for this aspect.[4] Such a committee generally comprises a number of people from different fields, who evaluate every study so as to balance the expected benefits and the potential risks to patients.

Ethics committee

The decision to undertake a clinical investigation cannot be left to the investigator alone. The proposed study should be judged by a group of informed individuals – the ethics committee. The committee should consist of experienced research workers, doctors of different specialties with expertise in patient care but not directly involved in the study, a nurse, a lawyer, a priest and a mother or layperson.[5,6] Guidelines for the composition of such a committee have been established; although these are not yet entirely satisfactory, they should help in organizing the group and checking its quality.[7-9] The role of this committee would be to analyze the validity of the aims of the study. It should assess whether the study would actually produce results relevant to patient care and weigh the expected benefit against the potential risks for the patients enrolled in the study. During the course of a clinical investigation, the benefit derived from the research by the patients studied might not be evident, except for closer monitoring. Smith[10] proposes the following:

> No treatment is without its dangers, and if doctors use treatments where they have no solid scientific evidence of benefit they are exposing patients to risk when there may not be benefit. There is also what might be called a breach of contract in that the patients assume that the doctors know that the treatment they are using is beneficial. That the doctors themselves may not understand that the evidence for the treatment they are using

is weak or non-existent seems to me to explain but not excuse the breach of contract. The lack of evidence of benefit also means that resources may be wasted on ineffective practices. Resources are always limited, and the lack of evidence means that we cannot concentrate them on treatments that are effective. Indeed, resources may be diverted from more effective uses either within or without the health-care system.

Therefore, it is also an ethical necessity to undertake research in order to provide more effective treatment to patients. No study should be undertaken only to satisfy human curiosity. This curiosity should always be accompanied by a wish to benefit the patients. Studies with no aim of improving medical care in the near or distant future should be rejected by the committee.This committee should favor studies aimed at assessing the short- and long-term effects of therapeutics, their validity and inocuity, in order to avoid jumping at the first opportunity with the empty belief that it may help the patients.[11] Finally, it is the role of this committee to protect the subjects from abuses and from futile studies. According to US federal law, to grant approval, the committee must assure itself that the following conditions are met:

1. the risks to the subjects are so outweighed by the sum of the benefit to the subjects and the importance of the knowledge to be gained as to warrant a decision to allow the subject to accept these risks;
2. the rights and welfare of any such subjects will be adequately protected;
3. legally, effective informed consent will be obtained by adequate and appropriate methods.[12]

However, in the case of research in intensive medicine, the application of these requirements creates a conflict. New insight should be brought to resolve this problem.[3, 11]

Requirements for good research

The first requirements for good clinical research are well-designed studies with a clear purpose, such as the understanding of a phenomenon which is often related to but hidden by others, or the effects of one therapeutic compared to another, and a well-defined endpoint. The necessity for a new study must be warranted and the design appropriate.[13] The benefit that would ensue should be clearly defined, in terms of care of patients, their welfare and outcome, or cost.[14]

Good research should consist of three phases:[1]

• The first phase should consist of *observation*, accumulation of facts and acquisition of expertise in the field.
• The second phase should describe the *hypothesis* on the mechanics leading to the phenomenon, the disease or the potential benefit of the therapeutics. This phase comprises experimental models in animals[15] and *in vitro* studies to confirm the hypothesis before bringing in human consideration.
• The third phase should consist of *modulation*, which implies that the investigators change one variable at a time to assess its effect, with the aim of substantiating the hypothesis.

The only way to answer questions correctly as to the usefulness and validity of a new therapy is to follow a rigorous diagram of research as proposed in Table 25.2. It will then be possible, from the results of these studies, to conclude the real clinical benefit or favorable cost-benefit of a new therapy. Appropriate ethics should be applied in order to answer the questions without harming the patients. General guidelines on research in the ICU have been issued by a council (Ethical Principles in Intensive Care) from the World Federation of Societies of Intensive and Critical Care Medicine [16] and are given in the Declaration of Helsinki.[17]

However, little benefit is to be expected from studies during the first two phases mentioned above. Indeed, neither the observation nor the hypothesis phase could improve the disease or change the outcome in the studied population. Here we must underline the notion of future benefit or social benefit as opposed to individual benefit. The social advantages must overwhelm the risks encountered by the patient enrolled in the research. At this stage, we should emphasize the time it has taken to develop a specific sense of ethics in the particular situation of intensive care medicine. Indeed, since ICU patients differ (they are unconscious, incompetent, dependent, facing death), since their diseases differ (they are critical, rapidly evolving, rapidly fatal), and the techniques applied to them differ (they are heavy, aggressive, supportive, rarely curative), ethics applicable in common medicine are probably not applicable in ICU clinical research.

Complexity of research in the ICU

Research in ICU patients presents many specific problems that are not encountered in other fields of medicine and are responsible for very specific ethical considerations.[3, 18, 19] Physicians working in this branch of medicine are aware of the multiple disturbances caused by critical illness and the difficulties this creates in testing new hypotheses. Many variables need to be

Table 25.2 The ideal scheme of scientific approach to a disease

Means	Approach
	Observation
Clinical observations	Phenomena
Additional exams	Natural clinical course
Histopathology	
	↓
	Hypothesis
Animal models	Risk factors leading to the disease
in vitro studies	Assessment of the factors involved in the course of the diseas
Basic science	Understanding of the pathophysiology
	Assessment of the mechanisms leading to the expected outcome
	Development of the rationale for potential therapeutics
	↓
	Modulation
	Therapeutic interventions
New therapeutic in healthy volunteers	• Assessment of the toxicity/secondary effects of a new treatment
Uncontrolled studies in disease	• Applicability of the treatment in disease and its efficacy
Double blind, placebo-controlled studies in disease	• Comparison with existing therapeutics

considered at the same time in the same patient, and one patient is never identical to another. Moreover, according to age, chronic health state and severity of disease, patients should be stratified theoretically into several subgroups. The acute character of care is induced by the rapidity of clinical evolution, yet the speed of evolution is not uniform among patients. Furthermore, so many variables move at the same time, and not necessarily in one direction, that modification of one variable rarely occurs. The criteria of uniformity for inclusion in a study is rarely fulfilled. How then can we assume that the results obtained are applicable to all patients? From this concept, one easily resorts to case-to-case management, a method which is the exact opposite of what is expected from good research. This problem, commonly encountered in clinical research, may be overcome by increasing the specificity of the inclusion criteria and applying strict treatment protocols.

This requirement, however, raises the problem of the number of cases. No study can pretend to be of any interest if an insufficient number of patients has been examined. When a large number of patients is required, the time necessary to enrol them must be considered. If a study needs too much time to be completed (i.e. many years), the results may not be relevant because of the evolution of knowledge in physiopathology; also the emergence of new therapeutic modalities may have changed the original concept. Moreover, research workers are under constant pressure to show results, otherwise they are threatened with noncontinuation of funding. This often prompts those most eager to do well to enlarge (even unconsciously) the study population to

an extent which creates biases in the final results. This problem is acute in intensive care medicine since most of the studied diseases are rare in terms of community, and furthermore intensive care units are often small. Consequently, how can one be sure that the results obtained are directly applicable to other patients, even if they were true for the majority of patients in the study? Multicenter studies offer one possibility of overcoming this problem. However, the definitions and inclusion criteria have to be very precise and clear to avoid inhomogeneity due to different views in different centers. The acceptability of such a protocol by every institutional research board and ethics committee is a problem.[20, 21]

The four basic principles of medical ethics are:

• maximization of benefit to the patient;
• miminization of harm to the patient;
• individual right of the patient to self-determination;
• maximization of benefit to society.[22]

However, it is quite evident, at least in research areas, that the first statement may sometimes contradict the last statement, and vice versa.[22] Indeed, a studied population might receive a new treatment which ends up being proved to be deleterious. This population did not take profit from the maximization of benefit nor from the minimization of harm to the patient, but would have contributed to the maximization of benefit to society. In contrast, in the case of an uncontrolled study, patients would receive the potentially beneficial therapy for maximization of benefit to themselves, but would not necessarily contribute to the maximization of benefit to society.

Therefore, before a therapeutic agent or therapy is accepted as being useful, studies must be undertaken. It should be mentioned here that, unfortunately, research groups and medical journals systematically fail to publish negative data, which demonstrates a great lack of objectivity and wastes time and resources, since many groups may repeat the experiments that still produce negative results. Some therapeutics under investigation do not produce the expected results or, even worse, they may induce adverse effects harmful to the patient. From the ethical point of view, other patients should not be subjected to the same type of study.

In an earlier section (**Requirements for good research**), three phases of clinical research were mentioned. Critical care research often leaps from the above-mentioned first phase of *observation* to the third of *modulation*, while basic scientists for their part struggle to understand the phenomena. Basic scientists at least have the advantage of dealing with experimental models that can be easily controlled, and are not concerned with the logistic and ethical problems related to clinical studies. However, the relevance and applicability to human disease of experimental study results are questionable.[5] The reasons why the conditions for this second hypothesis phase are rarely fulfilled in intensive care research are obvious. First, time is lacking: critically ill patients evolve quickly and even die rapidly. Phenomena occurring in these patients develop quickly and are therefore difficult to catch and understand step by step. Second, multiple factors intervene at the same time so that analysis of the implication of one of them in the course of the disease is difficult. Third, ethical considerations lead physicians erroneously to try the newest therapeutic without proof of benefit. The third phase of *modulation* has its own difficulties in intensive care medicine. It is impossible to change only one factor at a time in the clinical arena since patients evolve at their own pace and the variables are difficult to regulate.

The principle of three phases of research can be easily applied, for example, in infectious disease studies: in the first phase, the symptoms of the specific infectious disease would be defined; in the second phase the bacteria responsible for the disease would be identified and the specific antibiotic developed; in the third phase the drug would be administered and compared with another known antibiotic therapy to confirm the superiority of the new drug. This kind of study is understandable and acceptable by everybody and would be unlikely to be of ethical concern even for non-physicians. The reason for this easy acceptability in terms of ethics is that infection in this case is an entity well-known to everybody, even to laymen, so that the aim of such a study – the assessment of the efficacy of a new antibiotic therapy – would be clearly understood. The results may be rapidly interpretable, and finally the aim of such a study is directly related to the benefit it will bring to the patient.

Many other fields of critical care medicine are less straightforward. The purpose of studies in these fields is not always as evident as in the case of infection and a potential therapeutic, and possibly not directly and immediately related to welfare of the patient. The reasons why so many studies lack the first two phases which could substantiate their hypothesis are unfeasibility or difficulties closely related to ethical problems. Indeed, if a patient or their next of kin is willing to try a new drug which might improve their outcome or save their life, the patient will not necessarily agree to undergo supplementary and sometimes invasive procedures without any direct personal benefit. Furthermore, the patient might be concerned about possible complications due to those procedures and would not understand the potential benefit for other patients in the future. This is probably a natural human reaction, especially in situations of great distress often experienced by our ICU population. They should not be reproached for such a reaction nor should they be obliged to participate in such a study. However, this is one of the problems we are facing when conducting a purely investigational study.

One of the most debated subjects is *informed consent*. Some authors have even stated that the consent might be a barrier to research.[23,24] Since then, many suggestions have been made to bypass this problem.[25,26] In many countries, the law requires that a clinical study is conducted only after approval by the patient. However, this criteria is difficult to fulfil in the ICU population of patients who are unconscious either because of disease or because of the sedation enabling them to understand the necessary aggressive therapies. This situation represents one of the four exceptions cited in the literature where informed consent is not obligatory: indeed the US Food and Drug Administration regulations contain a provision that would permit subjects to receive experimental resuscitation therapy without informed consent if the following four conditions are met:

1. the human subject is confronted by a life-threatening situation;
2. informed consent cannot be obtained from the subject because of an inability to communicate with, or obtain legally effective consent from the subject;
3. time is not sufficient to obtain consent from the subject's legal representative;
4. there is no alternative generally recognized therapy that provides an equal or greater likelihood of saving the life of the subject.[27]

One way of overcoming the problem of informed consent is to obtain consent from a family member or next of kin. However, in the context of critical illness, it often happens that they do not want to assume any responsibility in the medical management of their relative. They are so concerned about the outcome of the disease that they cannot objectively judge the rightness of such a demand. In addition, it is doubtful whether any consent given under these conditions is of real legal value; people who care for a relative would never refuse anything to the doctors in charge of him or her because, even subconsciously, they would feel that their refusal might compromise the care of the patient.[28]

Another exception which allows physicians to undertake a study without the consent of the patient is the waiving of the right to make decision or the patient's clearly expressed preference that the physician make the decision.[29] This exception cannot be applied in the case of members of the patient's family.

A third possibility which would allow the physician to circumvent the need for informed consent is when the disclosure of the gravity of the disease and the risks related to the innovative therapy or the study is likely to cause a patient physical harm or distress; this situation is called the therapeutic privilege. The next of kin consulted with regard to undertaking a study in an ICU are in an emotionally stressful situation and it should be the concern of the physician not to add to their distress. This is a major ethical problem in clinical investigation in the ICU and in many countries there is no legal written text to which the physician may refer (for instance in Switzerland). Lidz proposed in his article on ethics in clinical research the establishment of a good relationship between the physician and the patient.[30] He is probably right in his claim that when communication has been good between the two partners, there should be no problem in gaining consent, since the patient would have sufficient confidence in his doctor that he would agree to his proposal without hesitation. However, the situation in ICU is slightly different since the therapeutics provided for this particular medical care assume a character of urgency, where it is essential to establish rapidly some kind of patient–physician relationship. Abramson *et al.* report an interesting alternative to informed consent in case of emergency medicine: deferred consent.[31] The therapeutic protocol or investigation under study is begun as soon as judged necessary by the physician; the informed consent is obtained whenever possible from the members of the family thereafter. The family have the opportunity to withdraw the patient from the study if they are not convinced of the utility of the study or do not agree with the ongoing investigation. Although this way of circumventing the rigorous procurement of an informed consent is attractive, it must be emphasized that no legal basis exists for such an approach.

Another interesting proposal regarding this problem in emergency situations was made by Grim, who suggested a 'two-step' consent.[32] The patient is asked if he or she accepts the proposed studied therapeutic as a first step. When the clinical situation has improved, a proposal is made to continue to participate in the study, which means undergoing another examination or intervention – the second step. Despite its potential interest, this approach also needs to be approved by law.

The reason for obtaining informed consent should not be forgotten. This procedure is designed to protect the patient from medical abuse. Indeed, signing the informed consent means that the patient or their surrogate has been informed of the potential benefit of the investigation or a new therapeutic as well as its side effects, that he or she accepts the risks related to such a study and thus would not complain about any eventual negative effects, complications, etc. due to the investigation. This implies that patients or members of their family are taking a full part in the management of the patient. To play a full part in making any decision, clear understanding and complete knowledge of the alternatives are necessary; however, medical science is not part of common knowledge. Therefore, how can a patient in such a particular and vulnerable situation as in an ICU be asked if the proposed treatment is convenient for him? How can the patient make such a decision in only a few minutes, since events are so rapid in an ICU? It is only by providing enough information and trying to establish a real climate of confidence that in the future the general public will be ready to sign the informed consent with real responsibility.[3]

How to achieve good standards in research

Good standards in clinical research begin with a clear definition of the requirements of the study. Ethics is one of the most important issues, although one of the most difficult to define and to teach. It is not sufficient to be a good physician; the researcher must also be capable of conducting a study that will help to improve patient care in the future. The primary requirement is education of the physicians themselves. It is a frequent practice in the USA that every physician beginning a career in any branch of medicine participates in a research activity. However, this is not a common rule in all countries, nor in small hospitals, and the word research sometimes sounds out of place. In this context where physicians have not been well enough prepared to undertake any research, it is not surprising that patients are even less ready than the physicians to take part in a clinical study. Thus if research is to be done well, training institutions must ensure that all students are involved with research at least once during their training.[33, 34] This must be an integral part of their education.[35]

The second requirement for achieving good standards in research is the education of the subjects of research, i.e. the general population. People need to recognize that medical science is not as infallible as was once thought and that physicians do not have all the answers – they do not have the power of healing any disease. The general population must accept the idea that physicians are also human beings and are therefore capable of making mistakes, and that responsibility must be shared by all, including the individual patient, their family, the community and even the politicians. They must learn to participate in research – not passively, acting as guinea pigs, but as active partners concerned about the future welfare of society.[36] The corollary of this is that everyone should feel concerned about medicine and its development. It is medical practitioners' role to provide adequate information to foster the general population's awareness of the necessity as well as the utility of research. When this aim is achieved on general basis, then patients will be ready to take a full part in research as motivated and informed individuals.

References

1. Moore FD. The desperate case : CARE (costs, applicability, research, ethics). *J Am Med Assoc* 1989; **261**: 1483–4.
2. Parillo JE. Research in critical care medicine : present status of critical care investigation. *Crit Care Med* 1991; **19**: 569–77.
3. Iserson KV, Mahowald MB. Acute care research : is it ethical? *Crit Care Med* 1992; **20**: 1032–7.
4. Kirkman E, Little R. The organisation of experimental studies related to intensive care. *Intensive Care World* 1991; **8**: 116–19.
5. Dobb GJ. Research in intensive care medicine. *Intensive Care World* 1991; **8**: 115.
6. Lock St. Monitoring research ethical committees. The profession must establish effective mechanisms with teeth, before the government imposes them. *Br Med J* 1990; **300**: 61–2.
8. Moodie PCE, Marshall T. Guidelines for local research ethics committees. *Br Med J* 1992; **304**: 1293–5.
9. Moodie PCE. The role of local research ethics committees. *Br Med J* 1992; **304**: 1129–30.
10. Smith R. The ethics of ignorance. *J Med Ethics* 1992; **18**: 117–18.
11. Abramson NS, Meisel A, Safar P. Informed consent in resuscitation research. *J Am Med Assoc* 1981; **246**: 2828–30.
12. Protection of Human Subjects. Code of Federal Regulation, title 45, pt 46.
13. Carpenter LM. Is the study worth doing? *Lancet* 1993; **342**: 221–3.
14. American College of Physicians. American college of physicians Ethics Manual. Part 2: The physician and society; research; life-sustaining treatment; other issues. *Ann Intern Med* 1989; **111**: 327–35.
15. Loeb JM, Hendee WR, Smith SJ, Schwarz MR. Human vs animal rights. In defense of animal research. *J Am Med Assoc* 1989; **262**: 2716–20.
16. The World Federation of Societies of Intensive and Critical Care Medicine. Suter PM. Introduction: Ethical principles in intensive care. Council WFSICCM: Ethical guidelines. *Intensive Cri Care Digest* 1992; **11**: 40–1.
17. Declaration of Helsinki, adopted by the 18th World Medical Assembly, Helsinki, Finland, 1964, and revised by the 29th World Medical Assembly, Tokyo, Japan, 1975.
18. Luce JM. Conflicts over ethical principles in the intensive care unit. *Crit Care Med* 1992; **20**: 313–15.
19. Park GR. Ethical and moral difficulties with trials in critically ill patients. *Intensive Care World* 1989; **6**: 11–12.
20. Benster R, Pollock A. Ethics and multicentre research projects. *Br Med J* 1992; **304**: 1696.
21. Horwitz R, Cheetham CH. Ethics and multicentre research projects. *Br Med J* 1992; **304**: 1446.
22. Boissaubin EV, Dresser R. Informed consent in emergency care: illusion and reform. *Ann Emergency Med* 1987; **16**: 62/89–67/94.
23. Fost N. Consent as a barrier to research. *New Engl J Med* 1979 **300**: 1272–3.
24. Relman AS. The ethics of randomized clinical trials: two perspectives. *New Engl J Med* 1979; **300**: 1272–4.
25. Zelen M. A new design for randomized clinical trials. *New Engl J Med* 1979; **300**: 1242–5.
26. Rosner F. The ethics of randomized clinical trials. *Am J Med* 1987; **82**: 283–90.
27. Department of Health and Human Services, Food and Drug Administration. Protection of human subjects: informed consent. *Federal Register* 1981; **46**: 8942–79.
28. Buchanan AE, Brock DW (eds). *Deciding for others: The Ethics of Surrogate Decision Making*. Cambridge: Cambridge University Press, 1990.
29. Meisel A. The *exception* to informed consent doctrine: striking a balance between competing values in medical decisionmaking. *Wis Law Res* 1979; 413–88.
30. Lidz CW, Appelbaum PS, Meisel A. Two models of implementing imformed consent. *Arch Intern Med* 1988; **148**: 1385–9.
31. Abramson NS, Meisel A, Safar P. Deferred consent. A new approach for resuscitation on comatose patients. *J Am Med Assoc* 1986; **255**: 2466–71.
32. Grim PS, Singer PA, Gramelspacher GP, Feldman T, Childers RW, Siegler M. Informed consent in emergency research. Prehospital thrombolytic therapy for acute myocardial infarction. *J Am Med Assoc* 1989; **262**: 252–5.
33. Arias IM. Training basic scientists to bridge the gap between basic science and its application to human disease. *New Engl J Med* 1990; **321**: 972–4.
34. Neale G. The place of research in the training of a physician. *J Roy Coll Physicians* 1991; **25**: 188–90.
35. Smith R. Being bullish about medical research. The need to accept concentration. *Br Med J* 1989; **298**: 544–5.
36. Herz DA, Looman JE, Lewis SK. Informed consent: is it a myth? *Neurosurgery* 1992; **30**: 453–8.

CHAPTER 26

Medico-Legal Aspects of Critical Care

United Kingdom
JENNY L URWIN
Decisions concerning medical treatment   367
Competent patients   372
Incompetent patients   373
Is feeding a medical treatment?   377
Do not resuscitate orders   378
Prospects for reform   378
References   380

United States of America
MARSHALL B KAPP
The regulation of critical care   382
Medical malpractice   383
Risk management and related issues   387
Conclusion   389
References   389

United Kingdom

JENNY L URWIN

Advances in the treatment and care of critically ill patients now enable many lives to be sustained for longer than was the case 40 years ago. An inevitable side effect of this development is, for some unlucky patients, the prolongation of the dying process and subsequent loss of dignity. This has focused attention on the legal rights of patients to exercise their autonomy and to decide on the nature and extent of their treatment. Patients are asserting the right to die with dignity. Medical decision making is now being questioned and has become more susceptible to legal challenge. For example, the Court of Appeal in *Re T*[1] was called upon to make a declaration about the lawfulness of administering a blood transfusion to an unconscious Jehovah's Witness who had earlier refused her consent to the procedure. In addition, questions concerning the criminal liability of health care professionals arise when termination of life-sustaining treatment results in the death of the patient. Deficiencies and uncertainties in the law in respect of decision making on behalf of those unable to make decisions for themselves have introduced further complexities and difficulties in relation to the medical treatment of incompetent patients.

The confusion surrounding the treatment of the critically ill and dying is exacerbated by misunderstanding of the many complicated legal issues involved. It still proves necessary to analyze cases in foreign jurisdictions, in particular the USA, although care must be taken in relying on American precedents. Many such American cases are founded on American Constitutional law and the right of privacy and, as a consequence, the principles they establish cannot simply be transferred and applied unequivocally into English common law.

Compared to ten years ago, there is now quite a body of jurisprudence on these medico-legal issues emerging in the UK, the most significant of these being *Airedale National Health Service Trust v Bland*,[2] the first 'right to die' case in the UK. The modern-day rights debate reveals an increasing awareness of patients' rights in respect of their medical treatment.

Decisions concerning medical treatment

One preliminary question is whether a patient can demand that *all* available treatment should be provided whatever the costs or benefits?

There are no circumstances in which a patient can *insist* that doctors exceed their normal duty. In *Re J*[3] a baby suffered severe and permanent brain damage and was likely to develop serious spastic quadriplegia. He would be blind and deaf and unlikely ever to speak or develop intellectual abilities. He was expected to die before late adolescence, but was neither on the point of death or dying. It was held that in exercising its inherent jurisdiction to protect the interests of minors, a court should never indirectly or directly order a medical practitioner to treat the minor in a manner contrary to the practitioner's duty. That duty was to treat the patient in accordance with the doctor's own best clinical judgment, notwithstanding that other practitioners might have formed a different judgment. Consequently, once a doctor has performed his or her duty of care, the patient cannot demand more in excess of that duty.

The predominant legal issues posed by the care of the critically ill relate mainly to the nature and extent of the treatment provided. Questions of criminal liability arise where withdrawal of medical treatment accelerates the death of a patient. Will the administration of pain-killing drugs, which have the effect of shortening the life of the patient, expose health care professionals to allegations of homicide? Similarly, where an artificial lung ventilator is switched off at the request of the patient, does the doctor commit the offence of aiding and abetting suicide, or alternatively murder or manslaughter?

LIFE-SHORTENING TREATMENT

No person may, for any reason, kill or assist suicide. Under English law, any person who intentionally and unlawfully takes the life of another commits murder; if the killing is done negligently or recklessly this is manslaughter. The definition of murder requires only that there is some acceleration of death; it makes no difference that the victim is already suffering from a fatal disease or injury.[4] All attempts to legalize active euthanasia have failed. In the Netherlands, an informal agreement between the authorities and the medical profession allow active euthanasia to take place as long as certain guidelines are adhered to. Despite this, euthanasia has never been legalized.[5]

In England, any doctor who commits an act of 'mercy-killing' or active euthanasia will expose himself or herself to liability under the criminal law.[6] *R v Adams*[6] provides one exception to this. The case was concerned with the administration of pain-killing but life-shortening drugs by a doctor to an 81-year-old woman. The allegation was that Dr Adams had administered such large quantities of drugs, particularly heroin and morphia, that he must have known the result would have been the death of his patient. Devlin J (as he then was) directed the jury that murder was an act or series of acts which were intended to kill and did in fact kill. It did not matter that the patient's death was inevitable and that her days were numbered but that, if her life was shortened by weeks or months, it was just as much murder as if it was cut short by years. He emphasized that there was no special defense that could be employed because a doctor acted mercifully to shorten life. Nonetheless, he continued:

> But that does not mean that a doctor aiding the sick and dying has to calculate in minutes or hours, or perhaps in weeks or days, the effect on a patient's life of the medicines which he administers. If the first purpose of medicine – the restoration of health – can no longer be achieved, there is still much for the doctor to do, and he is entitled to do all that is proper and necessary to relieve pain and suffering even if measures he takes may incidentally shorten life by hours or perhaps even longer.

The law has introduced a clear distinction between the active ending of life, and using means for the relief of suffering which may, as a side effect, shorten life.[8] Therefore, if medication used to relieve pain has the secondary result of cutting short the patient's life span there will be no criminal liability. The circumstances are very different where the dose is administered with the intention that the patient should die. This is murder. In *R v Cox*[9] Dr Cox was convicted of attempted murder[10] having, admittedly, injected a lethal dose of potassium chloride into his terminally ill patient, Lillian Boyes, who died almost instantly. Mrs Boyes had declined further medical treatment, except for pain-killers, 5 days before her death and she had repeatedly asked Dr Cox and others to kill her because she found her situation intolerable. Evidence was given that potassium chloride was not an analgesic and had no curative properties and further that the quantity of neat potassium chloride injected into Mrs Boyes was in fact a fatal dose. In Ognall J's summing up to the jury he drew the following crucial distinction:

> Is it proved that in giving that injection, in that form and in those amounts, Dr Cox's primary purpose was to bring the life of Lillian Boyes to an end?
> If it was, then he is guilty. If, on the other hand, it was, or may have been, his primary purpose in acting as he did to alleviate the pain and suffering, then he is not guilty. That is so even though he recognised that, in fulfilling that primary purpose, he might or even would hasten the moment of her death.
> That is the crucial distinction in this case. In short it is the question of primary purpose ... If Dr Cox's primary purpose was to hasten her death, then he is guilty.[11]

It does not matter by how much or by how little a person's death is hastened or intended to be hastened. Indeed, Lillian Boyes was only hours and possibly minutes away from death when she received her first injection, not containing potassium chloride, earlier that morning. The crucial point is that it is unlawful to hasten death, no matter by how short a period.

It may be asked whether any exemplary motives which a doctor might have in committing euthanasia, such as the relief of intolerable pain and suffering, are relevant to the question of criminal liability.[12] In *R v Arthur* Farquharson J said that it was accepted that the doctor had acted from the highest motives, but directed the jury that 'however noble his motives were ... that is irrelevant to the question of your deciding what his intention was.'[13] The fact that a doctor was acting to alleviate pain and suffering affords no defense to a murder charge. The conviction of Dr Cox underlines the principle that a doctor's motives, however honorable, afford no defense. If Dr Cox's primary intention was to end his patient's life, the fact that he had enabled her to die in peace and with dignity was irrelevant. Ognall J formed the opinion that if Dr Cox's primary intention was to bring about his patient's death, there could be no doubt that 'he was prompted only by his personal distress, the distress of Mrs Boyes's family and her own frequently expressed wish to have her journey through this veil of tears brought to an end.'[14] This, however, did not afford him a defense to the charge brought, though of course it was highly relevant to any sentence to be passed after a guilty plea was returned.

Albeit a doctor acts in the ordinary course of medical practice, this, again, would not provide any defense where the act was intended to hasten death.[15]

Further, consider the scenario where a patient begs a relative or her doctor to end her life quickly and painlessly because she can no longer endure the lack of dignity and suffering. Can the patient's consent to being killed in these circumstances excuse the actions of the accused? The simple answer is no. Mrs Boyes on numerous occasions begged both Dr Cox and other doctors to end her suffering. This fact is irrelevant to the question of criminal liability. Under English Law, no person can consent to their own death so as to provide a defense to murder.[16]

It has become customary for a relative to plead diminished responsibility in cases of euthanasia and mercy-killing which, if successful, reduces a murder charge to a conviction for manslaughter.[17] This, in turn, allows the judge discretion in sentencing. It is unlikely, however, that the court would accept such a plea from a health care professional.

R v Cox was approved by the House of Lords in *Bland*. Lord Goff stated:

> It is not lawful for a doctor to administer a drug to his patient to bring about his death, even though that course is prompted by a humanitarian desire to end his suffering, however great that suffering may be: see *R v Cox*.[18]

Although the judges drew a distinction between cases in which a doctor decided not to provide, or to continue to provide, treatment or care for a patient and those in which the doctor decided to actively bring the patient's life to an end by administering a lethal dose, they recognized the illogicality of distinguishing between the two scenarios.

> It is true that the drawing of this distinction may lead to a charge of hypocrisy, because it can be asked why, if the doctor, by discontinuing treatment, is entitled in consequence to let his patient die, it should not be lawful to put him out of his misery straight away, in a more humane manner, by a lethal injection, rather than let him linger on in pain until he dies.[19]

However, it was also made clear that any changes in or reform of the law was a matter for Parliament, and not for the courts.

More problematic is the case where a doctor leaves a large quantity of drugs at the disposal of the patient in the knowledge or strong suspicion that they will be used to cause death. Potentially, this is the criminal offense of aiding and abetting suicide. It would, of course, be open to the accused to argue that the intention was, for example, to ease the pain of the patient and leave the question of *mens rea* to the jury. Nonetheless, this approach inevitably leads to uncertainty and an element of gamble on the accused's part. In *Beecham's case*[20] Lesley Ann Pratt, suffering the terrible consequences of multiple sclerosis, asked her father to assist her in a third attempt to commit suicide. He helped her connect a pipe to a car exhaust and once she finally died called the police. He admitted the offense, saying, 'I did it because that is what she wanted. I didn't stop her because I love her.' Beecham was convicted of aiding and abetting suicide and given a 12 month suspended sentence.

Any doctor supplying the means for a patient to take his or her own life, likewise, faces the possibility of prosecution and criminal conviction. However, the standard of proof required is high. It must be shown that the doctor had supplied the drugs to a patient, known at the time of the supply to be contemplating suicide, with the intention of assisting and encouraging that patient to commit suicide by those means, and further that that patient was in fact assisted and encouraged by the supply of the drugs to commit or attempt to commit suicide.[21]

'PULLING THE PLUG'

Artificial ventilation may be a necessary step in the treatment of a critically ill patient. Where a patient is dependent on artificial ventilation, he or she will die if the ventilator is switched off. Does such an action fall within the definition of prohibited killing or is it permitted due to compliance with the patient's wishes?

The basic principle is that no act of murder is committed if the patient is already brain stem dead at the time the ventilator is switched off. The definition of brain stem death allows a person to be declared dead despite the existence of a heartbeat or breathing maintained by artificial means. Termination of life-support, where the patient is found to be brain stem dead, does not break the chain of causation between the initial injuries or illness and death.[22] It follows that the doctor is not responsible for the patient's death.

The difficulties emerge where the patient concerned is not brain stem dead. Questions of criminal liability arise in two separate legal situations. The first is where the patient has requested termination of the treatment; the second, where the respirator is turned off without the consent of the patient. What law governs the situation where a competent adult decides he or she wishes to have life-sustaining artificial ventilation discontinued?

Due to the absence of English cases in point, it is necessary to consider relevant American authorities. In *Satz v Perlmutter*,[23] an elderly man, still mentally competent, was terminally ill and dependent on a ventilator in hospital. At one point he had tried to remove the equipment from his trachea. This patient sought the court's approval to have the ventilator disconnected. Although removal of this life-support would hasten death, it was decided that the right to refuse treatment also included the right to discontinue it. The court in *Re Conroy*,[24] though primarily concerned with the treatment of an incompetent patient, also considered the legal issues in relation to competent patients. It was stated that a competent person, generally, has the right to decline any medical treatment initiated or continued.[25] Both these cases identified four state interests that may limit a person's right to refuse medical treatment: preserving life, protecting innocent third parties, safeguarding the integrity of the medical profession, and preventing suicide.

The interest in preserving life embraces two separate but related concerns: the preservation of the life of the particular patient, and the preservation of the sanctity of all life. A distinction is drawn between the state's interest when the affliction is curable, and where the issue is how long and at what cost to the individual life may be briefly extended. In *Satz v Perlmutter* the patient's condition was terminal and life-expectancy, even with the artificial ventilation, was short. Consequently, the state interest did not interfere with the patient's right of self-determination. Schrieber J in *Re Conroy* also stated that where a case does not involve the protection of the life of someone other than the decision maker, the state's interest in preserving the life of the competent patient generally gives way to the patient's much stronger personal interest in directing the course of his or her own life. It was also recognized by the judges in *Bland* that the principle of sanctity of life was not an absolute one.[26]

Secondly, the state interest in protecting innocent third parties who may be harmed by the patient's decision may override a patient's autonomy. An example may be where the patient's decision results in the financial and emotional abandonment of minors.

Safeguarding the integrity of the medical profession is the third interest. Ethical criteria which bind health care professionals are not particularly threatened by the refusal to continue with life-saving treatment as medical intervention is not ethically required at all costs.

Finally, the state has an interest in the prevention of suicide. In the USA, the general view is that declining life-sustaining treatment should not be seen as an attempt to commit suicide. Refusing medical intervention merely allows the disease to take its natural course; if death were eventually to occur, it would be the result, primarily, of the underlying disease, and not the result of the self-inflicted injury. In addition, people who refuse life-sustaining medical treatment may not harbor a specific intent to die.[27] They may fervently wish to live but free of unwanted medical technology and protracted suffering:

> The testimony of Mr. Perlmutter ... is that he really wants to live, but [to] do so, God and Mother Nature willing, under his own power.[28]

This issue materialized again in the Canadian case, *Nancy B v Hotel-Dieu de Quebec*.[29] Nancy B suffered from Guillan–Barré syndrome – a neurological disorder that left her incapable of movement – which meant she could only breathe with the aid of a ventilator. If she remained on the ventilator she could live a long time; without it her life would be brief. Notwithstanding this debilitating disease, Nancy B's intellectual and mental competence were unaffected. She commenced an action against the hospital and her physician to require them to comply with her decision to refuse further treatment. Permission was given to cease treatment with the ventilator at the time chosen by Nancy B. Dufour J stated that the person who would have to stop Nancy B's ventilator in order to allow nature to take its course would not commit a crime. Neither would there be an act of suicide.

> Homicide and suicide are not natural deaths, whereas in the present case, if the plaintiff's death takes place after respiratory support is stopped at her request, it would be the result of nature taking its course.

In any English case where the patient requests that the 'plug is pulled,' the predominant question would be whether the doctor is liable for aiding and abetting his patient's suicide contrary to section 2(1) Suicide Act 1961. It may be maintained, as in the US cases, that there was no intention on the part of the patient to die. On the contrary, she wished to live, albeit without medical intervention and without prolonged indignity and suffering. This being the case, there could be no suicide to aid and abet. Alternatively, the rather artificial 'acts versus omissions' argument could be advanced – that switching off the life-support machine is an omission. Once categorized as a failure to treat there is no liability, as only an act may be an abetment.[30] Thirdly, it may be argued that the doctor is only aiding and abetting the *decision* to forgo further treatment. It follows that the switching-off does not facilitate the suicide, but the decision.[31] Finally, the use of a ventilator could be classified as an 'extraordinary measure.' The fact that the patient has asked for its withdrawal absolves the doctor from a duty to continue treatment and he or she may discontinue it.[32]

English law recognizes the principle that competent patients have the right to refuse life-sustaining treatment. In *Bland* it was acknowledged that a patient is completely at liberty to decline treatment, even if the result of the patient doing so will be that he or she will die.[33] Lord Goff stated that there was no question of the patient having committed suicide in such circumstances and therefore no question of a doctor having aided and abetted the patient in doing so.[34]

But might the withdrawal of a life-support machine constitute murder? Has the doctor done an *act* which killed the patient? In another US case, *Barber v Superior Court*,[35] a doctor faced a murder charge after a comatose patient was removed from a ventilator and intravenous feeding was stopped, only nursing care being provided to preserve the dignity of the patient. The lower court ruled that this constituted murder. However, the appeal court avoided such a conclusion, albeit by applying artificial arguments. It was held that, although the removal of the life-support machine was done intentionally and with the knowledge that death would ensue, it was not an unlawful intentional killing. The court drew a distinction between acts and omissions; the withdrawal of life-supporting treatment characterized as the omission to provide further treatment. The life-support devices were compared to the manual administration of treatment, so that disconnecting the devices was like withholding manual treatment.[36]

Finding the withdrawal of artificial respiration to be an omission means there is no liability under criminal law, unless it is found that there is a duty to act. Once it is established that treatment is futile there is no duty on a doctor to act:

> Whether the patient is competent and refuses further treatment, or incompetent, a doctor is under no duty to continue treatment once it has proved to be ineffective.[37]

When a patient is expected to die within a few weeks or months, priorities change; the primary aim becomes to ensure that their remaining life is as comfortable as possible, not to preserve life at all costs.[38] Naturally, if the doctor has a duty to treat, and fails to do so, he or she will be liable whether the act is classified as an omission or not.

Alternatively, artificial ventilation could be categorized as an 'extraordinary' measure, as opposed to an 'ordinary' one. The law does not require a doctor to perform the unreasonable or extraordinary. Unfortunately, the distinction between ordinary and extraordinary measures is a difficult concept to apply – labelling a treatment extraordinary begs the very question. Penicillin may once have been seen as extraordinary, is it now? Is artificial ventilation always an extraordinary measure? Clearly, determining which category a particular treatment falls into depends on the specific circumstances of the case in question. In differing medical and factual situations the same treatment, whether artificial ventilation or the use of antibiotics, can be either extraordinary or ordinary. Each individual case must be considered in isolation.

The Canadian decision of *Nancy B* also lends support to the view in *Barber* that there would be no criminal liability for a doctor who disconnected the life-support at the patient's request. The Supreme Court of Quebec resolved that the patient's death was a natural one. It is likely that an English court would likewise follow the decision in *Barber* if faced with a similar situation. Lord Browne-Wilkinson in *Bland* was clear that in any ordinary case of murder by a positive act of commission, the consent of the victim is no defense.[39] However, where there is a charge of murder by omission to do an act and the act omitted could only be done with the patient's consent, refusal by the patient to provide such consent does, indirectly, provide a defense to a charge of murder.[40] Lord Goff agreed that the discontinuance of life-support could be properly categorized as an omission:

> Discontinuation of life support is, for present purposes, no different from not initiating life support in the first place. In each case, the doctor is simply allowing the patient to die in the sense that he is desisting from taking a step which might, in certain circumstances, prevent his patient from dying as a result of his pre-existing condition; and as a matter of general principle an omission such as this will not be unlawful unless it constitutes a breach of duty to the patient.[41]

Notwithstanding this, where respiration is stopped without the knowledge and consent of a competent patient, any exemplary motives of ending pain and suffering will not avail a doctor charged with homicide. If done with the necessary knowledge and intent, this would be murder.

The withdrawal of ventilation from incompetent patients also raises questions of criminal liability for homicide. In *Quinlan*[42] there was held to be no civil or criminal liability on the part of the participant in withdrawing the life-support system from Karen Quinlan, who was in a chronic and persistent vegetative state. The arguments advanced above in defense of allegations of murder where life-sustaining treatment is withdrawn from competent patients will similarly apply in relation to incompetent patients.[43] In *Bland* the question before the court was whether it would be lawful to discontinue artificial life-support, hydration and nutrition, from Tony Bland who was in a persistent vegetative state, and consequently incompetent, but whose brain stem was not dead. According to English Law he was therefore still technically alive. The judges drew a distinction between acts and omissions and unanimously reached the decision that withdrawal of artificial feeding was an omission and thereby lawful.

Competent patients

REFUSAL OF LIFE-PROLONGING TREATMENT

Where a patient is competent to decide whether to consent to treatment or not, and is in a life-threatening condition, does he or she have the legal right to refuse life-prolonging treatment? Alternatively, it may be asked whether a competent, unwilling adult can be required to undergo life-saving treatment. Every adult has the inviolable right to self-determination. It was clearly stated by Cardozo J in the American case of *Schloendorff v Society of New York Hospital*[44] that:

> Every human being of adult years and sound mind has a right to determine what shall be done with his own body.

It follows that any intentional touching of a patient by a doctor without the patient's consent is, *prima facie*, a battery.[45] Hence, if an adult patient positively forbids a particular treatment, a doctor acts unlawfully if he or she administers it. The doctor could be prosecuted for assault,[46] or, more likely, face a civil action for battery.

The legal position was outlined by Lord Bridge in *Sidaway*:

> It is clearly right to recognise that a conscious adult patient of sound mind is entitled to decide for himself whether or not he will submit to a particular course of treatment proposed by the doctor, most significantly surgical treatment under general anaesthesia.[47]

Therefore, where a patient's life is not in jeopardy, if a doctor undertakes treatment without the patient's consent, the doctor has committed an unlawful act which will give rise to civil and criminal liability.

Does the legal position remain the same where the situation is life-threatening; is a doctor entitled or, moreover, obliged to administer treatment irrespective of the patient's wishes? *Leigh v Gladstone*[48] is often cited in support of the view that a doctor is obliged to treat in order to prevent death occurring, despite the patient's refusal. In this case Mrs Leigh was force-fed while serving a prison sentence for her suffragette activities. She brought an action claiming damages for assault. Lord Alverstone directed the jury that:

> It was the duty, both under the rules and apart from the rules, of the officials to preserve the health and lives of the prisoners, who were in the custody of the Crown.[49]

The assumption seems to be that having a duty to treat also imposes a power to do so, even without consent. If this proved to be correct, massive inroads would be carved into the right of self-determination. Such an unacceptable conclusion has provoked extensive criticism of this solitary decision.[50] In fact, it is no longer policy to force-feed prisoners,[51] and it is doubtful whether this case still represents the law. It may be possible to distinguish the case on the grounds that, at the time the decision was made, suicide was still a crime and the forced-feeding was justified to prevent the commission of a crime under section 3 Criminal Law Act 1977. Indeed, Lord Keith in *Bland* expressly recognized that the principle of the sanctity of life was not absolute and did not authorize forcible feeding of prisoners on hunger strike.[52]

The overwhelming view is that the general principle – touching without consent is unlawful – applies to life-threatening situations. The patient has an absolute right of self-determination. This is supported not only by the BMA guidelines on the treatment of Jehovah's Witnesses but also by the decision in *Re T*.[53] T was brought up by her mother, a fervent Jehovah's Witness, but was not herself Jehovah's Witness. At 34 weeks into her pregnancy T was involved in a car accident. She was admitted to hospital, where she was treated with painkillers and antibiotics for pneumonia. She went into labor and was to have a cesarian section. After a visit by her mother, who as a Jehovah's Witness would not accept transfusions of blood or blood derivatives, T indicated that she did not want a blood transfusion. She signed a form of refusal of consent to blood transfusions. T's condition deteriorated to the extent that she was no longer conscious. Her father and the father of the baby applied to the court for a declaration as to whether it would be lawful to administer a blood transfusion. Ward J decided that although T was capable of reaching a decision as to her treatment, her refusal did not cover the emergency which had arisen, and in the circumstances it would be lawful for the hospital to administer blood to her if that was in her best interests. The Court of Appeal affirmed Ward J's decision. Lord Donaldson MR's judgment did not attack the principle that patients have the right to refuse treatment. He clearly stated that an adult who suffered from no mental incapacity had an absolute right to choose whether to consent to medical treatment, to refuse it or to choose one rather than another of the treatments offered. The only possible qualification being where the choice may lead to the death of a viable fetus. This right to choose existed notwithstanding that the reasons given were rational, irrational, not known or nonexistent and notwithstanding the very strong public interest in preserving the life and health of all citizens. However, the court ultimately overruled T's refusal because she was found to lack the requisite capacity in the circumstances of the emergency that had arisen. This, seemingly, was because of the influence of her mother and because T may have been lulled into a false sense of security about the availability of alternative treatments. It appears that the court made the decision to overrule T's refusal because of the particular circumstances of that case.

The decision in *Re T* has confirmed the basic principle of self-determination in life-sustaining situations as did the Canadian court in *Malette v Schuman*.[54] Here a doctor was held liable in battery for transfusing an unconscious Jehovah's Witness against her clearly expressed pre-incompetence wishes.

> A competent adult is generally entitled to reject a specific treatment or all treatment, or to select an alternate form of treatment, even if the decision may entail risks as serious as death and may appear mistaken in the eyes of the medical profession or of the community ... If the doctor were to proceed in the face of a decision to reject the treatment, he would be civilly liable for his unauthorised conduct notwithstanding his justifiable belief that what he did was necessary to preserve the patient's life or health.[55]

The House of Lords in *Airedale NHS Trust v Bland* has confirmed a patient's right to autonomy.[56] In determining the lawfulness of withdrawing treatment from an incompetent patient, they confirmed without hesitation the, generally, inviolable right of self-determination of a competent patient. It was reaffirmed that it would be unlawful, so as to constitute both a tort and the crime of battery, to administer medical treatment to an adult who is conscious and of sound mind without his or her consent. Such a person is at liberty to refuse treatment even if the consequence would be that that person would die as a result. Health care professionals are best advised not to administer any medical treatment, life-saving or otherwise, to a competent adult who has refused consent. Failure to respect a patient's refusal could lead to action in battery.

Re T provides a caveat. There is the problem that a patient may be found to be incompetent on the basis that he or she has refused treatment. There is no universal test for competency, or rather capacity to consent, in English law.[57] But in the context of medical treatment, Bristow J in *Chatterson v Gerson*[58] stated that for a patient to give a valid consent she must be informed 'in broad terms of the nature and purpose of the treatment.' Therefore patients must be deemed competent if they are informed and understand in broad terms the nature and purpose of the particular treatment they are to receive. It is the doctor who determines whether or not a patient has the capacity to consent to treatment.[59] A refusal could be used as evidence of irrationality and

incompetence, particularly in the context of life-saving treatment.[60] Lord Donaldson in *Re T* outlined some guidelines for doctors to follow when a patient refuses life-saving treatment. A doctor is required to give careful and detailed consideration to the patient's capacity to decide on his or her treatment at the time when the decision was made. The more serious the decision, the greater the capacity required. If the patient did not have the requisite capacity, doctors were free to treat the patient in what they believed to be his or her best interests. Doctors had to consider whether the patient's capacity or will had been overborne and the patient might not mean what he or she said. They had to consider the true scope and basis of the patient's decision and whether at the time it was made it was intended to apply to a different situation. It might have been so intended, or it might have been of more limited scope or been based on false assumptions.

While patients maintain an absolute right to refuse life-saving treatment, doctors must ensure the refusal is genuine, taken after full consultation about the consequences, and not made under any undue influence from others. If in any doubt as to the effect of the purported refusal, where failure to treat threatened the patient's life or irreparable damage to his or her health, doctors should ask the courts to intervene.

Concern has been expressed that doctors are now faced with an impossibly difficult task. How far are they supposed to investigate the capacity of a patient and whether he or she has been exposed to undue influence? How do doctors decide what is undue influence? These guidelines could also undermine patients' rights by questioning patient capacity only when a refusal challenges the views of doctors. Competency should be scrutinized in *all* circumstances, not just when considered irrational. It is important that a lower standard for testing capacity to consent is not applied when treatment is refused, as opposed to when there is agreement.

Incompetent patients

Problems of medical decision making become more acute where patients are mentally incapacitated because their present wishes cannot be ascertained. Few effective legal mechanisms exist for resolving any problems that arise. Inadequacies in the present law have led to the Law Commission setting up a review of the civil law relating to mental incapacity, the present procedures available for making decisions on behalf of mentally incapacitated people, and some of the options for reform.[61] At present, any medical treatment, however trivial, given to a patient who cannot provide a valid consent is technically an assault, unless it falls under the doctrine of necessity. Moreover, it is not clear who can reach decisions on behalf of mentally incapacitated adults. There is little guidance on the extent of the authority of health care professionals to act or decide on behalf of those mentally incapacitated. The dilemma of balancing the need to maximize the autonomy of the mentally incapacitated with providing sufficient protection against abuse and exploitation increases the complications.[62]

Procedures in the USA allow a guardian to be appointed who, by applying the substituted judgment test, can make medical decisions on behalf of an incompetent adult.[63] For example, a family member was appointed guardian in both the *Quinlan* and *Cruzan*[64] cases. The substituted judgment test involves an evaluation of how the incompetent patient would decide if he or she could make the choice. As stated in *Re Conroy*:[65]

> The goal of decision-making for incompetent patients should be to determine and effectuate, insofar as possible, the decision that the patient would have made if competent.

Recognition that conclusive evidence of a patient's desires was not always available led to the formulation of three separate tests in *Conroy*. First, the subjective test provides that if there is clear evidence that a patient would have refused a particular treatment, for example in the form of a living will, then it is unlawful to continue. Second, where there is no such unequivocal evidence but there is some 'trustworthy evidence,' then treatment can be withheld if the burdens outweigh the benefits. This is the limited objective test. Finally, the pure objective test states that in the absence of any evidence, treatment can only be withheld if it will 'clearly and markedly outweigh the benefits the patient derives from life.'

It must be recognized that although there have been many cases decided in the USA which may provide guidance to English courts, many of the principles formulated are founded on American constitutional law and the American right of privacy.[66] These principles cannot simply be transferred and applied unequivocally in a common law jurisdiction. The legal context will also differ where a legal guardian has been appointed by a US court to make medical decisions on behalf of an incompetent adult. There is no comparative power in England to appoint such a guardian.[67]

In the absence of a legal decision maker for mentally incapacitated adults in the UK, may a doctor treat or withhold treatment from such a patient? In the recent decision of *F v West Berkshire Health Authority*[68] it was held that adult incompetent patients could lawfully only receive treatment in their best interests. An application was made to the court for a declaration that the termination of a mentally handicapped adult's pregnancy and her sterilization were not unlawful. In granting the declaration, Lord Brandon stated:

> . . . a doctor can lawfully operate on, or give other treatment to, adult patients who are incapable, for one reason or another, of consenting to his doing so, provided that the operation or other treatment concerned is in the best interests of the patient.[69]

Although the House of Lords ruled that it had no jurisdiction to require doctors to apply to the court for a declaration, it was of the opinion that where the treatment was of a serious nature then 'it was highly desirable as a matter of good practice' to involve the court. Treatment was held to be in a patient's best interests only if it was life-saving, or carried out to improve or avoid deterioration of physical or mental health. It is for doctors to decide, in accordance with accepted standards of practice, what is in a patient's best interests. It follows that if life-sustaining treatment will not prevent deterioration of, or improvement in health, then it will not be in the patient's best interests. Past authority suggests that where patients are permanently comatose or in a persistently vegetative state it is not in their best interests to keep them alive indefinitely.[70]

The law in England has now been established by the House of Lords in *Airedale National Health Service Trust v Bland*.[71] In this case, a declaration was sought by Airedale NHS Trust that it would be lawful to withdraw life-sustaining treatment (including nutrition and hydration) from Tony Bland, who had been crushed in the disaster at Hillsborough. As a consequence he had suffered catastrophic and irreversible brain damage and was suffering from the condition known as persistent vegetative state. This meant that whilst his brain stem remained alive and functioning, the cortex of his brain had lost its function and activity. The result was that Tony was capable of breathing unaided but could not see, hear, taste or smell. He could not speak or feel emotion. The space where the brain should have been was a mass of watery fluid. All the medical witnesses were agreed on the diagnosis. As Tony was incapable of swallowing he was fed by means of a nasogastric tube, his bowels were emptied by enema and his bladder drained by a catheter. He had been subject to repeated bouts of infection which were treated with antibiotics.

Sir Stephen Brown P at first instance declared that it was lawful to discontinue life-sustaining treatment. The withdrawal of such treatment was in accordance with good medical practice and was, in the clinical judgment of the doctor responsible for the patient, in the patient's best interests. This decision was confirmed by the Court of Appeal. The Official Solicitor, acting as Guardian ad Litem on behalf of Tony Bland, appealed to the House of Lords where their Lordships were unanimous in upholding the declarations given.

The judges relied on the decision in *F v West Berkshire Health Authority*.[72] All agreed that the appropriate test of a doctor's duty was the 'best interests' test. They stated that the issue requiring determination was not whether it was in the best interests of Tony Bland that he should die but whether it was in his best interests that his life should be prolonged by the continuance of medical treatment. Despite unanimously endorsing the best interests test as the appropriate test to be applied, the judges differed in their interpretation of its application.

To Lord Goff the question was whether or not the patient would benefit from the prolongation of life. He drew a distinction between two different situations. On the one hand, there were cases in which, in light of all the circumstances, it may be judged that it was not in the best interests of the patient to initiate or continue life-prolonging treatment and, on the other hand, there were cases in which, so far as the living patient was concerned, the treatment was of no benefit to him because he was totally unconscious and there was no prospect of any improvement in his condition. In the former case, a decision was reached by weighing up the relevant considerations. In the latter case, of which Tony Bland's condition was an example, there was no balancing act to be performed. In this case, Lord Goff considered treatment inappropriate. It would have no therapeutic purpose and would be futile, the patient being unconscious with no prospect of any improvement. Both Lord Lowry and Lord Browne-Wilkinson agreed with Lord Goff's interpretation of the best interests test; the question being whether the patient would benefit from the treatment.

In contrast, Lord Mustill and Lord Keith took the view that the best interests test was determined by weighing up the benefits and burdens of treatment against those of nontreatment; continued existence against the absence of it. This approach, however, could result in someone effectively deciding whether a person should live or die.[73] The implications of determining the test in this way were avoided by their Lordships, who concluded that as there was no hope of recovery in Tony's case, as he had no cognitive capacity, it could not matter whether he lived or died. Termination of his life could not be in his best interests nor, however, could prolongation of his life. In short, they found he had no interests.

In addition, the *Bolam* test[74] was seen as a relevant factor in deciding whether or not a doctor should continue to treat in a patient's best interests. The question was whether the decision was reached in accordance with a practice accepted at the time as proper by a responsible body of medical opinion, notwithstanding that other doctors held different opinions. It was for the doctor having responsibility for the care of Tony Bland, supported by doctors of unrivalled experience and professional standing, to decide in accordance with good medical practice and in accordance with the best interests of Tony Bland himself, that the artificial feeding regime be withdrawn.

The appropriateness of applying this test where declarations as to the lawfulness of a proposed course of action are concerned, is dubious. As Lord Mustill pointed out:

> I venture to feel some reservations about the application of the principle of civil liability in negligence laid down in *Bolam v Friern Hospital Management Committee* to decisions on 'best interests' in a field dominated by the criminal law. I accept without difficulty that this principle applies to the ascertainment of the medical raw material such as diagnosis, prognosis and appraisal of the patient's cognitive functions. Beyond this point, however, it may be said that the decision is ethical, not medical, and that there is no reason in logic why on such a decision the opinions of the doctors should be conclusive.[75]

Decisions about the critical care of patients and the lawfulness of withholding life-prolonging treatment are decisions involving not just medical questions but also issues of law, practice and, importantly, ethics. These are issues about which doctors do not have greater claims to professional expertise than any other professional body. It should not be the case that the medical profession can determine questions having such legal and moral significance.

It was clear from the evidence given that Tony Bland did not at any time before the disaster give any indication of his wishes should he find himself in such a condition. However, his family agreed that the feeding tube should be removed and felt that this was what Tony would have wanted. In the absence of any evidence from a patient that he or she would have wanted treatment withheld, the courts would have to proceed on the basis of a purely objective test, i.e. decide whether or not treatment should be given in the best interests of the patient. However, both Lord Mustill and Lord Goff went further and rejected the 'substituted judgment test' as having any place in English Law.[76]

Admittedly, despite its apparent attraction, the substituted judgment test can pose many problems in practice.[77] It is more difficult to apply in the case of a person who has never been capable of his own decision making, for example a child or mentally handicapped adult. There are problems in deriving meaning from views a patient would have had if he or she was competent. Any decision made will be tainted with some consideration of what is in the patient's best interests, thereby leaving little to distinguish the best interests test from the substituted judgment test.[78] However, it seems that their Lordships' rejection of the test as having any place in English law may be based on a misunderstanding of its nature. Lord Goff based his premise on the decision in *F v West Berkshire Health*

Authority[79] where a straightforward best interests test was adopted. However, it should be noted that this case was concerned with the treatment of a mentally handicapped child. The substituted judgment test, therefore, could not be appropriate in any event as the patient had never been competent to express an opinion or view.

Lord Mustill drew a distinction between sentient persons unable to communicate and insentient persons. In respect of the latter, he took the view that as the patient could not know there was a choice to be made, to ask him whether he would choose to have his life terminated was meaningless. With respect, Lord Mustill seems to have missed the point. The substituted judgment test involves another making the decision by stepping into the shoes of the patient; it is not based on the patient's capability, or not as the case may be, in making his own decisions at the time in question.

On one view of the decision in *Re J*,[80] it would appear that the court applied the substituted judgment test in determining whether a seriously brain damaged minor, who had twice been ventilated when his breathing stopped, should be reventilated when he suffered a further collapse. The court held that where the minor suffered from physical disabilities so grave that his life would from his point of view be so intolerable if he were to continue living that he would choose to die if he were in a position to make a sound judgment, the court could direct that life-saving treatment need not be given. This would apply even though the child was not on the verge of death or dying. Lord Donaldson MR emphasized that the problem must not be looked at from the point of view of the decider but from the assumed point of view of the patient. If this view is correct, application of the substituted judgment test in these circumstances would be misplaced as the patient in question was never competent. The alternative view is that the Court of Appeal was simply asserting that the best interests test requires the decision maker to take into account the particular circumstances of the patient and was not in fact applying the substituted judgment test at all.[81]

Whatever the correct view of this particular case, there is and should be a place for the substituted judgment test in English Law. In the appropriate circumstances, for example, in the case of a previously competent patient where there is sufficient and trustworthy evidence, the test can be applied effectively to evaluate and ascertain what is in the patient's best interests. Here the test is easier to employ as there are previous opinions and actions to review in order to evaluate the situation from the patient's standpoint. As the Law Commission reasoned:

> ... thinking oneself into the shoes of the person concerned and recognising the value we all place on personal preferences ... is a mark of respect for human

individuality which may have a value greater than its practical effect.

One final point to consider is whether *Bland* is to be applied in cases concerning the medical treatment of patients who are not insensate or are less insensate than Tony Bland was.[82] Lords Mustill and Browne-Wilkinson expressly restricted their decision to its particular facts, i.e. to the permanently insensate patient in a persistent vegetative state. The Court of Appeal in *Frenchay Healthcare NHS Trust v S*[83] is the first case to apply *Bland*. S was a young man who in June 1991 took a drug overdose which resulted in acute and extreme brain damage. He was initially fed through a nasogastric tube but this proved unsatisfactory so an operation was performed to insert a gastrostomy tube through the stomach wall and into his stomach. On 10 January 1994, the medical staff discovered that the tube had been dislodged. A further operation was needed to reinsert the tube but the consultant in charge recommended that it was in S's best interests for no action to be taken and that he be allowed to die naturally. The hospital applied to the court as a matter of urgency for a declaration authorizing the hospital not to replace the tube.

The declaration was granted at first instance. The Official Solicitor, as S's Guardian ad Litem, appealed to the Court of Appeal contending that, inter alia, the procedure adopted had deprived the Official Solicitor of a full and fair opportunity to explore the matter fully so as to ensure all the relevant material was before the court, and that the judge had attached too much importance to the doctor's judgment as to what was in S's best interests. The appeal was dismissed. S died shortly after the Court of Appeal hearing on 14 January.

There are a number of causes for concern, the first being that because the case was presented as an emergency, the Official Solicitor had no opportunity to gather independent evidence on S's behalf. It was envisaged in *Bland* that any application before the court should be preceded by a full investigation with an opportunity for the Official Solicitor to explore the situation fully, to obtain independent medical opinions and to ensure that all proper material was before the court. The Master of the Rolls rejected the Official Solicitor's proposition that the tube, or alternatively a nasogastric tube, could be reinserted to continue to feed S whilst independent evidence was collated and the matter investigated properly. As it has been argued reinsertion of a feeding tube scarcely represents an acute medical emergency.[84] Patients in a persistent vegetative state can become restless and tubes do, not infrequently, become dislodged. Considering the serious consequence of the declaration sought, the disadvantage of involving a doctor in reinserting the tube against his or her own medical judgment would be one acceptable in the patient's interests in the short term until the matter could be more fully investigated. If the doctor concerned was opposed to reinserting the tube, then another doctor could have been found to perform the operation of inserting a nasogastric tube temporarily.[85]

Secondly, there was evidence before the court that S had suffered acute and extreme brain damage. Although the consultant in charge of S took the view that S was in a persistent vegetative state, there was other medical evidence which revealed that S showed reflex response to stimuli. In addition, another consultant did not unequivocally diagnose persistent vegetative state. There was the suggestion that S may have felt distress and be suffering and he showed voluntary behavior, not least of which was pulling at the nasogastric tube and pulling out the gastrostomy tube. There appeared to be reason enough to question the diagnosis of persistent vegetative state, at least to the extent that the decision should have been postponed to allow for an independent investigation. The Official Solicitor queried whether the facts of S fitted that of Bland and drew attention to the inconsistencies. Sir Thomas Bingham recognized that the evidence was not as emphatic as in *Bland* but concluded that S was a person who had no conscious being at all, thereby following the reasoning in *Bland* that he no longer had any interests which counted in weighing up what was in his best interests.

Thirdly, Sir Thomas Bingham placed too much reliance on the opinion of the doctors as to what was in the best interests of S. He was clear that the ultimate decision as to what was in a patient's best interests was for the courts, but that the court should be reluctant to place those treating the patient in a position of having to carry out treatment which they considered to be contrary to the patient's best interests unless the court had real doubt about the reliability, bona fides, or correctness of the medical opinion in question.[86] Unfortunately, the *Bolam* test was applied in reaching the conclusion that the tube should not be reinserted. In effect, the decision made by the medical profession not to reinsert the feeding tube was sanctioned by the medical profession. It is not appropriate for the *Bolam* test to be the determining factor in deciding what is in the best interests of an incompetent patient in an application for a declaration as to the lawfulness or not of a proposed course of action. Doctors are deciding the lawfulness of their own actions. In *Frenchay NHS Trust v S* the decision reached was based on the medical opinion of S's consultant, together with supporting opinions from other doctors who had treated S in the past. The Master of the Rolls found their supporting evidence to be to the 'same effect' as the Consultant's. There were not two *independent* medical opinions supporting the consultant. Should we be leaving these decisions, involving not just medical issues of practice and opinion but also legal and ethical issues, to be determined by the medical profession?

Is feeding medical treatment?

Feeding has been distinguished from other medical treatments, often because it is seen as the basic form of humane care, without which the patient dies of starvation, not the underlying disease.[87] The case of *R v Arthur* first provoked public debate on the matter in the UK in relation to the neonatal care of a Down's syndrome baby. Dr Arthur had written in his notes 'Parents do not wish it to survive: nursing care only.' He was initially charged with murder, but the charge was reduced to attempted murder, of which he was acquitted.[88] The issue was also addressed in *Re C*[89] where it was held that there was no duty artificially to feed a dying baby. The court authorized treatment which would relieve the suffering of a severely handicapped and terminally ill baby but that it was not necessary either (a) to prescribe and administer antibiotics to treat any serious infection or (b) to set up intravenous fusions or nasal gastric feeding regimes for the minor. The opinion of the nursing staff that the aim of nursing care should be to ease suffering, rather than the short prolongation of life, was respected by the court. This case supports the view that artificial feeding, as distinguished from manual feeding, is within the definition of medical treatment. In addition:

> If there is no duty to treat such an infant, and treatment is defined as including administering foods or fluids artificially, it must follow that there is no duty to impose such treatment.[90]

The court in *Re J*,[91] although it did not expressly address the issue of feeding, extended the principle in *Re C* to the situation where the patient was neither on the point of death nor dying. It was held that the court could direct that treatment without which death would ensue from natural causes need not be given to prolong life. Although *Re C* and *Re J* were concerned with the treatment of minors, their similarity with some of the cases in the USA suggests that the principles they establish are likely to apply to the treatment of adults. The cases draw a distinction between manual feeding and drinking, and artificial methods of sustenance. Artificial feeding is seen in the same light as artificial respiration by the majority of American courts. If the means of artificial life-support, whether intravenous feeding or respiration, are withdrawn then the cause of death is the underlying illness.

In *Barber v Superior Court*[92] the Californian Appellate court said mechanical nutrition is like feeding only as a matter of 'emotional symbolism.' A more prolonged analysis in *Re Conroy*,[93] which concerned the treatment of a dying patient as in *Re C*, acknowledged the 'emotional symbolism' of food but noted that:

Analytically, artificial feeding by means of a nasogastric tube or intravenous infusion can be seen as equivalent to artificial breathing by means of a respirator. Both prolong life through mechanical means when the body is no longer able to perform a vital bodily function on its own.

Further, the medical procedures to provide nutrition and hydration are not free from risks or burdens for the patient.[94] For example, there is the possibility of contracting pneumonia or the unpleasantness of the technique may require restraint to be used to prevent the patient removing the tubing. For those patients unable to sense hunger and thirst dehydration may well not be distressing or painful and, indeed, the patient may be more comfortable without receiving nourishment.

The courts have resolved that the competent patient has the right to decline any treatment, including artificial feeding. In *Bouvia v Superior Court*[95] a competent and incurably ill patient, though not dying, had the right to refuse life-sustaining treatment. She was entitled to the immediate removal of the nasogastric tube involuntarily inserted into her body. The principles apply to those not in the process of dying, as in *Re J.*

Where the patient is incompetent, a balance must be drawn between the benefits and burdens to the patient. As Meyers concludes:

> Where it is relevant, the greater the physical and emotional invasiveness of the treatment sustaining life, including artificial feeding, and the more hopeless the prognosis for improvement in health, the less will be the obligation to do other than keep the patient comfortable by the use of misting and to provide the nourishment capable of being taken manually, not medically supplied.[96]

In *Cruzan*[97] the court authorized withdrawal of nutrition and hydration from a persistently vegetative woman which potentially could have sustained her for 30 years. The case seems to confirm the view that medical treatment includes nutrition and hydration – nowhere does the Supreme Court question it.

In *Bland*, although it was argued for the Official Solicitor that the provision of artificial feeding by means of a nasogastric tube was not medical treatment, the House rejected this proposition and declined to draw a distinction between medical treatment and feeding by artificial means. According to Lord Keith one had to look at the whole regime, which included artificial feeding, and that regime amounted to medical treatment and care.[98] Lord Goff saw artificial feeding, if not strictly speaking medical treatment, as part of a patient's medical care.[99] The ruling is the first in an English court which allows withdrawal of artificial nutrition and hydration from an adult patient in a persistent vegetative state.

However, it is important not to oversimplify the distinction between manual and mechanical feeding.

The balancing of benefits and burdens may lead to the conclusion that spoon feeding of a reluctant patient is invasive and therefore improper; tube feeding may be the appropriate method of care in other circumstances involving a different patient. The question remains what is in the best interests of the patient. It is important to recognize that in different circumstances artificial feeding may well be an appropriate form of treatment, withdrawal of which could amount to murder.

Do not resuscitate (DNR) orders

Health care professionals treating the critically ill are likely to be faced with the issue of resuscitating patients. Doctors are under a duty to take care of their patients, where the patient has not refused treatment, and may be civilly, or criminally, liable if they fail to do so.[100] Legal issues of patient autonomy are raised. What input should the patient have in the decision to impose DNR status? Research in the US indicates that although most patients who are designated DNR in the hospital are competent on admission, DNR orders are written at a time when the majority of patients are incapable of participating in the decision.[101] Should, therefore, resuscitation decisions be addressed on admission? At what point should the decision be made and how consistent is the patient's decision over time? In contrast to the USA, guidelines in England are less readily available and the issues treated in a secretive manner. The Royal College of Physicians guidelines on resuscitation state that it is inappropriate to attempt to resuscitate those patients whose lives are drawing naturally to a close because of irreversible disease.[102]

Prospects for reform

Since the decision in *Bland*, English law has provided some guidance in the area of critical care for both competent and incompetent patients, but there are still many problems and areas of uncertainty remaining. The House restricted its decision to the facts before it, i.e. in relation to the treatment of patients in a persistent vegetative state, and subsequent applications of the ruling have done little to solve the difficulties in this area. Moreover, the acute problems of decision making for incompetent adults are only likely to increase as technological advances in resuscitative medicine, respirators and artificial feeding all create the possibility of a 'living death.'

Health care professionals are in a difficult position,

having to make decisions with little guidance that may leave them vulnerable to legal proceedings. 'Allowing to die' legislation has been called for to clarify the situation and set out a framework within which the medical profession can work. However, voluntary euthanasia legislation arouses many difficulties of its own, not least of which are the problems in drafting. Would euthanasia really be voluntary? Or would the sick and elderly feel pressurized into taking such action?

There is at present no mechanism for helping in decision making or for appointing a substitute decision maker where mentally incapacitated adults cannot decide matters for themselves. One possible solution receiving increasing attention is advance directives.[103] Advance directives are a way for competent adults to maintain control over their medical treatment in the event they become incompetent. There are two forms of advance directive – living wills and enduring powers of attorney. A living will is a document which specifies the type of care a person wants should he or she become incompetent, usually that he or she should not be given 'heroic' or 'extraordinary' treatment. Under an enduring power of attorney a competent patient can nominate an agent to make decisions about the patient's health when the patient is no longer able to form his or her own judgment.

At present, living wills have no legal force in the UK. Consequently, a doctor cannot be required to follow such a directive. Cases in the USA, however, suggest that a patient's wishes expressed while competent may be relevant in deciding what treatment should be administered. In *Conroy* Garibaldi J considered that a living will could be evidence of a patient's wishes at common law. The likely approach of the English courts is to see the living will as directive only and to be taken into account when deciding what should be done in the patient's best interests. A health care professional acting in accordance with the directive is not assured immunity from civil or criminal liability, but it should serve as evidence of a patient's wishes and provide a legal justification in the event of such action.[104] The House of Lords in *Bland* stated that clear instructions given in advance that medical treatment should not be given reflected a person's right to self-determination and were valid.[105]

The general view is that enduring powers of attorney likewise have no validity in the UK. At common law an agent may be nominated by a competent person to act on his or her behalf but the agency will end as soon as the nominee becomes incompetent. Similarly, under the Powers of Attorney Act 1971 the agency terminates on incompetency. The Enduring Powers of Attorney Act 1985, likewise, provides no solution. Although the agency does not terminate on the onset of incompetency under the provisions of the Act, it is thought not to cover dealings with the principal's person, which includes

medical decisions. The powers under the 1985 Act are to deal with the principal's 'property and affairs' which, in a different context, has been interpreted by Ungoed-Thomas J to exclude the 'the management or care of the patient's person'.[106] Legislation would have to be enacted to give legal validity to either of these methods of advance directive.

There are many technical difficulties with advance directives. If the drafting of a will is too specific in its directions it may fail to cover the situation that arises; if too general, health care professionals are given a wide discretion. It could also be claimed that the person who falls under the jurisdiction of the advance directive is no longer the same person who originally wrote it. Nomination of a health care proxy can create its own specific problems. Although there is more flexibility to adapt to changing circumstances, an elderly person, for example, may have no-one they can elect to be their agent.

It may be questioned whether there will be great demand for living wills or powers of attorney. After all, only 50% of the population currently make out ordinary wills to operate on a contingency that will inevitably occur – death. Advance directives require contemplation of any number of possible events that may or may not strike down a currently healthy human being. This problem has been recognized in the USA where the Patient Self Determination Act was enacted in 1990 to ensure that any advance directive was made available to the health care professionals and if the patient had not made one, that he or she was made aware of their right to do so.[107] However, there may be a growing demand for the availability of directives. Research has recently been done amongst HIV and AIDS sufferers to determine whether there is a demand for such advance directives. A few observations of the data collected show an overwhelming support for the availability of living wills and almost all would consider appointing a health care proxy.[108]

Clearly, the doubts and uncertainties surrounding care of the critically ill need resolving. Do people have the right to direct their treatment in advance of their incompetency? What procedure can be used to decide matters on behalf of an incompetent patient, and by whom? These complex legal issues will continue to arise and require clarification. The practice of applying to the court for declaratory relief considered by the House in *F v West Berkshire Health Authority* has been endorsed by Lord Keith and Lord Goff in *Bland*[109] as the appropriate procedure until a body of experience and practice has built up which would then obviate the need for an application in every case. There is, however, concern that the general position at present is unsatisfactory.[110] *Frenchay Healthcare NHS Trust v S* has clearly highlighted just some of the many difficulties and issues that remain unresolved. Lord Browne-Wilkinson in *Bland* was in no doubt that the development of new law and decisions on the legal issues raised by advances in medical technology were matters for Parliament and not the courts. A whole new area of legal, ethical, practical and social problems has arisen which cannot be dealt with adequately on an *ad hoc* basis. Any decisions made by judges on these issues will inevitably reflect their own moral stance, albeit society is so clearly divided in its moral standpoint. The present state of the law is unsatisfactory in dealing with such complex problems and highlights the necessity for these issues to be debated thoroughly in the public arena and explored by Parliament in depth.

References

1. *In Re T (Adult: Refusal of Treatment)* CA [1992] 3 WLR 782.
2. *Airedale National Health Service Trust v Bland* (1993) 4 Med LR 39; [1993] 1 All ER 821.
3. *Re J (A Minor) (Medical Treatment)* [1993] Fam 15; [1992] 4 All ER 614 (CA).
4. See *Dyson* [1908] 2 KB 454, per Alverstone CJ at 457.
5. See A report from the Netherlands. *Bioethics* 1987; **1**: 156.
6. Virtually all doctors prosecuted in recent times have ended in acquittal, perhaps revealing the reluctance of English juries to convict doctors of murder in the absence of the most compelling proof. See Gunn MJ, Smith JC. *Arthur's* Case and the Right to Life of a Down's Syndrome Child. *Criminal Law Rev* 1985; 705–15, and Comments on *Arthur's* case. *Criminal Law Rev* 1986; 383–90. However, see *R v Cox* (1992) 12 BMLR 38, where Dr Cox was convicted of attempted murder, contrary to the pattern to date.
7. *R v Adams* [1957] *Criminal Law Rev* 773.
8. This is the philosophical doctrine of double effect. See Glover, J. *Causing Death and Saving Lives*. Middlesex: Penguin Books, 1977: Ch. 6.
9. *R v Cox* (1992) 12 BMLR 38 (Winchester CC).
10. The charge brought against Dr Cox was one of attempted murder because the Prosecution could not exclude the possibility that Mrs Boyes died of natural causes between the actual injection of potassium chloride and death.
11. *Op. cit.*, at 41.
12. Skegg, PDG. *Law, Ethics and Medicine*. Oxford: Clarendon, 1988: 129–31. Smith JC, Hogan B. *Criminal Law*. London: Butterworths, 1992: 332. For an alternative view see Beynon H. Doctors as murderers. *Criminal Law Rev* 1982: 17–28.
13. Transcript, 26C-D.
14. *Op. cit.*, at 43.
15. Skegg, *op. cit.*, 1988: 131.
16. Criminal Law Revision Committee, Fourteenth Report, *Offences Against the Person*. Cmnd. 7844; 1980, para. 126; see also *R v Croft* [1944] 1 KB 295.
17. This allows the judge discretion in sentencing in place of the obligatory life sentence for murder. See Leng R.

Mercy killing and the CLRC. *New Law J* 1982; **132**: 76–8.
18. *Op. cit.*, per Lord Goff at 867; and see Lord Mustill at 890.
19. *Op. cit.*, per Lord Goff at 867.
20. *Daily Telegraph*, 18 February 1988. Horder J. Mercy-killings – some reflections on Beecham's case. *J Criminal Law* 1988: 309–14.
21. *Attorney General v Able* [1984] 1 All ER 277.
22. *R v Malcherek, R v Steel* [1981] 2 All ER 422, [1981] 1 WLR 690, CA.
23. *Satz v Perlmutter* (1978) 362 So 2d 162.
24. *Re Conroy* 486 A 2d 1209 (1985) (New Jersey Supreme Court).
25. The New Jersey Supreme Court in *Re Farrell* 529 A 2d 404 (1987) subsequently applied this principle expressed by Schrieber J in the case of a competent patient.
26. *Op. cit.*, per Lord Keith at 861; per Lord Goff at 865–6; per Lord Mustill at 891.
27. *Re Conroy, op cit.*; *Satz v Perlmutter, op cit.*
28. *Satz v Perlmutter, op cit.*
29. *Nancy B v Hotel-Dieu de Quebec et al.* (1992) 86 D.L.R. 385.
30. Williams, G. Euthanasia. *Medico-legal Journal*, 1973; **41**: 14 at 20–1.
31. See Kennedy, I. The Legal Effect of Requests by the Terminally Ill and Aged not to receive further Treatment from Doctors. *Criminal Law Rev* 1976; 217 at 226–8.
32. Kennedy, *ibid.*, at 228.
33. *Op. cit.*, per Lord Keith at 860; Lord Mustill at 889. See Wells C. Patients, consent and criminal law. *J Social Welfare Family Law* 1994: 65–78 for a differing view.
34. *Op. cit.*, per Lord Goff at 866.
35. *Barber v Superior Court* (1983) 195 Calif. Rptr. 484.
36. See also Beynon H. *op. cit.*, 1982; 17 at 21.
37. Brazier M. *Medicine, Patients and the Law*. London: Penguin Books, 1992: 454.
38. Twycross RG. Debate: euthanasia – a physician's viewpoint. *J Med Ethics* 1982; **8**: 86–95.
39. See *R v Cox, op. cit.*
40. *Op. cit.*, at 882.
41. *Op. cit.*, at 867–8.
42. *Re Quinlan* 355 A 2d 647 (1976).
43. See Kennedy I. Switching off life support machines: the legal implications. *Criminal Law Review* 1977: 443–52. See also Skegg PDG. The termination of life-support measures and the law of murder. *Modern Law Review* 1978; **41**: 423–36.
44. *Schloendorff v Society of New York Hospital* (1914) 211, NY 125.
45. See Brazier M. *op. cit.*, 1992; Ch. 4.
46. Williams G. *op. cit.*, 1973; **41**: 14 at 24.
47. *Sidaway v Board of Governors of the Bethlem Royal Hospital and the Maudsley Hospital* [1985] 2 WLR 480; 502.
48. *Leigh v Gladstone* (1909) 26 TLR 139.
49. *Ibid.*, at 142.
50. Zellick G. The legality of enforced therapy. *Public Law* 1976: 153–87. Kennedy I. *op. cit.*, 1976 at 227.
51. Announced by Mr Roy Jenkins, then Home Secretary, 17 July 1974. 877 Debs., col. 451.

52. *Op. cit.*, at 861.
53. *In Re T (Adult: Refusal of Treatment)* CA [1992] 3 WLR 782.
54. *Malette v Schuman* (1987) 47 DLR (4th) 18; (1990) 67 DLR (4th) 321.
55. *Ibid.*, per Robins JA at 328.
56. *Op. cit.*, per Lord Keith at 860, per Lord Goff at 866, per Lord Browne-Wilkinson at 881–2, per Lord Mustill at 889.
57. For a more comprehensive discussion on competency and consent see Brazier M. Competence, consent and proxy consents. In Brazier M, Lobjoit M (eds) *Protecting the Vulnerable: Autonomy and Consent in Health Care.* London: Routledge & Kegan Paul, 1991: 34.
58. *Chatterson v Gerson* [1981] QB 432.
59. Kennedy I, Grubb A. *Medical Law: Text and Materials.* London: Butterworths, 1994: 123–51.
60. See Buchanan AE, Brock DW. *Deciding for Others: The Ethics of Surrogate Decision Making.* Cambridge: Cambridge University Press, 1989: 58. Brock advocates treatment refusals should reasonably serve to trigger a competence evaluation, though should not be a basis or evidence for the finding of incompetence.
61. The Law Commission. *Mentally Incapacitated Adults and Decision-making: An Overview.* Consultation Paper No. 119. London: HMSO.
62. *Ibid.*
63. The *Quinlan* case is an example of a guardian authorising withdrawal of treatment.
64. *Op. cit.*; *Cruzan v Director, Missouri Department of Health* 110 S.Ct. 2841 (1990).
65. *Op. cit.*
66. See *Re Quinlan, op. cit.*
67. The Mental Health Act allows treatment of a mentally disordered person without their consent under Part 4 but only deals with treatment of the specific mental disorder suffered, not, for example, any additional physical problem. Similarly, the guardianship provisions are no help. It is arguable that the ancient *parens patriae* jurisdiction continues in existence, giving the crown jurisdiction over the mentally disordered. However, the court is unlikely to exercise this power at the present time. See *T v T* [1988] 2 WLR 189, per Wood J.; Hoggett B *Mental Health Law.* London: Sweet & Maxwell, 1990. Centre of Medical Law and Ethics and Age Concern. *The Living Will: Consent to Treatment at the End of Life – A Working Party Report*, 1988.
68. *Re F* [1990] 2 AC 1, sub nom *F v West Berkshire Health Authority* [1989] 42 All ER 545, HL.
69. *Ibid.*, at 551.
70. *Re C (A Minor) (Wardship: Medical Treatment)* [1989] 3 WLR 240; *Lim v Camden & Islington Area HA* [1974] 1 QB 196 (Lord Denning MR). *Airedale NHS Trust v Bland. Op. cit.*
71. *Op. cit.*
72. *Op. cit.*
73. Kennedy, I & Grubb, A. *Op. cit.*, at 1225.
74. *Bolam v Friern Hospital Management Committee* [1957] 2 All ER 118.
75. *Op. cit.*, at 895.
76. *Op. cit.*, per Lord Goff at 872–3 and Lord Mustill at 892.
77. See The Law Commission *Mentally Incapacitated Adults and Decision-making: An Overview*, para. 4.23.
78. See Mason JK. Master of the balancers: non consensual treatment under the mantle of Lord Donaldson. *Juridical Rev* 1993: 115.
79. *Op. cit.*
80. *Re J* [1990] 3 All ER 930.
81. See Kennedy I, Grubb A. *op. cit.* 1994 at 293.
82. See Kennedy I, Grubb A. *op. cit.*, 1994:1231–8; Stone J. Withholding life-sustaining treatment: the ultimate decision. *New Law J* 1994: 205–6.
83. *Frenchay Healthcare NHS Trust v S* [1994] 2 All ER 403.
84. Stone J. *op. cit.*, at 206. See Mason JK, McCall Smith RA. *Law and Medical Ethics.* London: Butterworths, 1994: 344 for a contrary view.
85. *Op. cit.*, at 412–3. Lord Waite rejected this approach.
86. *Op. cit.*, per Sir Bingham MR at 412.
87. See generally, Lynn, J. *By No Extraordinary Means: The Choice to Forgo Life-Sustaining Food and Water.* Indiana University Press, 1986.
88. See Mason JK, McCall RA. *Law and Medical Ethics.* London: Butterworths, 1994: 151; Brahams D. Putting *Arthur's* case in perspective. *Criminal Law Review* 1986: 387–9; Gunn MJ, Smith JC. *op. cit.*, 1985: 705–15.
89. *Re C (A Minor) (Wardship: Medical Treatment)* [1989] 2 All ER 782.
90. See Brazier M. *op. cit.*, 1992: 455.
91. *Re J (A Minor) (Wardship: Medical Treatment)* [1990] 3 All ER 930.
92. *Op. cit.*, p. 488.
93. *Op. cit.*, p. 1236.
94. Lynn J, Childress JF. Must patients always be given food and water? In *By No Extraordinary Means*, 1986: Ch. 5, 49–51.
95. *Bouvia v Superior Court* (1986) 179. Cal. App. 1127.
96. Meyers D. *The Human Body and the Law.* Edinburgh: Edinburgh University Press, 1990: 320.
97. *Cruzan v Director, Missouri Department of Health* 110 S.Ct. 2841 (1990).
98. *Op cit.*, at 861.
99. *Op cit.*, at 871.
100. Brazier M. *op. cit.*, 1992: 459.
101. Bedell SE., *et al.* Do-Not-Resuscitate orders for critically ill patients in the hospital: how are they used and what is their impact? *J Am Med Assoc* 1986; **256**: 233–7.
102. A Report of the Royal College of Physicians. Resuscitation from cardiopulmonary arrest: Training and organisation. *J Roy Coll Physicians, Lond* 1987; **21**: 175–82 at 181.
103. See *The Living Will, op. cit.* and for a general discussion Brennan C. The right to die. *New Law J* 1993: 1041–42.
104. See The President's Commission Report. Deciding to Forgo Life-Sustaining Treatment, 1983: 139–41; *The Living Will, op. cit.*, at 48.
105. *Op. cit.*, per Lord Keith at 860; per Lord Goff at 866; per Lord Mustill at 892.
106. *Re W (E.E.M.)* [1971] Ch. 123: 142–3.
107. For a discussion of some of the problems of this Act see

the paper presented by Eby MA. The Patient Self Determination Act: The Medical Miranda. The First UK
Forum on Health Care Ethics, 1992.
108. The results of this research are to be published in a
report by Ms Schlyter. Paper presented at the First UK
Forum on Health Care and Ethics, 1992 by The Terrence
Higgins Trust Living Will Project *Advance Directives
and AIDS*.
109. *Op. cit.*, at 862 & 874.
110. *Op. cit.*, per Lord Lowry at 876; Lord Browne-Wilkinson at 878–80; Lord Mustill at 889.

United States of America

MARSHALL B KAPP

Critical care medicine in the USA today is practiced
within a highly regulated environment. This chapter
first explores this regulatory climate in terms of external
controls on practice exerted by public and private third-
party entities. It next focuses on the foundations and
ramifications of medical malpractice litigation initiated
by individual patients against specific health care
providers. Finally, a variety of formal strategies for
identifying, avoiding, or managing possible legal risks
in critical care are outlined.

The regulation of critical care

The USA has a federal government system, in which the
central government and the 50 individual states exercise
concurrent or simultaneous authority over many aspects
of health care, including the regulation of hospitals
within which critical care is delivered to patients. The
most prominent form of hospital regulation taking place
at the state level is that of institutional licensure.

Every state legislature has enacted a statute requiring
hospitals to satisfy specific structural (e.g. nurse to
patient ratios, equipment, room size, medical staff
bylaws) and process (e.g. assurance of patient rights)
standards in order to receive a legal license or permission to operate.[1] A hospital license is time-limited and
must be renewed periodically. Some states deem a
hospital's compliance with standards set by the Joint
Commission on Accreditation of Healthcare Organizations (JCAHO), discussed below, to satisfy their
licensure requirements.

A second important source of hospital regulation is
found in the hospital Conditions of Participation[2]
promulgated by the federal Health Care Financing
Administration (HCFA), which is the part of the

Department of Health and Human Services (DHHS)
that has responsibility for managing the Medicare[3] and
Medicaid[4] financing programs. Virtually all US hospitals are economically dependent upon these government
financing programs for, respectively, the elderly and the
poor, and hence have little practical choice about
complying with the structural and process requirements
upon which participation in Medicare and Medicaid are
conditioned.

However, over 90% of the almost 7000 US hospitals
bypass direct government enforcement of Conditions of
Participation by meeting the hospital accreditation
standards set by the Joint Commission on Accreditation
of Healthcare Organizations (JCAHO).[5] JCAHO is a
private, nongovernmental consortium consisting of the
American Hospital Association, Canadian Hospital
Association, American Medical Association, American
College of Surgeons and American College of Physicians. It publishes, and directly surveys for compliance
with, extensive quality standards, including requirements pertaining particularly to intensive care (for
example, a mandate that 'Special care units are
designed and equipped to facilitate the safe and effective care of patients' and that 'Each special care unit is
organized as a physically and functionally distinct
entity with controlled access'). Institutions voluntarily
meet these standards in order to obtain accreditation. In
addition to prestige that helps attract patients and staff,
JCAHO accreditation also confers on hospitals 'deemed
status' that obviates the need for the hospital to
separately pass a Conditions of Participation inspection
by the government.

An additional source of nongovernmental regulation
of health care delivery, which exerts an extensive
impact, stems from private third-party insurance
requirements regarding utilization review (UR). In the
USA today, most nonroutine medical interventions
(such as placement of a patient in a critical care unit) are
scrutinized by insurers for necessity and appropriateness; this scrutiny may occur on a prospective,
retrospective, or concurrent basis, and nonpayment for
the service results upon a finding that the service was
unnecessary or inappropriate.

Many corporations in the USA self-insure for health
purposes, that is, they provide health insurance for their
employees, retirees, and dependents by reimbursing
providers directly from a set-aside fund rather than by
paying premiums to purchase coverage from a commercial insurer. Self-insured companies often utilize the
services of private UR firms, sometimes called Fourth-
Party Audit Organizations,[6] to evaluate whether
providers deserve to be paid for specific services. For
patients who are covered by government financing
programs, including Medicare and Medicaid, Peer
Review Organizations (PROs)[7] are private organizations that contract with the government to conduct UR
for program beneficiaries.

The upshot of the pervasive atmosphere of UR is a constant pressure on American physicians and institutional administrators to justify the necessity and appropriateness of services, including critical care and its various components, prescribed for individual patients, lest financial payment be denied. This aspect of a health care system where costs continue to rise inexorably has the intended effect of placing limitations on the range of clinical choices available to physicians, with a clear bias for treating patients as nonintensively as possible as early as safety will permit.

Medical malpractice

The US medical malpractice system,[8] in which instances of iatrogenic injury frequently are dealt with through civil lawsuits brought by or on behalf of injured individual patients against health care providers who are alleged to have acted negligently, exerts a powerful influence on the conduct of physicians in the US. One outgrowth of the malpractice anxiety among American physicians is – at least according to physician reports[9] – the common practice of 'defensive medicine' or the overuse of medical tests and procedures more to bolster the physician's eventual legal position than to medically benefit the patient.[10]

Most medical malpractice claims are predicated on the theory of negligence. Negligence is an unintentional, but nonetheless legally culpable, tort. A tort, in turn, is a civil wrong, predicated on some basis other than a contract; in the case of medical malpractice, the theoretical basis for the tort of negligence is the fiduciary or trust relationship that exists between physician and patient under which the physician is obligated to act always in the patient's best interests.

ELEMENTS OF NEGLIGENCE

In any negligence lawsuit, the plaintiff who is seeking damages must prove by a preponderance of the evidence (i.e. by showing that it is more likely or probable than not) that four distinct elements are present. Failure to suitably establish the existence of any one of these elements means that the entire claim will be dismissed.

The initial element that a plaintiff/patient in a medical malpractice action must establish is that the defendant/physician owed the plaintiff a duty. This burden of proof is met by showing that a professional/patient relationship had been created between the two parties. The applicable duty owed is defined by a particular standard of care, namely, the obligation that the physician had and used that degree of knowledge and skill commonly possessed and used by other competent, prudent peers of the physician in similar circumstances.

Thus, a physician's professional conduct is ordinarily judged against that of his or her peers in the same specialty; a critical care specialist would be held to the standards commonly exercised by others with similar training whose practices entail similar patients and situations. The locality rule, under which a physician's conduct was compared only to that of similar specialists in the same geographic locality, has been abandoned by now in virtually all US jurisdictions. Its place has been taken by a national standard of care,[11] in which the performance of an intensivist in Dayton, Ohio may be compared to that of an intensivist in New York, Philadelphia, or anywhere else in the USA. Besides its obvious ramifications for physicians' training and continuing education responsibilities, movement to a national standard of care has vastly expanded the pool of potential expert witnesses available for a plaintiff to call to testify at trial and to educate the jury about the applicable standard of care under the circumstances.

The second element that must be proven in order for a malpractice claim to succeed is that the defendant/physician violated or deviated from the acceptable standard of care. A breach of duty may occur at any time during the physician/patient relationship. It may consist of nonfeasance (failing to do something that one should have done), malfeasance (doing something that one should not have done), or misfeasance (doing something that one was supposed to do, but doing it improperly).

Third, a successful plaintiff/patient must show that he or she suffered some actual injury of the type that the tort system is equipped to compensate monetarily. Money damages are intended to compensate or make whole the harmed plaintiff. They may be measured by tangible out-of-pocket expenses or lost opportunities (pecuniary or special damages) or by intangible pain and suffering (nonpecuniary or general damages). In rare cases (especially extraordinary in the critical care context), where the physician's misconduct was intentional or reckless, a court may award punitive or exemplary damages – over and above compensatory damages – for the purpose of deterring similar wrongdoing in the future.

Finally, negligence doctrine requires that the injury incurred by the plaintiff/patient be proximately caused by the physician's violation of duty. Put differently, plaintiff recovery depends on adducing proof that the defendant/physician's deviation from acceptable professional standards not only was a 'cause in fact' of the patient's injury (*sine qua non* or 'but for' the deviation there would have been no injury) but that this deviation be the most direct or closest cause of the injury.

INFORMED CONSENT

Decisionally capable patients

The well-established legal concept of informed consent is founded on the fundamental ethical precepts of autonomy ('self-rule' or self-determination concerning one's own bodily integrity) and beneficence (properly informed patients ordinarily will make what for them is the best decision).[12] Lawsuits brought in the first three-quarters of the twentieth century growing out of medical interventions conducted in the absence of informed consent were predicated on the theory of battery, or intentional, offensive, unconsented-to touching of another. Most cases in this category initiated since the mid-1970s, however, are framed as negligence actions in which the physician has failed in the fiduciary or trust obligation to inform the patient sufficiently as part of the authorization process.[13]

To be counted as legally effective and binding, the patient's consent to diagnostic or therapeutic intervention must meet three conditions (unless an exception such as a life-threatening emergency is present).[14] These elements of effective consent are voluntariness, knowledge, and decisional capacity.

First, valid consent is voluntary rather than forced in nature. The patient (or proxy acting on the patient's behalf) must retain the power to ultimately say yes or no regarding the available medical options.

Next, by definition informed consent must be based on sufficient communication of information to the patient. The majority US (as well as UK)[15] standard of information disclosure is professionally-oriented, inquiring whether the type and amount of information disclosed by the physician to the patient or proxy fell within the usual information-sharing practices of other prudent physicians in the same specialty in similar situations. Almost half the states, though, hold to a more patient-oriented approach, mandating physicians to share all the information that the patient would want to know under the circumstances. The patient-oriented standard focuses on materiality, since it compels the disclosure of all information that would be material – that is, which might make a difference – to an average, reasonable patient.

Regardless of the precise quantity of information disclosure required in one's specific jurisdiction, a variety of particular kinds of information must be included in the physician's disclosure responsibilities. These items consist of: the nature or diagnosis of the patient's medical problem; likely prognosis with and without treatment; general description of the proposed intervention; expected (but not promised) benefits of treatment; viable alternatives; and reasonably foreseeably risks of the different alternatives. Further, many patients want to know ahead of time the financial implications of their medical decisions.

The third essential element of legally effective consent is adequate mental and emotional capacity on the part of the decision maker to engage in a rational decision making process. This aspect of consent can be especially troublesome in critical care delivery.

It is important for physicians and other health care providers to avoid confusing written consent forms with legally effective informed consent. The piece of paper is not equivalent to the process. True informed consent is the process of mutual communication and ultimate patient (or surrogate) choice.[16] The document itself is merely a receipt or evidence helping to show that the process of communication really took place. Certainly, such proof may be essential to the physician who is called upon to defend against a claim of unconsented-to intrusion into the patient's bodily integrity, by creating a legal presumption that the patient did give properly informed consent. However, where the process of information exchange actually was inadequate, the plaintiff may overcome or rebut the positive presumption created by the consent form. While broad, general consent forms found in many hospitals are all right for authorizing routine, nonintrusive medical interventions, more individually tailored and informative forms are advisable for interventions that are intrusive or that carry a higher risk than those encountered in everyday life, and a specific written consent form surely is advisable where an experimental or innovative therapy is involved.

Applying these general principles in the critical care context is somewhat complicated by the fact that intensive care interventions for unstable patients often are more nearly continuous than discrete events. Informed consent requirements are pertinent any time the physician wishes to do anything (i.e. engage in any 'intervention') to a patient. For quasi-ongoing interventions, informed consent must be secured at the commencement of treatment, and the patient or surrogate has the right to withdraw permission at any subsequent time.

Most interventions in critical care would be labelled (from a patient's perspective, at least) as risky or invasive. Thus, careful documentation of express consent in this environment should be made for most things done to the patient. The physician should keep in mind, though, that the requirement of an informed consent process itself applies with full force irrespective of a medical intervention's level of risk or invasiveness.

Decisionally incapable patients

Minor children (defined by almost all the states for medical purposes as people under the age of 18) are legally presumed to be incapable of giving effective informed consent or refusal for their own medical care. Unless some exception based on the minor's 'emancipated' or 'mature' status is applicable, the general rule is that the natural parent or court-appointed guardian (in some jurisdictions the nomenclature is 'conservator') is legally authorized to act as medical decision maker.[17] People older than 18 (i.e. adults), conversely, are legally presumed to be capable of making their own medical decisions.[18] In critical care, a significant proportion of patients are so ill and debilitated that they cannot at the time make and express treatment choices based on participation in a rational thought process of understanding and weighing information about the relative risks and benefits of various alternatives.[19]

Theoretically, the level of mental capacity necessary for the patient to validly decline a recommended medical intervention ought to be identical or similar to the level necessarily for effective consent to the intervention. In practice, however, physicians usually only raise the capacity issue formally in the case of patient refusal. Ideally, a working assessment of the patient's decisional capacity, which may fluctuate widely over time due to a constellation of natural and medically induced factors, is being conducted at least implicitly by the attending physician every time the patient is seen. This inquiry should be an innate, even if unstated, component of every physician–patient contact. Where the patient's decisional capacity is seriously questioned, a more concentrated inquiry needs to be conducted. Where the patient really falls within a gray zone, placement of written evaluations concerning capacity in the patient's medical records by consultants who have examined the patient specifically for this purpose is good risk management for the physician proposing the intervention, who is the one responsible in the final analysis for assuring informed consent. Correctly or not, the legal system (here meaning the judiciary) affords psychiatrists and psychologists a good deal of deference as consultant capacity evaluators.

For patients who are functionally unable to engage in a rational decision making process, the legal presumption of capacity is rebutted or overcome. Informed consent still remains necessary prior to specific medical interventions for patients in this category. However, the consent for cognitively incapacitated patients must be obtained from a surrogate or proxy who is acting as the patient's spokesperson. There are several approaches to proxy medical decision making currently found in the law.

In the past decade and a half, more than half the states have enacted 'family consent statutes,'[20] which enumerate relatives in a priority order who have legal authority to make medical decisions for an incapacitated family member. Some of these pieces of legislation purport to limit the kinds of decisions that families may make for the incapacitated patient without judicial approval, but these limitations may be constitutionally suspect.[21] Advance medical directives, especially the durable power of attorney for health care, may be employed by

currently capable persons to designate their own proxies in the event of future incapacity. Concerned parties may initiate a formal guardianship or conservatorship proceeding (depending on one's jurisdiction), in which the probate court finds the patient (the ward) to be decisionally incapacitated (i.e. incompetent) and appoints another person (the guardian or conservator of the person) to act as the proxy decision maker.

Even where there exists no particular legislative enactment, advance directive, or judicial order empowering the family, the physician ordinarily relies on family members to make surrogate choices for an incapacitated patient. This informal process of relying on 'next of kin,' even outside of specific legal authorization, works fine in the vast majority of circumstances where the family members agree on a course of conduct both among themselves and with the health care team, and they appear to be acting consistently with the patient's personal values and preferences (a 'substituted judgment' standard) or the patient's best interests.

LEGAL RESPONSIBILITY AND VICARIOUS LIABILITY

The physician may be held legally liable to a patient, for substandard professional care and/or conducting a medical intervention without effective consent, on a personal liability theory. Personal liability is the doctrine that holds an individual responsible for his or her own acts and omissions. It is a basic premise of the US legal system that each of us may be held accountable for things we personally do or fail to do. Thus, for example, the physician who prescribes the wrong drug or dosage for a patient may be found personally liable if the error constituted a deviation from the acceptable standard of practice. Similarly, a nurse who administers a drug through an improper route or using an incorrect dosage may be found personally liable for his or her mistake.

In addition to claims that may arise from an individual's personal conduct, that individual's supervisors and employer may also encounter vicarious liability for the individual's misconduct.[22] It is important to emphasize that the possible presence of vicarious liability in no way reduces the potential personal liability of anyone for improper personal conduct. Put differently, vicarious liability may be imposed in addition to or on top of, rather than in place of, a negligent party's personal liability.

Under the principles of agency, which is a part of contract law that embodies the concept of 'master' (employer, supervisor, principle) and 'servant' (employee, supervisee, agent), a 'master' is civilly responsible for injuries to the person or property of third persons occasioned by the negligence of a 'servant' that occurred within the scope of that 'servant's' employment definition. Vicarious liability is a doctrine that also applies to intentional as well as negligent wrongdoing of the subordinate, but only in those situations where the superior should have reasonably foreseen the intentional misdeed.[23]

The concept of vicarious liability has a number of implications in the critical care context. First, under a specific subset of vicarious liability known as *respondeat superior* (literally, 'let the master answer'), the hospital may be found legally answerable for negligent acts or omissions committed by nurses, technicians, physicians (e.g. house staff), or other personnel who are employed directly by the hospital.

Second, under the related doctrine of corporate liability, a hospital has certain duties to carefully screen, monitor, and supervise independent contractors with whom the hospital has a business relationship, most notably private physicians with admitting and treating medical staff privileges at the hospital. Corporate responsibility encompasses, at the least:

1. a duty to determine the professional knowledge, skills, and character of a physician before granting staff privileges;
2. a duty to evaluate the continuing professional abilities and performance adequacy of a physician before the periodic renewal of privileges; and
3. the duty to conduct ongoing assessments of a physician's abilities and performance.

The violation of any of these duties, where the direct or proximate result is foreseeable harm to a patient, may expose the hospital to possible liability. First, a hospital may be found negligent for granting staff privileges to a physician in the first place, if:

1. the criteria that were used to evaluate the applicant were insufficient to determine the applicant's competence and character;
2. the hospital knew (e.g. through information provided by the National Practitioner Data Bank[24] established by the Health Care Quality Improvement Act of 1986)[25] that the physician was incompetent or deficient in character; or
3. the hospital should have discovered by due diligence that the physician lacked adequate competence or character.

A hospital also may be found negligent for renewing or failing to limit privileges for a medical staff member who the hospital learns or should have learned was incompetent and/or performing inadequately. While the hospital administration cannot be expected to look constantly over the shoulder of every physician who renders care within its premises and to actively supervise every aspect of that care the moment that it is being provided, a general monitoring and review function

(part of a risk management system – see below) is essential.

A third implication of the vicarious liability doctrine concerns the potential answerability of the physician working in the critical care setting for the errors and omissions committed by personnel whom the physician is supposed to be supervising. Earlier legal principles that had been used to expand the reach of *respondeat superior*, including the 'borrowed servant' and 'captain of the ship' doctrines,[26] have now fallen into disfavor in the courts. However, a physician may still be held liable, on a case-by-case basis, if he or she really had the power and the duty to supervise and control an ancillary provider and failed to fulfill that responsibility properly, with resulting patient injury.

The concept of vicarious liability is especially relevant to critical care medicine, with its heavy reliance on an interprofessional team approach. The physician and other team members must understand their interdependent legal relationships and the implications of those relationships for assignment of tasks, oversight, reporting, communication, and problem resolution. The physician must function as the legal team leader, but without acting autocratically and thereby reducing the benefits of broad interprofessional contributions to patient care.

Written hospital protocols should spell out operational guidelines of the team and the individual physician's supervisory duties. In the case of multiple consultants for a particular patient, medical staff bylaws must specify the ongoing coordination and monitoring obligations of the attending physician. Consultants who are not hospital employees must be credentialed to practice within the hospital according to standards contained in the bylaws.

Where there is any confusion about allocation of responsibility for decisions or actions, development of a written institutional protocol should be considered. Courts usually afford health care institutions broad discretion in the creation, content, and enforcement of these sorts of protocols, provided that the policies and procedures aim toward assuring an acceptable level of patient care. JCAHO accreditation standards also define parameters for internal institutional protocols in many practice areas.

COST-CONTAINMENT AND MALPRACTICE EXPOSURE

The health care financing and delivery system in the USA is the source of much current public and professional consternation and recently was on the verge of significant modifications. This concern and the accompanying clamor for systemic reform resulted primarily from the astronomical rates at which the costs of providing health care to the American populace continue to rise; critical care services have contributed substantially to this cost explosion. Dissatisfaction with the high cost of health care is exacerbated by severe problems of access to the delivery system experienced by 35–40 million Americans without any health insurance.

Over the past decade a variety of cost-containment strategies have been attempted by the federal and state governments, private insurers, and employers who provide health benefits for their employees and retirees, and often for the dependents of their employees and retirees. These strategies – which no doubt will continue to be experimented with in some form well into the next decade – include different forms of rate-setting (e.g. Medicare's Prospective Pricing System (PPS) using Diagnosis Related Groups (DRGs)), utilization review done by Peer Review Organizations (PROs) or other entities, mandatory second opinions, and managed care arrangements such as Health Maintenance Organizations (HMOs), Independent Practice Associations (IPAs), and Preferred Provider Organizations (PPOs).

A number of medical practitioners, administrators, and scholarly commentators[27] have anxiously speculated that externally applied cost-containment pressures are likely to influence medical practice in a way that encourages undertreatment which might jeopardize patient welfare. It has been surmised further that bad patient outcomes resulting from stinting on care to save dollars is likely to expose physicians and other health care providers to an added degree of vulnerablility to malpractice suits, although some argue that the American courts simply will adjust (or 'ratchet down') the legally enforceable standards of care to be consistent with contemporary cost-containment influences.[28]

The real impact of cost-containment initiatives in the USA on the malpractice exposure of health care providers remains to be seen. Very few lawsuits specifically alleging substandard care as a result of cost containment pressures have been brought thus far, and the few that have materialized to this point have produced very unclear lessons.[29] This is an area that critical care professionals should follow over the coming years with particular interest, as large changes in the US health care system begin to unfold and many previous incentives in medical practice are challenged and reversed.

Risk management and related issues

DEFINITIONS AND CONTENT

In light of the pervasive legal climate described in this chapter, US institutions delivering critical care services definitely need to engage in a formal, comprehensive risk management strategy. A risk management program involves explicit mechanisms to identify, mitigate, and avoid potential problems that might result in legal, and therefore financial, loss to the institution. Special areas of concentration in a risk management program that is sensitive to critical care concerns would include specifications for the organization and administration of critical care units (CCUs), clarification of the assignments and obligations of the different professionals caring for critically ill patients, medical records, equipment maintenance and modification, equipment records, analysis of equipment malfunctions, incident or event reporting, trend analysis of unexpected (and hence legally dangerous) incidents,[30] and a plan for taking corrective action.

The physician must be familiar with the institution's risk management program and cooperate with it to make certain that critical care practices and potential problems are addressed in the quest for legal and financial loss avoidance or mitigation. The institutional risk manager, who often is an individual with some clinical background, should be seen as a partner in pursuit of the common objective of delivering, and if necessary proving after-the-fact, quality patient care.

DOCUMENTATION

Good documentation of patient care is an indispensable component of any worthwhile risk management program. Accurate, complete, timely recordkeeping is imperative to providing competent clinical care, and producing acceptable (that is, unsurprising) medical outcomes is the best way for health care providers to avoid lawsuits. Additionally, if allegations of substandard care are made, the physician's best (and often only) defense will rest with the quality of documentation that he or she can bring forward to explain and justify decisions made and actions taken. Not incidentally, institutional licensure, voluntary accreditation, and third-party reimbursement depend in large part on information reflected in medical records.

Documentation is particularly important in critical care, where patient conditions frequently change rapidly, many different professionals may be involved in patient treatment, cost considerations always lurk,[31] and choices (like limiting the application of life-sustaining devices) may be controversial. In addition to completeness, accuracy (i.e. truthfulness), and timeliness, other watchwords of documentation ought to be legibility, corrections that are made in a clear and unambiguous fashion, and objectivity (i.e. not using the medical record as an outlet to editorialize about the patient or other members of the health care team).

Associated with the topic of documentation is the issue of confidentiality. The physician and rest of the interprofessional team must be wary of unauthorized disclosures of personal information about the patient. Questions about the sharing of medical information with third parties in specific circumstances should be directed to the facility's medical records department or legal counsel.

What about a patient or surrogate's own right of access to the information contained in the medical record, in light of the fact that the tangible document has been created as a business record by, and is the property of, the health care institution? In the USA, this right of access is guaranteed, at least for in-hospital care, by the federal Privacy Act for federal facilities (e.g. military, Veterans Affairs, prisons), and by state statute and JCAHO standards in most private and state or local government institutions. Patients or their surrogates request access to records often and for many reasons, ranging from sheer curiosity to serious questioning of quality of care. A physician who learns that a patient or surrogate has requested access to records should use this request as an opportunity to foster his or her relationship with the patient or surrogate, by offering to explain the record and answer questions, rather than reacting with a defensive posture that may reinforce any negative predilictions or doubts held by the patient or surrogate.

CLINICAL PRACTICE PARAMETERS

An important recent development in US medicine has been the strong push in the last few years toward the formal creation, dissemination, and enforcement of explicit clinical practice guidelines or parameters that would guide the decisions and actions of physicians and other health care providers.[32,33] Medical societies,[34] governmental agencies such as the federal Agency for Health Care Policy and Research, and insurers are utilizing a variety of approaches to the development of practice parameters for medical diagnosis and intervention, including formal consensus development, evidence-based guideline development, and explicit guideline enumeration.[35] The number and variety of practice parameters has burgeoned in response to the wide national variations in medical practice patterns (a phenomenon that certainly characterizes critical care medicine), without corresponding differences in clinical outcomes, that have been documented by health services researchers.

Several commentators have expressed serious skepticism about the probable impact of practice parameters, surmising that they will be used extensively in a negative manner in medical malpractice litigation.[36,37] Others, however, have suggested that practice parameters will – if anything – exert a salutary effect on both malpractice avoidance and defense, as well as cost-

containment.[38,39] President Clinton has expressed a strong interest in this topic, and increased emphasis on practice parameters is likely to be an integral part of whatever health care delivery and financing reforms take place over the next decade in the USA.

INSTITUTIONAL ETHICS COMMITTEES – LEGAL IMPLICATIONS

In the critical care context, difficult questions relating to the initiation, continuation, withholding, or withdrawal of life-sustaining medical treatments (LSMT) arise daily. One mechanism that a growing number of health care institutions have put into place since the mid-1970s to assist in dealing with perplexing legal and ethical dilemmas is the institutional ethics committee (IEC), also referred to as a bioethics committee.[40] This development has been given a major push recently by insertion into the JCAHO's *Accreditation Manual for Hospitals* of a mandate for hospitals to have some formal mechanism available for resolving questions relating to the use of LSMTs for particular patients.

There is no single model for the composition and operation of an IEC, but the general idea is to create a multidisciplinary, interdisciplinary body bringing together a broad array of expertise, experience, and philosophical perspectives (including that of the community and consumer) that is available to the health care institution and its staff in ethical matters.[41] An IEC could be involved in any combination of policy making, educational, or individual case consultation activities concerning ethical aspects of patient care. In addition to helping the hospital satisfy JCAHO standards, IECs can also assist with the policy making and staff and community education requirements imposed by the Patient Self-Determination Act (PSDA)[42] passed by Congress in 1990 to deal with advance medical directives (e.g. living wills and durable powers of attorney for health care) and decision making concerning LSMT. Regarding case consultation, an IEC may be involved concurrently or retrospectively. IECs offer advice, rather than binding holdings, to the involved parties. IECs vary significantly over operational issues surrounding who may or who must bring a case before the IEC and under what circumstances.[43]

Despite the potential benefits of IEC development and implementation for many health care providers, a host of legal, ethical, and administrative questions arise whose answers either depend on particular state law or, more likely, have not yet been determined. Most basically, what is the relationship between the IEC's ethics focus and its potential risk management role, and how can (should?) an institution prevent the latter role from totally dominating the former? Should the institutional risk manager/attorney be a member of the IEC, and if so, what role should that person play to prevent institutional interests from overwhelming the patient's interests when there is a tension between the two? What recordkeeping and reporting practices are advisable if an institution is worried about the legal issues of possible discoverability and testimonial privilege for IEC records and reports? Structurally, should the IEC be a committee of the medical staff or of the governing board? What are the confidentiality considerations, in the sense of IEC access to patient records with and without patient or surrogate permission? What weight do and should courts give IEC recommendations? Thus far, courts have shown great respect for IECs as sources of guidance. No court has imposed any legal liability on an IEC or its members, or on any health care institution or professional who followed an IEC's advice, but the question of potential liability for IEC-related activity is one that continues to concern many members and sponsoring institutions.[44]

Conclusion

Critical care physicians and other professionals in the USA are influenced in their everyday practice by the extensive legal environment within which they provide care. This chapter has attempted to briefly sketch out some of the more salient aspects of this legal climate and their ramifications for the choices made and actions taken within the critical care provider–patient relationship. Included are some suggested strategies for addressing the challenges of modern critical care medicine while operating within contemporary US societal norms, expectations, and enforcement processes.

References

1. Miller RD. *Problems in Hospital Law*, 5th edn. Rockville, MD: Aspen Publications, 1986: 42–45.
2. 42 United States Code Part 482 (1986).
3. Title 18, Social Security Act, 42 United States Code § 1395.
4. Title 19, Social Security Act, 42 United States Code § 1396.
5. Joint Commission on Accreditation of Healthcare Organizations. *Accreditation Manual for Hospitals.* Chicago: JCAHO, 1994.
6. Hershey N. Fourth-party audit organizations: practical and legal considerations. *Law, Medicine Health Care* 1986; **14**: 54–65.
7. 42 United States Code § 1320c (1994).
8. King JH, Jr. *The Law of Medical Malpractice*, 2nd edn. St Paul, MN: West Publishing Company, 1986.
9. Wiley J. The impact of judicial decisions on professional conduct: an empirical study. *Southern California Law Rev* 1981; **55**: 345–82.
10. Reynolds J, Rizzo A, Gonzalez ML. The cost of medical professional liability. *J Am Med Assoc* 1987; **257**: 2776–81.
11. *Brune* v. *Belinkoff*, 354 Mass. 102, 235 N.E.2d 793 (1968).
12. Faden RR, Beauchamp TL, King N. *A History and Theory of Informed Consent.* New York: Oxford University Press, 1986.
13. *Canterbury* v. *Spence*, 464 F.2d 772 (1972).
14. Meisel A. Exceptions to the doctrine of informed consent. *Wisconsin Law Rev* 1979; **1979**: 413–88.
15. Miller FH. Informed consent for the man on the Clapham Omnibus: an English cure for the American disease? *Western New England Law Rev* 1987; **9**: 169–90.
16. Katz J. *The Silent World of Doctor and Patient.* New York: Free Press, 1984.
17. Holder AR. Minors' rights to consent to medical care. *J Am Med Assoc* 1987; **257**: 3400–2.
18. Annas GJ, Densberger J. Competence to refuse medical treatment: autonomy v. paternalism. *Toledo Law Rev* 1984; **15**: 561–96.
19. Kapp MB. Evaluating decisionmaking capacity in the elderly: a review of recent literature. *J Elder Abuse Neglect* 1990; **2**: 15–29.
20. Areen J. Advance directives under state law and judicial decisions. *Law, Medicine Health Care* 1991; **19**: 91–100.
21. Kapp MB. State statutes limiting advance directives: death warrants or life sentences? *J Am Geriatrics Soc* 1992; **40**: 722–6.
22. Flamm MB. Health care provider as a defendant. In: American College of Legal Medicine (ed.) *Legal Medicine*, 3rd edn. St Louis: CV Mosby Company, 1995: 123–4.
23. Hollowell E. Liability for employees' intentional torts: a growing concern for hospitals. *Law, Medicine Health Care* 1984; **12**: 68–71, 79.
24. Mullan F, Politzer RM, Lewis CT, Bastacky S, Rodak J Jr, Harmon RG. The National Practitioner Data Bank – report from the first year. *J Am Med Assoc* 1992; **268**: 73–9.
25. Public Law No. 99–660, 100 Stat. 3784.
26. Southwick A. *The Law of Hospital and Health Care Administration*, 2nd edn. Ann Arbor, MI: Health Administration Press, 1988.
27. Hall MA. The malpractice standard under health care cost containment. *Law, Medicine Health Care* 1989; **17**: 347–55.
28. Morreim EH. Stratified scarcity: redefining the standard of care. *Law, Medicine Health Care* 1989; **17**: 356–67.
29. *Wickline* v. *California*, 192 Cal.App.3d 1630, 239 Cal.Rptr. 810 (1986).
30. Benesch K, Abramson NS, Grenvik A, Meisel A (eds). *Medicolegal Aspects of Critical Care.* Rockville, MD: Aspen Publishers, 1986.
31. Raffin TA, Shurkin JN, Sinkler W III. *Intensive care:*

Facing the Critical Choices. New York: WW Freeman & Company, 1989: Ch. 10.

32. Eddy DM. Practice policies – what are they? *J Am Med Assoc* 1990; **263**: 877–80.

33. Woolf SH. Practice guidelines: a new reality in medicine. I. Recent developments. *Arch Intern Med* 1990; **150**: 1811–18.

34. US General Accounting Office. *Practice Guidelines: the Experience of Medical Specialty Societies*. Washington, DC, GAO/ PEMD-91–11, February 1991.

35. Woolf SH. Practice guidelines: a new reality in medicine. II. methods of developing guidelines. *Arch Intern Med* 1992; **152**: 946–52.

36. Fletcher RH, Fletcher SW. Clinical practice guidelines. *Ann Intern Med* 1990; **113**: 645–6.

37. Anbar M. Guidelines for medical practice and the future of medicine. *Arch Intern Med* 1992; **152**: 266–7.

38. American Medical Association. *Legal Implications of Practice Parameters*. Chicago: AMA, 1990.

39. Havighurst CC. Practice guidelines as legal standards governing physician liability. *Law Contemporary Problems* 1991; **54**: 87–117.

40. Rosner F. Hospital medical ethics committees: a review of their development. *J Am Med Assoc* 1985; **253**: 2693–7.

41. American Medical Association, Judicial Council. Guidelines for ethics committees in health care institutions. *J Am Med Assoc* 1985; **253**: 2698–9.

42. Public Law No. 101–508, §4206, codified at 42 United States Code §1395cc(a)(1).

43. Gramelspacher GP. Institutional ethics committees and case consultation: is there a role? *Issues Law Medicine* 1991; **7**: 73–82.

44. Staubach SM. What legal protection should a hospital provide, if any, to its ethics committee and individual members? *Hospital Ethics Committee Forum* 1989; **1**: 209–20.

CHAPTER 27

Moral and Religious Dilemmas

K BOYD

Introduction   391
The special case of Jehovah's Witnesses   393
Allowing or assisting patients to die   396
References   398

Introduction

Not all ethical issues in critical care are moral dilemmas or involve religion. But a need for rapid decision making may provoke moral dilemmas, and when these are about matters of life and death, religion can be a significant factor. This chapter will discuss two very different aspects of this: first, the special case of Jehovah's Witnesses; and second, broader issues related to allowing or assisting patients to die. We begin however with some general observations about medico-moral dilemmas and religion.

Moral dilemmas, by definition, are choices between equally unsatisfactory options, each of which entails sacrificing something of great value – whether it be a human life which otherwise might have been saved, or an ethical principle (such as telling the truth or keeping promises) which ought to have been respected. One sign of a true moral dilemma is that, after deciding, we often feel not just regret, but remorse. Most moral choices, in critical care as in health care generally, are not of this kind. But sometimes they are, and religious beliefs can play a part in this.

Religious beliefs influence how countless people make sense of themselves and of life. Other people may disagree with a particular set of religious beliefs, but they cannot normally disprove them: there are rational criteria for determining the truth or falsity of factual claims, but no equivalent for the value-judgments on which religious claims are based. Others, of course,

may have a moral duty to try to dissuade or even restrain someone from acting on a religious belief if the action will harm third parties. But if the action harms only the believer, intervention is more difficult to justify. It is particularly difficult if the harm involved seems, to the believer, less than the harm they will incur (for example to their eternal destiny) by going against their religion's teaching. The fact that no-one can prove that the believer is wrong about this is a good reason for respecting strongly held religious beliefs, even when one cannot agree with them.[1]

But what if the reasons for not agreeing also are strongly held? And what if they too have religious origins? When a Jehovah's Witness refuses a life-saving blood transfusion, for example, not only his or her beliefs, but also those of the medical and other staff are involved. The Hippocratic tradition in medicine, religious in origin,[2] and deeply influenced by Islam and Christianity, requires doctors to 'maintain the utmost respect for human life.'[3] This duty is emphasized, if anything, even more strongly in Jewish medical ethics;[4] and the nursing profession, with a significant part of its background in religious orders, shares this commitment. Nor is it simply a matter of the dilemma for professional ethics. The personal religious beliefs of many doctors and nurses may well lead them to conclude that Jehovah's Witnesses are profoundly mistaken about the implications for their eternal destiny.

Religious tensions also are involved in the other main issue to be discussed in this chapter – that of allowing or assisting patients to die. For example, the reasons given by most patients requesting euthanasia in the Netherlands today – 'loss of dignity' or 'not dying in a dignified way'[5] – are little different from those of ancient Stoics like Marcus Aurelius and Seneca or later Renaissance and Enlightenment thinkers like Francis Bacon and David Hume.[6] To object that these are philosophical rather than religious reasons begs the question, since it is not always possible to distinguish, either in principle or in practice, between a religion and a philosophy of life: Eastern religion, for example, may lack the concept of God, while Humanism can claim to be counted among the world religions.[7] Protestant thinking in the Netherlands and other countries influenced by the Reformation, moreover, was also deeply influenced by Renaissance and Enlightenment philosophy; and two of England's best-known apologies for suicide were written by two of its most distinguished churchmen, Thomas More[8] and John Donne.[9]

The part played by religion in medico-moral dilemmas then, is considerably more complicated than may appear at first sight. It includes the uncompromising stand taken by the Jehovah's Witnesses on blood transfusion and the Roman Catholic church on abortion and euthanasia. But different conclusions about these questions can be reached from other religious premises; and when these conclusions are expressed in provisional or context-dependent terms, that too may reflect a religious point of view – either one which sees all human judgments, including ecclesiastical, as fallible, or one which believes that the individual's conscience should always be respected.

The involvement of religion in moral dilemmas is further complicated by the fact that beliefs vary not only between but also within religions. For example, in a recent American survey of the attitudes of critical care medicine professionals concerning foregoing life-sustaining treatments,[10] a 'higher percentage of Jewish respondents reported that they had withheld or withdrawn therapies compared with Catholics or adherents of other religions.' As the authors of the study comment, this was

> surprising given the major importance in Jewish law of preserving life and differentiations between withholding and withdrawing and the theological basis in Catholicism for differentiating between ordinary and extraordinary care.

An explanation of this surprising finding, the authors suggest, could be either that

> some Catholics may be less likely to act on this distinction because of the range of therapeutic options they personally consider to fall within the realm of the ordinary [or] that some respondents belonging to a particular faith may not necessarily adhere to its teachings in these matters.

These possible explanations, however, should probably also be seen in the light of three other factors:

1. that different branches of Judaism have different ways of defining the point at which there is no reasonable hope of a patient's recovery;[11]
2. that traditional Catholic teaching morally obliges individuals to do what they believe to be right, even if they are (from the Church's point of view) mistaken;[12] and
3. that the Hippocratic tradition emphasizes the medical duty not only to

> 'maintain the utmost respect for life', but also[13] to do away with the sufferings of the sick, to lessen the violence of their diseases, and to refuse to treat those who are over-mastered by their diseases, realising that in such cases medicine is powerless.

The complexity of religion's involvement in medico-moral dilemmas applies equally, of course, to the attitudes of patients. What counts as a religious belief, how fundamental it is for the religion concerned, and how the relation between official teaching and individual conscience is understood by the patient, are all significant factors. Clearly, given so many variables, it is unrealistic to expect doctors or nurses to be experts in comparative religion. They need, of course, to be aware of the kinds of issue which may have religious significance for certain patients – obvious examples are attitudes to religious observance, the body, clothing, the opposite sex, diet, animal tissue, drugs, alcohol, pain and its treatment, dying and the last offices.[14] But the significance of these issues in each case will depend on how each patient understands the teachings of their particular branch of their religion.

In most cases then, knowing about all the religious beliefs which might play a part in medico-moral dilemmas is less important than knowing how to encourage a relationship of partnership with the patient. Establishing a partnership – based on respect for autonomy and expressed though open dialogue[15] – is normally the most effective way of empowering a patient to make his or her religious wishes known and thus of empowering the professional to respond appropriately.

This is not possible, of course, in crises involving a hitherto unknown patient who is unconscious or otherwise unable to make his or her wishes known. In that case, a clinical judgment simply has to be made about what seem to be the patient's best interests. At such times or soon afterwards, if the patient's ability to make choices remains impaired, the balance of moral argument supports normal clinical practice. Those whose relationship with the patient 'is long-term and characterized by interdependence,' and whose own lives as well as the patient's may be affected by any choices made, should be consulted and, unless there seem to be reasons why the patient would not have wished this, involved in decision making.[16]

Medico-moral dilemmas involving religion, in other

words, can normally be avoided or resolved by good communication and respect for the autonomy and integrity of patients and their families. Most religions either have ways of interpreting traditional teaching to accommodate modern medical practice, or allow their members freedom of conscience. Thus with all but the strictest sects, patience and courtesy will normally lead to agreement on a mutually acceptable form of care and treatment, especially when the latter is life-saving.

The strictest sects, moreover, are remarkably few. One or two new religious movements have members who occasionally reject modern medicine[17] and Christian Scientists may refuse drugs.[18] But in practice, moral dilemmas involving patients who refuse potentially successful life-saving treatment are likely to arise only in the case of adult Jehovah's Witnesses, who in the UK now number about a quarter of a million people.

The special case of Jehovah's Witnesses

Jehovah's Witnesses, then, seem to be a special case – and in some respects a puzzling one. At the time of writing, the most recently reported death of a British Jehovah's Witness after refusing a blood transfusion was in early January 1993. The patient, a 45-year-old father of two, had been seriously injured in a motorway crash, but remained conscious. A spokesman of the Jehovah's Witnesses stated: 'We feel that blood is a very special category of substance. The Bible repeatedly enjoins people not to take blood into their bodies and we accept that.' The general manager of the hospital involved commented: 'Our policy is to respect the wishes of patients and their families in cases where they are able to make their wishes clear and we did not give him blood.'[19]

The comments of these two spokesmen make it sound as if this case creates no moral dilemma. When an adult patient, with the capacity to decide, refuses consent to treatment, the doctors involved are relieved of any responsibility to maintain life – or indeed from what in other circumstances would be a normal duty of medical care. But are the moral and religious issues really so clear-cut?

OTHER RELIGIOUS VIEWS

One reason for doubting this is that no major religion for which the Biblical scriptures are authoritative endorses the Jehovah's Witnesses' interpretation of the texts[20] on which their opposition to blood transfusion is based. For example, the prohibition of 'eating blood' in a literal sense is taken seriously by Judaism. But its

extension to blood transfusion contradicts the more basic principles which make Judaism view the gift of blood to save a neighbor's life as a religious obligation.[21] Again, many Islamic authorities now employ the principle of public benefit to interpret new ideas not referred to in the Qur'an and Oral tradition. These authorities state that not only organ transplants (to which *per se* Jehovah's Witnesses are not opposed) but also blood transfusions are[22]

> legitimate, despite the fact that spilling out of blood is forbidden by Islamic law. It is acceptable to donate blood because this does not harm the donor, analogous to wet-nursing which is allowed by Islamic law.

Charity and the public good are important also to Christians: and all of the churches regard Jehovah's Witnesses' emphasis on and interpretation of the texts concerned as arbitrary and mistaken.

THE ATTITUDE OF THE LAW

In the light of the religious consensus that Jehovah's Witnesses are mistaken in their interpretation of Scripture, what seems most puzzling is the law's attitude to refusal of life-saving treatment by adult Jehovah's Witnesses. (The law's attitude to the children of Jehovah's Witnesses is more understandable and will not be discussed in this chapter.) Why is this particular religious belief, so clearly rejected by other religious authorities, now so clearly defended in law as to discharge doctors of their normal responsibilities in a case like that just mentioned?

The law's answer appears to be that blood transfusion cannot be achieved without bodily invasion; and that without the consent of a patient capable of giving it, bodily invasion is not medical treatment but assault. On these grounds, the law respects the right to refuse treatment – as an English Appeal Court judge stated in an earlier case involving Jehovah's Witnesses – whether the reasons for refusing are 'rational, irrational, unknown or even non-existent.'[23]

But if the reasons for refusing treatment really are immaterial, is the law's attitude to Jehovah's Witnesses not even more puzzling? If the case mentioned above (a 45-year-old father of two, within 24 hours of involvement in a car crash) had not involved a Jehovah's Witness, could respecting the patient's refusal of treatment have been justified simply by saying that medical treatment without consent is assault? Or if the patient had refused treatment for 'reasons' which were 'irrational' or 'non-existent,' might not the psychological implications (of that logical contradiction in terms) have given most doctors reason to think that they would be failing in their normal duty of care if they did not seek a psychiatric opinion? Or again, if urgent life-saving treatment was necessary, might not the doctor's duty be analogous to that recommended in current ethical guidelines in the case of clinical depression – namely 'that clinicians identify and treat conditions that transiently impair decision-making capacity before deciding to withhold or withdraw life-sustaining therapy'?[24] The moral argument in this case, indeed, might be even more compelling than in that of depression, since there is some evidence to suggest that, among the elderly for example, depressed patients who refuse life-sustaining therapy may have reasons for doing so which are not irrational.[25]

A MORAL ARGUMENT

There is also a further moral argument. The philosophical principle underlying the right to refuse treatment is that of respect for autonomy. But should one respect the autonomy of someone who proposes to exercise it in a way which means that they will then inevitably lose the power to exercise it? A Committee of the European Parliament, for example, has put this argument (in relation to euthanasia) in the following way.[26]

> It is quite clear that freedom presupposes the right to life. In the context of physical life, death is the exact opposite of freedom, the end of freedom. Freedom cannot negate itself: it is therefore not admissible to become a slave. For that reason, in the event of a suicide attempt, a person who intervenes, even by force, to prevent this act . . . is not robbing but restoring that individual's freedom.

This argument is very persuasive – if only because many would-be suicides have survived to thank those who saved them. So might not a doctor 'who intervenes, even by force' to give a necessary blood transfusion to a nonconsenting Jehovah's Witness be 'not robbing but restoring that individual's freedom'?

An objection to the Committee's argument however is that it fails to take account of the fact that some reasons for committing suicide may be judged more reasonable than others: much depends on the intentions and circumstances of the person concerned; and in practice it may be possible to distinguish between a 'rational suicide' and a 'cry for help' – either from the individual's previously expressed wishes or, if their wishes are unknown, by the care which they have taken to avoid having the attempt detected. Similar considerations apply to the Jehovah's Witness – who is concerned not, like the Committee, with 'the context of physical life,' but with that of his eternal destiny. The moral grounds for respecting his wishes are, as already suggested, that he believes he has good reasons for refusing life-saving treatment and because no-one else is in a better position than he is to judge this.

This moral argument is very different however from saying that the right to refuse treatment should be respected regardless of the reasons. It is difficult therefore to escape the conclusion that the reason why the law respects the wishes of Jehovah's Witnesses is not simply because medical treatment without consent is assault, but because of the ease with which the particular treatment to which Jehovah's Witnesses object can be identified. In this respect, the statement quoted above by the hospital general manager seems disingenuous. 'Our policy is to respect the wishes of patients and their families in cases where they are able to make their wishes clear', obscures the issue. It sounds as if it applies to any patient's capacity to make and communicate a decision. But in practice, their well-known and very clear wishes about a specific medical procedure set Jehovah's Witnesses apart from almost all other patients.

MORALITY, LAW AND POLICY

From the point of view of ethics, this legal expedient clearly is unsatisfactory, and a further question arises. If the intentions and circumstances of the Jehovah's Witness patient are what morally (even if not legally) justify respect for his refusal of life-saving treatment, are not the intentions and circumstances of the doctors involved also relevant to any definition of their acts? There is, after all, something offensive to common sense in the description of a medical act, whereby someone's life and health are saved, as 'assault'; and only in the law's totally decontextualized view could it be so radically distorted and misrepresented.

Why does the law do this? The historical reasons are perhaps sufficiently explained in Maine's dictum:[27]

> Analogy, the most valuable of instruments in the maturity of jurisprudence, is the most dangerous of snares in its infancy. Prohibitions and ordinances, originally confined, for good reasons, to a single description of acts, are made to apply to all acts of the same class, because a man menaced with the anger of the gods for doing one thing, feels a natural terror in doing any other thing which is remotely like it.

But as this suggests, the analogy may no longer be appropriate when the actions of doctors towards their patients are governed and regulated in many other ways than by the criminal law.

The question of doctors' intentions and circumstances is not raised here in order to argue that they should be allowed to give blood transfusions to Jehovah's Witnesses against their well-considered wishes. The 'other ways' in which doctors are governed and regulated include medical ethics – in which the basic principles[28] of beneficence and nonmaleficence cannot be allowed simply to override the equally basic principle of respect for autonomy. As long as adult Jehovah's Witnesses capable of making decisions for themselves refuse to have blood transfusions, their autonomy must be respected. But the duty to respect the autonomy of these patients does not abrogate their doctors' continuing and equally important duties of beneficence and nonmaleficence towards them. This undoubtedly creates a genuine moral dilemma for doctors, which cannot be dissolved by invoking a 'policy' of respecting 'the wishes of patients and their families when they are able to make their wishes clear.'

The fourth basic principle of medical ethics – that of justice or fairness – also is relevant. It means that if the religious wishes of Jehovah's Witnesses are to be respected, so too should those of any other patient. The practical implications can be illustrated by advice given to the growing number of Tibetan Buddists in the West by one of their most respected teachers. Bearing in mind the spiritual significance for Buddists of dying in silence and serenity, and of their bodies remaining undisturbed thereafter, he writes:[29]

> If you can, you should arrange with the doctor to be told when there is no possibility of the person recovering, and then request to have them moved to a private room, if the dying person wishes it, with the monitors disconnected. Make sure that the staff knows and respects the dying person's wishes, especially if he or she does not wish to be resuscitated, and make sure that the staff knows too to leave the body undisturbed after death for as long as possible.

CURRENT GUIDELINES

In Britain, medico-moral dilemmas raised by Jehovah's Witnesses were made no easier by guidelines issued by the Court of Appeal in July 1992. These stated:[30]

> Where an adult patient had refused to consent to treatment which in the clinical judgement of the doctors was necessary, the doctors should consider (1) whether the patient's capacity to make the decision had been affected by the effects of shock, pain or drugs; (2) whether the patient's capacity had been overborne by outside influences; and (3) whether the patient's decision had been intended to apply to the particular circumstances which had arisen.

These guidelines derive from the case of a patient, Miss T, who, although not a Jehovah's Witness, had signed a form of refusal of consent to blood transfusion, but under the influence of her mother (a 'fervent' believer) and in circumstances when she was not fully aware of the consequences. In Miss T's case, the reasoning behind the Court's guidelines led it to decide that it was not unlawful for the hospital to administer blood. But that reasoning may be more difficult for doctors to apply in other cases.

Difficulty is likely to arise because all the questions which the guidelines ask doctors to consider are matters of judgment. The first is probably the least contentious, since answering it is mainly a matter of medical judgment. But the third poses potentially quite undecidable questions; and with reference to religion, the second – 'whether the patient's capacity has been overborne by outside influence' – is the most difficult to answer. Expecting doctors to disentangle 'outside' influences from the complex psychological web of a patient's relationship with religion, especially when some of the strands are familial, may be asking the impossible. It seems, indeed, tantamount to asking them to be judges of the sincerity of their patients' beliefs – a role for which doctors neither are nor should be qualified. They may need to make their own tentative judgments when discussing with patients – or, when the patient cannot participate in decision making, to determine what is in the patient's best interest, or who is best placed to interpret the patient's wishes. But this is a very different matter from having to make particular judgments in the shadow of the law's decontextualized view of medical treatment without consent as assault. To require doctors to make formal judgments of this kind, which might later be cited in court, can only encourage defensive medical practice.

WRITING AND SOCIAL CHANGE

One reason why the law privileges Jehovah's Witnesses has already been suggested by quoting Maine's observation about laws 'originally confined, for good reasons, to a single description of acts' being 'made to apply to all acts of the same class' – hence the conflation of medical treatment and assault insofar as each involves bodily invasion.

A further aspect of this question is explored by the anthropologist J Goody, who points out that writing (among other factors) has played an important part in 'the decontextualization or generalization of norms,' not only in law, but also in religion.[31] A society without writing has greater freedom to reconcile conflicting interests of the kind discussed above both because it is not tied to the letter of a law, and because it has no concept of 'a' religion, let alone 'religions' as distinct from its whole way of life. This flexibility is particularly useful, of course, at times of social change. But written records make convenient forgetting, necessary for compromise, more difficult. Law, Goody observes, is now no longer where the 'simple person' thinks it should be, 'in conscience and public opinion, in custom, and sound human understanding,' but in books;[32] and historically because varying interpretation of the authoritative religious Book led to dissent, 'given literate expression, even dissent established its own tradition.'[33]

Against this background, the legal problems created by Jehovah's Witnesses can be seen as symptomatic of a literate society whose circumstances have changed (by the innovation of blood transfusion), but in which the written traditions of both the law and dissent stand in the way of any accommodation to that change. In such circumstances, Goody points out, 'some means has to be found of deliberately altering (or ignoring) the [existing legal] code.'[34] He then cites the three ways in which Maine stated that this could be done: by Legal Fictions, by Equity and by Legislation.[35] We shall return to these below.

Allowing or assisting patients to die

PARLIAMENTARY RESPONSE TO RECENT LEGAL CASES

A need for legal accommodation to changing circumstances has been increasingly perceived in relation to the ethics of allowing or assisting patients to die. Matters were brought to a head in Britain, during 1992, by the conviction for attempted murder of a rheumatologist (Dr Nigel Cox) who gave a dying patient a lethal injection of potassium chloride, and by the courts allowing the doctors of a patient in the persistent vegetative state (Mr Anthony Bland) to discontinue artificial feeding. In the final judgment on the latter case, by the House of Lords, Lord Mustil stated[36] that it emphasized 'the distortions of a legal structure which is already both morally and intellectually misshapen' and that the

> whole matter cries out for exploration in depth by Parliament and then for the establishment by legislation not only of a new set of ethically and intellectually consistent rules, distinct from the general criminal law, but also of a sound procedural framework within which the rules can be applied to individual cases. The rapid advance of medical technology makes this an ever more urgent task ...

No such authoritative comment was made in the case of Dr Cox. But the moral incongruity, for many people, of his conviction was illustrated by three members of the jury which found him guilty weeping when the verdict was announced,[37] and by the subsequent decision of the General Medical Council not to impose any sanction upon him.[38]

The Parliamentary response to these events was set up, in February 1993, a House of Lords committee:[39]

> To consider the ethical, legal and clinical implications of a person's right to withhold consent to life-prolonging treatment, and the position of persons who are no longer able to give or withhold consent. To consider whether and in what circumstances actions that have as

their intention or a likely consequence the shortening of another person's life may be justified on the grounds that they accord with that person's wishes or with that person's best interests; and in all the forgoing considerations regard is to be paid to the likely effects of changes in law or medical practice on society as a whole.

These terms of reference thus include not only withholding or withdrawing treatment, but also euthanasia and possibly assisted suicide, acts permitted under certain circumstances in the Netherlands, and which there are continuing attempts to legalize in the USA. As the experience of these and other countries suggests, the influence of religion is likely to play a significant part in determining whether any 'new set of ethically and intellectually consistent rules' and 'sound procedural framework' which might be proposed by the House of Lords committee will successfully pass into legislation. (See Note Added in Proof, p. 398.)

RELIGIOUS LIMITATIONS TO CHANGE

The possibility of religious agreement with any 'new set of ethically and intellectually consistent rules' is likely to be limited by the different ways in which the major religions interpret their authoritative written texts. On some issues, change is possible. For example, some Catholics have claimed that withdrawing artificial feeding from a patient in the persistent vegetative state is forbidden by the commandment 'Do not kill,' and have supported this by pointing to the symbolic significance of feeding those who cannot feed themselves. But other Catholics now see this as a overly legalistic reading of the commandment, and argue that it has to be understood in the context both of more general scriptural teaching and of the intentions and circumstances of the act. Thus, they write that to 'persist in indiscriminately using such gestures can convey stupidity and cruelty, not compassion and love.'[40] Other religious traditions argue in their own ways. Those Islamic authorities who employ the principle of public benefit to interpret new ideas not referred to in the Qur'an and Oral tradition, for example, have already been mentioned.

Accommodating religious tradition to new practices is more difficult however when the practice can be very clearly identified with what is unequivocally forbidden in authoritative written texts. The Qur'an, for example, prohibits not only murder, but also suicide, leading an Islamic authority to state that 'euthanasia is 100 percent not accepted in Islam, for mercy reasons or anything.'[41] The same is not true, on the other hand, of suicide in the Christian scriptures. As David Hume remarked, 'There is not a single text of Scripture which prohibits it.'[42] What Hume's observation excludes, however, are all the authoritative non-Scriptural texts of the Roman

Catholic Church which prohibit not only suicide, but also, and increasingly in recent years, euthanasia. Like Jehovah's Witnesses on blood transfusion, Roman Catholic authorities have drawn a very firm line indeed at 'intentional direct killing,' and it is difficult to imagine any circumstances in which they would be prepared to consider as justifiable 'actions that have as their intention ... the shortening of another person's life.'

How is it then that in a country like the Netherlands, a substantial minority of whose population is Roman Catholic, this (at least officially) new practice is now permitted? Leaving aside the traditional importance of individual freedom of conscience among Roman Catholics, part of the answer may be that significant objections have not been raised by the majority Reformed Churches.[43] Their interpretation of Scripture, unconditioned by the detailed commentary of authoritative non-Scriptural texts, has to take seriously an observation of the kind made by Hume – and having done so, to take into account the kind of contextual considerations which now lead some Roman Catholics to regard withholding or withdrawing treatment as acceptable in certain circumstances.

Despite this, of course, euthanasia has not been legalized in the Netherlands, where it remains a potentially criminal act unless carried out according to very specific guidelines. This suggests that the Netherlands has responded to changing circumstances (medicine's ability to keep people alive and Dutch public opinion) by opting for the first of Maine's categories – a legal fiction, or 'assumption which conceals or affects to conceal, the fact that a rule of law has undergone alteration, its letter remaining unchanged, its operation being modified.'[44] If the diagnosis, by Lord Mustil, of the present English law as 'both morally and intellectually misshapen' is accurate, a similar palliative measure may be the most that will be achieved in Britain also. A legislative cure, in terms of 'a new set of ethically and intellectually consistent rules,' simply does not seem possible as long as a substantial proportion of the population continues to subscribe to Roman Catholic, Islamic and other religious objections to euthanasia.

RELIGION AND EQUITY

Religious objections to euthanasia, however, are unlikely to silence those who argue that it is sometimes morally justifiable for doctors to assist a patient's death, and that the law should recognize this. Assisting death may be justifiable, they argue, when this is what the patient truly wishes, and when all other means of relieving pain or suffering have been exhausted.[45] Nor is this argument likely to be silenced by medical claims that such occasions can be avoided by better management of terminal pain. This is not only because even the best medical management may sometimes fail to relieve intense and unremitting pain. It is also in some cases because, from the patient's own deeply considered point of view, rooted in the experience of a lifetime, the most appropriate way of ending their suffering is by being allowed or assisted 'to give up the ghost.'[46]

As this use of religious language implies, it is a mistake to see religious pressures operating only on one side of the dilemma which confronts medicine, the law and society in the current debate about the ethics of allowing or assisting patients to die. The dilemma, acknowledged in the House of Lords reference to 'the likely effects of changes in law or medical practice on society as a whole,' is created by the law's inability to guarantee that sufficient safeguards can be built into any legislation allowing medically assisted death.

The crucial question here is often represented in terms of whether or not to cross a moral boundary. On one side of that boundary the ground is clearly marked on ethical charts which show where it is safe to walk – not prolonging life by disproportionate or extraordinary means of medical treatment; treating terminal pain and suffering with pain-relieving drugs even if their use shortens the patient's life. On or near the boundary is the difficult but not impossible equation of artificial nutrition and hydration with extraordinary means of medical treatment, at least for patients in the persistent vegetative state. But beyond this is unknown territory: ending a patient's suffering at the patient's request by directly and intentionally ending the patient's life, some argue, is the fatal first step on a slippery slope. Once medically assisted death is legalized, doctors will have less incentive to explore all the alternatives, vulnerable patients (particularly the frail elderly) will feel or be pressurized to ask for it, and it will then be but a short step to involuntary euthanasia.

Representing these issues simply in terms of whether or not to cross this moral boundary, however, is not necessarily the most adequate way of understanding them. For many doctors, nurses and clergy with pastoral responsibility, it will seem an ethically impoverished description of the choice actually facing many patients and practitioners. Crucial variables missing from it are the uniqueness and the fallibility of the individuals involved. When a moral dilemma about allowing or assisting a patient to die arises, legal and ethical analysis, the law and official guidelines, can go a long way towards informing those involved about what are the best (or 'least worst') ways of resolving this kind of dilemma. But precisely because it is this particular dilemma, they cannot predetermine which way to choose on this occasion. That remains a matter for fallible human judgment, which will inevitably be influenced by the character of and relationships between the doctors, nurses, patients and families involved.

This has significant implications for society's choice of legislative cures or palliation for its 'morally and intellectually misshapen' laws. Whether these remain as they are or are changed, the moral claims of individual patients and of society will inevitably depend, for justice to be done to them, on the degree of maturity of judgment of individual doctors and nurses, and on how this is encouraged by means of education, peer-review and professional association. Attending to these factors is essential in order to serve the best interests of those most intimately affected by the outcome of the present debate – whatever its outcome may be. Attending to these factors is also a religious requirement, since religion is concerned not just with what is right or wrong (expressed at present mostly in terms of caution about euthanasia), but also with encouraging what is good in human character.

In this respect, Maine's third way of accommodating the law to changing circumstances is suggestive. 'Equity,' Maine states, is 'any body of rules existing by the side of the original civil law, founded on distinct principles and claiming incidentally to supersede the civil law in virtue of a superior sanctity inherent in these principles.'[47] Leaving aside the technical aspects of this concept, it seems clear that many people in Britain, observing the *Bland* and *Cox* cases, felt that judgments made in the intimacy of professional relationships embodied rules and principles of superior sanctity to those of a law which identified assault as the base line for medical treatment. The law, in other words, was intruding in matters on which the professionals, patients and families concerned were better judges.

Feelings of this kind, clearly, are an inadequate basis on which to decide how the present debate about legislation should be resolved. As the Netherlands' choice of a legal fiction – and of course the frequently invoked example of Nazi Germany – imply, the possibility of medical treatment becoming a form of assault can never be excluded, and therefore the possibility of legal prosecution must always be retained in the background. But that acknowledged, the most important question in the foreground remains how those who are (in Sir Thomas Browne's words) 'capable of goodnesse' and might be 'railed into vice' can 'as easily be admonished into virtue.'[48]

Lord Mustil's call for 'a new set of ethically and intellectually consistent rules' perhaps underestimates the limitations of human rationality; and indeed Maine may have been correct to remark on 'the exaggerated respect which is ordinarily paid to the doubtful virtue of consistency.'[49] But the notion of 'a sound procedural framework ... distinct from the general criminal law ... within which ... rules can be applied to individual cases' is already familiar to doctors in the process of confidential review of perinatal and perioperative deaths; and an appropriate extension of this kind of procedure could help to bridge the gap between the respective requirements of the law and of medico-moral judgment in individual cases. Such procedures, indeed, have already been advocated by at least one group from within the Church of England.[50]

Procedural frameworks alone, however, will not provide sufficient public reassurance that justice is being done to the interests both of individual patients and of society in the difficult area of moral dilemmas related to allowing or assisting patients to die. Medicine and the professions related to it also need to be seen to be helping their members become more responsive to the wishes of their increasingly well-informed patients and their families. How to improve the quality of professional education and communication thus is perhaps the greatest single challenge in this area.[51]

Note Added in Proof

Since this chapter was written, the House of Lords committee mentioned in the text has published its report.[52] This strongly endorses 'the right of the competent patient to refuse consent to any medical treatment, for whatever reason,' and recommends 'that there should be no change in the law to permit euthanasia.' Subsequently, the English Law Commission published an important report on Mental Incapacity.[53] This recommends that 'advance refusal of treatment' should have recognized legal status and that a judicial forum with powers related to health care matters should be created.

References

1. Wreen MJ. Autonomy, religious values, and refusal of lifesaving medical treatment. *J Med Ethics* 1991; **17**: 124–30.
2. Edelstein L. *Ancient Medicine*. Baltimore: Johns Hopkins Press, 1967: 3–63.
3. Declaration of Geneva, 1948. Mason JK, McCall Smith RA. *Law and Medical Ethics*. London: Butterworths, 1991: 440.
4. Jakobovits I. *Jewish Medical Ethics*. New York: Bloch Publishing Company, 1959: 49ff.
5. van der Maas PJ, van Delden JJM, Pijnenborg L. *Euthanasia and other Medical Decisions Concerning the End of Life*. Amsterdam: Elsevier, 1992: 44–5.
6. Cowley LT, Young E, Raffin TA. Care of the dying: an ethical and historical perspective. *Crit Care Med* 1992; **20**: 1473–82.
7. Larue GA. *Euthanasia and Religion. A Survey of the Attitudes of World Religions to the Right-to-die*. Los Angeles: Hemlock Society, 1985: 127–31.
8. More T. *Utopia* (1516). London: JM Dent & Sons Ltd, 1951.

9. Donne J. *Biathanatos* (1647). New York: Garland Publishing, Inc, 1982.

10. The Society of Critical Care Medicine Ethics Committee. Attitudes of critical care medicine professionals concerning forgoing life-sustaining treatments. *Crit Care Med* 1992; **20**: 320–5.

11. Hamel R, DuBose ER. *Active Euthanasia, Religion, and the Public Debate.* Chicago: Park Ridge Center, 1991: 48.

12. McDermott T. *St Thomas Aquinas, Summa Theologiae, A Concise Translation.* London: Methuen, 1991: 196f. [I.19.5–6].

13. Hippocrates (Jones WHS trans). *The Art.* London: Heinmann, 1959: 193.

14. Sampson C. *The Neglected Ethic: Religious and Cultural Factors in the Care of Patients.* London: McGraw-Hill Book Company (UK) Ltd, 1982: 10–14.

15. Institute of Medical Ethics Working Party on the Ethical Implications of AIDS. AIDS and the Ethics of Medical Care and Treatment. *Q J Med* 1992; NS 83, **302**: 419–26.

16. Jecker NS. *Aging and Ethics.* Clifton, New Jersey: Humana Press, 1991: 199–216.

17. Barker E. *New Religious Movements, A Practical Introduction.* London: Her Majesty's Stationery Office, 1989: 62.

18. See ref. 14: 93–5.

19. News Item. Jehovah's Witness dies after refusing blood transfusion. *The Independent.* 8 January 1993: 5.

20. Genesis 9: 3–4; Leviticus 17: 10–14; Deuteronomy 12: 33; Acts 15: 28–9.

21. See ref. 4: 285.

22. Rispler-Chaim V. Islamic medical ethics in the 20th century. *J Med Ethics* 1989; **15**: 203–8.

23. Tan YH. Law Report: Decision on treatment did not cover emergency. *The Independent.* 31 July 1992: 22.

24. Lee MA. Depression and refusal of life support in older people: an ethical dilemma. *J Am Geriatrics Soc* 1990; **38**: 710–14.

25. Lee MA, Ganzinin L. Depression in the elderly: effect on patient attitudes toward life-sustaining therapy. *J Am Geriatrics Soc* 1992; **40**: 983–8.

26. Committee on Legal Affairs and Citizens Rights. Draft Opinion on the motion for a resolution on counselling for the terminally ill. Strasbourg: European Parliament, 1991, 12 September: 8f.

27. Maine HS. *Ancient Law* (1861). USA: Dorset Press, 1986: 16.

28. Gillon R. *Philosophical Medical Ethics.* Chichester: John Wiley & Sons, 1986.

29. Rinpoche S. *The Tibetan Book of Living and Dying.* London: Rider, 1992: 186.

30. See ref. 23.

31. Goody J. *The Logic of Writing and the Organization of Society.* Cambridge: Cambridge University Press, 1986: 12.

32. *Ibid*: 164.

33. *Ibid*: 31.

34. *Ibid*: 136.

35. *Ibid*: 138f.

36. House of Lords Judgement. *Airedale NHS Trust (Respondents) v. Bland (Acting by his guardian ad litem) (Appellant).* London: House of Lords 1993, 4 Feb: 39.

37. Dyer C. Rheumatologist convicted of attempted murder. *Br Med J* 1992; **305**: 731.

38. Dyer C. GMC tempers justice with mercy in Cox case. *Br Med J* 1992; **305**: 1311.

39. Warden J. Lords focus on medical ethics. *Br Med J* 1993; **306**: 541.

40. British Medical Association Medical Ethics Committee. *Discussion Paper on Treatment of Patients in Persistent Vegetative State.* London: British Medical Association, 1992: 17.

41. See ref. 11: 51.

42. Hume D. *On Suicide* (1777) in *Hume on Religion.* London: Collins, 1963: 262.

43. de Wachter MAM. Euthanasia in the Netherlands. *Hastings Center Report* 1992; **22** (2): 23–30.

44. See ref. 27: 21f.

45. Institute of Medical Ethics Working Party on the Ethics of Prolonging Life and Assisting Death. Assisted death. *The Lancet* 1990; **336**: 610–13.

46. St John's Gospel 10: 30.

47. See ref. 27: 23.

48. Browne T. *Religio Medici* (1643) in *Sir Thomas Browne: Selected Writings.* London: Faber & Faber, 1968: 72.

49. See ref. 27:53.

50. News Item. Doctors' aid body mooted. *Church Times.* 9 October 1992.

51. Wojtas O. Day to day, a life worth living. *The Times Higher.* 5 March 1993.

52. House of Lords. *Report of the Select Committee on Medical Ethics.* London: HMSO, 1994.

53. Law Commission. *Mental Incapacity.* London: HMSO, 1995.

Index

Abbreviated Injury Scale (AIS) 280, 282
Abdominal radiology 115–18
Abscesses, intra-abdominal, radiology 117
A/C (assist/control) ventilation 141, 142
Accommodation requirements, ICUs 39–45, 61
ACEI (angiotensin converting enzyme inhibitors), renal function and 182
Activated partial thromboplastin time (APTT) 131
Acute lung injury (ALI), extrapulmonary gas exchange 151
Acute Physiology and Chronic Health Evaluation *see* APACHE systems
Acute renal failure (ARF) *see* Renal failure
Acute ventilatory failure (respiratory acidosis) 140
Admission criteria
    age 290
    children 293
    elective intensive care 291
    emergencies 292, 294, 344–5
    ethics of prioritization 331–41
    for monitoring 8, 291, 300
    patient outcome data 290
    policy making and policing 292–3
    scoring systems 53, 284, 290–1, 294, 301–5
    trauma 292
    underlying disease 291
    unit management 51–2, 53–4, 60
Adult respiratory distress syndrome (ARDS) 7, 110
Advance directives (living wills) 347–8, 379, 385
Advanced Trauma Life Support (ATLS) 24, 28
Aerosol masks, oxygen delivery 136
Aerosol therapy, bronchial hygiene 137–8, 139
Age factors
    admission criteria 290
    costs of care 7
    geriatric intensive care units 63, 67
    as measure of physiological reserve 278
    patient demographics 6
    quality of life 311
Air conditioning, building design 43
Aircraft, patient transfer 22, 26–8, 31–2
Airway management
    bedside services 45
    bronchial hygiene therapy 136–8
    initial treatment 28–9
    primary care in the field 24–5
    see also Ventilation
Airway pressure release ventilation (APRV) 143–4
AIS (Abbreviated Injury Scale) 280, 282
ALI (acute lung injury), extrapulmonary gas exchange 151
Allen's test, collateral circulation 93

Ambulances 22, 26–8, 30
American Society of Anesthesiologists (ASA) status 280
Amrinone, cardiac failure 159–60, 173
Anencephalic donors, ethics 358
Angiography 108
Angioplasty, percutaneous transluminal coronary (PTCA) 161–2, 170, 171
Angiotensin converting enzyme inhibitors (ACEI), renal function and 182
Antiasthmatics, aerosolized 139
Aorta
    dissection of 112
    intra-aortic balloon pumping 6, 115, 161, 171, 173
    radiology of aortic aneurysm 118
    shearing injury to 111–12
APACHE systems 279
    admission decisions and 290, 291
    age factors 278, 279, 290
    clinical audit 266, 270, 283
    data collection 53
    dynamic scoring 278, 285
    expenditure forecasting 16, 17, 338
    GCS component 279, 281
    mortality/survival prediction 279, 285, 302–3, 304, 306, 309
    multiple organ dysfunction 292
    need for 8
    physiological reserve 277–8, 291
    treatment limitation 285
Apnea 140
Appendicitis, radiology 117
APRV (airway pressure release ventilation) 143–4
APTT (activated partial thromboplastin time) 131
ARAS (atherosclerotic renal artery stenosis) 182
Architecture of ICUs 39–44, 61
ARDS (adult respiratory distress syndrome) 7, 110
ARF (acute renal failure) *see* Renal failure
Arterial catheterization 6, 92–3, 94–6, 97, 98–9, 100
Arterial oxygen, noninvasive monitoring 77–8, 78–9
Arterial pressure, invasive monitoring 84, 91–2
Arterial tonometry, blood pressure measurement 71
Arteriography (angiography) 108
Artificial hearts (TAHs) 164–5, 169, 170
ASA (American Society of Anesthesiologists) status 280
Aspiration, radiology 109–10
Assist/control (A/C) ventilation 141, 142
Assisted suicide 346
    ethical arguments 396–8
    legal aspects 368, 369, 396
Atherosclerotic renal artery stenosis (ARAS) 182

ATLS (Advanced Trauma Life Support) 24, 28
Australia
    intensive care costs 14
    medical staff 197–201
    nursing staff 217–22
    organ donation 353
    physical therapy 239–43
    witholding and withdrawing care 17

Bed capacity and occupancy 16–17
    accommodation requirements 40–3
    growth rates 12–13
    guidelines on 38
    international comparisons 4, 5, 6
    moral and economic issues 7–8, 12, 16
    rationalization 15
    staffing levels and 5, 37, 38, 39, 213–14
    supply and demand 16–17, 300
Bedside services, monitoring and management 40–1, 44–5, 131
Belgium, ICU staffing 224–5
Bile duct calculus, radiology 116–17
Bioethics committees 361–2, 388–9
Biomedical engineers *see* Clinical engineers
BIPAC (biphasic positive airway pressure) 144
Bladder, blunt trauma to, radiology 118
Blood glucose analyzers 130
Blood pressure
    ARF and 183–4
    invasive monitoring
        arterial catheterization 92–3, 94–6, 99
        central venous catheterization 93–4
        MAP to reflect cardiovascular stability 91–2
        Ppao and left ventricular preload 86–9, 95
    noninvasive measurement of 70–1
Blood samples, laboratory analysis 128–31
Blood transfusions *see* Intravenous infusions
Blood warmers 29
Bowel radiology 115–16
Brain laryngeal mask airway 25
Brain stem, injuries to 120
Brain stem death
    defining death 346–7
    organ donation
        admission criteria 292
        diagnoses 351–3
        elective ventilation 355–6
        incidence of 353–4
        religious objections 355
    witholding and withdrawing care 17, 352, 369
Breathing *see* Respiratory headings; Ventilation
Bronchial hygiene therapy 136–8
Bronchodilators, aerosolized 139
Bronchoscopes, bedside services 45
Buddhism 355, 395
Building design, ICUs 39–44, 61
Bumetanide, reversal of ARF 185
Burns units 62, 65

CABG (coronary artery bypass grafting) 162–3
Canada
    ICU personnel and training 207–11
    intensive care costs 14

    legal issues, witholding and withdrawing care 370, 371, 373
    physical therapy 234–6
    respiratory therapy 236–8
CAPD (continuous ambulatory peritoneal dialysis) 189
Capnography 78–9
Carbon dioxide
    extrapulmonary gas exchange 151–2; *see also* Respiratory support
    high frequency ventilation 145
    monitoring of 78–9, 84, 97–8
Cardioscint, cardiac function assessment 71–2
Cardiovascular disease and failure
    cardiogenic pulmonary edema, diffuse alveolar shadowing and 110
    cardiogenic shock
        coronary artery bypass grafting 162–3
        hemodynamic management of 171–3
        inotropic agents 158–60, 173
        intra-aortic balloon pumping 161, 171, 173
        pathophysiology of 156–7
        percutaneous transluminal coronary angioplasty 161–2, 170, 171
        predictors of 157
        prognosis after development of 157–8
        thrombolytic therapy 161, 172
        vasodilators 160–1, 172–3
        ventricular assist devices/total artificial hearts 163–71
    coronary care units 7, 12, 15, 63, 67–8, 68, 291
        postoperative 62, 65–6
    defibrillation 7, 23, 26
    definition of failure 54
    DNR (do not resuscitate) orders 345
    intra-aortic balloon pumping 6, 115, 161, 171, 173
    mediastinum, radiology 111–12
    positioning pacemaker electrodes 114–15
    post cardiac arrest, admission criteria 292
    primary care in the field 21, 26
    VAD as transplantation bridge 166, 169, 170
    ventilation and
        cardiac output reduction with PEEP 147
        cardiopulmonary reserves assessment 150
Cardiovascular monitoring 70–7
    invasive 82–101
        arterial catheterization 6, 92–3, 94–6, 97, 98–9, 100
        benefits of 85
        central venous catheterization 6, 93–4, 97, 98, 99–100, 114
        clinical practice recommendations 100–1
        future research 101
        MAP as reflection of cardiovascular stability 91–2
        oxygen delivery and consumption to describe metabolic status 90–1
        physiological variables derived from 84–5
        Ppao and left ventricular preload 86–9, 95
        rationale for 82–4
    noninvasive
        blood pressure 70–1
        Doppler ultrasound 73–6
        perfusion 72–3
        radionucleotide imaging 71–2
        thoracic bioimpedance 76–7
        transesophageal echocardiography 72

Case law
    Airedale NHS Trust v Bland 369, 371–2, 373, 374–7,
        378, 379–80, 396, 398
    Barber v Superior Court 371, 377
    Beecham 369
    Bolam v Friern Hospital Management Committee 375, 377
    Bouvia v Superior Court 378
    Chatterson v Gerson 373
    Cruzan v Director, Missouri Department of Health 346,
        374, 378
    F v West Berkshire Health Authority 374, 375–6, 379
    Frenchay Healthcare NHS Trust v S 376–7, 379
    Leigh v Gladstone 372
    Malette v Schuman 373
    Nancy B v Hotel-Dieu de Quebec 370, 371
    R v Adams 368
    R v Arthur 377
    R v Cox 368–9, 396, 398
    Re C (A Minor) (Wardship: Medical Treatment) 377
    Re Conroy 370, 374, 377–8, 379
    Re J (A Minor) (Medical Treatment) 367, 376, 377
    Re Quinlan 346, 371, 374
    Re T (Adult: Refusal of Treatment) 372–3, 395
    Satz v Perlmutter 370
    Schloendorff v Society of New York Hospital 372
    Sidaway v Bethlem Royal and Maudsley Hospital 372
Case reviews, clinical audit differentiated 266
Cast nephropathy 181
Catecholamines, cardiac failure 158–9, 173
Catholicism, religious dilemmas 392, 396, 397
CCUs *see* Coronary care units
Cell lysis, ARF secondary to 181
Central venous catheterization 6, 93–4
    indications for 97, 98, 99–100
    positioning of 114
Central venous pressure (CVP), monitoring 84, 93–4
Cerebral infarcts, radiology 121
Cervical injury *see* Spinal injury
Chemotherapy, specialist care units 66–7
Chest drains, tube positioning 114
Chest Pain Index 305
Chest physical therapy (CPT) 138, 228–9, 236
Chest wall, radiology of fractures in 113–14
Children
    informed consent 384–5
    pediatric ICUs 15, 62, 64, 292–3
    primary care, intraosseous infusions 26
    witholding and withdrawing care, legal aspects 367,
        375–6, 377
    see also Neonatal intensive care
Cholecystitis, radiology 117
Choledocholithiasis, radiology 116–17
Christian Scientists 355, 393
Circulatory management 7
    arterial catheterization and 99
    cardiogenic shock 172
    during transfers 29
    initial treatment 29
    primary care in the field 22, 25–6
    religious objections to blood transfusions 347, 372–3,
        391, 393–6
    reversal of ARF 184–5

Clinical audit 265–74
    audit costs 273–4
    audit cycle principles 266–9
    audit teams 267, 269
    case review differentiated 266
    change implementation 268–9, 272–3
    data collection and analysis 52–3, 268, 270–2, 273–4
    data set selection 268, 269–70
    definition 265
    future directions 274
    general principles for SCU development 60
    report evaluation 268–9, 272–3
    research differentiated 265
    resource management differentiated 266
    severity scoring and 266, 270, 282–3
    standard setting 267–8
    topic selection 267
Clinical engineers 5, 255–61
    certification and registration 258
    clinical measurements 259–60
    education and training 257–8
    ethics 259
    history 256–7
    safety 259
    standards 259
    technology management 258–9
    user training 260
Clinical research, ethics 360–6
    complexity of research 362–6
        informed consent 364–5
        research phases 364
        study population 363–4
        variables 362–3
    ethics committees 361–2
    need for research 360–1
    research standards 362, 365–6
Closed ICU model 12, 13, 15–16
CMV (control mode ventilation) 141
Coagulation analyzers 131
Cohort studies 318
Colloid solutions 25–6, 172
Computed tomography (CT) 108
Computer support, clinical audit 270–2
Confidentiality, legal aspects 387–8
Conjunctival oxygen tension (CjO2), cardiac output and
    oxygen delivery and 73
Continuous ambulatory peritoneal dialysis (CAPD) 189
Continuous positive airway pressure (CPAP) 143–4, 147,
    148–9
Contrast enhanced radiography 107–8
Control mode ventilation (CMV) 141
Coronary artery bypass grafting (CABG) 162–3
Coronary care units (CCUs) 7
    admissions for monitoring 291
    characteristics of 63, 67–8
    in development of ICUs 12
    or multidisciplinary ICUs 15
    postoperative 62, 65–6
Coronary Prognostic Index (CPI) 280, 283
Costs of care *see* Financial issues
CPAP (continuous positive airway pressure) 143–4, 147,
    148–9

CPT (chest physical therapy) 138, 228–9, 236
Creatinine, glomerular filtration rate and 182
Cricothyroidotomy, primary care in the field 25
Critical care, definitions and history 3, 11–12, 36–8, 197, 289–90, 297–8
Crystalloid solutions 25–6, 172
CT (computed tomography) 108
CVP (central venous pressure), monitoring 84, 93–4

De Bakey classification, dissection of aorta 112
Death
    brain stem death diagnosis 351–3
    definition of 346–7
Decompression sickness, air transfers and 32
DEF (DEFinitive methodology), trauma scoring 280
Defibrillation 7, 23, 26
Demographics, patient populations 6, 7–8, 13
Dependency scoring, nursing levels and 53, 213–14, 221–2, 283
    see also Severity scoring
Diagnosis Related Group (DRG) system 221–2, 283–4
Diagnostic coding systems *see* Severity scoring
Diagnostic technology, benefits and costs 318–19, 320, 326–7
Dialysis 187–90
    adequacy of 190
    anticoagulation during 190
    bedside services 45
    building design 43
    dialysate solutions 187, 188–9
    hemodialysis 7, 43, 187–8
    hemofiltration 45, 189–90
    membranes 188
    peritoneal 189
    specialist units 63, 66
    vascular access 188
Diaphragm, radiology 113
Dietitians 5, 51
Diffuse alveolar shadowing, causes of 110–11
Diffuse axonal injury, radiology 119
Direct mechanical ventricular actuation (DMVA) 166, 170–1
Discharge criteria 51, 52, 53–4
Diuretics, reversal of ARF 185
Divers, air transfers of 32
DNR (do not resuscitate) orders 345, 378
Dobutamine, cardiac failure 158, 160, 173
Dopamine
    cardiac failure 158, 173
    renal failure 185
Doppler ultrasound, cardiac output 73–6
DRG (diagnosis related group) system 221–2, 283–4
Drugs
    aerosolized bronchodilators and antiasthmatics 139
    analyzers 130
    pharmaceutical knowledge of IC staff 195
    pharmacists' role 5
    primary care in the field 22, 25
    randomized control trials 318
    in renal failure 180, 181, 190
    see also Clinical research, ethics
Dyspnea Index 305

ECMO (extracorporeal membrane oxygenation) 151
Edema, pulmonary, diffuse alveolar shadowing and 110
Education *see* Training and competency
Elective intensive care
    preoperative scoring systems 282
    selection criteria 291
Elective ventilation, organ donation 355–6
Electrical supply, building design 43, 44
Electrolytes
    ARF and 183, 185, 186; *see also* Dialysis
    electrolyte analyzers 129
Electromagnetic flowmeter (EMF), cardiac output 75
Emboli
    diffuse alveolar shadowing and 110
    pulmonary 6, 109
Emergencies
    admission criteria and decision making 291–2, 294, 344–5
    initial treatment in emergency room 28–30
    see also Primary care in the field
Endotracheal intubation
    positioning 114
    primary care in the field 23, 25
Engineers, in medicine 255–61
Enzyme analyzers 130
Equipment *see* Health care technology
Erythropoietin (EPO), ARF and 183
Ethics 7–8, 13–14
    bioethics committees 361–2, 388–9
    clinical engineering 259
    in clinical research 360–6
    legal issues 347–9, 367–80, 382–9
    moral dilemmas and religious beliefs 347, 355, 372–3, 391–8
    organ donation 350–9
    prioritization 331–41
    witholding and withdrawing care 344–9, 352, 367–80
Europe
    bed capacity and occupancy 4, 5, 6, 12–13
    Belgian ICU staffing 224–5
    EC requirements and guidelines
        nursing 223–4
        physiotherapy 250–4
    euthanasia 368, 391–2, 397–8
    French primary care system (SAMU) 21
    intensive care costs 14
    witholding and withdrawing care 348, 349
    see also UK
Euthanasia 17, 345–6
    legal aspects 349, 368–9, 379
    moral and ethical arguments 394, 396–8
Excretion urography (IVU), equipment 107
Extrapulmonary gas exchange 151–2

Face masks, oxygen delivery 135, 136
Families *see* Relatives
Fat embolism, diffuse alveolar shadowing and 110
Feeding *see* Nutrition
Financial issues 312, 315–27
    audit principles for SCU development 60
    benefit analysis and evaluation 317–20; *see also* Financial issues, cost-benefit analysis

Financial issues – *continued*
  calculating costs 321–2
  capital expenditure on equipment 44
  clinical audit differentiated from resource management
      266
  cost centres 16
  cost-benefit analysis 324–5, 335, 336–7, 338–40
  cost-control strategies 16–17
    malpractice lawsuits and 386–7
    moral and ethical dilemmas 7–8; *see also*
        Prioritization, ethics of
  cost-effectiveness analysis 323–4, 334
  cost-minimization analysis 323
  cost-utility analysis 325–6, 334–5, 338–40
  data collection 53, 60
  definitions 316–17
  demand 13, 16–17
  equipment 44
  expenditure forecasting, scoring systems 8, 281, 282,
      283–4, 337–8
  financial management by ICU staff 193–4
  ICU utilization 12–13
  reported costs 13–14
  standardization 14–16
  supply of resources 13, 16
Finapress, blood pressure measurement 71
Fire safety 44
Floor plans, ICU accommodation requirements 40–3
Fluid balance, ARF and 183, 184–5, 186
  see also Dialysis
Fluoroscopy 107–8
Food *see* Nutrition
France, primary care system (SAMU) 21
Frank–Starling relationship, cardiac pump function 86, 87
Frusemide, reversal of ARF 185
Funding *see* Financial issues

Gallbladder, cholecystitis, radiology 117
Gas supplies
  accommodation design 44
  in ambulances 22, 30
Gastrointestinal failure, definition of 54
Gastrointestinal hemorrhage, radiology 117
Gastrointestinal mucosal tonometry, cardiac function
    assessment and 72–3
General ICUs (GICUs)
  characteristics of 4, 62
  or specialist units 15, 56–7, 60–1, 64
Geriatric intensive care units 63, 67
Glasgow Coma Scale (GCS) 279, 280, 281
Glomerular filtration rate (GFR), reduction with renal
    failure 182–3, 190
Glomerulonephritis, ARF and 180, 185–6
'Goal directed' intensive care 291

HD (hemodialysis) 7, 43, 187–8
HDU *see* High dependency care
Head injury and disease
  brain damage, defining death 346–7
  brain stem 119–20
  hyperventilation for ICP control 140

  primary care
    laryngoscopy 25
    nasotracheal intubation 28–9
    transfer 26–7
  radiology 119–20
  see also Brain stem death; Persistent vegetative state
Health care systems, effects of IC on 299, 312–13, 338
Health care technology 5–6
  clinical engineers 255–61
  costs and consequences 315–27
    benefit evaluation and analysis 317–20
    calculating costs 321–2
    cost-benefit 324–5, 335, 336–7, 338–40
    cost-effectiveness 323–4, 334
    cost-minimization 323
    cost-utility 325–6, 334–5, 338–40
    definitions 316–17; *see also* Financial issues;
        Prioritization, ethics of
  maintenance 44, 51, 129, 259
  for monitoring and measurement 44–5
  practical skills required 194
  product liability 131, 259
  range of in ICUs 5–6
  replacement 44
  technical knowledge required 195
  technology management 258–9
  ventilators 45
Heart *see* Cardiovascular disease and failure; Cardiovascular
    monitoring
Helicopters *see* Aircraft
Hematological failure, definition of 54
Hematomas, radiology 119
Hemodialysis (HD) 7, 43, 187–8
Hemodynamic management, cardiogenic shock 171–3
Hemodynamic monitoring 7, 82–101
  arterial catheterization 92–3, 94–6, 97–9, 100
  benefits of 85
  central venous catheterization 93–4, 97, 98, 99–100
  future research 101
  MAP as reflection of cardiovascular stability 91–2
  oxygen delivery and consumption to describe metabolic
      status 90–1
  physiological variables derived from 84–5
  Ppao and left ventricular preload 86–9, 95
  rationale for 82–4
  recommendations for clinical practice 100–1
Hemodynamically mediated ARF 179–80, 185
Hemofiltration (HF) 45, 189–90
Hemoglobin, laboratory measurement of 130
Hemopump VAD 164, 169, 170
Hemorrhage
  arterial catheterization and 99
  gastrointestinal 117
  mediastinum 111
  pulmonary 111
  subarachnoid 120
Henderson–Hasselbach equation, cardiac function
    assessment and 73
Heparin, dialysis 185
Hepatic failure
  blunt trauma 118
  choledocholithiasis 116–17

definition of 54
liver transplants 66, 357
Hepatorenal syndrome (HRS) 179
Hetastarch, circulatory management 26
Heterografts 358
HF (hemofiltration) 45, 189–90
HFV *see* High frequency ventilation
High dependency care and step-down units
    characteristics of 62
    combined with ICU 213–14
    definitions 38, 289
    need for 8, 65
High frequency ventilation (HFV) 144–6
    clinical applications 145–6
    gas transport mechanisms 145
    high frequency oscillation 145
    high-frequency jet ventilation 145
    high-frequency positive pressure ventilation 144–5
Hippocratic tradition, medico-moral dilemmas 391, 392
HIV tests, organ donors 353
Hospital design, ICU accommodation 39–44, 61
Hospital structure, impact of critical care on 298–9
HRS (hepatorenal syndrome) 179
Humidification 43, 45, 136, 137
Hyperkalemia, in ARF 186
Hypertension, ARF and 183–4
Hypertonic saline, circulatory management 26
Hypothermia, with intravenous fluid infusion 29

IABP (intra-aortic balloon pumping) 6, 115, 161, 171, 173
ICD (International Classification of Diseases) systems 53,
    270
ICP (intracranial pressure), hyperventilation for control 140
IECs (institutional ethics committees) 361–2, 388–9
Illness, severity of *see* Severity scoring
Iloprost, renal failure 185
Imaging 6, 105–21
    abdomen 115–18
    cardiac function assessment 71–2
    cardiac output 73–6
    computed tomography 108
    contrast enhanced radiography 107–8
    head 119–21
    magnetic resonance imaging 108
    plain film radiography 105–7
    radionucleotide imaging 71–2, 108–9
    thorax 109–15
    ultrasound 73–6, 108
Impending ventilatory failure 140
IMV (intermittent mandatory ventilation) 141–2, 143
Incentive spirometry, bronchial hygiene therapy 137
Infarcts, radiology 109, 121
Infections
    building design and 44
    disease patterns 7
    specialist care units for infectious diseases 62
    unit management 53
Infusion pumps, bedside services 45
Inhalation therapy 231
    see also Respiratory therapy
Injury Severity Score (ISS) 21, 282, 283, 284
Inotropic agents

cardiac failure 158–60, 173
    renal failure 185
Institutional ethics committees (IECs) 361–2, 388–9
Intensive care, definitions and history 3, 11–12, 36–8, 197,
    289–90, 297–8
Intensivists 4, 12, 15–16
    Australia 197–8, 201
    Canada 207, 209–10
    termination of intensive care 17
    UK 193, 196
    USA 202–3, 204–6
Intermittent mandatory ventilation (IMV) 141–2, 143
Intermittent positive pressure breathing (IPPB) 138
International Classification of Diseases (ICD) systems 53,
    270
Intra-aortic balloon pumping (IABP) 6, 115, 161, 171, 173
Intracranial pressure (ICP), hyperventilation for control 140
Intraosseous infusions, circulatory management 26
Intravascular oxygenator (IVOX) 151–2
Intravenous infusions
    arterial catheterization and 99
    initial treatment 29
    primary care in the field 22, 25–6
    religious objections to blood transfusions 347, 372–3,
        391, 393–6
    reversal of ARF 184–5
    see also Nutrition, legal aspects of feeding
Intubation
    during air transfers 31–2
    initial treatment 28–9
    primary care in the field 22, 23, 25
    radiology for positioning 114
IPPB (intermittent positive pressure breathing) 138
Islam 355, 391, 393, 396
Isoproterenol, cardiac failure 159
ISS (Injury Severity Score) 21, 282, 283, 284
IVOX (intravascular oxygenator) 151–2
IVU (excretion urography), equipment 107

Jehovah's Witnesses, blood transfusions 373–4, 391, 393–6
Judaism 355, 391, 392, 393

Karnofsky index 280
Kidneys *see* Renal failure

Laboratory facilities 5–6, 123–32
    bedside services 131
    building design 43
    equipment 125, 128–31
    evaluation of standards 126, 128
    legal liability 131
    on-site 61, 123–4, 131–2
    organization and administration standards 124–5
    policies and procedures 125–6
    quality assurance procedures 126–8
    staff 124, 125, 126
Lactate analyzers 130
Laryngoscopy, head injuries and 25
Left ventricular (LV) preload
    pulmonary artery occlusion pressure and 86–9, 95
    see also Ventricular assist devices

Legal issues 348–9, 367–80, 382–9
    advance directives (living wills) 347–8, 379, 385
    autonomy (self-determination) principle 347, 372–3, 384
    DNR orders 378
    enduring powers of attorney 379, 385
    feeding 371–2, 376–7, 377–8
    incompetent patients 371–2, 373–7, 374, 379–80, 384–5
    informed consent 372–3, 384–5
        clinical research 364–5
    legal responsibility 385–6
    life-shortening treatment 368–9, 396–8
    life-support termination 369–72, 396
    malpractice 383–7
        cost-containment and malpractice exposure 386–7
        informed consent 384–5
        negligence 131, 256, 259, 383, 385–6
        vicarious liability 385–6
    organ donation 353, 354
        elective ventilation 356
        living donors 357
    reform prospects 378–80, 396–8
    refusal of treatment by patients 346, 369–71, 372–3,
        393–8
    regulation of care in US 382–3
    risk management 387–9
        clinical practice parameters 388
        definitions and content 387
        documentation 387–8
        ethics committees 388–9
    see also Case law
Levey–Jennings control chart 127
Life quality
    cost-utility analyses, QALYs 325–6, 334–5, 338–9
    as outcome measure 285, 301, 305–6, 309–11
Life-shortening treatment, legal aspects 368–9, 396–8
Life-support, withholding and withdrawing *see* Witholding
    and withdrawing care
Lighting, building design 43
Liver *see* Hepatic failure
Living wills 347–8, 379, 385
Location of ICUs 39–40, 61
Loop diuretics, reversal of ARF 185
Lungs *see* Pulmonary injury and failure
LV preload *see* Left ventricular (LV) preload

Magnetic resonance imaging (MRI) 108
Malpractice 383–7
    cost-containment and malpractice exposure 386–7
    informed consent 384–5
    negligence 131, 256, 259, 383, 385–6
    vicarious liability 385–6
Management
    accommodation design 41–3
    leadership and control of ICUs 12, 56–7, 60–1
    by medical staff 193–4
    nurse managers 213, 214–15
    patterns of 51–3
    protocol development 59–60
Mandatory minute ventilation (MMV) 144
Mannitol, reversal of ARF 185
MAP (mean arterial pressure), as reflection of
    cardiovascular stability 91–2

Marrow transplant units 62, 66–7
MAST (Military Anti-Shock Trousers) 26
Mediastinum, radiology 111–12
Medical engineers 255–61
Medical equipment *see* Health care technology
Medical ICUs (MICUs) 15, 66–8
Medico-legal issues *see* Legal issues
Mercy killing *see* Euthanasia
Metabolic failure, definition of 54
MMV (mandatory minute ventilation) 144
Mobile care
    air transfers 22, 26–8, 31–2
    land transfers 30
    preparation for transfer 29–30, 293–4
    primary care in the field 21, 22–6
    primary patient transfer 26–8
    road ambulances 22, 26
    sea transfers 30–1
    severity scoring and 283, 284
MOF *see* Multiple organ failure
Monitoring 5–6
    admission to ICUs for 8, 291, 300
    benefits and costs of monitoring technologies 319–20,
        323–4, 326–7, 339
    building design and 40, 44–5
    during transfers between hospitals 29, 283, 284
    initial treatment 29
    invasive hemodynamic 82–101
    noninvasive 70–9
    primary care in the field 23
Moral dilemmas 7–8, 355, 391–8
    blood transfusions 347, 391, 393–6
    prospects of legal reform 396–9
Mortality
    as outcome marker 278, 282–3, 285, 301, 304–9, 336–7
    risk assessment
        methods 279, 280–1, 301–5
        purpose of 301
        treatment limitation 285
        triage 284
Mortality Prediction Model (MPM) 8, 280, 281, 284, 290,
    291, 303–4
MRI (magnetic resonance imaging) 108
Multidisciplinary ICUs *see* General ICUs
Multidisciplinary teams, ICUs 5, 50–1, 202
Multiple organ failure (MOF)
    admission criteria 292
    definitions 38, 54
    incidence 7
    perfusion and cardiac function assessment 72
Myeloma cast nephropathy 181
Myocardial infarction, cardiogenic shock
    coronary artery bypass grafting 162–3
    hemodynamic management of 171–3
    inotropic agents 158–60, 173
    intra-aortic balloon pumping 161, 171, 173
    pathophysiology 156–7
    percutaneous transluminal coronary angioplasty 161–2,
        170, 171
    predictors 157
    prognosis 157–8
    thrombolytic therapy 161, 172

vasodilators 160–1, 172–3
ventricular assist devices/total artificial hearts 163–71

Nasal cannulae, oxygen delivery 135
Nasogastric tubes, positioning of 114
see also Nutrition, legal aspects of feeding
Nasotracheal intubation
cervical injury and 25
complications 28–9
initial treatment 28–9
Nebulizers 136
Neonatal intensive care
anencephalic donors 358
characteristics of 62
cost-benefit analysis 324–5, 339–40
extracorporeal membrane oxygenation 151
need for 15, 64
severity scoring, transfers and 284
survival rates 6–7
Nephritis, acute interstitial 180–1
Nephropathy, obstructive 181–2
Netherlands
euthanasia 368, 391–2, 397, 398
intensive care costs 14
Neurogenic pulmonary edema, diffuse alveolar shadowing
and 110
Neurological failure, definition of 54
Nitroglycerin
cardiac failure 161
renal failure 185
Nitroprusside
cardiac failure 160–1
renal failure 185
Noise abatement, building design 40
Noninvasive monitoring
cardiovascular system 70–7
respiratory system 77–9
Norepinephrine, cardiac failure 158–9, 173
Novacor left ventricular assist device (LVAD) 165, 169,
170
Nuclear medicine 71–2, 108–9
Nursing staff
Australia 217–22
Belgium 224–5
EC requirements and guidelines 223–4
international comparisons 5
UK 50–1, 212–17
building design and 40
required staffing levels 37, 38, 53, 213–15
skillmix 214
Nutrition
in ARF 186–7
dietitians 5, 51
ethics of discontinuation of feeding 346
legal aspects of feeding 371–2, 376–7, 377–8
parenteral 7
religious beliefs and 396

Office of Population Census and Studies Classification 4
(OPCS4) 53
Oncology, specialist care units 62, 66–7
Open ICU model 12, 13, 15–16

Organ donation 350–9
allocation of donated organs 358
anencephalic donors 358
brain stem death
admission criteria 292
diagnosis 351–3
elective ventilation 355–6
incidence of 353–4
religious objections to 355
donor organ shortfalls, causes 353–4
donors as vendors 357–8
fetus as donor 358
HIV testing of donors 353
living donors 357
medical contraindications 354–5
multiple organ donation 353, 355
non-heart beating cadaveric donors 356
opt in/out consent systems 354
organ retrieval 352, 353
payment for organs 357–8, 358–9
religious beliefs 355, 393
unused organs 355
xenografts 358
Organ System Failures (OSFs) 280, 281, 285
Organ transplant units *see* Transplantation units
Orotracheal intubation 25, 28
Osmotic diuretics, reversal of ARF 185
Outcome measures
admission criteria and 290
age and 278, 290
determining accuracy of 278–9, 300–1
financial implications 7–8
mortality/survival as 278, 282–3, 285, 301, 304–9,
336–7
quality of life as 285, 301, 305–6, 309–11
severity scoring and 284–5
Outcomes
classification schemes 301
critical care directed to 298
definitional problems 300
expenditure forecasting 315–16, 336–7, 340
scoring systems 281, 282, 283–4, 337–8
health care systems, effects of critical care 299
hospital organization, impact of critical care on 298–9
patient care and survival
classification schemes 301
goals of critical care 300–1
impact of critical care on 299–301
prediction 284–5
dynamic systems 278, 285
to explain outcome differences 282–3, 301, 304–5,
306–7
methods of 279–82, 290, 301–5; *see also* main entries
for named methods
severity scores required for 276–7
treatment limitation 285, 290–1
triage 284
unmeasured benefits/costs 311–12, 345
Oxygen
ambulance supplies of 22, 30
extrapulmonary gas exchange 151–2
see also Respiratory support

Oxygen metabolism
   invasive monitoring 84
      oxygen delivery measures and 90–1, 96, 100
      pulmonary artery catheterization (SvO2) 95–6, 100
   noninvasive monitoring 77–9
Oxygen therapy 133–6
   delivery systems 134–6
Oxygen transport
   cardiac function assessment and 72–3
   high frequency ventilation 145
   invasive monitoring 84
      metabolic status and 90–1, 96, 100

Pacemakers 7, 115
Pain
   indices of 305
   life-shortening treatment and 368–9
Paralyzing disease and injury
   skin breakdown 65
   witholding and withdrawing care 347
Parsonnet scoring system 282
Passive euthanasia 17, 345–6
PC-IRV (pressure control/inverse ratio ventilation) 143
PCPS (percutaneous cardiopulmonary support) 165–6, 170
PD (peritoneal dialysis) 189
Pediatric ICUs 15, 62, 64, 292–3
Pediatric Risk of Mortality (PRISM) 280, 290, 291, 303, 304
Pediatric trauma score (PTS) 280
PEEP (positive end expiratory pressure) 146–8, 149
Pentastarch, circulatory management 26
Perceived Quality of Life Scale (PQOL) 310
Percutaneous cardiopulmonary support (PCPS) 165–6, 170
Percutaneous transluminal coronary angioplasty (PTCA) 161–2, 170, 171
Perfusion
   cardiac function assessment 72–3
   reperfusion techniques in cardiac failure 161–3
Peritoneal dialysis (PD) 189
Persistent vegetative state
   advance directives and 348
   elective ventilation 356
   ICU rationing and 17
   legal aspects of witholding and withdrawing care 346, 371–2, 374–7, 378
   organ donation and 356, 358
Personnel
   advantages and disadvantages of ICUs 37
   Australia
      medical staff 198–201
      nursing staff 217–22
      physical therapy 242–3
   Belgium 224–5
   Canada 207–11
   EC requirements and guidelines
      nursing 223–4
      physiotherapy 250–4
   general principles for SCU development 58–9
   laboratories 124, 125
   multidisciplinary teams 4, 5, 51, 202

skillmix 214
skills required 193–4
stress reduction 40, 195–6
UK 45, 50–1, 193–6, 212–17
   physical therapy 249
   required staffing levels 37, 38, 53, 213–15
USA 4–5, 202–6
   physical therapy 229–30
   respiratory care 233–4
   see also Intensivists; Training and competency
Pharmacists 5, 53
Phosphodiesterase inhibitors, cardiac failure 159–60
Photo-plethysmographic method, blood pressure measurement 71
Physical therapy
   Australia 239–43
   Canada 234–6
   chest (CPT) 138, 228–9, 236
   European Community 251–4
   rehabilitation 228–9, 236, 249, 250
   services 51
   staffing 229–30, 242–3, 249
   training and competency 227–8, 234, 235–6, 239–42, 244–9, 250–4
   UK 244–51
   USA 226–30
   see also Respiratory therapy
Physiologic PEEP 149
Physiological and operative severity score (POSSUM) 280, 282
Physiological reserve, severity scoring 277–8, 291
Physiological Stability Index (PSI) 280, 283
Pierce–Donachy VAD 163–4, 168–9, 170
Plain film radiography, equipment 105–7
Plasma exchange, rapidly progressive glomerulonephritis (RPGN) 185–6
Pleural effusions
   chest drains 114
   radiology 113
Pneumomediastinum 112
Pneumonia, radiology 109
Pneumothorax
   chest drains 114
   radiology 113
Poisoning, specialist care units 63
Polygelatins, circulatory management 25–6
Positive airway pressure therapy 138–50
   continuous positive airway pressure 143–4, 147, 148–9
   positive end expiratory pressure 146–8, 149
   positive pressure ventilation
      full or partial support 140–1
      indications 138, 140
      initiation of 140
      modes of 141–6
   ventilator discontinuance 144, 149–50
Positive end expiratory pressure (PEEP) 146–8, 149
Positive pressure ventilation (PPV)
   full or partial ventilatory support 140–1
   indications 138, 140
   initiation of 140
   modes of 141–6
POSSUM 280, 282

Postural drainage therapy 138, 229
Power supplies, building design 43, 44
Ppa (pulmonary arterial pressure), monitoring 84, 94–6
Ppao *see* Pulmonary artery occlusion pressure
PPV *see* Positive pressure ventilation
PQOL (Perceived Quality of Life Scale) 310
Prehospital care *see* Primary care in the field
Pressure control/inverse ratio ventilation (PC-IRV) 143
Pressure support (PS) 142–3
Primary care in the field 21, 22–6
   airway management 24–5
   breathing 25
   circulatory management 25–6
   intubation 23, 25
   monitoring 23
   resuscitation bag 22
   temperature measurement 23
   training 23–4
   transfers 26–8, 283
   ventilation equipment 22, 23
Prioritization, ethics of 331–41
   choices 333
   costs and benefits 335, 336–7, 338–41
   efficiency 332–3
   heterogeneity 337–8
   mechanisms for setting of 333–4
   need for 332
   resource availability 332
   role of economic analysis in 334–5
PRISM (Pediatric Risk of Mortality) 280, 290, 291, 303, 304
Procedures room, building design 43
Product liability
   clinical engineers 256, 259
   laboratories 131
Prognosis *see* Outcomes, prediction
Prostacyclin 185
Protein analyzers 130
Protein metabolism, ARF and 182–3, 186–7
Protestantism 392
Prothrombin time (PT), measurement of 131
PS (pressure support) 142–3
PSI (Physiological Stability Index) 280, 283
Psychiatric intensive care units 63, 67
PT (prothrombin time), measurement of 131
PTCA (percutaneous transluminal coronary angioplasty) 161–2, 170, 171
PTS (Pediatric trauma score) 280
Pulmonary arterial pressure (Ppa), monitoring 84, 94–6
Pulmonary artery catheterization 94–6
   complications 6, 96
   indications for 97, 98–9, 100
Pulmonary artery occlusion pressure (Ppao) 84
   left ventricular preload and 86–9, 95
   pulmonary artery catheterization 94, 95
Pulmonary injury and failure
   diffuse alveolar shadowing 110, 111
   emboli and infarcts 6, 109
   extrapulmonary gas exchange 151–2
   lung transplants 357
   radiology 109–11
Pulmonary interstitial emphysema 111

Pulse oximetry, arterial oxygen saturation 77–8
Pulsus paradoxus, arterial catheterization and 99

Quality assurance 126–8
   control charts 127–8
   strategies for 14–17
   see also Clinical audit
Quality of life
   cost-utility analyses, QALYs 325–6, 334–5, 338–9
   as outcome measure 285, 301, 305–6, 309–11

Radiation protection, mobile X-ray equipment 107
Radiology 6, 105–21
   abdomen 115–18
   computed tomography 108
   contrast enhanced radiography 107–8
   head 119–21
   magnetic resonance imaging 108
   plain film radiography, equipment 105–7
   radionucleotide imaging 71–2, 108–9
   thorax 109–15
Radionucleotide imaging 71–2, 108–9
Radiotherapy, specialist care units 66–7
Randomized control trials (RCTs) 318
Rapidly progressive glomerulonephritis (RPGN) 180, 185–6
Rationing, health care *see* Prioritization, ethics of
Rebreathing systems, oxygen delivery 134, 135
Reception areas, building design 43
Records
   data collection 52–3, 60
   design of 45, 46–9
   legal aspects of risk management 387–8
   see also Clinical audit
Regionalization, IC services 14–15
Rehabilitation, physical therapy 228–9, 236, 249, 250
Relatives
   clinical research, consent to 364–5
   discharge criteria and 52
   family support teams 60
   legal issues
      access to medical records 388
      informed consent 384–5
      witholding and withdrawing care 369, 374, 375
   organ donation
      consents 352, 353, 354, 356, 357
      as live donors 357
   religious beliefs 392–3
   rooms for, building design 43
   witholding and withdrawing care
      decisions about 347–9
      legal aspects 369, 374, 375
Religious beliefs 347, 391–8
   blood transfusions 347, 372–3, 391, 393–6
   legal reform and 396–9
   organ donation 355
Renal failure
   acute intrinsic renal disease 180–1
   definition of 54
   dialysis 187–90
      bedside services 45
      building design 43
      specialist units 63, 66

Renal failure – *continued*
  diffuse alveolar shadowing and 110
  hemodynamically mediated ARF 179–80, 185
  incidence and mortality of ARF 178
  kidney transplants
    allocation of organs 358
    organ donations 357
    organ transplant units 66
  management of ARF (acute renal failure) 184–90
    ARF reversal 184–6
    conservative 186–7
    renal replacement therapy 187–90
  manifestations of 182–4
    glomerular filtration rate reduction 182–3, 190
    renal synthetic functions 183–4
    tubular function disturbance 183, 190
  obstructive nephropathy 181–2
  pre-existent renal disease 178–9
  radiology 117–18
  renovascular disease 182
Research, ethics 360–6
Resource allocation, financial *see* Financial issues
Respiratory acidosis (acute ventilatory failure) 140
Respiratory failure
  definition of 54
  with spinal cord injury 64–5
Respiratory monitoring 77–9
Respiratory support
  during transfers 29, 31–2
  elective ventilation, organ donation 355–6
  ethics of 'terminal weaning' 346
  extrapulmonary gas exchange 151–2
  initial treatment 29
  nonventilatory 133–8
  positive airway pressure therapy 138–50
  primary care in the field 22, 23, 25
  ventilatory *see* Ventilation
Respiratory therapy 5, 231–4, 236–8, 246–7, 250
  see also Bronchial hygiene
Resuscitation bag, primary care in the field 22
Rib fractures, radiology 113
Right ventricular (RV) ejection fraction, monitoring 84–5,
    96, 100
Risk management, legal aspects 387–9
Riyadh Intensive Care Programme (RIP) 279, 280, 281,
    292
Road ambulances *see* Ambulances
Roman Catholicism 392, 396, 397
RPGN (rapidly progressive glomerulonephritis) 180,
    185–6

Safety
  clinical engineering 259
  fire 44
Saline, hypertonic, circulatory management 26
SAPS *see* Simplified Acute Physiology Score
Scoring systems *see* Severity scoring
SCUs *see* Specialist care units (SCUs)
Sea transport 30–1
Secondment, personnel 59
Selection criteria *see* Admission criteria

Seminar rooms, building design 43
Sepsis
  ARF and 179–80, 185
  intra-abdominal, radiology 117
Sepsis score (SS) 280
Septic shock
  conjunctival oxygen tension (CjO2) and 73
  disease patterns 7
Severity scoring 276–85, 301
  admission decisions and 53, 284, 290–1, 294
  applications 282–5, 305
    clinical decisions 284–5
    explaining outcome differences 282–3, 304–5,
        306–7
    outcome prediction 284–5, 304–5
    research stratification 282
    resource utilization 281, 282, 283–4, 337–8
  clinical audit 266, 270
  dynamic 278, 285, 292
  ethics of prioritization and 337–8
  future developments 285
  measurement accuracy 278–9, 301
  methods of 279–82, 304–5; *see also* main entries for
      named methods
  need for measurement of 276–7
  primary care and 21
  quantification 277–8
    acute illness 277
    diagnoses 278
    physiological reserve 277–8
Shift systems, ICU management 196, 215, 223–4
Sickness Impact Profile (SIP) 280, 285, 310
SICUs (surgical ICUs) 15, 65–6
Simplified Acute Physiology Score (SAPS) 279–81, 290,
    291, 303
SIMV (synchronized intermittent mandatory ventilation)
    141–2, 143
Siting of ICUs 39–40, 61
Skin breakdown, spinal injury units 65
Skull fractures, radiology 119
Sodium nitroprusside, cardiac failure 160–1
Specialist care units (SCUs) 4, 15, 56–68
  general principles for development of 57–60
  integration into hospitals 60–1
  medical 15, 66–8
  surgical 15, 65–6
  types of 61–5
Spinal injury
  primary care
    airway management 25, 28
    transfers 26
  specialist units for 62, 64–5
Spleen, blunt trauma, radiology 118
SS (sepsis score) 280
Staff *see* Personnel
Standardization, strategies for 14–17
Starch solutions, circulatory management 26
Step-down units *see* High dependency care and step-down
    units
Sternal fractures, radiology 114
Storage space, accommodation design 40, 43, 44
Streptokinase, intravenous, in myocardial infarction 161

Stress reduction
    building design 40
    training 195–6
Subarachnoid hemorrhage 120–1
Subcutaneous oxygen tonometry 78
Suctioning, bronchial hygiene therapy 137
Suicide, ethical and legal aspects 346, 368, 369, 370–1, 394, 396–8
Surgical ICUs (SICUs) 15, 65–6
Survival, as outcome measure 281, 285, 301, 305–11, 336–7
Swan–Ganz catheters, positioning of 114
Symbion total artifical heart 164–5, 169, 170
Synchronized intermittent mandatory ventilation (SIMV) 141–2, 143
Syringe pumps, bedside services 45

TAHs *see* Total artificial hearts
Tamponade, pulsus paradoxus and arterial catheterization 99
Taylor dispersion 145
TBIP (thoracic bioimpedance), cardiac output 76–7
Technology *see* Health care technology
TED (transesophageal Doppler), cardiac output 74, 75
TEE (transesophageal echocardiography), cardiac function assessment 72
Temperature control, intravenous fluid infusions and 29
Temperature measurement
    primary care in the field 23
    toe, cardiac output and oxygen delivery and 73
Termination of care *see* Witholding and withdrawing care
Therapeutic Intervention Scoring System (TISS) 280, 281, 305
    clinical audit 270
    quality of survival 285
    resource management and 8, 16, 17, 53, 281, 283, 337–8
    technologic interventions 270
Therapeutic technologies, benefits and costs 317–18, 326
Thermodilution method, cardiac output assessment 95
Thoracic bioimpedance (TBIP), cardiac output 76–7
Thoracotomy 29
Thorax, imaging techniques 109–15
Thromboelastography 131
Thrombolytic therapy 161, 172
Time oriented score system (TOSS) 280
TISS *see* Therapeutic Intervention Scoring System
Toe temperature, cardiac output and oxygen delivery and 73
Tonometry 71, 72–3, 78
Total artificial hearts (TAHs) 164–5, 169, 170
Tracheostomy, complications 6
Tracheostomy collars, oxygen delivery 135
Tracheostomy tubes, positioning of 114
Training and competency
    Australia 199–201, 218–21, 239–42
    Belgium 224–5
    Canada 210–11, 234, 235–8
    caseload 'critical mass' 58–9
    of clinical engineers 257–8
    by clinical engineers 260
    cost awareness 16
    dedicated schemes 50, 196, 199–200, 202
    European Community 223, 250–4
    international comparisons 5

laboratory staff 126
medical staff 195–6, 199–201, 202, 204–6, 210–11
nursing staff 199–201, 214, 215–17, 218–21, 223, 224–5
phases of 59
physical therapy 226–8, 234, 235–6, 239–42, 244–9, 250–4
practical skills 194–5
primary care in the field 23–4
respiratory therapy 232, 236–8
secondment 59
teaching skills 195
UK 195–6, 214, 215–17, 244–9
USA 202, 204–6, 227–8, 232
Transcutaneous oxygen tension, cardiac output and oxygen delivery and 73
Transesophageal Doppler (TED), cardiac output 74, 75
Transesophageal echocardiography (TEE), cardiac function assessment 72
Transfers
    from emergency room to intensive care 29–30
    neonates 64
    policy making 293–4
    primary 22, 26–8
    severity scoring and 283, 284
    unit management for 52
Transplantation
    artificial organs 358; *see also* Total artificial hearts (TAHs)
    organ donation 292, 350–9
    VAD as bridge to cardiac transplants 166, 168–9, 170
    xenografts 358
Transplantation units
    characteristics of 62
    family support teams 60
    need for 66
    patient assessment 60
Transtracheal Doppler (TTD), cardiac output 74–5
Trauma Score (TS) 280, 282
Trauma scoring
    admission criteria 292
    systems 280
    see also named systems
Treatment room, building design 43
Triage *see* Admission criteria
TRISS system 280, 282, 283

UK
    history and definitions of intensive care 36–8
    legal issues 367–80
        DNR orders 378
        feeding 371–2, 377–8
        incompetent patients 371–2, 373–7
        life-shortening treatment 368–9, 396
        reform prospects 378–80, 396–8
        refusal of treatment by patients 369–71, 372–3, 393–4, 395
        terminating care 369–72, 396
    medical staff 37, 45, 50, 193–6
    nursing staff 50–1, 212–17
        building design and 40
        required staffing levels 37, 38, 53, 213–15
        skillmix 214

UK – *continued*
  organ donation
    brain stem death debate 352–3
    consent systems 354
    donor shortfalls 353–4
    donors as vendors 357–8
    elective ventilation 356
    permission for organ retrieval 353
  physical therapy 244–50
  primary care in the field 22, 23–4
  survey of IC provision 38–40
Ultrasound 73–6, 108
Uniscale, severity scoring 280, 285
Urea, glomerular filtration rate and 182
Urography (IVU), equipment 107
USA
  bed capacity and occupancy 12, 13
  clinical research, informed consent 364
  intensive care costs 13–14, 17
  legal issues 348–9, 382–9
    advance directives 379, 385
    autonomy (self-determination) principle 347, 372, 384
    cost-containment 386–7
    enduring powers of attorney 385
    feeding 377–8
    incompetent patients 374
    informed consent 384–5
    legal responsibility 385–6
    malpractice exposure 386–7
    negligence 383
    regulation of care 382–3
    risk management 387–9
    termination at patient's request 346, 370, 371
    vicarious liability 385–6
  organ donation
    consent systems 354
    donor shortfalls 354
    permission for organ retrieval 353
  personnel and training 4–5, 202–6, 229–30, 233–4
  physical therapy 226–30
  respiratory care 231–4
Utility rooms, building design 43

VADs *see* Ventricular assist devices
Vascular resistance, invasive monitoring 84
Vasodilators
  cardiac failure 160–1, 172–3
  renal failure 185
Ventilation
  bedside services 45
  building design 43
  continuous positive airway pressure 148–9
  discontinuance 144, 149–50
    legal aspects 369–72
    see also Witholding and withdrawing care, ethics
  during hospital transfers 29
  initial treatment 29
  organ donation 355–6
  positioning of tubes 114
  positive end expiratory pressure 146–8, 149
  positive pressure ventilation
    full or partial support 140–1

  indications 138, 140
  initiation of 140
  modes of 141–6
  primary care in the field 22, 23, 25
  with spinal cord injuries 64–5
  ventilator choices 45
Ventricular assist devices (VADs) 163–71
  complications 170–1
  indications 166
  outcomes 168–70
Ventricular preload
  central venous catheterization 94, 99
  pulmonary artery occlusion pressure and 86–9, 95
Ventricular pump function, invasive monitoring 84
Venturi mask, oxygen delivery 135–6
Vitamin D, ARF and 183
Volume expanders 25–6, 172

Waiting rooms, building design 43
Ward rounds, unit management 53
Wedge pressure 95
Weighing scales, bedside services 45
Winching operations, aircraft transfers 27–8
Wisconsin Ischemic Heart Index 304
Witholding and withdrawing care
  brain stem death 17
    legal aspects 369
    organ donation 352
  ethics 344–9
    death defined 346–7
    decision-makers 347–9, 374, 375–7, 379
    definition 346
    institutional ethics committees 388–9
    international differences 348–9
    need for withholding and withdrawing treatment 345–6
    patients' request for 347, 348–9, 393–8
  legal issues 367–80
    advance directives (living wills) 347–8, 379
    autonomy (self-determination) principle 347, 372–3
    DNR orders 378
    enduring powers of attorney 379
    feeding 371–2, 376–7, 377–8
    incompetent patients 371–2, 373–7, 379–80
    institutional ethics committees 388–9
    international differences 348–9, 369–72
    life-shortening treatment 368–9, 396–8
    life-support termination 369–72, 396
    reform prospects 378–80
    refusal of treatment by patients 369–71, 372–3, 393–8
    see also Case law
  unit management 52, 53–4
Wriggler's sign, bowel perforation 115

X-ray units, mobile 105–7
  battery-operated 106
  capacitor discharge units 106
  radiation protection 107
  technique 106–7
Xenografts 358